Esophageal Squamous Cell Carcinoma

Yuko Kitagawa
Hirofumi Kawakubo • Satoru Matsuda
Editors

Esophageal Squamous Cell Carcinoma

Diagnosis and Treatment

Third Edition

Springer

Editors
Yuko Kitagawa
Department of Surgery
Keio University School of Medicine
Shinjuku, Tokyo, Japan

Hirofumi Kawakubo
Japanese Foundation for Cancer Research
Cancer Institute Hospital
Tokyo, Japan

Satoru Matsuda
Department of Surgery
Keio University School of Medicine
Shinjuku, Tokyo, Japan

ISBN 978-981-92-2610-8 ISBN 978-981-92-2611-5 (eBook)
https://doi.org/10.1007/978-981-92-2611-5

Previously published by SpringerNature (same language)

This Springer imprint is published by the registered company Springer Nature Singapore Pte Ltd.
The registered company address is: 152 Beach Road, #21-01/04 Gateway East, Singapore 189721, Singapore

Contents

Epidemiology

1

Taiki Yamaji and Shoichiro Tsugane

1.1 Esophageal Cancer in the World and Japan

1.1.1 Esophageal Cancer in the World: Burden, Geographical Difference and Trends

1.1.1.1 Global Burden and Geographical Difference (Global Cancer Observatory, https://gco.iarc.fr/)

Esophageal cancer is the 11th most common cancer worldwide, with 511,054 new cases (2.6% of the total) estimated in 2022, and the seventh most common cause of death from cancer with 445,391 deaths (4.6% of the total). These figures encompass both adenocarcinoma and squamous cell carcinoma types. More than 80% of esophageal cancer cases and deaths occur in developing countries.

The incidence rates of esophageal cancer vary internationally more than nine-fold in men (age-standardized incidence rate to the World population (ASR) 12.2 per 100,000 in Eastern Asia compared to 1.3 in Western Africa), and more than 20-fold in women (ASR 6.3 per 100,000 in Eastern Africa compared to 0.27 in Polynesia) (Fig. 1.1). The highest incidence rates in men are observed in Malawi, Bangladesh, and Mongolia (ASR 21.5, 20.6, and 19.7 per 100,000, respectively), while the highest incidence rates in women are seen in Malawi, Mongolia, and Kenya (ASR 15.4, 12.6, and 12.2 per 100,000, respectively). Despite being a developed country, Japan exhibits relatively high incidence rates (ASR 7.8 per 100,000 in men and 2.3 in women).

Esophageal cancer is more common among men than women in general. Of note, it is approximately 3.5 times more common among men in Japan and approximately 8 times more common among men in Korea. These differences in sex ratio may suggest different etiologies by region. In Japan and Korea, tobacco smoking and

T. Yamaji (✉) · S. Tsugane
National Cancer Center Institute for Cancer Control 5-1-1 Tsukiji, Chuo-ku, Tokyo, Japan
e-mail: tyamaji@ncc.go.jp

Y. Kitagawa et al. (eds.), *Esophageal Squamous Cell Carcinoma*,
https://doi.org/10.1007/978-981-92-2611-5_1

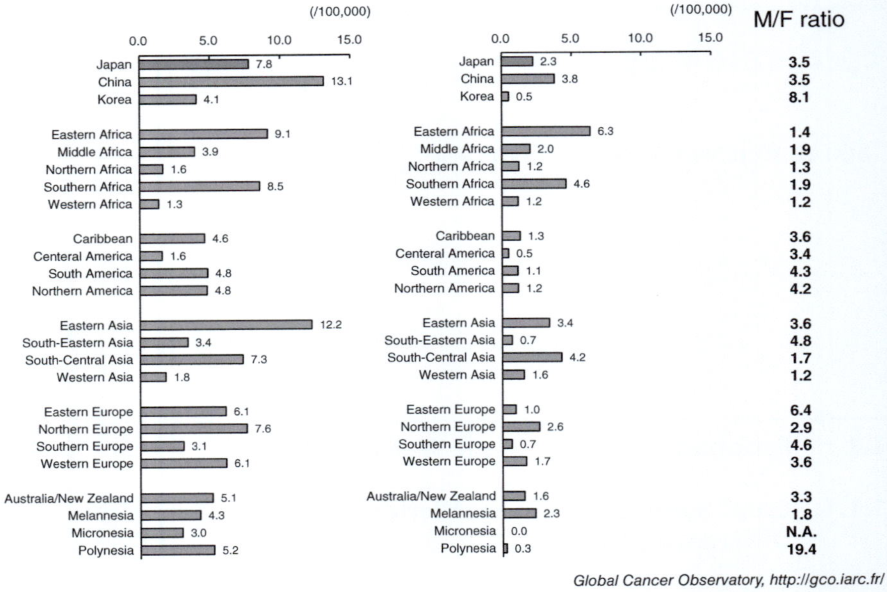

Fig. 1.1 Age-standardized incidence rate (World population) of esophageal cancer in the world (2022)

alcohol consumption are assumed to be major causes of esophageal cancer and the predominant incidence rate among males is associated with much higher prevalence of smoking of tobacco and alcohol use among men versus women. In Eastern and Southern Africa, an important risk factor, in addition to tobacco smoking and alcohol consumption, is thought to be nutrient deficiency such as vitamins and micronutrients, which occurs equally in both men and women. However, the apparent reason of geographic variations is unspecified.

1.1.1.2 Histological Type [3]

In those high-incidence regions that provide information on histological type, approximately 80–90% are squamous cell carcinomas (Fig. 1.2). This is in contrast to some lower-risk populations, such as Caucasian Americans and Europeans, where adenocarcinomas are predominant. For example, in the USA, SEER (Non-Hispanic White) indicated ASR 5.2 in men where 75% of cases are coded as adenocarcinoma as opposed to 15% as squamous cell carcinoma. In contrast, Hiroshima, Japan, indicated ASR 12.4 in men where only 7% as adenocarcinoma as opposed to 85% as squamous cell carcinoma.

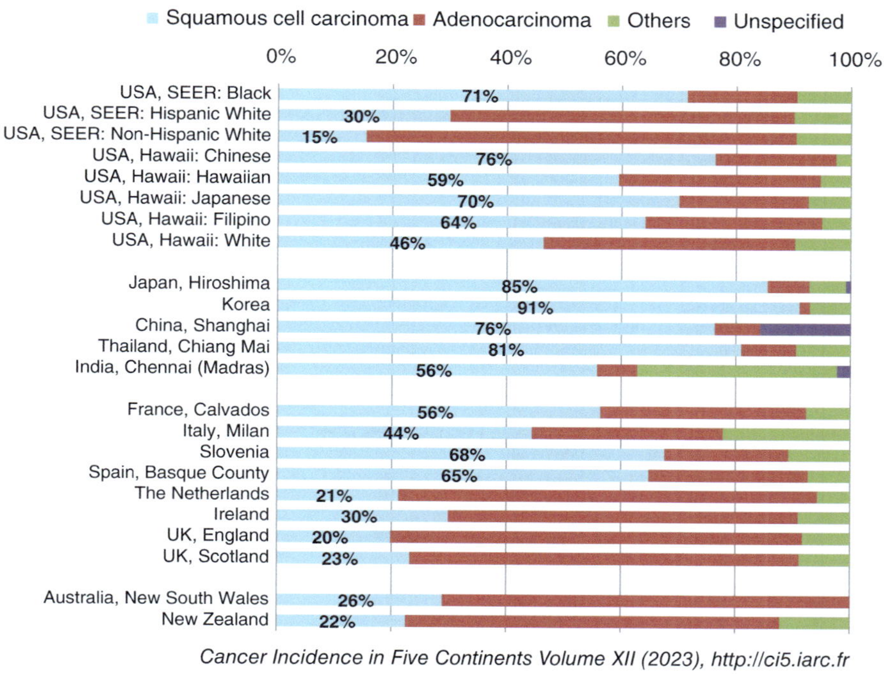

Fig. 1.2 Esophageal cancer—histological distribution % (2013–2017) [3]

1.1.2 Esophageal Cancer in Japan (Cancer Information Service, https://ganjoho.jp)

In 2023, 8647 men and 2103 women died from esophageal cancer, representing 3.9% and 1.3% of total cancer death in men and women, respectively. Mortality rates increased with age rapidly after 45–49 years (Fig. 1.3). The mortality rate of esophageal cancer is estimated to be 0.6% in men and 0.1% in women up to 80 years, increasing to 1.0% in men and 0.2% in women over lifetime. Regarding incidence, 21,150 men and 4925 women were estimated to be diagnosed with esophageal cancer in 2021 and probability of esophageal cancer diagnosis was 1.9% in men and 0.4% in women up to 80 years, increasing to 2.5% in men and 0.5% in women for lifetime. Five-year survival rates were 40.6% in men and 45.9% in women who were diagnosed with esophageal cancer in 2009–2011 based on the population-based cancer registry.

The incidence in both sexes has been observed to increase in number since 1960 due to the aging of the Japanese population (Fig. 1.4, Left), while age-standardized mortality rates have tended to decrease in both males and females (Fig. 1.4, Right). Histological distribution trends were analyzed using eight population-based cancer registries with high level of reliability from 1993 to 2001 [15] and the Miyagi Prefectural Cancer Registry from 2000 to 2015 (Fig. 1.5). Squamous cell carcinoma

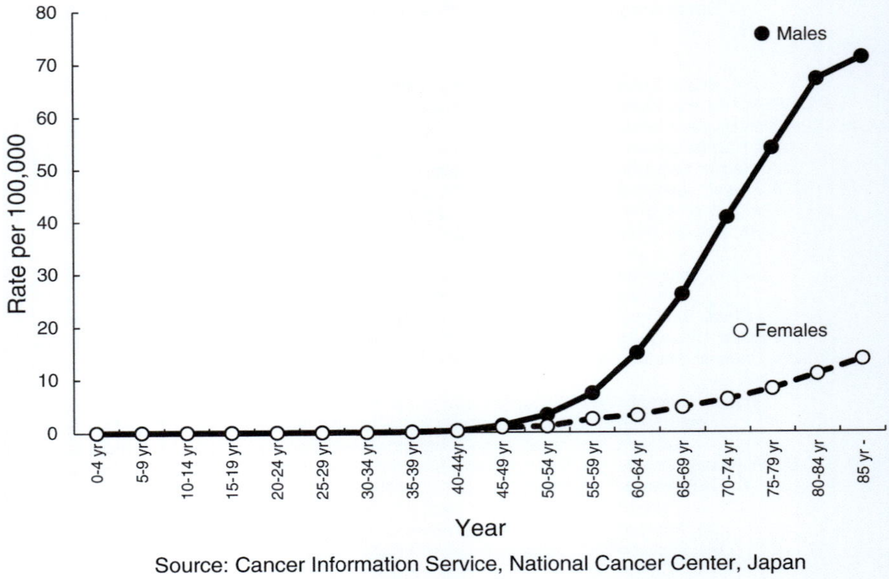

Fig. 1.3 Age-specific mortality rate of esophageal cancer in Japan (2023)

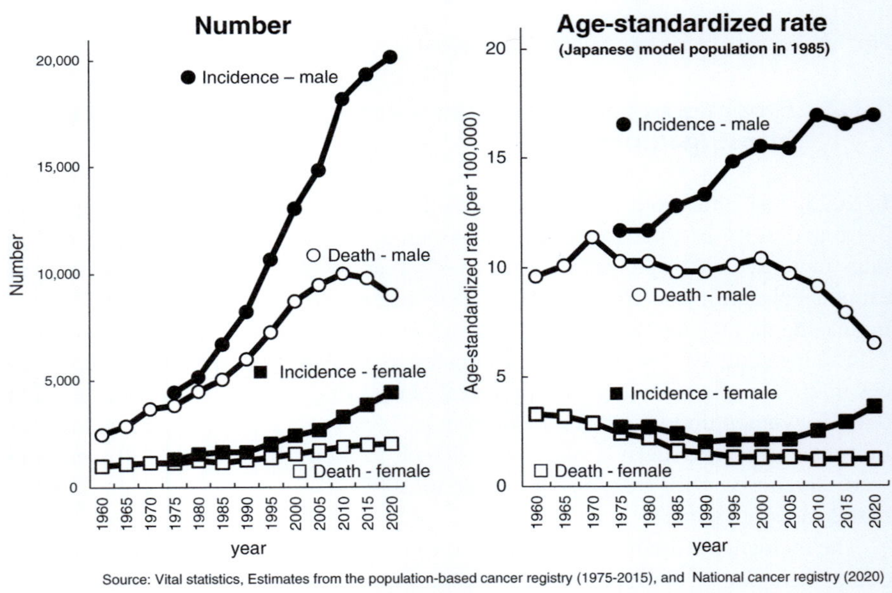

Fig. 1.4 Time trends in the incidence and mortality of esophageal cancer in Japan

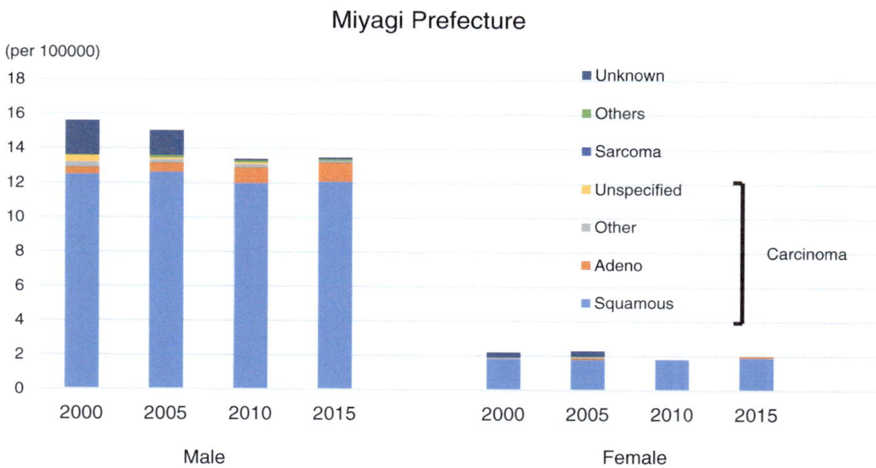

Cancer Incidence in Five Continents Volume IX (2007), X (2012), XI (2017), XII (2023), http://ci5.iarc.fr

Fig. 1.5 Time trends in the age-standardized incidence rate (World population) of esophageal cancer by histological subtype in Japan [3]

was the predominant type of esophageal cancer in Japan, and a remarkable increase in adenocarcinoma was not observed until 2015. Disparity in the classification of esophageal and gastric cardia adenocarcinoma may have led to underestimation of esophageal adenocarcinoma incidence.

1.2 Risk Factors

Established risk and protective factors for esophageal cancer are listed according to level of certainty (Table 1.1). Tobacco smoking and alcohol consumption are convincing risk factors for esophageal cancer, especially squamous cell carcinoma [4, 5, 15]. Acetaldehyde associated with consumption of alcoholic beverages has also been judged as convincing risk factor for esophageal squamous cell carcinoma [6]. Very hot beverages including, but not limited to, mate, a traditional herbal beverage consumed in parts of South America, has been identified as a probable cause of esophageal squamous cell carcinoma [7]. Physical activity and vegetables may prevent both types of esophageal cancer [16].

1.2.1 Tobacco Smoking and Alcohol Consumption

The main risk factors for esophageal squamous cell carcinoma (ESCC) are tobacco smoking and alcohol consumption, which in individual studies have been found to account for 75–90% of cases [1]. The risk of esophageal cancer increases rapidly

Table 1.1 Established risk and protective factors for esophageal cancer

Evidence	Risk factors	Protective factors
Convincing	Tobacco smoking[a] Alcohol consumption[b,e] (squamous cell carcinoma) Acetaldehyde associated with consumption of alcoholic beverages[a] Body fatness[b] (adenocarcinoma)	–
Probable	Mate[b] (squamous cell carcinoma) Very hot beverages including, but not limited to, mate[c] (squamous cell carcinoma)	–
Limited-suggestive	Processed meat[b] (squamous cell carcinoma)	Physical activity[b] Vegetables[b] Fruit[b] (squamous cell carcinoma)

[a]IARC monograph on the Evaluation of Carcinogenic Risks to Humans, Volume 100E (2012) [6]
[b]World Cancer Research Fund/American Institute for Cancer Research. Continuous Update Project Expert Report 2018
[c]IARC monograph on the Evaluation of Carcinogenic Risks to Humans, Volume 116 (2018) [7]
[d]IARC monograph on the Evaluation of Carcinogenic Risks to Humans, Volume 83 (2003) [4]
[e]IARC monograph on the Evaluation of Carcinogenic Risks to Humans, Volume 96 (2007) [5]

with the amount of both tobacco smoking and alcohol consumption, with no evidence of any threshold effect for either.

In Japan, four cohort studies and 11 case–control studies tested the association between tobacco smoking and esophageal cancer risk [13]. With the exception of three case–control studies, all cohort studies and eight case–control studies showed strong positive associations and dose–response relationships. Meta-analysis of 12 studies indicated that the summary estimate for current and former smokers relative to lifetime nonsmokers was 3.73 (95% confidence interval (CI), 2.16–6.43) and 2.21 (95% CI, 1.60–3.06), respectively. Similarly four cohort studies and nine case–control studies tested the association between alcohol consumption and esophageal cancer [12]. With the exception of three case–control studies, all cohort studies and six case–control studies showed strong positive associations and dose–response relationship. Meta-analysis of 12 studies indicated that the summary estimate for ever drinkers relative to never drinkers was 3.30 (95% CI, 2.30–4.74) and 3.36 (95% CI, 1.66–6.78), respectively, across the four studies adjusted for smoking.

We examined the effect of tobacco smoking and alcohol consumption on ESCC in a large-scale population-based cohort study [9]. A total of 44,970 middle-aged and older Japanese men were followed up for up to 14 years, and a total of 215 cases of ESCC were newly diagnosed among participants during this time. Regular alcohol consumers of 150–299 and ≥300 g ethanol/week had a 2.59- (95% CI, 1.57–4.29) and 4.64-fold (95% CI, 2.88–7.48) higher risk of ESCC than nondrinkers, respectively (p for trend = 0.001). Past smokers as well as current smokers had a higher risk than never-smokers. Among current smokers, pack-year and cigarettes per day were also associated with the incidence of ESCC, with risk increasing in a dose-dependent manner (p for trend = 0.001). With regard to the interaction of tobacco smoking (pack-years: <40 vs. ≥40) and alcohol consumption (ethanol g/week: <300

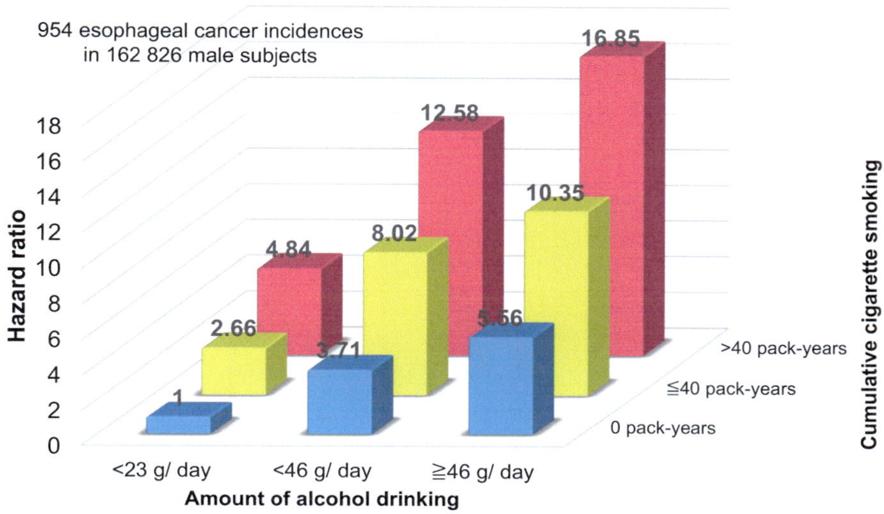

Fig. 1.6 Cumulative cigarette smoking, amount of alcohol drinking, and their interaction for the risk of esophageal cancer—a pooled analysis using eight large-scale population-based cohort studies in Japan [14]

vs. ≥300), no statistically significant results were identified (p for interaction = 0.70). Similarly, a pooled analysis of eight large-scale population-based cohort studies in Japan did not find a significant interaction between cigarette smoking and alcohol consumption on the multiplicative scale [14]. More importantly, however, the pooled analysis did reveal an interaction on the additive scale, suggesting a potential biological interaction between the two factors (Fig. 1.6).

1.2.2 Genetic Susceptibility to Tobacco Smoking and Alcohol Consumption

Regarding genetic susceptibility, esophageal cancer does not exhibit any strong familial aggregation and genetic studies of esophageal cancer have instead focused on genes such as cytochrome P 450 (CYP), glutathione-S-transferase (GST), alcohol dehydrogenase (ADH), and acetaldehyde dehydrogenase (ALDH), which metabolize suspected tobacco- and alcohol-derived carcinogens. No consistent findings have emerged for tobacco-derived pathways, although the majority of studies have been limited in sample size.

Conversely, strongly significant effect modifications have been observed with ADH1B and ALDH2 genotype. Among those with ADH1B who have the His allele, approximately 95% of Japanese and 10–20% of Caucasians show a rapid increase of blood acetaldehyde due to the high alcohol metabolizing activity of the ADH1B enzyme, compared with those who have the Arg allele. Among those with ALDH2

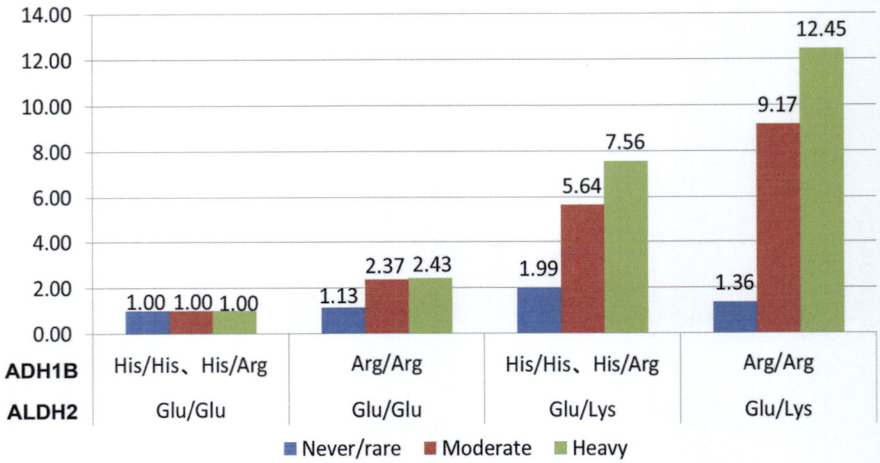

Fig. 1.7 Risk of esophageal cancer associated with combinations of alcohol dehydrogenase (ADH)-1B and aldehyde dehydrogenase (ALDH)-2 genotypes [19]

Lys allele, approximately 50% of Japanese and <10% of Caucasians show a higher concentration of blood acetaldehyde after alcohol consumption compared to those who have the ALDH Glu allele due to the low catalytic activity of ALDH2 enzyme.

A meta-analysis of 19 case–control studies was conducted to evaluate the effect of alcohol consumption modification by ADH1B and ALDH2 polymorphism, to the risk of esophageal cancer [19]. The majority of the studies focused on ESCC and was conducted in Asian populations. A meta-analysis of 13 case–control studies on ADH1B showed that ADH1B*1/*1 (Arg/Arg) increased the risk of esophageal cancer among never/rare [odds ratio (OR) = 1.56 (95% CI, 0.93–2.61)], moderate [2.71 (95% CI, 1.37–5.35)], and heavy alcohol consumers [3.22 (95% CI, 2.27–4.57)], compared with ADH1B*2/*2 (His/His). Similarly, a meta-analysis of 18 case–control studies on ALDH2 showed that ALDH2*1/*2 (Glu/Lys) increased the risk among never/rare [1.28 (95% CI, 0.91–1.80)], moderate [3.12 (95% CI, 1.95–5.01)], and heavy [7.12 (95% CI, 4.67–10.86)] alcohol consumers, compared with ALDH2*1*1 (Glu/Glu). The analysis of combined effects of ADH1B and ALDH2 genotypes showed that ADH1B*1/*1 plus ALDH2*1/*2 was associated with the highest risk of esophageal cancer among heavy drinkers [12.45 (2.9–53.46)] (Fig. 1.7), but no significant increase in risk was seen among never/rare drinkers. Recent large-scale genome-wide gene–alcohol consumption interaction analysis of ESCC in China also showed that drinkers with both of the ADH1B and ALDH2 risk alleles experienced a fourfold increase in risk compared to drinkers without the aforementioned risk alleles, while no increased risk was observed among nondrinkers [17].

Numerous experimental studies have also reported that acetaldehyde has a cytotoxic, genotoxic, mutagenic, and clastogenic potential. In fact, acetaldehyde can cause DNA–protein crosslinks, DNA strand breaks, DNA adducts, sister chromatid exchanges, chromosomal aberrations, and micronuclei in eukaryotic cells in vitro. In addition, acetaldehyde can induce DNA–protein crosslinks, sister chromatid exchanges, and chromosomal aberrations in rodents in vivo [5].

Based on sufficient evidence both in humans and experimental animals for the carcinogenicity of acetaldehyde, the International Agency for Research on Cancer (IARC) Working Group on the Evaluation of Carcinogenic Risks to Humans has concluded that acetaldehyde associated with the consumption of alcoholic beverages is carcinogenic to humans and causes cancers of the esophagus [6].

1.2.3 Fruit and Vegetable Intake

Although the tobacco smoking and alcohol consumption are the primary lifestyle risk factors for esophageal cancer, dietary factors are also likely to be important [16]. Intake of fruit and vegetables appears to have a protective effect. Although the relationship for particular types of fruits and vegetables is unclear, citrus fruits and green leafy vegetables appear to possess greater effects than other families of fruits and vegetables.

The Research Group for the Development and Evaluation of Cancer Prevention Strategies in Japan evaluated that fruit and vegetable intake probably prevent esophageal cancer based on systematic review of epidemiologic evidence among the Japanese population (unpublished data, available at http://epi.ncc.go.jp/can_prev/). Seven studies, two cohort and five case–control studies, tested the association of esophageal cancer prevention with fruit intake and all studies showed a significant protective effect. Eight studies, three cohort and five case–control studies, tested the association with vegetable intake as a whole, as well as green–yellow or cruciferous vegetables. The majority of studies showed significant relationship between the intake of such vegetables and esophageal cancer prevention. However, residual confounding by tobacco smoking and alcohol consumption cannot be ruled out even after adjusting for and stratified by these variables. Both of the variables are strong risk factors for esophageal cancer as well as correlate with the amount of fruit and vegetable intake. The casual association between such lifestyle behaviors and esophageal cancer should be investigated further.

We examined the effect of fruit and vegetable intake on ESCC in a large-scale population-based cohort study (Fig. 1.8) [18]. An increase in consumption of total fruit and vegetables by 100 grams per day (g/day) was associated with an 11% decrease in the incidence of ESCC (95% CI, 1–21%). In particular, a higher intake of cruciferous vegetables was associated with a significant decrease in risk (hazard ratio per 100 g/day: 0.44; 95% CI, 0.23–0.82). Stratified analyses revealed that the beneficial effect of fruits and vegetables was observed regardless of smoking of tobacco and alcohol use; however, it did not completely offset the harmful effects of smoking of tobacco and alcohol consumption.

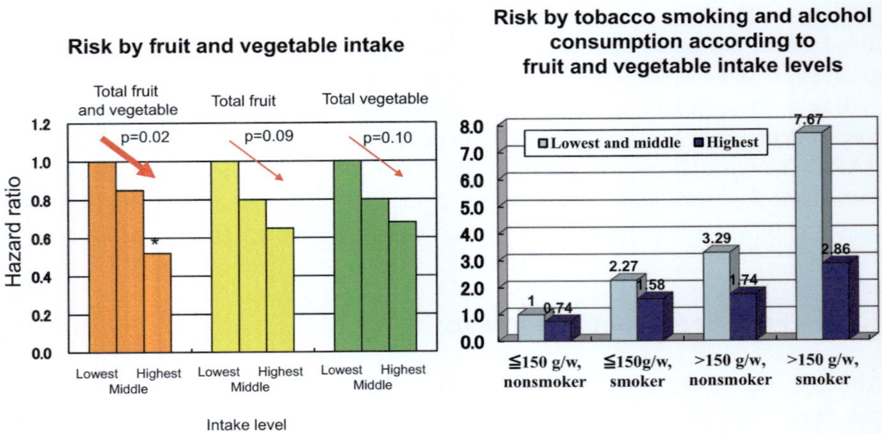

Fig. 1.8 Fruit, vegetable intake, and subsequent risk of esophageal squamous cell carcinoma—JPHC study [18]

1.2.4 Mate and Hot Beverages

Regarding the consumption of hot mate, a traditional herbal beverage consumed in parts of Southern Brazil, Argentina, and Uruguay, there appears to be a strong association with consumption of the beverage and development of esophageal squamous cell carcinoma. Meta-analysis of five case–control studies, all adjusted for smoking, showed a summary estimate of 1.16 (95%CI, 1.07–1.25) per cup/day. Mate is typically consumed very hot through a metal straw. This can cause burns in the esophagus and repeated damage of this nature can lead to cancer, although some have proposed that this may also be a result of chemical carcinogenesis from the composition of mate.

In addition to hot mate, there are several studies that show high-temperature drinks and foods are associated with the increased risk of esophageal squamous cell carcinoma, although some studies have not adequately adjusted for tobacco smoking and alcohol consumption. A recent systematic review has reported an overall OR of 2.28 (95% CI, 1.62–3.22) for the association between the consumption of hot beverages (other than mate) or food and risk of squamous cell carcinoma [2]. When the analysis was repeated in 11 studies with adjustment for smoking and alcohol consumption, the OR for all hot beverages (including mate) and food was 2.39 (95% CI, 1.71–3.22). Of interest, there was no statistically significant association with esophageal adenocarcinoma according to the meta-analysis of four studies (OR, 0.78; 95% CI, 0.45–1.35). Based on limited but suggestive evidence not only in humans for the carcinogenicity of drinking very hot beverages but also in experimental animals for the carcinogenicity of very hot water at 65 °C or above, the IARC Working Group on the Evaluation of Carcinogenic Risks to Humans has concluded that drinking very hot beverages at temperatures above 65 °C is probably carcinogenic to humans and may lead to squamous cell carcinoma of the esophagus [7].

The Research Group for the Development and Evaluation of Cancer Prevention Strategies in Japan evaluated that intake of hot tea and food is likely to have increased the risk of esophageal cancer based on systematic review of epidemiologic evidence (two cohort and three case–control studies) among the Japanese population (unpublished data, available at http://epi.ncc.go.jp/can_prev/). A cohort study showed an increased risk of 1.6-fold (95% CI, 1.2–2.0) for consumption of hot tea (drinking green tea at high temperatures) in comparison with not-hot tea (drinking green tea at moderate temperatures) [11], while another cohort showed that green tea consumption was significantly associated with an increased risk of esophageal cancer [10].

1.2.5 Causes of Esophageal Cancer in Japan

We estimated the population attributable fractions (PAFs) of esophageal cancer attributable to known risk factors from relative risks derived primarily from Japanese pooled analyses (e.g., tobacco smoking), the JPHC study (e.g., alcohol consumption, fruit and vegetables), and the prevalence of exposure in the period around 1990 [8]. PAFs of tobacco smoking, alcohol consumption, insufficient intake of vegetables and fruit were estimated to be 58.9%, 53.8%, 10.4%, and 10.9% in men and 14.7%, 28.9%, 10.4%, and 10.9% in women, respectively. Thus, 88% of esophageal cancer in men was estimated to be avoidable by lifestyle improvement such as quitting smoking, refraining from too much alcohol consumption, and sufficient intake of fruit and vegetables, after considering combined effect of risk factors. The corresponding statistic for women was estimated at 52%. Therefore, esophageal cancer can be regarded as a lifestyle-related disease.

Diet, nutrition, physical activity, and esophageal cancer [16]. Available at dietandcancerreport.org

References

1. Adami HO, Hunter DJ, Trichopoulos D. Textbook of cancer epidemiology. Oxford: Oxford University Press; 2002.
2. Andrici J, Eslick GD. Hot food and beverage consumption and the risk of esophageal cancer: a meta-analysis. Am J Prev Med. 2015;49:952–60.
3. Bray F, Colombet M, Mery L, Piñeros M, Znaor A, Zanetti R, Ferlay J, editors. Cancer incidence in five continents, Vol. XI, IARC Scientific Publication No. 166. Lyon: International Agency for Research on Cancer; 2017. Available from: http://ci5.iarc.fr. Accessed 1 Mar 2019
4. IARC Working Group on the Evaluation of Carcinogenic Risks to Humans. IARC monographs on the evaluation of carcinogenic risks to humans, Volume 83; Tobacco Smoke and Involuntary Smoking. Lyon: International Agency for Research on Cancer; 2004.
5. IARC Working Group on the Evaluation of Carcinogenic Risks to Humans. IARC monographs on the evaluation of carcinogenic risks to humans, Volume 96; Alcohol consumption and ethyl carbamate. Lyon: International Agency for Research on Cancer; 2010.

6. IARC Working Group on the Evaluation of Carcinogenic Risks to Humans. IARC monographs on the evaluation of carcinogenic risks to humans, volume 100E; a review of human carcinogens. Part E: personal habits and indoor combustions. Lyon: International Agency for Research on Cancer; 2012.
7. IARC Working Group on the Evaluation of Carcinogenic Risks to Humans. IARC monographs on the evaluation of carcinogenic risks to humans, volume 116; drinking coffee, mate, and very hot beverages. Lyon: International Agency for Research on Cancer; 2018.
8. Inoue M, Sawada N, Matsuda T, et al. Attributable causes of cancer in Japan in 2005—systematic assessment to estimate current burden of cancer attributable to known preventable risk factors in Japan. Ann Oncol. 2012;23:1362–9.
9. Ishiguro S, Sasazuki S, Inoue M, et al. Effect of alcohol consumption, cigarette smoking and flushing response on esophageal cancer risk: a population-based cohort study (JPHC study). Cancer Lett. 2009;275:240–6.
10. Ishikawa A, Kuriyama S, Tsubono Y, et al. Smoking, alcohol drinking, green tea consumption and the risk of esophageal cancer in Japanese men. J Epidemiol. 2006;16:185–92.
11. Kinjo Y, Cui Y, Akiba S, et al. Mortality risks of oesophageal cancer associated with hot tea, alcohol, tobacco and diet in Japan. J Epidemiol. 1998;8:235–43.
12. Oze I, Matsuo K, Wakai K, et al. Alcohol drinking and esophageal cancer risk: an evaluation based on a systematic review of epidemiologic evidence among the Japanese population. Jpn J Clin Oncol. 2011;41:677–92.
13. Oze I, Matsuo K, Ito H, et al. Cigarette smoking and esophageal cancer risk: an evaluation based on a systematic review of epidemiologic evidence among the Japanese population. Jpn J Clin Oncol. 2012;42:63–73.
14. Oze I, Charvat H, Matsuo K, et al. Revisit of an unanswered question by pooled analysis of eight cohort studies in Japan: does cigarette smoking and alcohol drinking have interaction for the risk of esophageal cancer? Cancer Med. 2019;8:6414–25.
15. Shibata A, Matsuda T, Ajiki W, Sobue T. Trend in incidence of adenocarcinoma of the esophagus in Japan, 1993-2001. Jpn J Clin Oncol. 2008;38:464–8.
16. World Cancer Research Fund/American Institute for Cancer Research. Continuous Update Project Expert Report 2018. Diet, nutrition, physical activity and oesophageal cancer. 2018. Available from: dietandcancerreport.org. Accessed Mar 2019.
17. Wu C, Kraft P, Zhai K, et al. Genome-wide association analyses of esophageal squamous cell carcinoma in Chinese identify multiple. Nat Genet. 2012;44:1090–8.
18. Yamaji T, Inoue M, Sasazuki S, et al. Fruit and vegetable consumption and squamous cell carcinoma of the esophagus in Japan: the JPHC study. Int J Cancer. 2008;123:1935–40.
19. Yang S-J, Yokoyama A, Yokoyama T, et al. Relationship between genetic polymorphisms of ALDH2 and ADH1B and esophageal cancer risk: a meta-analysis. World J Gastroenterol. 2010;16:4210–20.

Pathology

2

Yoko Tateishi and Yukihiro Nakanishi

2.1 Definitions

According to the Japanese Classification of Esophageal Cancer [1–3] and the World Health Organization (WHO) Classification of Tumors of the Digestive System [4], esophageal squamous cell carcinoma (ESCC), superficial esophageal cancer, early esophageal cancer, and advanced esophageal cancer are defined as follows:

Squamous cell carcinoma: a malignant epithelial tumor with squamous cell differentiation, microscopically characterized by keratinocyte-like cells with intercellular bridges and/or keratinization and/or stratified squamous differentiation [1–4].

Early esophageal cancer: an esophageal cancer whose invasion is limited to the mucosa irrespective of the presence or absence of lymph node or distant organ metastasis [1–4].

Superficial esophageal cancer: an esophageal cancer whose invasion is limited to the mucosa or submucosa irrespective of the presence or absence of lymph node or distant organ metastasis [1–4].

Advanced esophageal cancer: an esophageal cancer whose invasion extends into or beyond the muscularis propria irrespective of the presence or absence of lymph node or distant organ metastasis [1–4].

Y. Tateishi
Department of Pathology, Yokohama Municipal Citizen's Hospital,
Yokohama, Kanagawa Prefecture, Japan
e-mail: yo04-tateishi@hosp.city.yokohama.lg.jp

Y. Nakanishi (✉)
Department of Pathology, Moffitt Cancer Center, Tampa, FL, USA

Department of Pathology and Cell Biology, School of Medicine University of South Florida,
Tampa, FL, USA
e-mail: Yukihiro.nakanishi@moffitt.org

Y. Kitagawa et al. (eds.), *Esophageal Squamous Cell Carcinoma*,
https://doi.org/10.1007/978-981-92-2611-5_2

Fig. 2.1 Classification of the depth of invasion

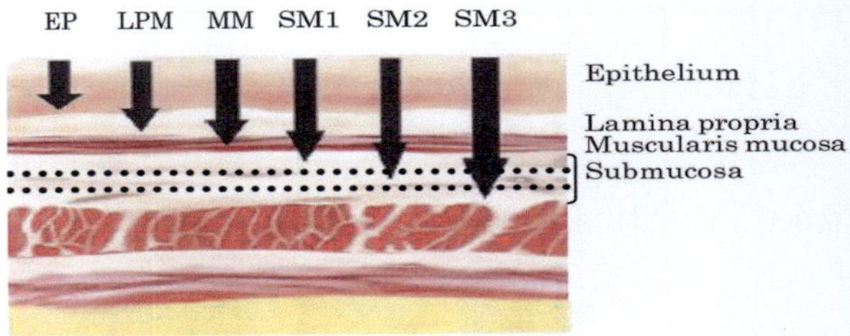

Mucosal cancer and submucosal cancer are subclassified into three categories, respectively, based on the depth of cancer invasion [1–3]: "T1a-EP" for intraepithelial carcinomas/carcinoma in situ, "T1a-LPM" for tumors invading the lamina propria, "T1a-MM" for tumors in contact with or invading the muscularis mucosae, "T1b-SM1" for tumors invading the upper third of the submucosa, "T1b-SM2" for tumors invading the middle third of the submucosa, and "T1b-SM3" for tumors invading the lower third of the submucosa (Fig. 2.1). In endoscopically resected specimens, "T1b-SM1" is defined as a carcinoma that infiltrates the submucosa up to 200 μm below the lower border of the muscularis mucosae, and "T1b-*SM2*" is defined as a carcinoma that infiltrates more than a depth of 200 μm in the submucosa [1–3], since the entire thickness of the submucosal layer is unknown in endoscopically resected specimens. Superficial esophageal squamous cell carcinoma is classified into *Tis* (high-grade dysplasia/carcinoma in situ), *T1a* (tumor invades the lamina propria or muscularis mucosae), or *T1b* (tumor invades the submucosa) by the American Joint Committee on Cancer (AJCC) [5] and the Union for International Cancer Control (UICC) TNM Classification [6].

2.2 Macroscopic Features

2.2.1 Handling of Specimens

The proper handling of a specimen by a competent pathologist is the most important step to render an accurate diagnosis and to generate a comprehensive pathology report that will help determine patient management and prognosis. The resected esophagus should be opened along the longitudinal line on the opposite side of the deepest cancer invasion. The specimens should be stretched out to approximate the length to what is in the patient's body, and should be pinned out on flat boards with the mucosal side up before fixation. After applying iodine solution on the esophageal mucosa, superficial esophageal cancers should be sectioned in its entirety [1–3]. Endoscopically resected specimens should be sectioned serially at 2–3 mm intervals parallel to a line that includes the closest part between the margin of the specimen and of the neoplasm, so that both lateral and vertical margins are assessed [1–3] (Fig. 2.2a, b). Spraying the mucosa with iodine solution is the standard method for gross examination of the specimens with abnormal squamous lesions. Iodine staining method significantly improves delineation of abnormal squamous lesions (Fig. 2.3a, b). Glycogen in the normal squamous epithelium interacts with

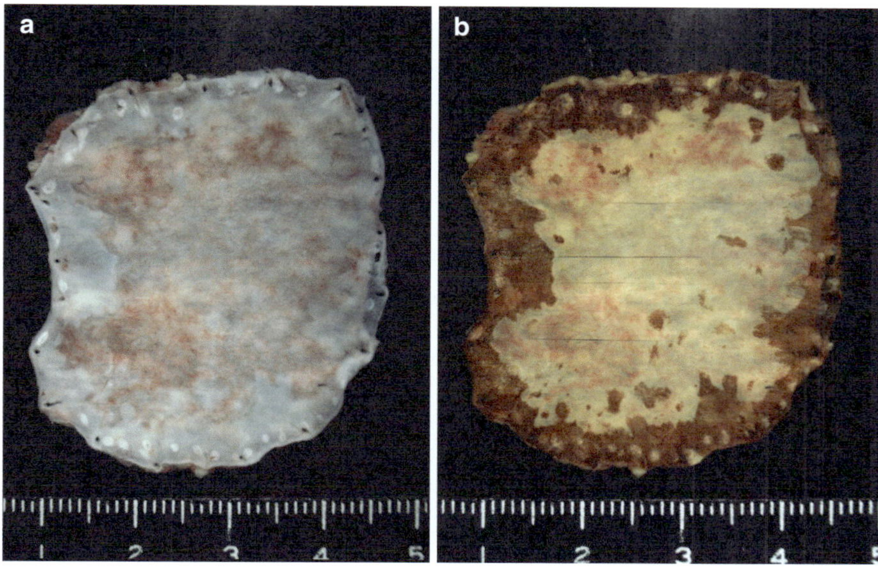

Fig. 2.2 (**a**) A 0-IIc type superficial esophageal carcinoma resected by endoscopic submucosal dissection (ESD). (**b**) After fixation and iodine staining, the specimen was sectioned serially at 2–3 mm intervals

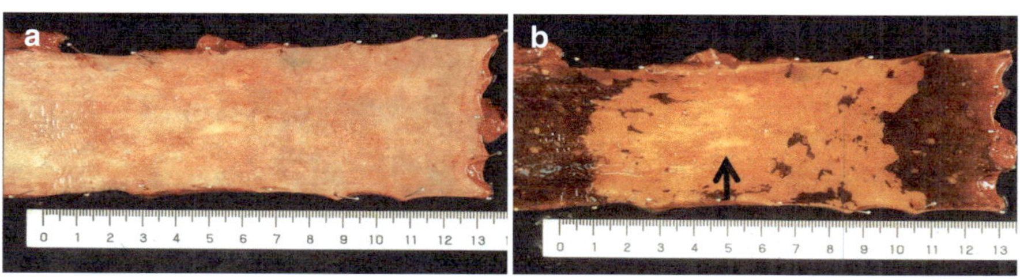

Fig. 2.3 (**a**) A shallow depressed lesion (0-IIc type) resected by esophagectomy. (**b**) Iodine staining clearly revealed an unstained area. This 0-IIc type cancer showed submucosal invasion in the whitish discolored area (arrow). This cancer can be also classified as a superficial spreading type, which is defined as a superficial esophageal cancer with more than 5 cm superficial spreading

iodine and shows a brown color. Whereas in abnormal squamous mucosa, including areas of squamous intraepithelial neoplasia/dysplasia, squamous cell carcinoma, atrophy, epidermization/epidermal metaplasia, parakeratosis, and esophagitis, the squamous epithelium often loses glycogen, and remains partially or totally unstained [7–12]. Glandular mucosa, including normal gastric mucosa, gastric heterotopia, and Barrett's mucosa, also appears unstained [13]. Foci of glycogenic acanthosis appear overstained [10].

2.2.2 General Features

Squamous cell carcinoma can occur in any portion of the esophagus but is most common in the middle third [14]. Superficial esophageal cancers appear as pink-tan or gray-white, shallow depressions, plaque-like thickenings or elevations of the mucosa. Advanced esophageal cancers grow into exophytic or ulcerated masses and obstruct the lumen.

2.2.3 Superficial Esophageal Cancer

Superficial esophageal cancers are classified as subtypes of Type 0, and further subclassified into three major types including Type 0-I, Type 0-II, and Type 0-III, based on the presence of elevation and depression [1–4] (Fig. 2.4). Type 0-I is a superficial and protruding type and includes Type 0-Ip, which is pedunculated, and Type 0-Is, which is sessile. Type 0-II is a superficial and flat type and is further subclassified into three subtypes, namely Type 0-IIa, which is slightly elevated up to 1 mm in height, Type 0-IIb, which is completely flat, and Type 0-IIc, which is slightly depressed (Fig. 2.3a, b). Type 0-III is a superficial and excavated type.

Type 0-Ip cancer is most typically seen in esophageal carcinosarcoma/spindle cell squamous cell carcinoma/sarcomatoid carcinoma (Fig. 2.5) [15]. Type 0-IIc cancer is most common in superficial esophageal cancers [16, 17]. Type 0-IIb cancer is almost always mucosal cancer, whereas Type 0-IIc cancer consists of squamous cell carcinoma, showing a wide range of cancer invasion depth from mucosal to submucosal invasion [17, 18]. More protruded (Type 0-I) or more depressed (Type 0-III) lesions are associated with deeper invasion in the submucosa [17, 18]. This applies particularly when the lesion has a mixed morphologic pattern. Many superficial esophageal cancers show combined types, e.g., a shallow depression and a sessile protrusion, 0-IIc + "0-Is" (Fig. 2.6). In the combined types, the type occupying the larger area is described first, followed by the next type according to the Japanese classification of esophageal cancer [1–3]. Double quotation marks (" ") are placed around the macroscopic tumor type that has the deepest tumor invasion.

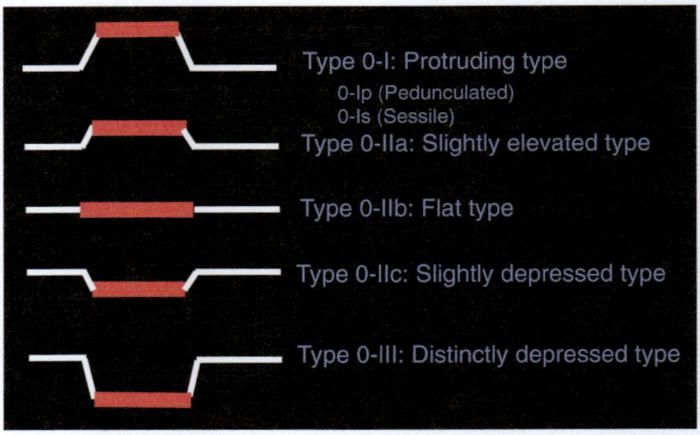

Fig. 2.4 Macroscopic classification of superficial esophageal cancer

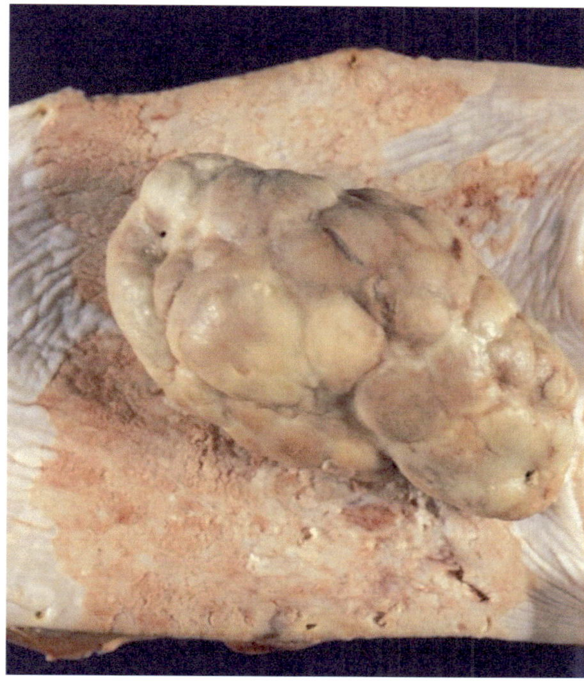

Fig. 2.5 A typical 0-Ip type superficial esophageal cancer (carcinosarcoma), which appears as a large polypoid tumor with a smooth surface and prominent lobulation. The stalk is very small and narrow, and not visible in this picture. Erosive superficial squamous cell carcinoma surrounding the polypoid tumor is also noted

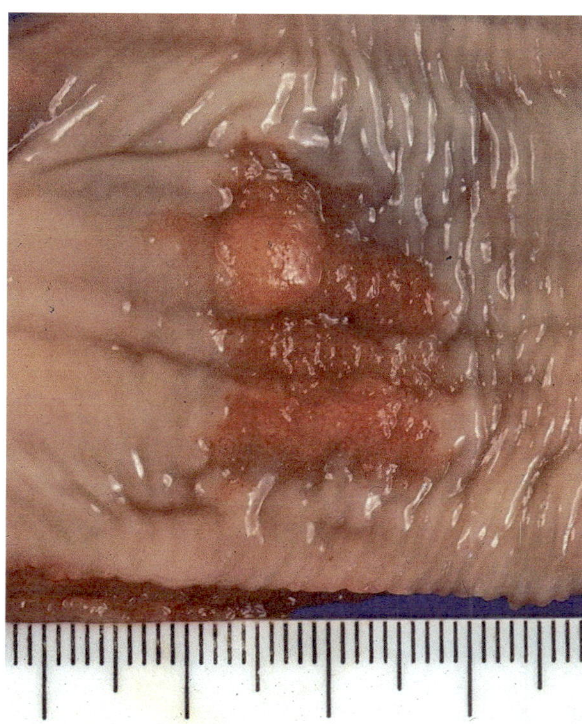

Fig. 2.6 A 0-IIc + "0-Is" type superficial esophageal cancer. The sessile portion (0-Is type) showed a deepest cancer invasion

2.2.4 Advanced Esophageal Cancer

Advanced esophageal cancers are classified into five types [1–4]. Type 1 tumor is defined as a protruding tumor (Fig. 2.7a). Type 2 tumor is defined as an ulcerative and localized tumor characterized by an ulcerated tumor with a sharply demarcated raised border (Fig. 2.7b). Type 3 tumor is defined as an ulcerative and infiltrative tumor characterized also by an ulcerated tumor, but shows infiltration into the surrounding wall, making the tumor border rather unclear (Fig. 2.7c). Type 4 tumor is defined as a diffusely infiltrating tumor in which ulceration or protrusion is usually not a prominent feature (Fig. 2.7d). A Type 5 tumor is defined as a tumor that cannot be classified into any of these types. Type 5 tumor is further classified into two subtypes: Type 5a (unclassified type without treatment) and Type 5b (unclassified type after treatment). Superficial esophageal cancer can be found at the periphery of an advanced tumor. When an advanced type is mixed with a superficial type, the advanced type is described first without placing double quotation marks [1–3]. The macroscopic classification of ESCC can be applied to all esophageal adenocarcinomas.

The two most frequent types of advanced cancers are Types 2 and 3 [16]. A protruding type tumor is usually found to be a carcinosarcoma/spindle cell squamous cell carcinoma/sarcomatoid carcinoma, squamous cell carcinoma, or malignant melanoma [15]. A protruding type tumor, especially showing a subepithelial growth, is usually composed of a small cell neuroendocrine carcinoma, basaloid squamous cell carcinoma, or lymphoepithelioma-like carcinoma/esophageal carcinoma with lymphoid stroma [19].

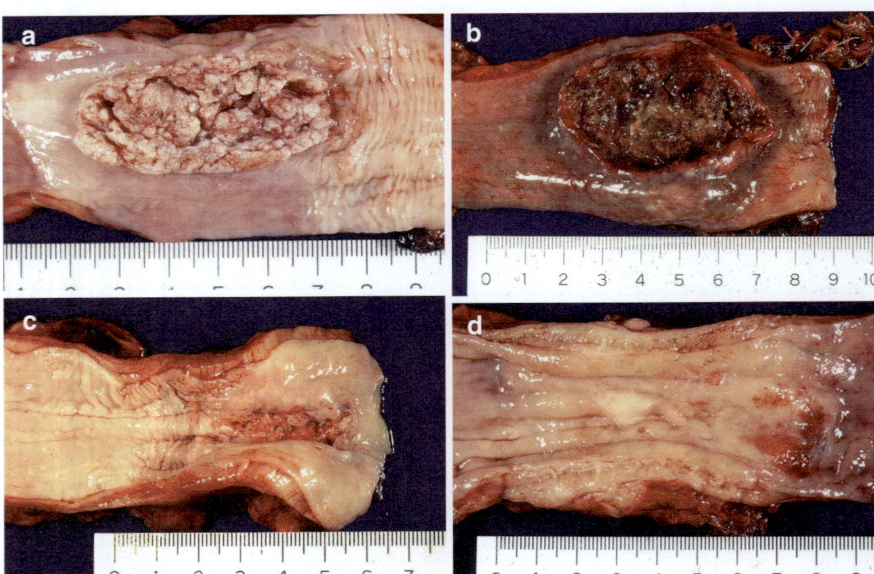

Fig. 2.7 (**a**) Type 1 tumor (a protruding tumor); (**b**) Type 2 tumor (an ulcerated tumor with a sharply demarcated raised border); (**c**) Type 3 tumor (an ulcerated tumor with an unclear border); (**d**) Type 4 tumor (a diffusely infiltrating tumor)

2.2.5 Multicentric Squamous Cell Carcinoma (Field Cancerization)

The presence of other cancers synchronously or metachronously associated with esophageal carcinoma is relatively common. According to the comprehensive registry of esophageal cancer in Japan, up to 47% of patients with esophageal carcinoma had synchronous or metachronous carcinoma at another sites including the stomach, head and neck, colon/rectum, and lung in this descending order [16]. Up to 20% of patients with ESCC had synchronous or metachronous multiple primary cancers of the esophagus [16]. ESCC, especially multicentric squamous cell carcinoma, is often associated with multiple small areas unstained with Lugol's iodine observed in the mucosa surrounding esophageal carcinomas (Fig. 2.8) [8]. Patients with head and neck squamous cell carcinoma, who have a high risk for ESCC, have also been reported to be frequently associated with multiple Lugol-voiding lesions [8, 20, 21]. The incidence of multiple Lugol-voiding lesions has been reported to be associated with the development of multiple primary cancers in the upper aerodigestive tract and the patients' tobacco and alcohol consumption [8]. Also, male sex and alcohol-degrading enzyme ADH1B and ALDH2 genotypes have been reported to be associated with an increased risk for multiple Lugol-voiding lesions of the esophageal mucosa in patients with ESCC [22]. Therefore, iodine staining method is useful not only for optimal visualization of esophageal squamous mucosal abnormalities but also for detecting groups at high risk of multicentric cancer in the upper aerodigestive tract. Although staining esophageal mucosa with iodine solution has not often been used by endoscopists and pathologists in North America, iodine staining is the necessary diagnostic method for ESCC.

2.2.6 Risk Factors

Risk factors include alcohol [23], alcohol-degrading enzyme genotype [24], tobacco use [23], history of upper aerodigestive tract cancer [23], Achalasia (Fig. 2.9) [23], severe caustic injury [23], frequent consumption of very hot beverages [25], prior radiation therapy to the mediastinum [26], non-epidermolytic palmoplantar

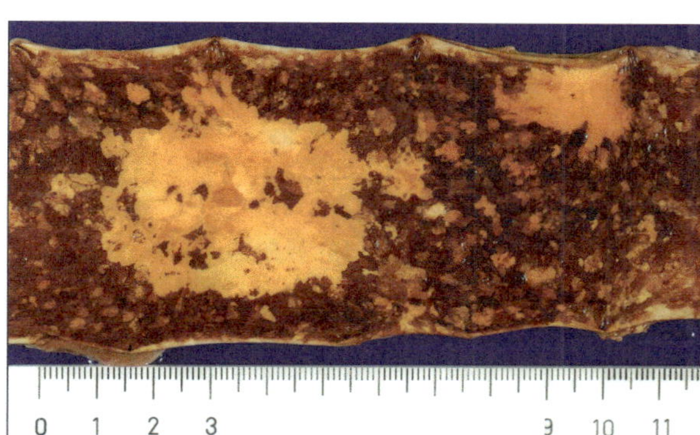

Fig. 2.8 Iodine staining clearly reveals two unstained cancerous areas. In addition to the cancerous areas, there are multiple small iodine-unstained areas in the mucosa surrounding the cancerous lesions

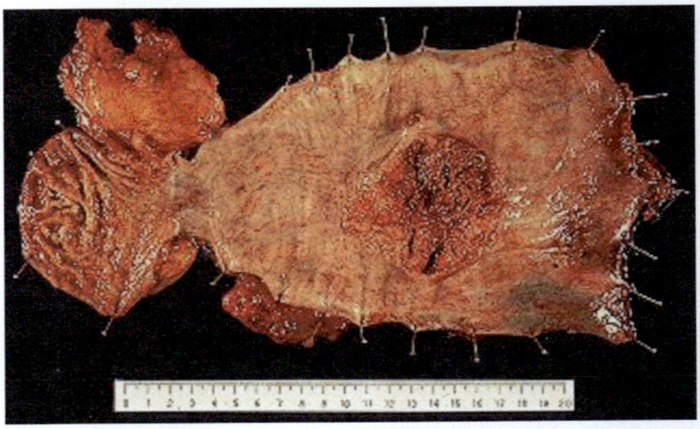

Fig. 2.9 A Type 2 advanced esophageal cancer developed in Achalasia

keratoderma (tylosis), [23] Plummer-Vinson syndrome [27], nutrition (e.g., nitrosamines in pickled or moldy foods) [28], celiac sprue [29], lichen planus [30], and human papilloma virus [31].

2.3 Microscopic Features

2.3.1 General Features

The histology of ESCC is similar to that of squamous cell carcinomas of other sites with enlarged, often vesicular nuclei and eosinophilic opaque cytoplasm. Variable amounts of keratinization with intercellular bridges and stratified squamous differentiation are observed depending on tumor differentiation grade. The neoplastic cells form variably-sized irregular tumor nests with variable amount of desmoplastic stromal reaction and inflammatory response [32]. The desmoplastic stromal reaction is one of the histological hallmarks of invasive carcinoma and is composed of activated fibroblasts with enlarged nuclei, inflammatory cells, and capillary proliferation. This stromal reaction results from a complex interaction between infiltrating cancer cells and the host. Zonal squamous differentiation with keratinization and vague palisading of basaloid tumor cells in the periphery of tumor nests recapitulate the organization of normal stratified squamous epithelium (Fig. 2.10). According to the Japanese classification of esophageal cancer [1–3], well-differentiated squamous cell carcinoma is characterized by extensive keratinization and stratified squamous differentiation, whereas poorly differentiated squamous cell carcinoma shows a nest or sheet-like growth pattern with minimal keratinization. Moderately differentiated squamous cell carcinoma lies between these two (Fig. 2.10). The WHO classification states that grading is based on the degree of cytological atypia, and the presence of keratinization. Both the Japanese and the WHO classifications include no special reference to the ratio of keratinization [1–4]. No widely-accepted, well-tested grading system has been established. Although both the Japanese and the WHO classifications classify squamous cell carcinomas into well-differentiated (grade 1), moderately differentiated (grade 2), and poorly

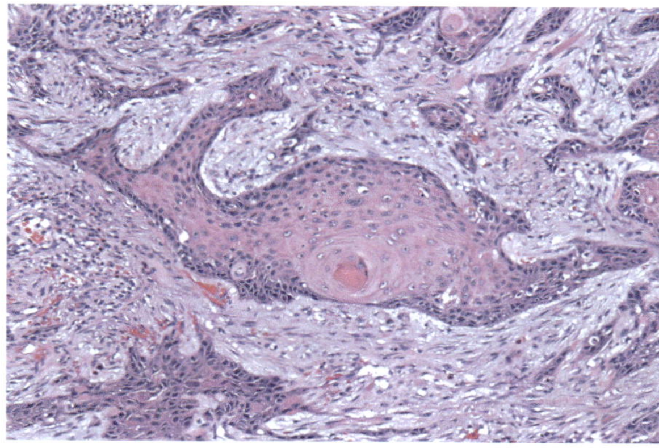

Fig. 2.10 Moderately differentiated squamous cell carcinoma with stratified squamous differentiation and keratinization. The desmoplastic stromal reaction, one of the histological hallmarks of invasive carcinoma, is noted

differentiated (grade 3), the WHO classification recommends a two-tiered system (grade 1–2 vs grade 3), because the pathological distinction between grade 1 and grade 2 often shows high interobserver variation. Most of ESCCs show a characteristic histomorphology, so that the diagnosis might be unproblematic. The differential diagnosis of squamous cell carcinoma, especially poorly differentiated type, in a biopsy or surgical specimen includes squamous epithelium with reactive changes, undifferentiated carcinoma, neuroendocrine carcinoma, poorly differentiated adenocarcinoma, salivary gland-type carcinoma, pseudoepitheliomatous hyperplasia (e.g., pseudoepitheliomatous hyperplasia associated with granular cell tumor [33]), radiation effect, hyperplastic polyp of the esophagogastric junction [34], malignant melanoma, and metastatic tumor. Immunohistochemistry (e.g., p40, p63, and cytokeratin 5/6) can provide assistance in the differential diagnosis, as well as review of imaging studies. The main differential diagnosis of squamous cell carcinoma in a biopsy specimen is usually a squamous epithelium with reactive changes.

2.3.2 Microvessel Morphology (Vascular Classification)

In superficial ESCC, the morphology of intrapapillary capillary loops (IPCLs), a microvascular structure within the lesion, is utilized to assess the extent of the lesion and predict the depth of invasion. These vascular patterns are evaluated by endoscopic observation using narrow-band imaging (NBI). According to the classification of the Japan Esophageal Society, vascular patterns are categorized into Type A (normal to low-grade atypia) and Type B (B1–B3), which indicate neoplastic changes [3, 35]. Type B1 consists of fine, loop-like vessels structurally resembling normal IPCLs and is typically associated with T1a-EP/LPM lesions. Type B2 is characterized by dilated and irregular vessels and is typically associated with T1a-MM/T1b-SM1 lesions. Type B3 shows marked dilation and is typically associated with T1b-SM2 or deeper lesions. In carcinoma in situ, Type B1 vessels appear elongated and dilated, whereas in invasive carcinoma, thick and irregular vessels corresponding to Type B2 are observed in the stroma surrounding tumor nests.

2.4 Tumor Spread

ESCC shows unique patterns of tumor spread including ductal/glandular involvement, diffuse pagetoid spread, and intramural metastasis like those frequently seen in other organs such as uterine cervix and nipple.

2.4.1 Superficial Esophageal Cancer

ESCC begins as an in situ carcinoma and spreads both horizontally and vertically. Squamous cell carcinoma in situ is characterized by well-demarcated border and a high cellularity with a loss of the basal layer. Initial invasion into the lamina propria is characterized by the downward growth of neoplastic squamous epithelium without prominent desmoplastic stromal reaction. It is a distinctive feature of ESCC that lymph node metastasis occurs early in the course of the disease. The abundant lymphatic channels in the lamina propria and submucosa of the esophagus are responsible for the high frequency of lymph node metastasis [36, 37]. All submucosal tumors have a substantial risk of lymph node metastasis [17, 18, 38].

2.4.1.1 Ductal/Glandular Involvement

The esophageal submucosal glands are considered to be a continuation of the minor salivary glands and scattered throughout the entire esophagus. Squamous cell carcinoma in situ can extend into the ducts of the submucosal glands. Ductal/glandular involvement has often been observed in superficial squamous cell carcinoma of the esophagus, with an incidence of 21.3–38.1% [39–41]. Maximum tumor size has been reported to be associated with the presence of ductal/glandular involvement by multivariate analysis, indicating that ductal/glandular involvement develops in association with horizontal tumor growth [39, 41]. According to the Japanese classification of esophageal cancer, tumors with ductal/glandular involvement that extends to the submucosa but does not definitely invade the submucosal stroma should not be classified as submucosal carcinoma [1–3]. However, even in mucosal carcinoma, there exists a possibility of incomplete clearance of the tumor tissue by endoscopic resection or endoscopic ablation therapy due to the presence of ductal/glandular involvement extending to the submucosal layer or reaching the end portions of esophageal glands [41]. Also, it is very important to judge accurately whether a small cancerous nest in the submucosal layer in an endoscopically resected specimen is ductal/glandular involvement, direct tumor invasion, or lympho-vascular invasion in deciding the necessity for additional surgical resection based on the histopathologic findings in endoscopically resected specimens. Immunohistochemistry (e.g., CD31, D2–40) and elastic stain can be helpful in the differential diagnosis, as well as deeper cut sections.

2.4.1.2 Diffuse Pagetoid Spread

Occasionally, squamous cell carcinoma cells exhibit a pagetoid pattern of growth. However, diffuse pagetoid spreading of squamous cell carcinoma in situ of the esophagus is very rare and is characterized by the pronounced pagetoid spread of squamous cell carcinoma [42–44]. Pagetoid spread of squamous cell carcinoma in situ and true Paget's disease are very similar histologically.

2.4.2 Lymph Node Metastasis in Patients with Superficial Esophageal Cancer

The proportion of patients with superficial ESCC and lymph node metastasis has been reported to be 39–54%, whereas the proportion of patients with superficial ESCC invading the lamina propria mucosae (LPM) and lymph node metastasis is only 1.4–4.0% [17, 18, 45, 46]. The risk of lymph node metastasis is surprisingly high when it reaches the muscularis mucosae (MM: 5.0–18.0%) or the superficial submucosa (SM1: 26.5–53.9%) [17, 18, 45, 46]. Consequently, intraepithelial carcinoma (EP) or carcinoma invading the lamina propria is generally treated by endoscopic resection [1–3]. Tumors with an estimated depth of invasion of MM or SM1 without lymph node metastasis on diagnostic imaging studies are considered to have a relative indication for endoscopic resection, whereas tumors with an estimated depth of invasion of SM2 or SM3 have no indication for endoscopic resection [1–3]. However, clinical diagnosis of the depth of invasion is not always accurate. One of the major advantages of endoscopic resection is to recover a specimen for histopathologic analysis, which helps to make a clinical decision for further therapy after endoscopic resection. Previous studies have reported that lymphatic invasion was significantly associated with lymph node metastasis in patients with superficial ESCC in a multivariate analysis [45–47].

2.4.3 Advanced Esophageal Cancer

Advanced esophageal cancers may invade surrounding structures including the trachea, lung, aorta, mediastinum, and pericardium. Distally located tumors often invade the stomach. Metastases to distant organs are frequent, particularly to the liver and lung [16].

2.4.3.1 Intramural Metastasis

Metastasis from an esophageal carcinoma to the esophagus or stomach is termed intramural metastasis. Intramural metastasis has often been found in the resected esophagus, with an incidence of 3.9–15% [48–50]. Patients with intramural metastasis have a higher frequency of lymph node metastasis and liver recurrence than those without intramural metastasis [50]. Intramural metastasis is more predictive of a worse prognosis than local recurrence [48].

2.4.3.2 Prognostic Factors

Clinicopathologic prognostic factors include TNM stage [1–3], lymph node metastasis [51, 52], tumor invasion depth [51, 52], lympho-vascular invasion [52], intramural metastasis [48, 50, 52], tumor vascularity [53], infiltrating growth pattern [54], inflammatory response [54, 55], tumor budding [56], tumor nest configuration [32], extranodal spreading [57], epithelial–mesenchymal transition phenotype [58]. pathologic response to neoadjuvant therapy [59], completeness of surgical resection [51], patient's general health condition [60], and PD-1 and PD-L1 expression level [61]. Most of these studies have shown no significant influence of tumor differentiation grade on survival. Among these clinicopathologic prognostic factors, the number of metastasis-positive lymph nodes is a simple and reliable prognostic factor [62, 63]. In patients with tumor limited to the submucosal layer, even with tumors located in the mid- and lower esophagus, lymph node metastasis was frequent in the upper mediastinum and perigastric area [64]. Isolated distant lymph node involvement from superficial esophageal cancer is thus not necessarily a sign of advanced disease [64]. The most predictive factor for patient's survival is not the area of involved nodes, but the number of involved nodes [65, 66]. Numerous genomic and epigenomic aberrations are involved in the development of ESCC [67–69]. Most of them are involved in signal transduction, regulation of transcription, cell cycle, cell apoptosis, hypermethylation in CpG islands, and immune cell-specific gene. Such markers may have potential implications in early detection of tumorigenesis and prediction of metastasis and survival.

2.4.3.3 PD-L1 Evaluation

When administering immune checkpoint inhibitors (ICIs), such as nivolumab or pembrolizumab, PD-L1 expression is assessed by immunohistochemistry using scoring systems such as the Combined Positive Score (CPS) and the Tumor Proportion Score (TPS). In general, tumors with high PD-L1 expression—typically defined as CPS $\geq$10—tend to show a better response to ICI-based therapies [70]. However, clinical *PD-L1* efficacy has also been demonstrated regardless of PD-L1 expression status, and combined regimens with chemotherapy are increasingly recommended as standard first-line treatment [71].

2.5 Precursor Lesion (Squamous Dysplasia/Intraepithelial Neoplasia)

Precursor lesion is named as dysplasia, and also referred to as intraepithelial neoplasia [1–4]. Squamous dysplasia/intraepithelial neoplasia is defined as a neoplastic lesion with architectural and cytological abnormalities [1–4]. Squamous dysplasia/intraepithelial neoplasia is characterized by nuclear atypia and abnormal epithelial maturation with well-demarcated border (Fig. 2.11). Although the 12th edition of the Japanese Classification of Esophageal Cancer has abolished the two-tier subclassification of low grade and high grade, the WHO Classification of Tumors of the Digestive System still maintains the two-tier subclassification [3, 4].

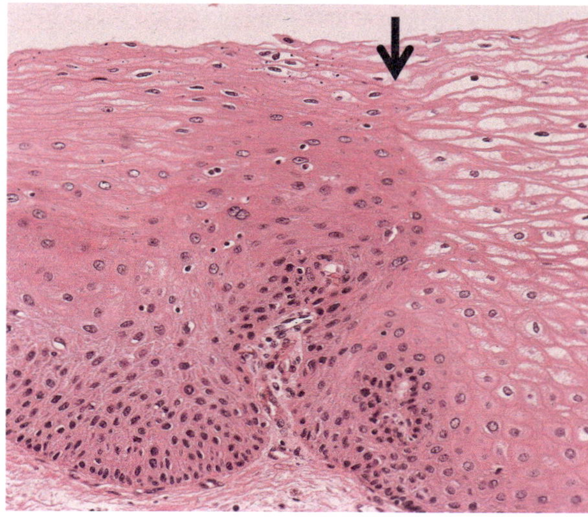

Fig. 2.11 Increased cellularity, mild nuclear atypia, and hyperchromasia are evident, which can be regarded as dysplasia (low-grade intraepithelial neoplasia). The abrupt transition of squamous cells (right) to atypical squamous cells (left) is noted. Arrow indicates the border between normal squamous epithelium and dysplastic squamous epithelium

In low-grade intraepithelial neoplasia, the architectural and cytological abnormalities are confined to the lower half of the epithelium. In high-grade squamous dysplasia/intraepithelial neoplasia, the abnormalities involve the upper half of the epithelium. High-grade dysplasia/intraepithelial neoplasia is also diagnosed when severe cytological atypia is present regardless of the extent of epithelial involvement. Full thickness involvement of the squamous epithelium, called squamous cell carcinoma in situ in Japan, is considered synonymous with high-grade intraepithelial neoplasia (high-grade dysplasia) in North America and Europe based on their similar histologic appearance and risk of progression into invasive ESCC [4, 72]. Japanese pathologists diagnose carcinoma solely on the basis of the architectural and cytological changes observed without requiring histological evidence of invasive growth, whereas pathologists in North America and Europe define carcinoma as one that has histological evidence of invasive growth [4, 73, 74].

The differentiation of squamous dysplasia/intraepithelial neoplasia from reactive change is sometimes challenging. The abrupt transition of the normal squamous cells to atypical squamous cells may serve as a diagnostic indicator for squamous dysplasia/intraepithelial neoplasia (Fig. 2.11). Immunohistochemistry for Ki-67 and p53 is also adjunctively available in the diagnosis of squamous dysplasia/intraepithelial neoplasia [75].

2.6 Tumor Response to Neoadjuvant Therapy

Tumor response to neoadjuvant therapy has been identified as an important prognostic factor. [59] Histopathologic changes induced by neoadjuvant therapy include eosinophilic cytoplasm, nuclear enlargement or shrinkage, cytoplasmic or nuclear vacuolation, apoptosis, necrosis, free keratin pearls/debris, foreign body giant cell reaction, dystrophic calcification, atypical fibroblast, fibrosis, and vascular alterations such as myxoid or hyaline intimal changes, capillary dilation, organized thrombi, and obliterative endoarteritis [4]. Despite degenerative changes, tumor cells that are judged to retain proliferative capacity must be evaluated as viable cancer cells. The extent of tumor regression is graded based on histologic examination by subjectively comparing the amount of residual tumor with the amount of therapy-induced fibrosis. [1–4, 76] The Japan Esophageal Society classifies therapeutic effect into four grades: Grade 0 (no effect), Grade 1 (residual tumor in ≥2/3 of the lesion), Grade 2 (residual tumor in ≥1/3 but <2/3 of the lesion), and Grade 3 (complete response with no detectable cancer cells) [3]. In contrast, the Mandard classification, widely used in Western countries and primarily applied to adenocarcinoma, stratifies tumor regression into five tiers: TRG 1 (complete response with no residual cancer cells) to TRG 5 (no response) [76].

2.7 Variants

The subtypes of ESCC include basaloid squamous cell carcinoma, carcinosarcoma/spindle cell squamous cell carcinoma/sarcomatoid carcinoma, adenosquamous carcinoma, and verrucous carcinoma.

2.7.1 Basaloid Squamous Cell Carcinoma

Basaloid squamous cell carcinoma is an uncommon variant of squamous cell carcinoma with a male predominance, accounting for approximately 2–5% of primary esophageal malignancies [4, 14, 77–79]. It is histopathologically distinct from squamous cell carcinoma, and is characterized by a poor degree of differentiation and high proliferative activity [78]. Histologically, typical basaloid squamous cell carcinomas are composed of relatively uniform, small, round-to-oval cells with scant cytoplasm forming large solid tumor nests with comedo-like necrosis (Fig. 2.12). The tumor nests contain eosinophilic hyaline material, suggesting a basement membrane-like substance. Basaloid squamous cell carcinoma has a wide variation of histological features including solid nest, cribriform pattern, microcyst, trabecular nest, and ductal differentiation [77]. Basaloid squamous cell carcinoma with salivary-type differentiation, mimicking the histologic features of epithelial–myoepithelial carcinoma of the salivary gland, has also been reported [80]. Areas of squamous intraepithelial neoplasia or invasive squamous cell carcinoma are often observed [79, 81]. Biopsy specimens are taken from superficial areas of a tumor. Therefore, many cases of basaloid squamous cell carcinoma of the esophagus are reportedly diagnosed as squamous cell carcinoma preoperatively. Basaloid squamous cell carcinoma could be mistakenly diagnosed as adenocarcinoma, adenoid cystic carcinoma, undifferentiated carcinoma, or neuroendocrine carcinoma if a

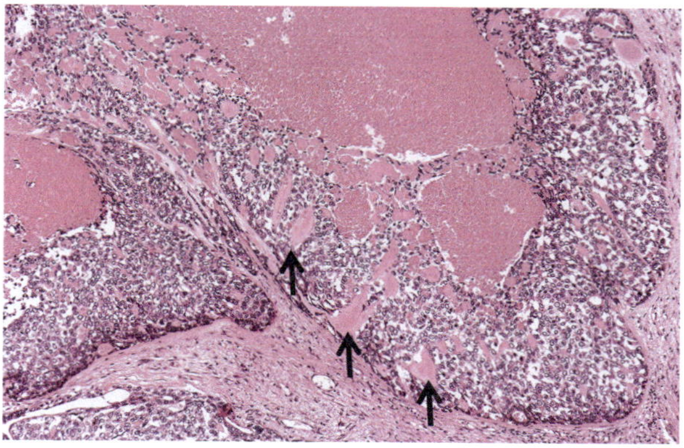

Fig. 2.12 Typical histologic features of basaloid squamous cell carcinoma. Relatively uniform neoplastic cells with scant cytoplasm form large solid tumor nests with comedo-like necrosis. The tumor nests contain eosinophilic hyaline material, suggesting a basement membrane-like substance (arrows)

biopsy sample contains the components of ductal differentiation, cribriform pattern, sold nest, or trabecular nest, respectively [77, 82].

2.7.2 Carcinosarcoma/Spindle Cell Squamous Cell Carcinoma/ Sarcomatoid Carcinoma

Carcinosarcoma/spindle cell squamous cell carcinoma/sarcomatoid carcinoma is a rare variant of squamous cell carcinoma and accounts for approximately 1.0% of primary esophageal malignancies [14]. Histologically, carcinosarcoma/spindle cell squamous cell carcinoma/sarcomatoid carcinoma is composed of a proliferation of spindle-shaped sarcomatous tumor cells and squamous cell carcinoma forming tumor nests (Fig. 2.13) [4]. The spindle-cell component may show osseous, cartilaginous, and skeletal-muscle differentiation. Therefore, this tumor can be regarded as carcinosarcoma with biphasic differentiation. Immunohistochemically, spindle-shaped sarcomatous tumor cells may display various degrees of epithelial differentiation. Almost all reported cases of esophageal carcinosarcoma/spindle cell squamous cell carcinoma/sarcomatoid carcinoma have been macroscopically polypoid, and rarely show an ulcerated appearance [15]. Grossly, esophageal carcinosarcoma/spindle cell squamous cell carcinoma/sarcomatoid carcinoma shows a typical 0-Ip type superficial esophageal cancer, which appears as a large polypoid tumor with a smooth surface and prominent lobulation (Fig. 2.5). The stalk is usually very small and narrow. This tumor shows such characteristic macroscopic features that one can easily recognize its histologic type. Superficial-type squamous cell carcinoma is often found in the mucosa surrounding a polypoid carcinosarcoma/spindle cell squamous cell carcinoma/sarcomatoid carcinoma (Fig. 2.5). Patients with carcinosarcoma become symptomatic early because of their large polypoid mass. Therefore, the overall prognosis of the patients with carcinosarcoma has been reported to be better than that of the patients with conventional squamous cell carcinoma [83].

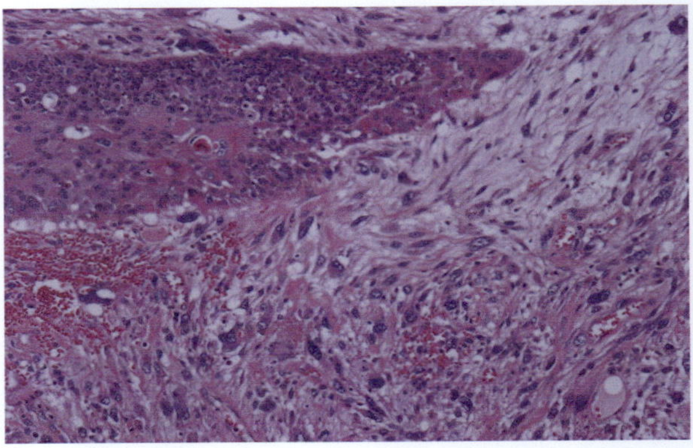

Fig. 2.13 Carcinosarcoma/spindle cell squamous cell carcinoma/sarcomatoid carcinoma with biphasic differentiation composed of both spindle-shaped sarcomatous tumor cells and squamous cell carcinoma forming tumor nests

2.7.3 Adenosquamous Carcinoma

Adenosquamous carcinoma is a rare variant of squamous cell carcinoma. According to the previous reports, approximately 1.0% of resected esophageal cancers are diagnosed pathologically as adenosquamous carcinoma [14, 84, 85]. Microscopically, it consists of coexisting elements of infiltrating squamous cell carcinoma and adenocarcinoma (Fig. 2.14). According to the Japanese Classification of Esophageal Cancer, adenosquamous carcinoma of the esophagus is defined as having at least 20% of each of squamous cell carcinoma and adenocarcinoma elements on routine microscopic examination, using hematoxylin and eosin staining [1–3]. The WHO classification, however, states simply that adenosquamous carcinoma has a significant squamous carcinomatous component that is intermingled with tubular adenocarcinoma elements, with no special reference to the ratio of these two components [4]. Although some previous reports of esophageal adenosquamous carcinoma have indicated that these tumors show highly aggressive biological behavior, other previous reports showed that such patients had a significantly better outcome or had no significant difference in survival time compared with patients with squamous cell carcinomas or adenocarcinomas [84–90]. The median age at presentation, the location, and macroscopic features of adenosquamous carcinomas were similar to those of squamous cell carcinomas [84, 85].

2.7.4 Verrucous Carcinoma

Verrucous carcinoma is an extremely rare, highly differentiated variant of squamous cell carcinoma. Verrucous carcinoma grows slowly and locally, and only rarely metastasizes [1–3, 91, 92]. It is generally an exophytic and warty in appearance, and demonstrates blunt papillary projections of highly differentiated squamous cells with a pushing margin. Therefore, the diagnosis of verrucous carcinoma is particularly challenging due to its bland histologic features. A superficial biopsy is usually not sufficient to make a definitive diagnosis.

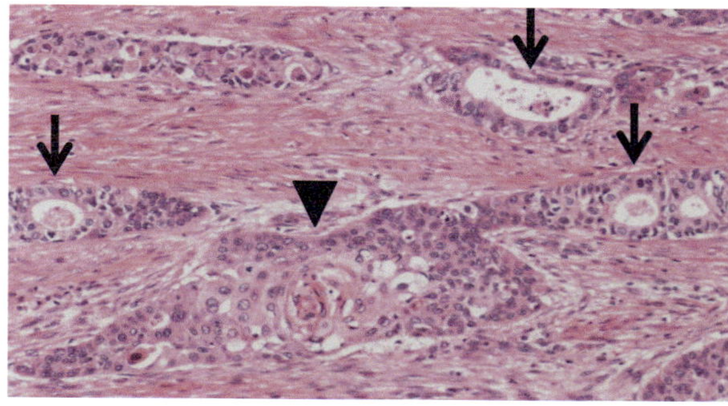

Fig. 2.14 Adenosquamous carcinoma containing coexisting elements of infiltrating squamous cell carcinoma (arrow head) and adenocarcinoma (arrows)

References

1. Japan Esophageal Society. Japanese classification of esophageal cancer, English version. Kanehara, Tokyo; 2015.
2. Japan Esophageal Society. Japanese classification of esophageal cancer, 12th edition: part 1. Esophagus. 2024;21:179–215.
3. Japan Esophageal Society. Japanese classification of esophageal cancer, 12th edition: part II. Esophagus. 2024;21:216–69.
4. Odze RD, Cree IA, Klimstra DS, et al., editors. WHO classification of tumours. Digestive system tumours. 5th ed. Lyon: IARC Press; 2019.
5. Amin MB, et al., editors. AJCC cancer staging manual. 8th ed. New York: Springer; 2017.
6. Brierley JD, Gospodarowicz MK, Wittekind C, editors. TNM classification of malignant Tumours. 8th ed. Oxford: Wiley-Blackwell; 2017.
7. Dawsey SM, Fleischer DE, Wang GQ, et al. Mucosal iodine staining improves endoscopic visualization of squamous dysplasia and squamous cell carcinoma of the esophagus in Linxian, China. Cancer. 1998;83:220–31.
8. Nakanishi Y, Ochiai A, Yoshimura K, et al. The clinicopathologic significance of small areas unstained by Lugol's iodine in the mucosa surrounding resected esophageal carcinoma: an analysis of 147 cases. Cancer. 1998;82:1454–9.
9. Nakanishi Y, Ochiai A, Shimoda T, et al. Epidermization in the esophageal mucosa: unusual epithelial changes clearly detected by Lugol's staining. Am J Surg Pathol. 1997;21:605–9.
10. Mori M, Adachi Y, Matsushima T, et al. Lugol staining pattern and histology of esophageal lesions. Am J Gastroenterol. 1993;88:701–5.
11. Park JY, Kim DM, Min BH, et al. Esophageal parakeratosis mimicking endoscopic appearance of superficial esophageal neoplastic lesion such as dysplasia. Dig Endosc. 2012;24:117–9.
12. Yoshikawa I, Yamasaki M, Yamasaki T, et al. Lugol chromoendoscopy as a diagnostic tool in so-called endoscopy-negative GERD. Gastrointest Endosc. 2005;62:698–703.
13. Boyce HW. Barrett esophagus. Endoscopic findings and what to biopsy. J Clin Gastroenterol. 2003;36(Suppl. 1):S6–S18.
14. Watanabe M, Toh Y, Ishihara R, et al. Comprehensive registry of esophageal cancer in Japan, 2015. Esophagus. 2023;20:1–28.
15. Raza MA, Mazzara PF. Sarcomatoid carcinoma of esophagus. Arch Pathol Lab Med. 2011;135:945–8.
16. Ide H, Ozawa S, Matsubara H, et al. Comprehensive registry of esophageal cancer in Japan, 2000. Esophagus. 2009;6:27–47.
17. Participants in the Paris Workshop. The Paris endoscopic classification of superficial neoplastic lesions: esophagus, stomach, and colon. Gastrointest Endosc. 2003;58(Suppl 6):S3–S43.

18. Kodama M, Kakegawa T. Treatment of superficial cancer of the esophagus: a summary of responses to a questionnaire on superficial cancer of the esophagus in Japan. Surgery. 1998;123:432–9.
19. Takubo K. Pathology of the esophagus. 3rd ed. Tokyo: Wiley; 2017.
20. Muto H, Katada C, Yokoyama T, et al. Field effect of alcohol, cigarette smoking, and their cessation on the development of multiple dysplastic lesions and squamous cell carcinoma: a long-term multicenter cohort study. Gastro Hep Adv. 2022;15:265–76.
21. Hori K, Katada C, Okada H, et al. Association between continuous cessation or reduction of drinking alcohol and improvement of multiple dysplastic lesions in patients with esophageal squamous cell carcinoma after endoscopic resection. Esophagus. 2024;21:31–40.
22. Cui R, Kamatani Y, Takahashi A, et al. Functional variants in ADH1B and ALDH2 coupled with alcohol and smoking synergistically enhance esophageal cancer risk. Gastroenterology. 2009;137:1768–75.
23. Hirota WK, Zuckerman MJ, Adler DG, et al. ASGE guideline: the role of endoscopy in the surveillance of premalignant conditions of the upper GI tract. Gastrointest Endosc. 2006;63(4):570–80.
24. Tajiri A, Ishihara R, Sakurai H, et al. Clinical features of superficial esophagus squamous cell carcinoma according to alcohol-degrading enzyme ADH1B and ALDH2 genotypes. J Gastroenterol. 2022;57:630–9.
25. Islami F, Boffetta P, Ren JS, et al. High-temperature beverages and foods and esophageal cancer risk—a systemic review. Int J Cancer. 2009;125:491–524.
26. Morton LM, Gilbert ES, Hall P, et al. Risk of treatment-related esophageal cancer among breast cancer survivors. Ann Oncol. 2012;23:3081–91.
27. Anderson SR, Sinacori JT. Plummer-Vinson syndrome heralded by postcricoid carcinoma. Am J Otolaryngol. 2007;28:22–4.
28. Abnet CC, Arnold M, Wei WQ. Epidemiology of esophageal squamous cell carcinoma. Gastroenterology. 2018;154:360–73.
29. Landgren AM, Landgren O, Gridley G, et al. Autoimmune disease and subsequent risk of developing alimentary tract cancers among 4.5 million U.S. male veterans. Cancer. 2011;117:1163–71.
30. Chandan VS, Murray JA, Abraham SC. Esophageal lichen planus. Arch Pathol Lab Med. 2008;132:1026–9.
31. Bauer AH, Alkhateeb KJ, Agoston AT, et al. Transcriptionally active human papillomavirus infection in a minority of esophageal squamous cell carcinomas in North America. Am J Surg Pathol. 2024;48:883–9.
32. Nakanishi Y, Ochiai A, Kato H, et al. Clinicopathological significance of tumor nest configuration in patients with esophageal squamous cell carcinoma. Cancer. 2001;91:1114–11120.
33. Lack E, Worsham F, Callihan M, et al. Granular cell tumor: a clinicopathologic study of 110 patients. J Surg Oncol. 1980;13:301–6.
34. Abraham S, Singh V, Yardley J, et al. Hyperplastic polyps of the esophagus and esophagogastric junction. Am J Surg Pathol. 2001;25:1180–7.
35. Oyama T, Inoue H, Arima M, et al. Prediction of the invasion depth of superficial squamous cell carcinoma based on microvessel morphology: magnifying endoscopic classification of the Japan Esophageal Society. Esophagus. 2017;14:105–12.
36. Weinberg JA. Lymphatics of the esophagus. In: Haagensen CD, Feind CR, Herter FP, Slanetz Jr CA, Weinberg JA, editors. The lymphatics in cancer. Philadelphia: Saunders; 1972.
37. Rice TW, Zuccaro G, Adelstein DJ, et al. Esophageal carcinoma: depth of tumor invasion is predictive of regional lymph node status. Ann Thorac Surg. 1998;65:787–92.
38. Kitagawa Y, Uno T, Oyama T, et al. Esophageal cancer practice guidelines 2017 edited by the Japan esophageal society: part 2. Esophagus. 2019;16:25–43.
39. Tajima T, Nakanishi Y, Tachimori Y, et al. Significance of involvement by squamous cell carcinoma of the ducts of esophageal submucosal glands. Cancer. 2000;89:248–54.
40. Nishimaki T, Tanaka O, Suzuki T, et al. Tumor spread in superficial esophageal cancer: histopathologic basis for rational surgical treatment. World J Surg. 1993;17:766–72.

41. Wang WL, Chang IW, Hsu MH, et al. Risk factors and pathological characteristics for intraductal tumor spread of submucosal gland in early esophageal squamous cell neoplasia. Sci Rep. 2020;10:6860.
42. Chu P, Stagias J, West AB, et al. Diffuse pagetoid squamous cell carcinoma in situ of the esophagus. Cancer. 1997;79:1865–70.
43. Ishihara A, Mori T, Kono M. Diffuse pagetoid squamous cell carcinoma of the esophagus combined with choriocarcinoma and mucoepidermoid carcinoma: an autopsy case report. Path Int. 2002;53:147–52.
44. Miller TR, Zhang X, Ko HM, et al. Esophageal squamous cell carcinoma with pagetoid spread: a clinicopathologic study. Virchows Arch. 2025;486:313–22.
45. Eguchi T, Nakanishi Y, Shimoda T, et al. Histopathological criteria for additional treatment after endoscopic mucosal resection for esophageal cancer: analysis of 464 surgically resected cases. Mod Pathol. 2006;19:475–80.
46. Tajima Y, Nakanishi Y, Ochiai A, et al. Histopathologic findings predicting lymph node metastasis and prognosis of patients with superficial esophageal carcinoma: analysis of 240 surgically resected tumors. Cancer. 2000;88:1285–93.
47. Katada C, Yokoyama T, Hirasawa D, et al. Curative management after endoscopic resection for esophageal squamous cell carcinoma invading muscularis mucosa or shallow submucosal layer-multicenter real-world survey in Japan. Am J Gastroenterol. 2023;118:1175–83.
48. Kato H, Tachimori Y, Watanabe H, et al. Intramural metastasis of thoracic esophageal carcinoma. Int J Cancer. 1992;50:49–52.
49. Kuwano H, Nakajima M, Miyazaki T, et al. Distinctive clinicopathological characteristics in esophageal squamous cell carcinoma. Ann Thorac Cardiovasc Surg. 2003;9:6–13.
50. Ushimaru Y, Makino T, Tanaka K, et al. Clinical significance of intramural metastasis as an independent prognostic factor in esophageal squamous cell carcinoma. Ann Surg Oncol. 2023;30:5195–202.
51. Igaki H, Kato H, Tachimori Y, et al. Prognostic evaluation of patients with clinical T1 and T2 squamous cell carcinomas of the thoracic esophagus after 3-field lymph node dissection. Surgery. 2003;133:368–74.
52. Ide H, Nakamura T, Hayashi K, et al. Esophageal squamous cell carcinoma: pathology and prognosis. World J Surg. 1994;18:321–30.
53. Tanigawa N, Matsumura M, Amaya H, et al. Tumor vascularity correlates with the prognosis of patients with esophageal squamous cell carcinoma. Cancer. 1997;79:220–5.
54. Sarbia M, Bittinger F, Porschen R, et al. Prognostic value of histopathologic parameters of esophageal squamous cell carcinoma. Cancer. 1995;76:922–7.
55. Schumacher K, Haensch W, Roefzaad C, et al. Prognostic significance of activated $CD8^+$ T cell infiltration within esophageal carcinomas. Cancer Res. 2001;61:3932–6.
56. Miyata H, Yoshioka A, Yamasaki M, et al. Tumor budding in tumor invasive front predicts prognosis and survival of patients with esophageal squamous cell carcinomas receiving neoadjuvant chemotherapy. Cancer. 2009;115:3324–34.
57. Tanabe T, Kanda T, Kosugi S, et al. Extranodal spreading of esophageal squamous cell carcinoma: Clinicopathological characteristics and prognostic impact. World J Surg. 2007;31:2192–8.
58. Sung CO, Park CK, Kim SH, et al. Classification of epithelial-mesenchymal transition phenotypes in esophageal squamous cell carcinoma is strongly associated with patient prognosis. Mod Pathol. 2011;24:1060–8.
59. Sato Y, Mori K, Atsumi S, et al. Response to chemotherapy could predict the prognosis of esophageal squamous cell carcinoma treated with neoadjuvant docetaxel, cisplatin, and fluorouracil (DCF) followed by surgery: long-term results in a single institute. Esophagus. 2024;21:514–22.
60. Takagawa R, Kunisaki C, Makino H, et al. Efficacy of chemoradiotherapy with low-dose cisplatin and continuous infusion of 5-fluorouracil for unresectable squamous cell carcinoma of the esophagus. Dis Esophagus. 2009;22:482–9.

61. Matsubara Y, Toriyama K, Kadowaki S, et al. The impact of combined PD-L1 positive score on clinical response to nivolumab in patients with advanced esophageal squamous cell carcinoma. Esophagus. 2023;20:524–32.
62. Shimada H, Okazumi S, Shiratori T, et al. Impact of lymph node involvement in T2 or T3 thoracic esophageal squamous cell carcinoma. Hepato-Gastroenterology. 2009;56:1039–43.
63. Akutsu Y, Matsubara H. The significance of lymph node status as s prognostic factor for esophageal cancer. Surg Today. 2011;41:1190–5.
64. Tachimori T, Nagai Y, Kanamori N, et al. Pattern of lymph node metastases of esophageal squamous cell carcinoma based on the anatomical lymphatic drainage system. Dis Esophagus. 2011;24:33–8.
65. Rizk N, Venkatraman E, Park B, et al. The prognostic importance of the number of involved lymph nodes in esophageal cancer: implications for revisions of the American Joint Committee on Cancer staging system. J Thorac Cardiovasc Surg. 2006;132:1374–81.
66. Peyre CG, Hagen JA, DeMeester SR, et al. Predicting systemic disease in patients with esophageal cancer after esophagectomy: a multinational study on the significance of the number of involved lymph nodes. Ann Surg. 2008;248:979–85.
67. Liu Z, Zhao Y, Kong P, et al. Integrated multi-omics profiling yields a clinically relevant molecular classification for esophageal squamous cell carcinoma. Cancer Cell. 2023;41:181–95.
68. Chang J, Zhao X, Wang Y, et al. Genomic alterations driving precancerous to cancerous lesions in esophageal cancer development. Cancer Cell. 2023;41:2038–50.
69. Henick BS, Taylor AM, Nakagawa H, et al. Squamous cell cancers of the aero-upper digestive tract: a unified perspective on biology, genetics, and therapy. Cancer Cell. 2025;43:178–94.
70. Song Y, Zhang B, Xin D, et al. First-line serplulimab or placebo plus chemotherapy in PD-L1-positive esophageal squamous cell carcinoma: a randomized, double-blind phase 3 trial. Nat Med. 2023;29:473–82.
71. Doki Y, Ajani JA, Kato K, et al. Nivolumab combination therapy in advanced esophageal squamous cell carcinoma. N Engl J Med. 2022;386:449–62.
72. Taylor PR, Abnet CC, Dawsey SM. Squamous dysplasia—the precursor lesion for esophageal squamous cell carcinoma. Cancer Epidemiol Biomarkers Prev. 2013;22:540–52.
73. Schlemper RJ, Dawsey SM, Itabashi M, et al. Differences in diagnostic criteria for esophageal squamous cell carcinoma between Japanese and Western pathologists. Cancer. 2000;88:996–1006.
74. Itabashi M, Nasierowska-Guttmejer A, Shimoda T, et al. The importance of the concept and histological criteria of "intraepithelial squamous cell carcinoma" of the esophagus: in comparison between Western and Japanese criteria. Esophagus. 2017;14:333–42.
75. Wang WC, Wu TT, Chandan VS, et al. Ki-67 and ProEXC are useful immunohistochemical markers in esophageal squamous intraepithelial neoplasia. Hum Pathol. 2011;42:1430–7.
76. Mandard AM, Dalibard F, Mandard JC. Pathologic assessment of tumor regression after preoperative chemoradiotherapy of esophageal carcinoma: clinicopathologic correlations. Cancer. 1994;73:2680–6.
77. Kobayashi Y, Nakanishi Y, Taniguchi H, et al. Histological diversity in basaloid squamous cell carcinoma of the esophagus. Dis Esophagus. 2009;22:231–8.
78. Imamhasan A, Mitomi H, Saito T, et al. Immunohistochemical and oncogenetic analyses of the esophageal basaloid squamous cell carcinoma in comparison with conventional squamous cell carcinomas. Hum Pathol. 2012;43:2012–23.
79. Tripathi M, Swanson PE. Rare tumors of esophageal squamous mucosa. Ann N Y Acad Sci. 2016;1381:122–32.
80. Hishida T, Nakanishi Y, Shimoda T, et al. Esophageal basaloid carcinoma with marked myoepithelial differentiation. Pathol Int. 2002;52:313–7.
81. Sarbia M, Verreet P, Bittinger F, et al. Basaloid squamous cell carcinoma of the esophagus: diagnosis and prognosis. Cancer. 1997;79:1871–8.
82. Ishida H, Kasajima A, Yamauchi T, et al. A diagnostic pitfall; small cell carcinoma-like features in basaloid squamous cell carcinoma of the esophagus. Histol Histopathol. 2023;28:155–63.

83. Zhang B, Xiao Q, Yang D, et al. Spindle cell carcinoma of the esophagus: a multicenter analysis in comparison with typical squamous cell carcinoma. Medicine (Baltimore). 2016;95(37):e4768.
84. Yachida S, Nakanishi Y, Shimoda T, et al. Adenosquamous carcinoma of the esophagus. Oncology. 2004;66:218–25.
85. Ni PZ, Yang YS, Hu WP, et al. Primary adenosquamous carcinoma of the esophagus: an analysis of 39 cases. J Thorac Dis. 2016;8:2689–96.
86. Chen SB, Liu AT, Chen YP, et al. Surgical resection for esophageal adenosquamous carcinoma: an analysis of 56 cases. World J Surg Oncol. 2022;20:143–50.
87. Yendamuri S, Malhotra U, Hennon M, et al. Clinical characteristics of adenosquamous esophageal carcinoma. J Gastrointest Oncologia. 2017;8:89–95.
88. Chen SB, Weng HR, Wang G, et al. Primary adenosquamous carcinoma of the esophagus. World J Gastroenterol. 2013;19:8382–90.
89. Bombi JA, Riverola A, Bordas JM, et al. Adenosquamous carcinoma of the esophagus: a case report. Path Res Pract. 1991;187:514–9.
90. Lam KY, Dickens P, Loke SL, et al. Squamous cell carcinoma of the esophagus with mucin-producing component (muco-epidermoid carcinoma and adenosquamous carcinoma): a clinicopathologic study and a review of literature. Eur J Surg Oncol. 1994;20:25–31.
91. Isidro RA, Dong F, Hornick JL, et al. Verrucous carcinoma of the oesophagus is a genetically distinct subtype of oesophageal squamous cell carcinoma. Histopathology. 2025;79:642–9.
92. Cappellesso R, Coati I, Barzon L, et al. Human papillomavirus infection is not involved in esophageal verrucous carcinoma. Hum Pathol. 2019;85:50–7.

Diagnostic Imaging of Esophageal Cancer

3

Daisuke Tsurumaru, Yusuke Nishimuta, Yutaro Shimomura, Katsuya Nanjo, Masahiro Jinzaki, and Kousei Ishigami

3.1 Introduction

Esophageal cancer generally carries a poor prognosis, as many patients present with dysphagia, leading to diagnosis at an advanced stage. Treatment strategies vary considerably depending on the stage of the disease and range from minimally invasive endoscopic procedures to more invasive surgical resections, organ-preserving radiation therapy, and systemic chemotherapy. Therefore, providing optimal treatment tailored to each patient is essential, making accurate preoperative diagnosis critically important. Histologically, esophageal cancers are broadly classified into squamous cell carcinoma (SCC) and adenocarcinoma. As these two types differ in origin and risk factors, their incidence varies by country and region. This chapter focuses on squamous cell carcinoma, which demonstrates characteristic patterns of progression and imaging findings that are important to recognize. Radiologists play a pivotal role in the detection and staging of esophageal cancer. Current diagnostic modalities include barium esophagography, endoscopy, and endoscopic ultrasound (EUS), computed tomography (CT), magnetic resonance imaging (MRI), and ^{18}F-FDG (2-[18F]-fluoro-2-deoxy-D-glucose) positron emission tomography (PET). The appropriate use of these modalities is essential for determining the most suitable treatment plan for each patient [1]. Among these, CT is routinely used as the

D. Tsurumaru (✉) · Y. Nishimuta · Y. Shimomura · K. Nanjo · K. Ishigami
Department of Clinical Radiology, Graduate School of Medical Sciences, Kyushu University, Fukuoka, Japan
e-mail: tsurumaru.daisuke.931@m.kyushu-u.ac.jp; nishimuta.yusuke.021@m.kyushu-u.ac.jp; shimomura.yutaro.729@m.kyushu-u.ac.jp; nanjo.katsuya.410@m.kyushu-u.ac.jp; ishigami.kosei.581@m.kyushu-u.ac.jp

M. Jinzaki
Department of Radiology, Keio University School of Medicine, Shinjuku, Tokyo, Japan
e-mail: jinzaki@rad.med.keio.ac.jp

Y. Kitagawa et al. (eds.), *Esophageal Squamous Cell Carcinoma*,
https://doi.org/10.1007/978-981-92-2611-5_3

primary modality, while ^{18}F-FDG-PET provides valuable support, particularly in the assessment of lymph node metastases. Therefore, understanding the strengths and limitations of each imaging technique, the anatomy of the esophagus, and the patterns of disease progression is crucial. This chapter provides an overview of imaging-based knowledge of esophageal anatomy and the diagnostic imaging of esophageal squamous cell carcinoma, with reference to the 12th edition of the Japanese Classification of Esophageal Cancer and the 8th edition of the TNM Classification of Malignant Tumours [2, 3].

3.2 Anatomy of the Esophagus

3.2.1 Divisions of the Esophagus

Anatomical Definition of the Esophagus (Fig. 3.1)

The esophagus is a tubular structure that extends from the pharyngoesophageal junction to the esophagogastric junction (EGJ). It is anatomically divided into the cervical esophagus (Ce), thoracic esophagus (Te), and the esophagogastric junctional zone (Jz). The thoracic esophagus is further subdivided into the upper thoracic (Ut), middle thoracic (Mt), and lower thoracic (Lt) segments. The

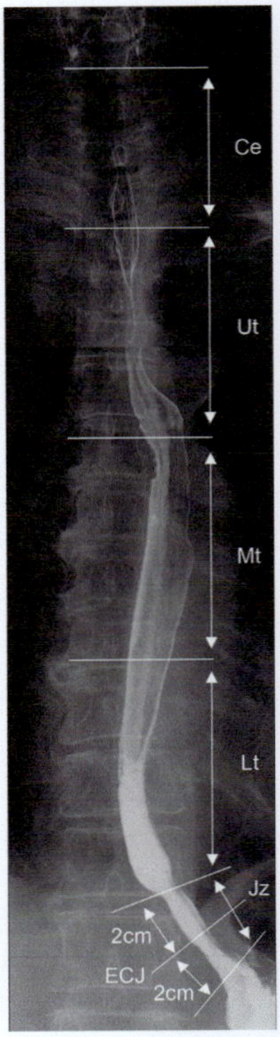

Fig. 3.1 Anatomical divisions of the esophagus. The esophagus is divided into the following segments: (1) Cervical esophagus (Ce): From the esophageal inlet to the upper border of the sternum. (2) Upper thoracic esophagus (Ut): From the upper border of the sternum to the tracheal bifurcation. (3) Middle thoracic esophagus (Mt): Proximal half of the segment between the tracheal bifurcation and the esophagogastric junction (EGJ). (4) Lower thoracic esophagus (Lt): From the lower border of Mt. to 2 cm above the EGJ. (5) Esophagogastric junctional zone (Jz): The region extending 2 cm above and 2 cm below the EGJ

cervical esophagus (Ce) extends from the pharyngoesophageal junction to the superior border of the sternum. The upper thoracic esophagus (Ut) extends from the superior border of the sternum to the tracheal bifurcation. The middle thoracic esophagus (Mt) corresponds to the proximal half of the segment between the tracheal bifurcation and the EGJ. The lower thoracic esophagus (Lt) extends from the distal edge of the Mt. to a point 2 cm above the EGJ. The esophagogastric junctional zone (Jz) is defined as the region spanning 2 cm above and 2 cm below the EGJ.

3.3 Imaging Diagnosis of T Stage

3.3.1 Depth of Wall Invasion

The depth of esophageal cancer invasion is classified as follows:

(12th edition of the Japanese Classification of Esophageal Cancer)
T1a: Tumor confined to the mucosa.
  T1a-EP: Carcinoma in situ (epithelium).
  T1a-LPM: Invading the lamina propria mucosae.
  T1a-MM: Invading the muscularis mucosae.
T1b: Tumor invading the submucosa (SM).

- T1b-SM1: Invasion into the upper third of the submucosa.
- T1b-SM2: Invasion into the middle third of the submucosa.
- T1b-SM3: Invasion into the lower third of the submucosa.

T2: Invasion into the muscularis propria.
T3: Invasion into the adventitia.
T4: Invasion into adjacent organs.
T3 is further subclassified clinically as follows:

- T3r: No invasion into adjacent organs observed on imaging (resectable).
- T3br: Invasion into the trachea, bronchi, or aorta cannot be ruled out (borderline resectable).

(TNM Classification of Malignant Tumours, eighth edition)
Tis: Carcinoma in situ/high grade dysplasia.
T1: Tumor invades lamina propria, muscularis mucosae, or submucosa.

- T1a: Tumor invades lamina propria or muscularis mucosae.
- T1b: Tumor invades submucosa.

T2: Tumor invades muscularis propria.
T3: Tumor invades adventitia.
T4: Tumor invades adjacent structures.

- T4a: Tumor invades pleura, pericardium, azygos vein, diaphragm, or peritoneum.
- T4b: Tumor invades other adjacent structures such as aorta, vertebral body, or trachea.

3.3.2 Esophagography

Barium esophagography is performed for the evaluation of esophageal cancer and enables not only detection and qualitative assessment (including depth of invasion) but also functional evaluation, such as identifying passage disturbances. Double-contrast barium studies are particularly useful for detecting subtle mucosal abnormalities, such as protrusions or depressions, and for assessing the depth of invasion using lateral views (Fig. 3.2) [4, 5]. In cases of obstruction or increased aspiration risk due to esophageal cancer, caution is required. Large-volume aspiration of barium sulfate can result in severe aspiration pneumonia. In such cases, low-osmolar, nonionic iodinated contrast agents, typically used in videofluoroscopic swallowing studies, are recommended [6]. If esophageal perforation is suspected, amidotrizoic acid (Gastrografin), an iodinated contrast agent, may be used (Fig. 3.3); however, due to its potential pulmonary toxicity, it should be administered with great caution and close monitoring of the patient's general condition [7].

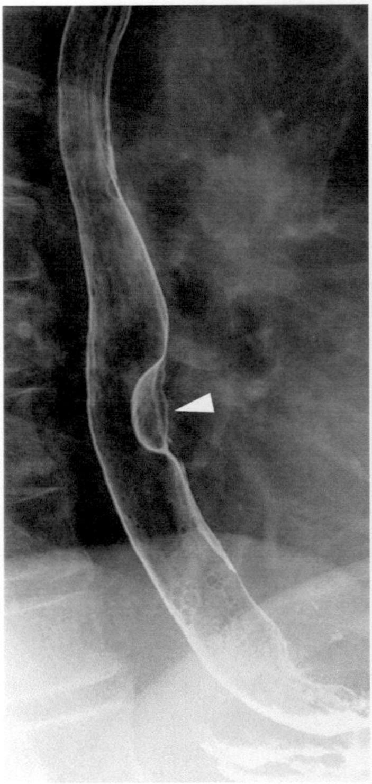

Fig. 3.2 Barium esophagography of superficial esophageal cancer. Lateral barium esophagography demonstrates a protruding lesion on the anterior wall of the middle thoracic esophagus, consistent with type 0-I superficial cancer (arrowhead). Mucosal distortion at the lesion's base suggests submucosal invasion

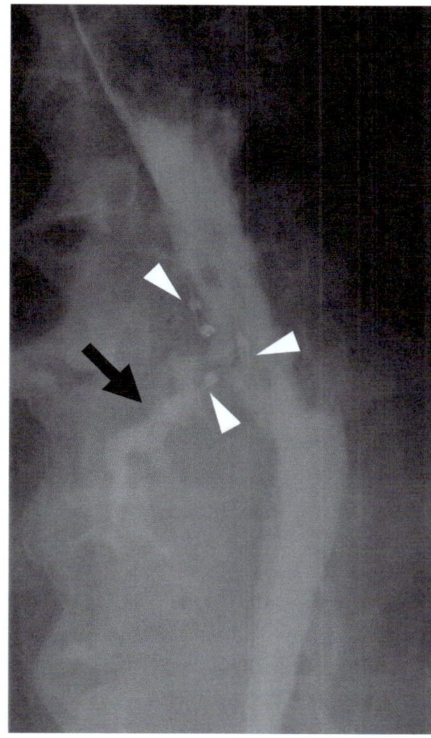

Fig. 3.3 Esophageal perforation caused by endoscopic submucosal dissection (ESD). Esophagography using Gastrografin shows extraluminal leakage of contrast medium (arrow). Endoscopic clips used to close the perforation during ESD are also visible (arrowheads)

3.3.3 CT

CT plays a crucial role in the detection and T-staging of esophageal cancer. With the advent of multi-detector CT, more accurate disease staging has become possible [8]. CT remains a cornerstone in the staging of newly diagnosed esophageal cancer and is further complemented by other modalities such as EUS and ^{18}F-FDG-PET. It is generally recommended as the initial imaging modality following pathological confirmation of esophageal cancer. CT is essential not only for assessing local tumor extension but also for evaluating lymph node involvement and distant metastases, making it an integral component of comprehensive oncologic staging.

3.3.3.1 CT Study Protocol and Optimal Phase for the Evaluation

Accurate T-staging is essential for determining appropriate treatment strategies. CT should be performed from the neck to the upper abdomen using intravenous contrast to ensure complete visualization of the esophagus and surrounding structures. For evaluation of the T factor, dynamic CT during the second arterial phase (approximately 35 s after the descending aorta reaches 200 Hounsfield units) provides optimal visualization [9, 10]. Early rim enhancement observed in the arterial phase is associated with T3/T4 lesions and may improve the accuracy of staging.

3.3.3.2 Diagnostic Criteria of Esophageal Cancer

Wall thickening greater than 5 mm is generally considered abnormal [11, 12]. In clinical practice, careful evaluation of wall thickness, lesion length, enhancement pattern, and associated findings such as obstruction or proximal dilatation is essential for interpretation. Conventional CT has limited ability to detect T1 lesions due to insufficient spatial resolution. Holscher et al. reported arterial phase CT sensitivities of 0% for T1a, 71.4% for T1b, 12.5% for T2, 89.5% for T3, and 100% for T4 [13], highlighting the need for complementary imaging modalities in early-stage disease. Dual-energy CT (DECT) is an advanced technique that uses two X-ray energy levels to provide more detailed tissue characterization than conventional CT. Recent advances in DECT have enhanced lesion visibility and T-staging accuracy by utilizing virtual monoenergetic imaging at 40 keV, which offers improved contrast and clearer delineation of tumor margins (Fig. 3.4) [14]. DECT also enables iodine mapping and material decomposition, providing functional information that complements anatomical evaluation.

Most esophageal cancers are diagnosed at an advanced stage and appear on CT as localized wall thickening or masses. Tumors that invade the adventitia without clear invasion of adjacent organs are classified as T3. T3 is further subdivided into cT3r (resectable) and cT3br (borderline resectable) according to the predictive resectability. Definite invasion of adjacent organs, including the pleura, pericardium, or diaphragm, is classified as cT4. When invasion of critical structures such as the trachea, bronchus, or aorta cannot be definitively ruled out but no overt cT4 features are observed, the tumor is considered cT3br (Fig. 3.5).

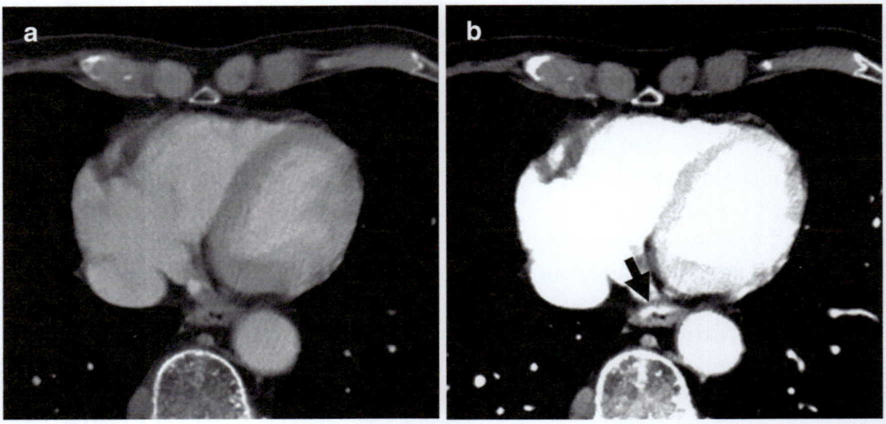

Fig. 3.4 Esophageal cancer in the lower thoracic esophagus (T1). Contrast-enhanced CT images of the lower esophagus. (**a**) Standard polyenergetic image fails to clearly visualize the tumor. (**b**) Virtual monoenergetic image at 40 keV clearly shows a high-density lesion (arrow) arising from the anterior esophageal wall

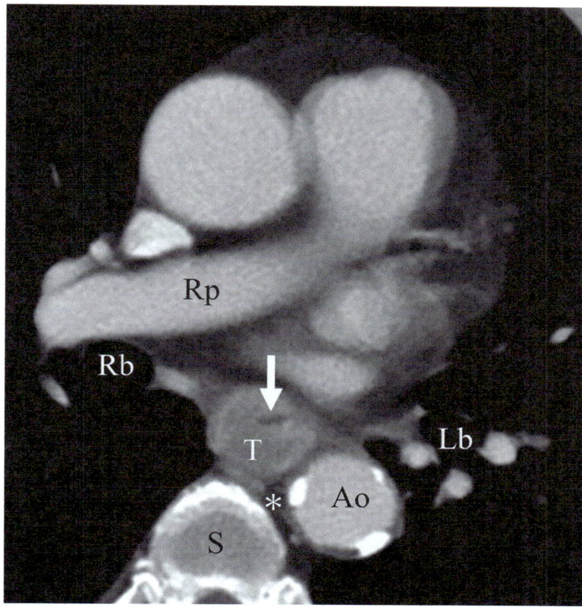

Fig. 3.5 Esophageal cancer in the middle thoracic esophagus (T3br). Contrast-enhanced axial CT image at the level of the middle thoracic esophagus. Asymmetrical wall thickening forms a soft tissue mass (T) in the distended middle thoracic esophagus. Narrowing esophageal lumen is identified as an eccentric area of air density (arrow). The fat plane around the esophagus is entirely preserved, and a triangular fat space (asterisk) among the esophagus, aorta (Ao), and spine (S) is also maintained. These findings exclude T4 disease with high degree of confidence. Lb: left main bronchus, Rb: right main bronchus, Rp: right pulmonary artery

3.3.3.3 Diagnostic Criteria for Tumor Invasion to Adjacent Structures

CT criteria for local invasion include the loss of fat planes between the tumor and adjacent mediastinal structures, as well as displacement or indentation of these structures [15, 16]. The reported sensitivity and specificity of CT for predicting mediastinal invasion are 88–100% and 85–100%, respectively. While the presence of a fat plane generally rules out invasion, its absence is not definitive. However, invasion is more likely if the fat plane is obliterated at the suspected site but remains intact above and below. Notably, fat plane obliteration can also result from prior radiotherapy or surgery. Lesions wider than 3.0 cm on CT are associated with a higher risk of extraesophageal spread [16]. Aortic invasion is suspected when the interface between the tumor and aorta lacks a clear layered structure, and the contact angle (Picus angle) is $\geq 110°$ with a craniocaudal length ≥ 10 mm, or 90–110° with ≥ 20 mm length (Fig. 3.6) [14]. Takashima et al. proposed an additional criterion: obliteration of the triangular fat space between the esophagus, aorta, and spine suggests aortic invasion. They reported MRI sensitivity and specificity of 100% and 86%, respectively, using this method; both CT and MRI offer comparable accuracy in assessing resectability [17]. Tracheal and

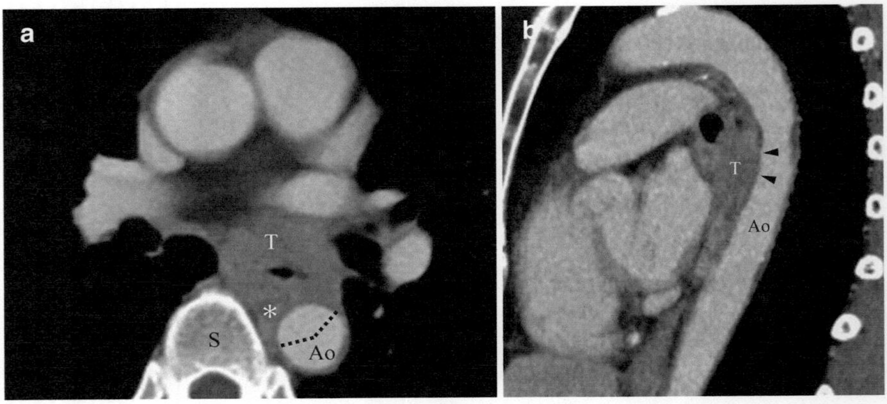

Fig. 3.6 Advanced esophageal cancer in the middle thoracic esophagus (cT4). (**a**) A contrast-enhanced axial CT image at the level of the tracheal bifurcation shows an infiltrative esophageal tumor (T) in the posterior mediastinum. The tumor is in direct contact with the anterior aspect of the descending aorta (Ao), with obliteration of the triangular fat space (asterisk) between the esophagus, aorta, and spine (S). The area of contact forms an arc of approximately 120°, exceeding 90°, as outlined by the dotted lines representing the "Picus angle." (**b**) The sagittal image demonstrates broad contact between the tumor (T) and the descending aorta (Ao), with complete obliteration of the intervening fat plane (arrowheads), strongly suggesting aortic invasion

bronchial invasion is diagnosed when the tumor disrupts the layered interface with the airway, or when there is airway compression, displacement, or luminal narrowing (Fig. 3.7). Definitive signs include tracheobronchial fistula or intraluminal tumor extension. Displacement or indentation of the posterior tracheal wall or bronchus also suggests invasion [18]. Bronchoscopy is helpful in conjunction with CT for accurate evaluation. Invasion into other structures includes gastric involvement, seen as a soft tissue mass extending into the gastric fundus, and pericardial invasion, indicated by pericardial thickening, effusion, or loss of the pericardial fat plane. These criteria are critical for staging and guiding treatment decisions.

3.3.4 MRI

MRI is a noninvasive, radiation-free imaging modality that provides excellent soft tissue contrast and is particularly useful for evaluating esophageal cancer, especially in anatomically complex regions such as the cervical esophagus and the esophagogastric junction. While CT and EUS remain the standard for staging, MRI has become increasingly valuable for local T-staging, supported by recent advances in motion-reduction techniques and image quality. The absence of ionizing radiation makes MRI suitable for repeated assessments, and its superior contrast resolution enables detailed visualization of esophageal wall layers, facilitating accurate localization and T-stage evaluation.

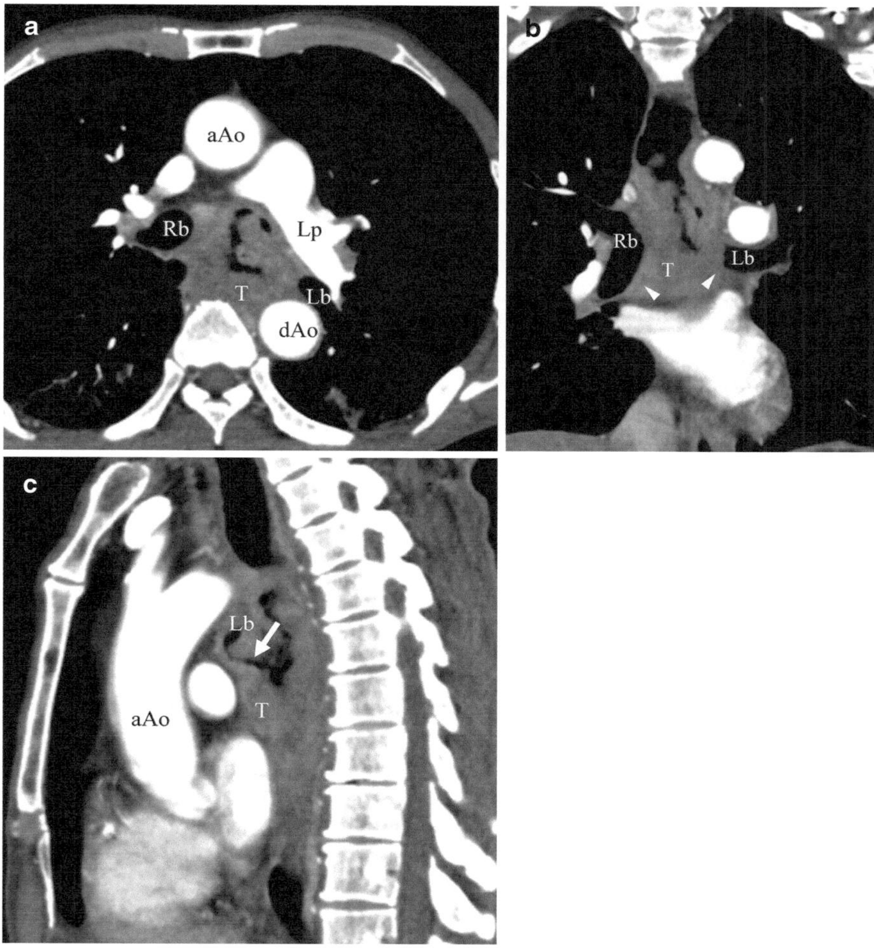

Fig. 3.7 Advanced esophageal cancer in the middle thoracic esophagus (cT4). Esophageal cancer (middle thoracic esophagus; cT4). Contrast-enhanced axial CT image below the tracheal bifurcation (**a**) and coronal image at the level of the tracheal bifurcation (**b**) show irregular and circumferential wall thickening of the esophagus representing esophageal cancer (T). An irregular interface between the tumor (T) and the air density within the bilateral main bronchi, along with diffusely infiltrative changes along both bronchi (arrows), strongly suggests bronchial invasion. The reformatted sagittal image (**c**) clearly depicts a fistula (arrow) between the tumor (T) and a posterior aspect of left main bronchus (Lb). aAo: ascending aorta, dAo: descending aorta, Lb: left main bronchus, Rb: right main bronchus, Rp: right pulmonary artery

3.3.4.1 Major Technical Developments and Protocols

Early applications of MRI in esophageal cancer were limited by motion artifacts caused by respiration, swallowing, and cardiac activity, particularly in the thoracic region. However, advancements such as electrocardiography gating, phased-array surface coils, and ultrafast gradient echo sequences have significantly improved both spatial and temporal resolution [19]. High-resolution T2-weighted fast spin echo sequences allow detailed visualization of the esophageal wall layers. Advanced turbo spin echo (TSE)-based motion correction methods help suppress respiratory motion artifacts, improving the detection of T3 lesions [20]. Diffusion-weighted imaging (DWI) assesses tumor cellularity and supports the detection of local invasion. Free-breathing radial three-dimensional gradient-echo sequences and multi-shot TSE are beneficial for patients who are unable to hold their breath, enhancing lesion conspicuity. Modern MRI protocols typically include axial and coronal T1-weighted images (pre- and postcontrast), high-resolution T2-weighted sequences, and DWI, often supplemented by free-breathing radial acquisitions to improve motion robustness.

3.3.4.2 Role in T-Staging

MRI has shown promising performance in the T-staging of esophageal cancer, particularly in distinguishing early-stage tumors (T1–2) from advanced-stage tumors (T3–4). Its key advantage lies in superior contrast resolution, which enables detailed evaluation of the esophageal wall layers and adjacent structures. In cervical esophageal cancer, T2-weighted axial images can clearly differentiate the hyperintense inner layer (mucosa/submucosa) from the hypointense outer layer (muscularis propria) (Fig. 3.8) [21]. T3 disease is characterized by involvement of the hypointense outer layer with preservation of tissue planes between the tumor and surrounding structures (Fig. 3.9), while T4 disease shows disruption of these planes due to direct invasion. Several studies have demonstrated that 3 T MRI using specific sequences outperforms CT and EUS in preoperative T-staging. In one prospective study, 3 T MRI achieved diagnostic accuracy rates of 95–96% compared to 80–82% for CT and 81–85% for EUS [22, 23]. Moreover, MRI has proven particularly valuable in assessing invasion of critical structures. For instance, it offers greater diagnostic accuracy than CT for evaluating thoracic aorta and tracheobronchial invasion—both key indicators of

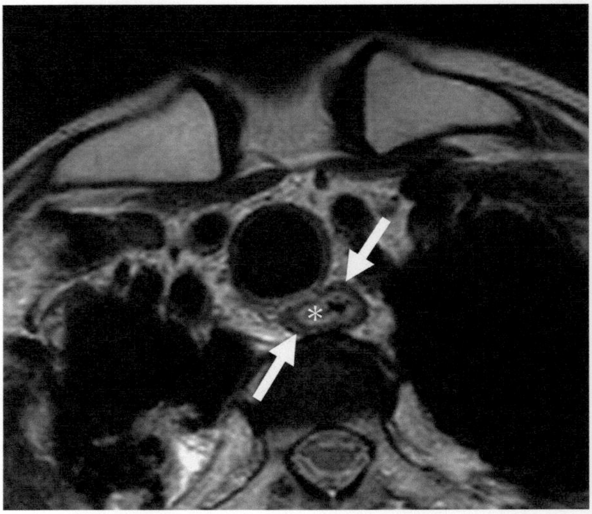

Fig. 3.8 Zonal anatomy of esophagus on MRI. Zonal anatomy of the esophageal wall on MRI. A T2-weighted axial image of the cervical esophagus reveals two different layers of the esophageal wall: the inner high-intensity layer (asterisk) and outer low-intensity layer (arrows), representing the mucosa/submucosa and muscularis propria, respectively. Tr: trachea

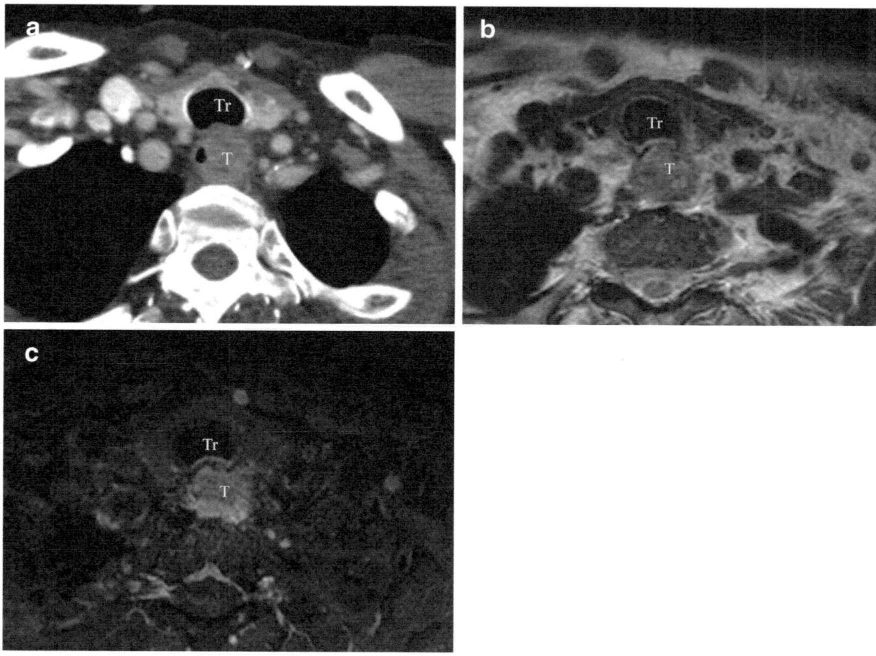

Fig. 3.9 Cervical esophageal cancer with borderline resectability (cT3br). (**a**) Contrast-enhanced CT, (**b**) T2-weighted axial MR image (T2WI), and (**c**) contrast-enhanced T1-weighted axial MR image (CE-T1WI) at the level of the cervical esophagus demonstrate asymmetric thickening of the esophageal wall (T). The primary lesion is in broad contact with the trachea (Tr), compressing its posterior wall; however, displacement, stenosis, and deformation of the trachea are relatively mild and smooth. On MRI, the tracheobronchial wall exhibits a two-layered appearance: the inner layer (mucosa and submucosa) shows hyperintensity on T2WI and higher signal intensity on CE-T1WI, whereas the outer layer (cartilaginous rings, intercartilaginous membrane, and adventitia) appears hypointense on both T1WI and T2WI, without obvious contrast enhancement. Part of the outer tracheal layer appears indistinct, making invasion radiologically indeterminate. Surgery was performed without preoperative therapy, and the pathological depth of invasion was confirmed as pT3

unresectability and important for determining definitive treatment strategies [24, 25]. MRI's ability to visualize organ layers and fat planes allows more confident differentiation between direct tumor invasion and inflammatory changes. Despite these advantages, MRI has limitations. It is more time-consuming than CT and susceptible to motion artifacts, especially near the diaphragm. Additionally, access to high-end MRI systems and advanced sequences may be restricted to tertiary care centers.

3.3.5 PET

PET is a unique imaging modality that visualizes the metabolic activity of tissues in contrast to CT and MRI, which primarily provide anatomical information. The most commonly used tracer, ^{18}F-FDG, accumulates in hypermetabolic malignant tumors, including esophageal cancer.

3.3.5.1 Role in T-Staging

^{18}F-FDG-PET is generally not suitable for determining the precise depth of tumor invasion (T staging) due to its limited spatial resolution; lesions smaller than 5 mm may go undetected [26]. Detection rates vary by tumor depth: 0% in pT1a (limited to the mucosa), 20% in pT1b (invading the submucosa), and nearly 100% in T2 or deeper tumors [27, 28]. Since ^{18}F-FDG-PET cannot clearly delineate esophageal wall layers or tumor margins, it is generally considered inappropriate for assigning specific T classifications. Additionally, false positives may occur due to FDG uptake associated with esophagitis or gastroesophageal reflux disease, reflecting active inflammation.

3.4 Imaging Diagnosis of N Stage (Lymph Node Metastasis)

Accurate evaluation of lymph node metastasis (N category) is essential for selecting an appropriate treatment strategy and predicting prognosis in esophageal cancer. The 12th edition of the Japanese Classification of Esophageal Cancer defines both the anatomical locations and the number of lymph node metastases [2, 3]. Nodal status is classified based on the number of metastatic regional lymph nodes. The definition of "regional" lymph nodes is based on clinical data showing that dissection of these nodal stations offers therapeutic benefit. Accordingly, regional lymph node metastasis is defined relative to the location of the primary tumor. For lymph node involvement outside the regional field, a distinction is made between nodal stations where surgical resection is expected to be beneficial (M1a) and all other distant lesions (M1b).

- NX: Regional lymph node status cannot be assessed.
- N0: No regional lymph node metastasis.
- N1: Metastasis in 1–2 regional lymph nodes.
- N2: Metastasis in 3–6 regional lymph nodes.
- N3: Metastasis in ≥7 regional lymph nodes.

3.4.1 CT

CT is the primary modality for evaluating nodal status. An understanding of the anatomical relations of the esophagus and adjacent structures is essential for accurate diagnosis (Fig. 3.10). A contrast-enhanced study with a slice thickness of ≤2.5 mm is recommended (2). Historically, diagnosis has relied primarily on lymph node size, with a short-axis diameter >10 mm in mediastinal or abdominal nodes typically considered positive [28]. Using this 10 mm threshold, reported sensitivity ranges from 30% to 60% and specificity from 60% to 80% [29–31]. Recent guidelines recommend a 6 mm cutoff, based on analyses that included nodes with a short-axis diameter ≥5 mm [2]. However, approximately one-third of metastatic nodes measure <5 mm, highlighting the limitations of size-based criteria. In addition to size, focal low-attenuation areas—suggestive of central necrosis or internal defects—strongly indicate metastasis, even in non-enlarged nodes [29].

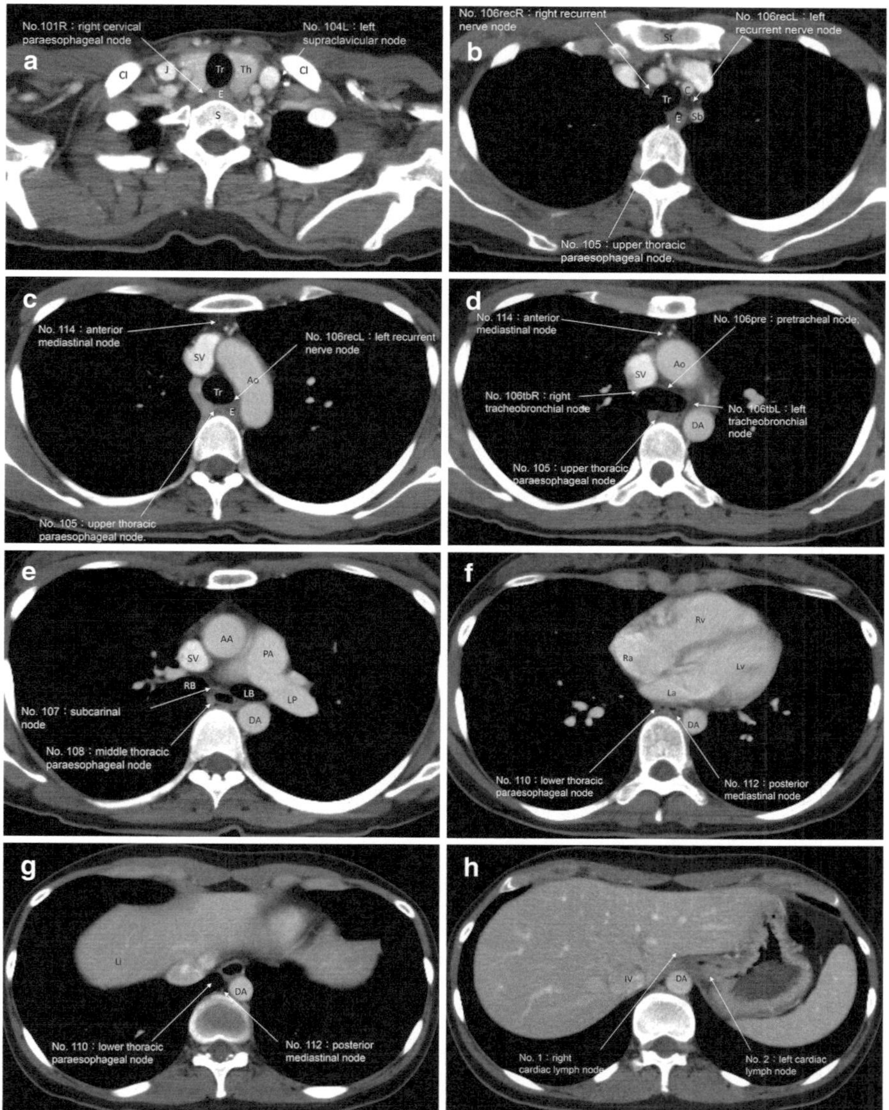

Fig. 3.10 An example of nodal group in the lower neck and mediastinum on CT. CT images at the levels of (**a**) the lower neck, (**b**) the superior mediastinum, (**c**) the aortic arch, (**d**) below the aortic arch, (**e**) below the tracheal bifurcation, (**f**) the inferior pulmonary vein, (**g**) just above the diaphragm, and (**h**) the gastric cardia. AA: ascending aorta, Ao: aortic arch, C: common carotid artery, Cl: clavicle, DA: descending aorta, E: esophagus, IV: inferior vena cava, La: left atrium, LB: left main bronchus, Li: liver, LP: left pulmonary artery, Lv: left ventricle, PA: pulmonary artery (main trunk), Ra: right atrium, RB: right main bronchus, S: spine, Sb: subclavian artery, St: sternum, SV: superior vena cava, Th: thyroid gland, Tr: trachea

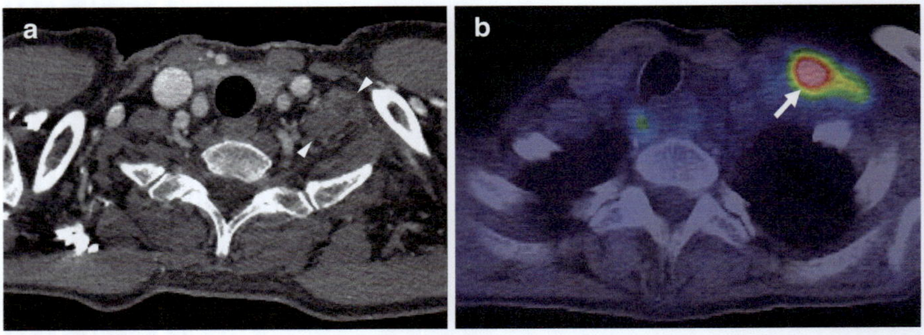

Fig. 3.11 Thoracic esophageal cancer with lymph node metastasis. (**a**) Contrast-enhanced CT reveals a soft-tissue density mass in the left supraclavicular fossa, consistent with lymph node metastasis from esophageal cancer (arrowheads). (**b**) ^{18}F-FDG-PET/CT demonstrates abnormal FDG uptake (arrow, SUVmax = 7.9) corresponding to the lymph node metastasis visualized on CT, strongly suggesting nodal involvement

3.4.2 PET/CT

^{18}F-FDG-PET/CT is a hybrid imaging modality that combines metabolic information from ^{18}F-FDG-PET with anatomical detail from CT, enabling a more accurate evaluation of lymph node metastases in esophageal cancer. It provides complementary information to CT alone, improving the detection of metastatic lymph nodes and enhancing diagnostic confidence in nodal staging. Meta-analyses report a sensitivity of 51% and a specificity of 84% for ^{18}F-FDG-PET, with sensitivity comparable to that of CT but superior specificity [32, 33]. The positive predictive value is generally higher than that of CT (Fig. 3.11). Diagnostic thresholds based on the maximum standardized uptake value (SUVmax) vary among institutions, as they are affected by factors such as blood glucose levels, scanning protocols, and equipment; thus, no universal standard exists. FDG uptake in mediastinal—particularly hilar—lymph nodes can also increase due to inflammatory conditions such as pneumonia or sarcoidosis, leading to false-positive results.

3.5 Imaging Diagnosis of M Stage (Distant Metastasis)

Distant metastasis is simply divided into M0 and M1 based on the presence of distant visceral metastasis, according to the 8th edition of the TNM Classification of Malignant Tumours [3].

- M0: No distant metastasis.
- M1: Distant metastasis.

In contrast, the 12th edition of the Japanese Classification of Esophageal Cancer defines distant metastasis to include both lymph node and visceral metastasis (refer

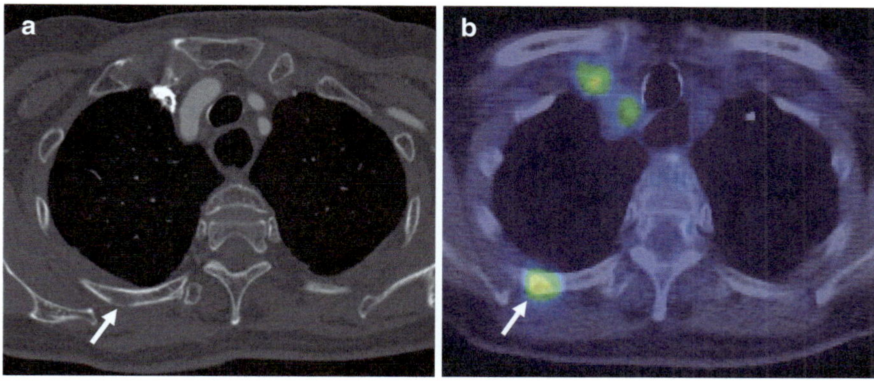

Fig. 3.12 Esophageal cancer with bone metastasis. (**a**) On contrast-enhanced CT using the bone window, an osteolytic bone metastasis is observed in the right fourth rib (→). (**b**) ^{18}F-FDG-PET/CT demonstrates abnormal FDG uptake corresponding to the lesion identified in image 5C is observed (SUVmax = 3.7) (→)

to the description of lymph node metastasis in the Sect. 3.4). Visceral metastasis is placed in M1b [2].

- MX: Distant organ or extra-regional lymph node metastasis cannot be assessed.
- M0: No metastasis to distant organs or to extra-regional lymph nodes.
- M1a: Metastasis to lymph nodes outside the regional field for which surgical removal is expected to yield some therapeutic effect.
- M1b: Metastasis to extra-regional lymph nodes other than those specified for M1a, or metastasis to any distant organ.

Distant metastases most commonly occur in the abdominal lymph nodes [33]. Hematogenous metastases in esophageal cancer frequently involve the liver, lungs, bones, adrenal glands, kidneys, and brain, in descending order of frequency [34, 35]. Contrast-enhanced CT is the most commonly used modality for detecting distant metastases, although its sensitivity is relatively low [17]. ^{18}F-FDG-PET serves as a valuable complementary tool, offering higher sensitivity in detecting distant disease (Fig. 3.12) [36]. ^{18}F-FDG-PET can reveal metastases in approximately 15% of patients who were previously considered free of distant disease based solely on conventional imaging findings [28, 37].

3.6 Evaluation of Response to Radiotherapy, Chemotherapy, and Chemoradiotherapy

In recent years, the development of numerous therapeutic agents has increased the importance of preoperative therapy, making imaging-based evaluation of treatment response increasingly crucial. Endoscopy and CT are the primary modalities used to

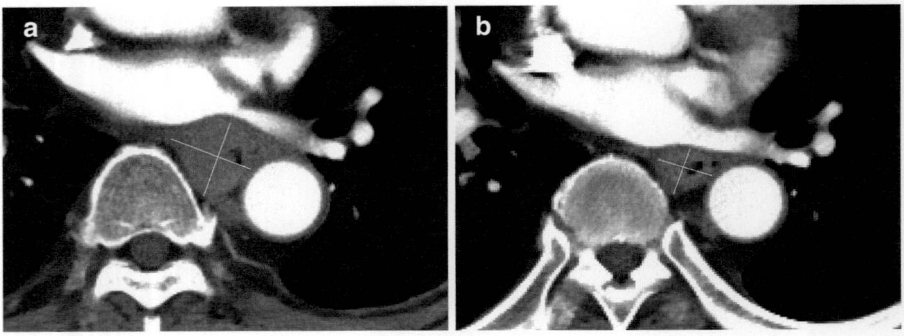

Fig. 3.13 Treatment response to chemotherapy for esophageal cancer (assessed by cross-sectional area on CT). (**a**) A tumor is observed in the thoracic esophagus, consistent with esophageal cancer. The cross-sectional area at the level of the maximum lesion on CT is used for evaluation (long diameter 28 mm × short diameter 27 mm = 756 mm^2). (**b**) After chemotherapy, the tumor shrunk. The cross-sectional area on CT (long diameter 19 mm × short diameter 16 mm = 304 mm^2) decreased by more than half

assess therapeutic effects [2]. For local evaluation, histological assessment via endoscopy and endoscopic biopsy is possible. In contrast, objective evaluation of macroscopic lesions and the progression of lymph node metastases relies on imaging modalities such as CT and ^{18}F-FDG-PET [38]. On CT, measurable lesions are assessed according to size criteria. The primary esophageal lesion is considered evaluable if its long-axis diameter is ≥20 mm, while lymph node metastases are considered evaluable if their short-axis diameter is ≥15 mm. When distinguishing the lesion from normal esophageal wall is challenging, evaluation based on the lesion's short-axis diameter may be used if separable; otherwise, the overall esophageal diameter on cross-sectional imaging can be measured (Fig. 3.13). ^{18}F-FDG-PET/CT visualizes glucose metabolism in tumors, providing functional information that reflects tumor proliferation. Metabolic parameters, such as the SUVmax, can serve as indicators of response to chemotherapy or radiation therapy [39]. However, according to the Japanese Classification of Esophageal Cancer, ^{18}F-FDG-PET/CT findings are regarded only as supplemental information and are not officially incorporated into response evaluation criteria [2].

References

1. Bruzzi JF, Munden RF, Truong MT, Marom EM, Sabloff BS, Gladish GW, Iyer RB, Pan TS, Macapinlac HA, Erasmus JJ. PET/CT of esophageal cancer: its role in clinical management. Radiographics. 2007;27(6):1635–52.
2. Japan Esophageal Society. Esophageal cancer treatment guidelines 2025. Japan Esophageal Society; 2025. https://www.jse.or.jp/guideline/esophageal-cancer. Accessed 9 July 2025
3. Brierley J, Gospodarowicz MK, Wittekind CH, editors. TNM classification of malignant tumours. 8th ed. Oxford, UK/Hoboken: Wiley; 2017.
4. Levine MS, Chu P, Furth EE, et al. Carcinoma of the esophagus and esophagogastric junction: sensitivity of radiographic diagnosis. AJR Am J Roentgenol. 1997;168:1423–6.

5. Levine MS, Halvorsen RA. Esophageal carcinoma. In: Core RM, Levine MS, Laufer I, editors. Textbook of gastrointestinal radiology. Philadelphia: WB Saunders Co; 1994.
6. Ghazanfar H, Shehi E, Makker J, Patel H. The role of imaging modalities in diagnosing dysphagia: a clinical review. Cureus. 2021;13(7):e16786.
7. Trulzsch DV, Penmetsa A, Karim A, Evans DA. Gastrografin-induced aspiration pneumonia: a lethal complication of computed tomography. South Med J. 1992;85(12):1255–6.
8. Kim TJ, Kim HY, Lee KW, et al. Multimodality assessment of esophageal cancer: preoperative staging and monitoring of response to therapy. Radiographics. 2009;29:403–21.
9. Umeoka S, Koyama T, Togashi K, et al. Esophageal cancer: evaluation with triple-phase dynamic CT—initial experience. Radiology. 2006;239:777–83.
10. Umeoka S, Okada T, Daido S, et al. "Early esophageal rim enhancement": a new sign of esophageal cancer on dynamic CT. Eur J Radiol. 2013;82:459–63.
11. Desai RK, Tagliabue JR, Wegryn SA, et al. CT evaluation of wall thickening in the alimentary tract. Radiographics. 1991;11:771–83.
12. Xia F, Mao J, Ding J, Yang H. Observation of normal appearance and wall thickness of esophagus on CT images. Eur J Radiol. 2009;72:406–11.
13. Holscher AH, Dittler HJ, Siewert JR. Staging of squamous esophageal cancer: accuracy and value. World J Surg. 1994;18:312–20.
14. Cheng F, Liu Y, Du L, et al. Evaluation of optimal monoenergetic images acquired by dual-energy CT in the diagnosis of T staging of thoracic esophageal cancer. Insights Imaging. 2023;14:33.
15. Picus D, Balfe DM, Koehler RE, et al. Computed tomography in the staging of esophageal carcinoma. Radiology. 1983;146:433–8.
16. Lefor AT, Merino MM, Steinberg SM, et al. Computerized tomographic prediction of extraluminal spread and prognostic implications of lesion width in esophageal cancer. Radiology. 1989;171:290.
17. Takashima S, Takeuchi N, Shiozaki H, et al. Carcinoma of the esophagus: CT vs MR imaging in determining resectability. AJR Am J Roentgenol. 1991;156:297–302.
18. Lehr L, Rupp N, Siewert JR. Assessment of resectability of esophageal cancer by computed tomography and magnetic resonance imaging. Surgery. 1988;103:344–50.
19. Riddell AM, Richardson C, Scurr E, et al. The development and optimization of high spatial resolution MRI for imaging the oesophagus using an external surface coil. Br J Radiol. 2006;79:873–9.
20. Riddell AM, Allum WH, Thompson JN, et al. The appearances of oesophageal carcinoma demonstrated on high-resolution, T2-weighted MRI, with histopathological correlation. Eur Radiol. 2007;17:391–9.
21. Van Rossum PSN, van Hillegersberg R, Lever FM, et al. Imaging strategies in the management of oesophageal cancer: what's the role of MRI? Eur Radiol. 2013;23:1753–65.
22. Guo J, Wang Z, Qin J, et al. A prospective analysis of the diagnostic accuracy of 3T MRI, CT and endoscopic ultrasound for preoperative T staging of potentially resectable esophageal cancer. Cancer Imaging. 2020;20:64.
23. Zhang F, Qu J, Zhang H, et al. Preoperative T staging of potentially resectable esophageal cancer: a comparison between free-breathing radial VIBE and breath-hold Cartesian VIBE, with histopathological correlation. Transl Oncol. 2017;10:324–31.
24. Zhao K, Chu F, Wang Z, et al. Aorta and tracheobronchial invasion in esophageal cancer: comparing diagnostic performance of 3.0-T MRI and CT. Eur Radiol. 2023;33:4962–72.
25. Harino T, Yamasaki M, Murai S, et al. Impact of MRI on the post-therapeutic diagnosis of T4 esophageal cancer. Esophagus. 2023;20:740–8.
26. Rice TW. Clinical staging of esophageal carcinoma. CT, EUS, and PET. Chest Surg Clin N Am. 2000;10:471–85.
27. Kato H, Miyazaki T, Nakajima M, et al. The incremental effect of positron emission tomography on diagnostic accuracy in the initial staging of esophageal carcinoma. Cancer. 2005;103:148–56.

28. Flamen P, Lerut A, Van Cutsem E, et al. Utility of positron emission tomography for the staging of patients with potentially operable esophageal carcinoma. J Clin Oncol. 2000;18:3202–10.
29. Ojiri H. Diagnostic imaging of the esophageal cancer. In: Ando N, editor. Esophageal squamous cell carcinoma. Singapore: Springer; 2020. p. 35–61.
30. Block MI, Patterson GA, Sundaresan RS, et al. Improvement in staging of esophageal cancer with the addition of positron emission tomography. Ann Thorac Surg. 1997;64(3):770–7.
31. Kato H, Kuwano H, Nakajima M, et al. Comparison between positron emission tomography and computed tomography in the assessment of esophageal carcinoma. Cancer. 2002;94(4):921–8.
32. Van Vliet EP, Heijenbrok-Kal MH, Hunink MG, et al. Staging investigation for oesophageal cancer: a meta-analysis. Br J Cancer. 2008;98(3):547–57.
33. Van Westreenen HL, Westerterp M, Bossuyt PM, et al. Systematic review of the staging performance of 18F-fluorodeoxyglucose positron emission tomography in esophageal cancer. J Clin Oncol. 2004;22(18):3805–12.
34. Quint LE, Hepburn LM, Francis IR, et al. Incidence and distribution of distant metastases from newly diagnosed esophageal carcinoma. Cancer. 1995;76:1120–5.
35. Mandard AM, Chasle J, Marnay J, et al. Autopsy findings in 111 cases of esophageal cancer. Cancer. 1981;48:329–35.
36. Flanagan FL, Dehdashti F, Siegel BA, et al. Staging of esophageal cancer with 18F-fluorodeoxyglucose positron emission tomography. AJR Am J Roentgenol. 1997;168:417–24.
37. Downey RJ, Akhurst T, Ilson D, et al. Whole-body 18FDG-PET and the response of esophageal cancer to induction therapy: results of the prospective trial. J Clin Oncol. 2003;21:428.
38. Eyck BM, Onstenk BD, Noordman BJ, et al. Accuracy of detecting residual disease after neoadjuvant chemoradiotherapy for esophageal cancer: a systematic review and meta-analysis. Ann Surg. 2020;271(2):245–56.
39. Rebollo Aguirre AC, Ramos-Font C, Villegas Portero R, et al. 18F-fluorodeoxiglucose positron emission tomography for the evaluation of neoadjuvant therapy response in esophageal cancer: systematic review of the literature. Ann Surg. 2009;250(2):247–54.

Endoscopic Diagnosis

4

Ryu Ishihara

4.1 Introduction

The development of endoscopic techniques for detecting esophageal squamous cell carcinomas (ESCCs) began with the introduction of pan-endoscopy in 1973. This procedure enabled comprehensive visualization of the digestive tract, from the esophagus to the second portion of the duodenum, establishing a foundation for the screening and identification of ESCCs.

Two major advancements have since revolutionized the detection of ESCCs. The first was the adoption of image enhancement technologies. Iodine staining, introduced in the late 1970s, significantly improved visualization of esophageal lesions, including superficial cancers. However, its use was limited by mucosal irritation, often resulting in retrosternal discomfort or pain. In 2003, narrow-band imaging (NBI), a noninvasive optical enhancement technology, was developed, offering superior visualization of surface and microvascular structures in the esophagus without significant discomfort [3]. NBI has become a valuable tool for detecting early-stage ESCCs.

The second advancement was magnifying endoscopy. Emerging around 1990s, this technology enabled detailed visualization of superficial ESCCs. By the late 1990s, magnification of 80-fold or greater became available, with widespread adoption following its integration with NBI in the early 2000s. Advances in this technology now allow detection of small intramucosal ESCCs, measuring only a few millimeters. These techniques facilitate optical diagnosis of ESCCs by highlighting changes in microvascular structures.

Endoscopes equipped with advanced imaging technologies are now widely used for detecting, characterizing, and staging ESCCs. These innovations have also improved the identification of high-risk individuals based on characteristic findings associated with ESCCs and enabled precise evaluation of esophageal

R. Ishihara (✉)
Department of Gastrointestinal Oncology, Osaka International Cancer Institute, Osaka, Japan

Y. Kitagawa et al. (eds.), *Esophageal Squamous Cell Carcinoma*,
https://doi.org/10.1007/978-981-92-2611-5_4

subsites. Furthermore, endoscopic ultrasound (EUS) provides higher sensitivity than computed tomography (CT) for detecting lymph nodes in the periesophageal region. Together, these advancements have established endoscopy as an indispensable diagnostic modality, particularly for evaluating superficial ESCCs. This section provides a comprehensive overview of the current state of endoscopic diagnosis for ESCCs.

4.2 Diagnosis of Esophageal Subsites

Esophagectomy and chemoradiotherapy are the mainstays of treatment for ESCC. The extent of lymphadenectomy during esophagectomy and the radiation field in chemoradiotherapy are determined based on the tumor's esophageal subsite, such as the cervical esophagus, upper thoracic esophagus, middle thoracic esophagus, or lower thoracic esophagus [14, 15]. While the anatomical landmarks of these subsites have been well-defined, their corresponding endoscopic landmarks were not thoroughly investigated until recently.

A recent study utilizing EUS has elucidated the correlation between anatomical and endoscopic landmarks [9]. For instance, the lower end of the pyriform sinus corresponds to the pharynx–cervical esophagus junction (Fig. 4.1a), while the lower end of the compression caused by the left main bronchus marks the upper-middle thoracic esophagus junction (Fig. 4.1b). The average distances from the superior incisors to these landmarks were measured as follows: 16.9 ± 1.7 cm for the pharynx–esophagus junction, 21.7 ± 1.9 cm for the cervical–upper thoracic esophagus junction, and 29.0 ± 1.9 cm for the upper-middle thoracic esophagus junction.

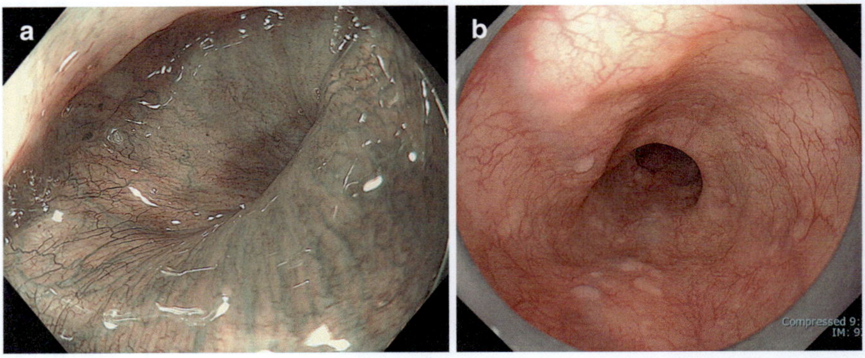

Fig. 4.1 (**a**) The lower end of the pyriform sinus, corresponding to the pharynx–cervical esophagus junction. (**b**) The lower end of the compression caused by the left main bronchus, corresponding to the upper-middle thoracic esophagus junction

4.3 Identification of High-Risk Individuals

Key risk factors for ESCC include alcohol consumption, smoking, and aldehyde dehydrogenase deficiency [7, 22]. These factors not only promote carcinogenic transformation but also induce mucosal changes in the esophagus, oral cavity, pharynx, and upper aerodigestive tract, as described by the "field cancerization theory" [25]. Among these changes, melanosis (Fig. 4.2a) and whitish epithelium in the soft palate (Fig. 4.2b, c) have been shown to correlate with ESCC risk [4, 28, 29].

Melanosis, often resulting from chronic exposure to alcohol and smoking, is commonly observed at the junction of the hard and soft palate, pharynx, and esophagus [29]. Approximately 31% of ESCC patients exhibit melanosis in the soft palate, which is associated with an increased risk of ESCC [4, 28].

Similarly, whitish epithelium, regarded as a broader form of leukoplakia, is linked to alcohol consumption, smoking, or chronic irritation of the oral mucosa [1]. This finding is observed in approximately 13% of ESCC patients and is also associated with elevated ESCC risk [28].

The soft palate is easily accessible during endoscopic examinations, and changes such as melanosis and whitish epithelium are readily identifiable. When these findings are detected, thorough evaluation of the esophagus is imperative to identify potential ESCCs.

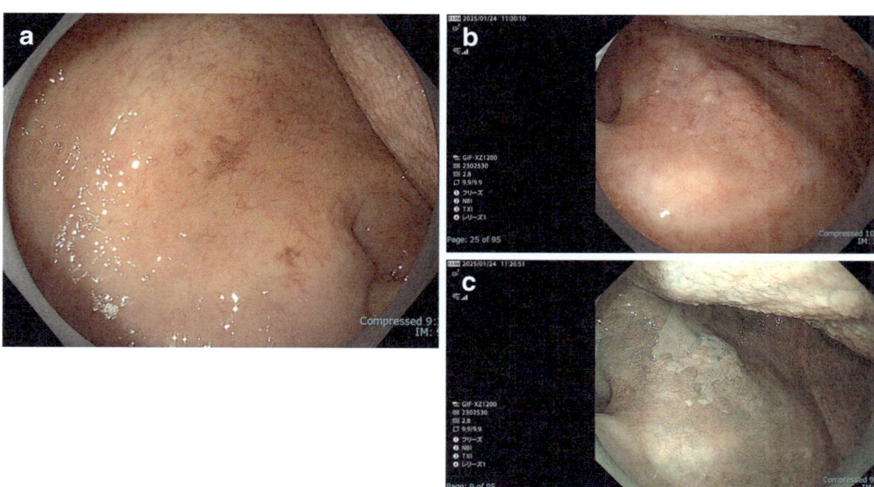

Fig. 4.2 (**a**) Melanosis in the soft palate, which has been shown to correlate with esophageal cancer risk. (**b**) Whitish epithelium on white-light imaging in the soft palate, which has been shown to correlate with esophageal cancer risk. (**c**) Whitish epithelium on narrow-band imaging in the soft palate

4.4 Detection

4.4.1 Observation Method

The visibility of superficial ESCCs is closely associated with the degree of air insufflation within the esophagus. Full air insufflation, which distends the esophageal walls, facilitates a comprehensive view of the entire esophagus but often reduces the visibility of cancerous lesions (Fig. 4.3a) [11]. Conversely, deflation of the esophagus, allowing the walls to relax, enhances the contrast between cancerous lesions (Fig. 4.3b)—appearing as brownish areas or areas of background coloration (Fig. 4.3c)—and the surrounding normal tissue. This relaxed state also permits closer examination of the esophageal wall, improving the detection of characteristic dot-like vascular patterns associated with superficial ESCCs. Therefore, observing the esophagus in a deflated condition is recommended to optimize the early detection of superficial ESCCs.

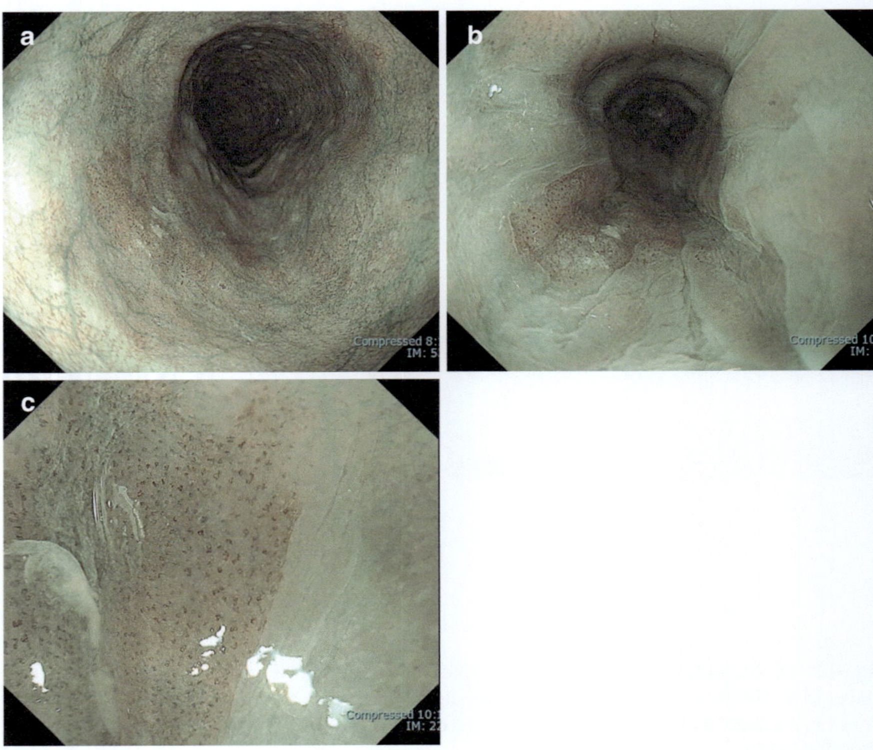

Fig. 4.3 (**a**) Reduced visibility of a cancerous lesion by full air insufflation. (**b**) Enhanced visibility of a cancerous lesion by deflation of the air. (**c**) Background coloration

4.4.2 White-Light Endoscopy

Advanced esophageal cancer typically presents with prominent features, such as elevated protrusions, extensive wall rigidity, and crater formation, making lesions readily identifiable with standard white-light endoscopy (WLE) (Fig. 4.4). In contrast, early-stage ESCC may exhibit subtle findings, including slight redness, loss of mucosal luster, and areas of reduced vascular permeability. These subtle changes are challenging to detect using standard WLE, limiting its utility in identifying superficial ESCCs and its precursors.

4.4.3 Iodine Staining

Iodine chromoendoscopy, a dye-based image-enhanced endoscopy, significantly improves the detection of ESCCs by highlighting abnormal areas. Glycogen-rich normal esophageal squamous cells readily take up iodine, while glycogen-poor neoplastic cells show reduced iodine uptake, resulting in iodine-unstained areas. This technique offers strong contrast between cancerous and noncancerous mucosa, making it a highly sensitive method for detecting ESCCs.

Patients with multiple iodine unstained lesions (patchy distributions of weak or absent iodine staining) throughout the esophagus are considered to have increased carcinogenic potential in both the pharynx and esophagus. This finding serves as a valuable indicator for identifying individuals at high risk of developing metachronous esophageal and pharyngeal cancers following endoscopic resection [12]. However, iodine staining has limitations, including low specificity, as inflammatory esophageal mucosa can also remain unstained. Moreover, the use of iodine spray can lead to adverse events, such as iodine hypersensitivity, laryngitis, pneumonitis, chest discomfort, and nausea [16].

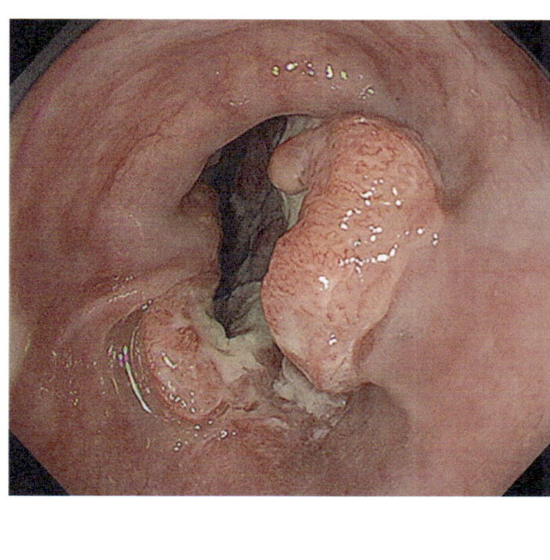

Fig. 4.4 Advanced esophageal cancer

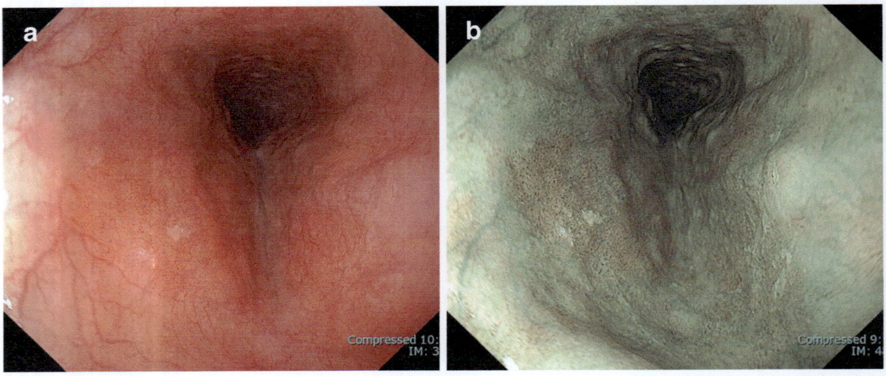

Fig. 4.5 (**a**) Esophageal cancer on white-light imaging. (**b**) Esophageal cancer on narrow-band imaging. Narrow-band imaging can enhance the surface and microvascular structures of esophageal cancer

4.4.4 Optical Image-Enhanced Endoscopy

The utility of optical image-enhanced endoscopy, including NBI and blue laser imaging (BLI), in diagnosing ESCC has been increasingly recognized worldwide. NBI employs specific wavelengths of blue (415 nm) and green (540 nm) light to provide enhanced visualization of the surface and microvascular structures (Fig. 4.5a, b) [3]. Blue light highlights the superficial mucosa, while green light penetrates deeper layers, allowing detailed examination of microvascular structures and epithelial patterns. NBI is easily activated during routine endoscopy with the press of a button, imposing minimal additional burden on the patient.

Studies have demonstrated that NBI outperforms standard WLE in sensitivity for detecting superficial ESCC [20], with diagnostic accuracy comparable to that of iodine chromoendoscopy [26]. As a result, NBI is now considered the standard imaging modality for the early detection of superficial ESCCs. Similarly, BLI uses laser technology to transmit light at wavelengths of 410 and 450 nm and provides similar sensitivity to NBI for the detection of superficial ESCCs [13].

4.5 Characterization

4.5.1 Non-magnifying Endoscopy

Superficial ESCCs are frequently identified as brownish areas during observation with non-magnifying NBI or BLI. Magnified close-up imaging of these areas often reveals well-demarcated background discoloration and dot-like vessels, enabling a definitive diagnosis of ESCCs.

4.5.2 Iodine Staining

Iodine staining is a highly sensitive method for detecting superficial ESCCs, but its low specificity limits its ability to differentiate between cancerous and noncancerous lesions. The "pink-color sign," a phenomenon characterized by a distinct color change from yellow to pink within 2–3 min after iodine application, has proven valuable for identifying malignant lesions (Fig. 4.6a, b). This sign significantly enhances the diagnostic specificity for ESCC [10, 24].

4.5.3 Magnifying Observation

Magnified observation facilitates detailed examination of blood vessels, allowing for the diagnosis of ESCCs based on the Japan Esophageal Society classification criteria. Type B1 vessels, indicative of superficial ESCCs, are characterized by dilation, tortuosity, caliber irregularity, and morphological heterogeneity of the intraepithelial papillary capillary loop (IPCL). These features are strongly associated with lesions confined to the epithelium (EP) or lamina propria mucosae (LPM). Conversely, Type A vessels, which lack these features, are more commonly observed in noncancerous lesions, such as intraepithelial neoplasia (Fig. 4.7a).

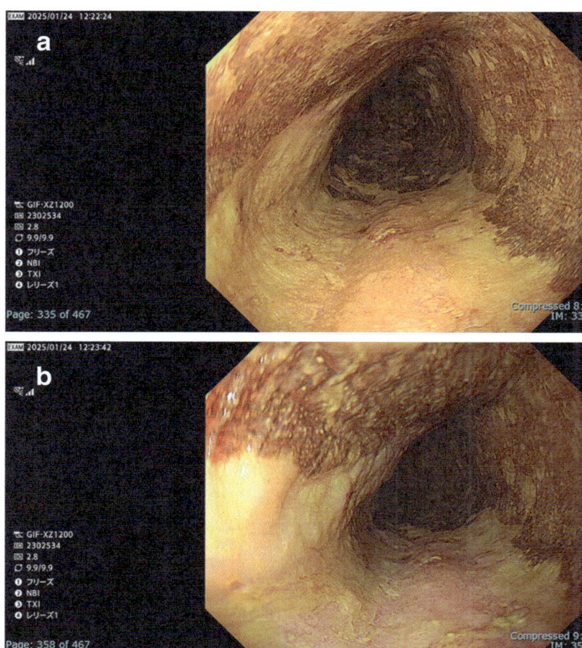

Fig. 4.6 (**a**) Esophageal cancer immediately after spraying iodine solution. (**b**) Color change from yellow to pink within 2–3 min after iodine application

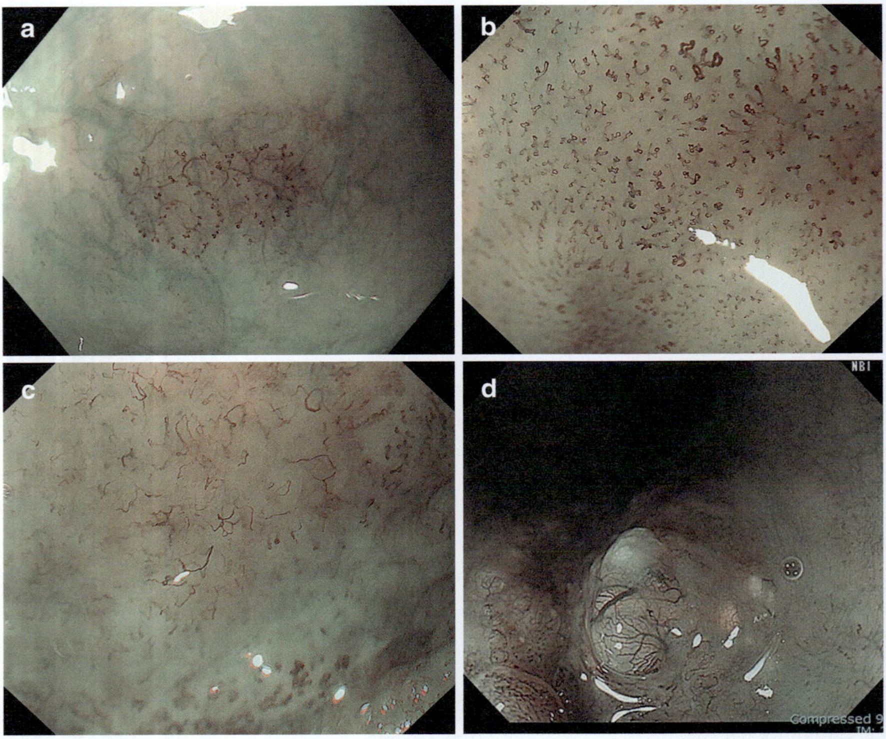

Fig. 4.7 (**a**) Type A vessels, which show some but not all of the following four features: dilation, tortuosity, caliber irregularity, and morphological heterogeneity. (**b**) Type B vessels, which show all of the following four features: dilation, tortuosity, caliber irregularity, and morphological heterogeneity. Type B1: Type B vessels with loop-like formation. (**c**) Type B vessels without loop-like formation. (**d**) Type B vessels with highly dilated vessels, whose calibers appear to be more than three times that of usual B2 vessels

4.5.4 Endocytoscopy

Advanced ultra-high magnification technologies, including confocal endoscopy [5] and endocytoscopy (ECS) [18], enable detailed visualization of cellular structures within the superficial epithelial layer. ECS, combined with methylene blue staining, provides high-resolution images comparable to histology, facilitating real-time optical biopsies and lesion characterization [6]. ECS has demonstrated high sensitivity and specificity for characterizing superficial ESCC [17, 19].

4.6 Staging

4.6.1 Non-magnifying Endoscopy

Cancer invasion depth is initially assessed using non-magnifying WLE, focusing on surface irregularities, lesion stiffness, and thickness. Lesions with an almost flat or slightly uneven surface (≤1 mm elevation) are typically categorized as submucosa (SM)1 or less invasive. Conversely, lesions with >1 mm elevation or thickness are diagnosed as SM2.

To evaluate lesion stiffness, the esophageal lumen is observed while varying air insufflation or deflation, carefully noting morphological changes. Lesions exhibiting no morphological alterations despite air volume changes are considered stiff, indicating potential deep invasion. In contrast, lesions showing significant morphological changes suggest superficial-layer confinement. For more detailed assessment, magnifying endoscopy is used to refine the evaluation of suspected deep invasion.

4.6.2 Magnifying Endoscopy

Magnifying endoscopy, particularly with NBI, is utilized for areas suspected of deeper invasion based on non-magnifying endoscopy findings. The Japan Esophageal Society classification [21] guides endoscopic staging by analyzing changes in microvascular structures.

Type B1 (Fig. 4.7b) vessels or AVA-small: Indicates EP/LPM cancer.

Type B2 (Fig. 4.7c) vessels or AVA-middle: Indicates MM/SM1 cancer.

Type B3 (Fig. 4.7d) vessels or AVA-large: Indicates SM2 cancer.

4.6.3 EUS

EUS uses high-frequency ultrasound (20–30 MHz) to delineate the wall structure of the gastrointestinal tract and adjacent organs, enabling precise assessment of invasion depth in superficial ESCCs. Effective visualization requires eliminating air between the probe and the lesion, achieved through methods such as water immersion, gel application, or the soft balloon technique. The esophageal wall typically appears as nine distinct layers under optimal resolution. Diagnostic criteria for staging include:

EP/LPM cancer: No disruption in the inner three layers (3/9 layers).

MM/SM1 cancer: Disruption of the inner three layers, with no tumor echo in the fourth layer (4/9 layers).

SM2 cancer: Tumor echo present in the fourth layer (4/9 layers) (Fig. 4.8).

EUS is performed following non-magnifying or magnifying endoscopy to supplement the evaluation. A multicenter prospective study [8] reported diagnostic

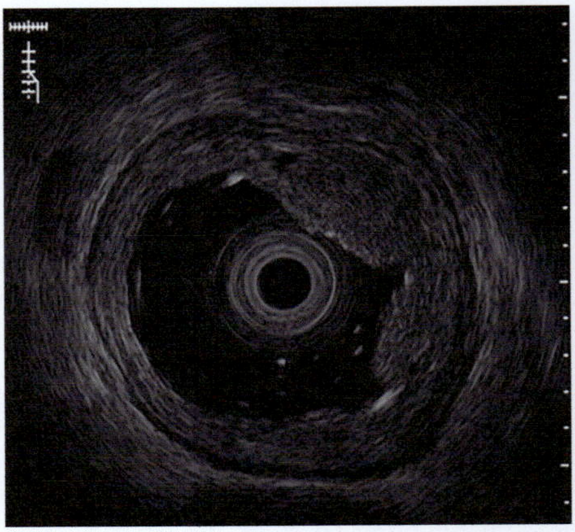

Fig. 4.8 Tumor echo present in the fourth layer (4/9 layers)

accuracies of 72.9% and 74.0% for distinguishing EP/LPM/MM/SM1 cancers from SM2 or more advanced cancers, with and without EUS, respectively. The findings suggested that incorporating EUS did not significantly enhance diagnostic accuracy. Moreover, EUS was associated with a 6.6% increase in overdiagnosis, defined as an overestimation of the cancer's depth, which could lead to unnecessary overtreatment. This limitation highlights the need for judicious use of EUS in clinical practice.

4.7 Diagnosis of Lymph Node Metastasis by EUS

In the pretreatment staging and post-treatment surveillance of ESCCs, accurate evaluation of lymph node metastases in the cervical, mediastinal, and abdominal regions is crucial. In Japan, CT and fluorodeoxyglucose positron emission tomography (FDG-PET) are the primary imaging modalities for assessing lymph node metastases, but EUS is also employed in select cases. EUS enables detailed visualization of lymph nodes in the cervical, mediastinal, and abdominal regions using specialized equipment. Suspicious lymph nodes identified via EUS can be sampled using EUS-guided fine-needle aspiration, allowing for histological confirmation of metastasis.

A meta-analysis comparing the diagnostic performance of EUS, CT, and FDG-PET [27] reported sensitivities of 80%, 50%, and 57%, respectively, and specificities of 70%, 83%, and 85%, respectively. These findings underscore EUS's high sensitivity, particularly for detecting small lymph nodes. However, the lower specificity of EUS compared to CT and FDG-PET highlights the potential for false-positive findings, as not all lymph nodes detected via EUS are metastatic. Understanding these strengths and limitations is essential for integrating EUS with other imaging modalities to optimize diagnostic accuracy in clinical practice.

4.8 Computer-Aided Diagnosis

Significant advancements have been made in diagnostic imaging for ESCCs, yet the interpretation of endoscopic images continues to rely heavily on individual expertise. To address variability in diagnostic accuracy among endoscopists, computer-aided diagnosis systems powered by artificial intelligence (AI) have emerged as transformative tools for reducing inter- and intra-observer variability.

In the context of ESCCs, AI applications span the entire diagnostic workflow in clinical practice. AI systems can assist in detecting lesions during non-magnifying endoscopy, distinguishing cancerous from noncancerous lesions during magnifying endoscopy, and assessing invasion depth in cancerous lesions. Current AI algorithms have demonstrated diagnostic performance comparable to, or even exceeding, that of expert endoscopists in controlled laboratory settings [2, 23]. Moreover, clinical studies have shown that integrating AI into practice significantly reduces missed diagnoses of ESCCs [30]. The future implementation of thoroughly trained AI systems holds substantial promise for achieving reliable, efficient, and early detection of ESCCs. These advancements have the potential to complement expert judgment and improve diagnostic accuracy, ultimately contributing to better clinical outcomes.

References

1. Arduino PG, Bagan J, El-Naggar AK, Carrozzo M. Urban legends series: oral leukoplakia. Oral Dis. 2013;19(7):642–59. https://doi.org/10.1111/odi.12065.
2. Fukuda H, Ishihara R, Kato Y, Matsunaga T, Nishida T, Yamada T, Ogiyama H, Horie M, Kinoshita K, Tada T. Comparison of performances of artificial intelligence versus expert endoscopists for real-time assisted diagnosis of esophageal squamous cell carcinoma (with video). Gastrointest Endosc. 2020;92(4):848–55. https://doi.org/10.1016/j.gie.2020.05.043.
3. Gono K, Obi T, Yamaguchi M, Ohyama N, Machida H, Sano Y, Yoshida S, Hamamoto Y, Endo T. Appearance of enhanced tissue features in narrow-band endoscopic imaging. J Biomed Opt. 2004;9(3):568–77. https://doi.org/10.1117/1.1695563.
4. Hirata K, Yokoyama A, Nakamura R, Omori T, Kawakubo H, Mizukami T, Maruyama K, Kanai T, Yokoyama T. Soft palatal melanosis, a simple predictor for neoplasia in the upper aerodigestive tract in Japanese alcoholic men. Cancer Sci. 2017;108(5):1058–64. https://doi.org/10.1111/cas.13207.
5. Inoue H, Igari T, Nishikage T, Ami K, Yoshida T, Iwai T. A novel method of virtual histopathology using laser-scanning confocal microscopy in-vitro with untreated fresh specimens from the gastrointestinal mucosa. Endoscopy. 2000;32(6):439–43. https://doi.org/10.1055/s-2000-654.
6. Inoue H, Kazawa T, Sato Y, Satodate H, Sasajima K, Kudo SE, Shiokawa A. In vivo observation of living cancer cells in the esophagus, stomach, and colon using catheter-type contact endoscope, "Endo-Cytoscopy system". Gastrointest Endosc Clin N Am. 2004;14(3):589–94., x–xi. https://doi.org/10.1016/j.giec.2004.03.013.
7. Ishiguro S, Sasazuki S, Inoue M, Kurahashi N, Iwasaki M, Tsugane S, JPHC Study Group. Effect of alcohol consumption, cigarette smoking and flushing response on esophageal cancer risk: a population-based cohort study (JPHC study). Cancer Lett. 2009;275(2):240–6. https://doi.org/10.1016/j.canlet.2008.10.020.

8. Ishihara R, Mizusawa J, Kushima R, Matsuura N, Yano T, Kataoka T, Fukuda H, Hanaoka N, Yoshio T, Abe S, Yamamoto Y, Nagata S, Ono H, Tamaoki M, Yoshida N, Takizawa K, Muto M. Assessment of the diagnostic performance of endoscopic ultrasonography after conventional endoscopy for the evaluation of esophageal squamous cell carcinoma invasion depth. JAMA Netw Open. 2021;4(9):e2125317. https://doi.org/10.1001/jamanetworkopen.2021.25317.
9. Ishihara R, Tani Y, Okubo Y, Asada Y, Ueda T, Kitagawa D, Ninomiya T, Tamashiro A, Yoshii S, Shichijo S, Kanesaka T, Yamamoto S, Takeuchi Y, Higashino K, Uedo N, Michida T. Endoscopic landmarks corresponding to anatomical landmarks for esophageal subsite classification. DEN Open. 2024;4(1):e273. https://doi.org/10.1002/deo2.273.
10. Ishihara R, Yamada T, Iishi H, Kato M, Yamamoto S, Yamamoto S, Masuda E, Tatsumi K, Takeuchi Y, Higashino K, Uedo N, Tatsuta M, Ishiguro S. Quantitative analysis of the color change after iodine staining for diagnosing esophageal high-grade intraepithelial neoplasia and invasive cancer. Gastrointest Endosc. 2009;69(2):213–8. https://doi.org/10.1016/j.gie.2008.04.052.
11. Iwatsubo T, Ishihara R, Yamasaki Y, Tonai Y, Hamada K, Kato M, Suzuki S, Kono M, Fukuda H, Shimamoto Y, Nakagawa K, Ohmori M, Arao M, Matsuno K, Iwagami H, Inoue S, Nakahira H, Matsuura N, Shichijo S, et al. Narrow band imaging under less-air condition improves the visibility of superficial esophageal squamous cell carcinoma. BMC Gastroenterol. 2020;20(1):389. https://doi.org/10.1186/s12876-020-01534-2.
12. Katada C, Yokoyama T, Yano T, Kaneko K, Oda I, Shimizu Y, Doyama H, Koike T, Takizawa K, Hirao M, Okada H, Yoshii T, Konishi K, Yamanouchi T, Tsuda T, Omori T, Kobayashi N, Shimoda T, Ochiai A, et al. Alcohol consumption and multiple dysplastic lesions increase risk of squamous cell carcinoma in the esophagus, head, and neck. Gastroenterology. 2016;151(5):860–869 e867. https://doi.org/10.1053/j.gastro.2016.07.040.
13. Kawada K, Arima M, Miyahara R, Tsunomiya M, Kikuchi M, Yamamoto F, Hoshino A, Nakajima Y, Kinugasa Y, Kawano T. Effect of adding magnifying BLI, magnifying NBI, and iodine staining to white light imaging in diagnosis of early esophageal cancer. Endosc Int Open. 2021;9(12):E1877–85. https://doi.org/10.1055/a-1583-9196.
14. Kitagawa Y, Ishihara R, Ishikawa H, Ito Y, Oyama T, Oyama T, Kato K, Kato H, Kawakubo H, Kawachi H, Kuribayashi S, Kono K, Kojima T, Takeuchi H, Tsushima T, Toh Y, Nemoto K, Booka E, Makino T, et al. Esophageal cancer practice guidelines 2022 edited by the Japan esophageal society: part 1. Esophagus. 2023a;20(3):343–72. https://doi.org/10.1007/s10388-023-00993-2.
15. Kitagawa Y, Ishihara R, Ishikawa H, Ito Y, Oyama T, Oyama T, Kato K, Kato H, Kawakubo H, Kawachi H, Kuribayashi S, Kono K, Kojima T, Takeuchi H, Tsushima T, Toh Y, Nemoto K, Booka E, Makino T, et al. Esophageal cancer practice guidelines 2022 edited by the Japan esophageal society: part 2. Esophagus. 2023b;20(3):373–89. https://doi.org/10.1007/s10388-023-00994-1.
16. Kondo H, Fukuda H, Ono H, Gotoda T, Saito D, Takahiro K, Shirao K, Yamaguchi H, Yoshida S. Sodium thiosulfate solution spray for relief of irritation caused by Lugol's stain in chromoendoscopy. Gastrointest Endosc. 2001;53(2):199–202. https://doi.org/10.1067/mge.2001.110730.
17. Kumagai Y, Kawada K, Higashi M, Ishiguro T, Sobajima J, Fukuchi M, Ishibashi K, Baba H, Mochiki E, Aida J, Kawano T, Ishida H, Takubo K. Endocytoscopic observation of various esophageal lesions at x600: can nuclear abnormality be recognized? Dis Esophagus. 2015;28(3):269–75. https://doi.org/10.1111/dote.12183.
18. Kumagai Y, Monma K, Kawada K. Magnifying chromoendoscopy of the esophagus: in-vivo pathological diagnosis using an endocytoscopy system. Endoscopy. 2004;36(7):590–4. https://doi.org/10.1055/s-2004-814533.
19. Morita S, Goda K, Yano T, Kaise M, Kato M, Inoue H, Niwa Y, Kodashima S, Miyahara R, Ochiai A, Ikegami M, Hamatani S, Shimoda T, Ohkura Y, Aida J, Nakanishi Y, Yoshimura K, Ishikawa H, Takubo K, Muto M. Multicenter prospective in vivo study of an endocytoscope system (ECS) for superficial esophageal cancer. J Gastroenterol. 2021;56(9):808–13. https://doi.org/10.1007/s00535-021-01810-2.

20. Muto M, Minashi K, Yano T, Saito Y, Oda I, Nonaka S, Omori T, Sugiura H, Goda K, Kaise M, Inoue H, Ishikawa H, Ochiai A, Shimoda T, Watanabe H, Tajiri H, Saito D. Early detection of superficial squamous cell carcinoma in the head and neck region and esophagus by narrow band imaging: a multicenter randomized controlled trial. J Clin Oncol. 2010;28(9):1566–72. https://doi.org/10.1200/JCO.2009.25.4680.
21. Oyama T, Inoue H, Arima M, Momma K, Omori T, Ishihara R, Hirasawa D, Takeuchi M, Tomori A, Goda K. Prediction of the invasion depth of superficial squamous cell carcinoma based on microvessel morphology: magnifying endoscopic classification of the Japan esophageal society. Esophagus. 2017;14(2):105–12. https://doi.org/10.1007/s10388-016-0527-7.
22. Secretan B, Straif K, Baan R, Grosse Y, El Ghissassi F, Bouvard V, Benbrahim-Tallaa L, Guha N, Freeman C, Galichet L, Cogliano V, WHO International Agency for Research on Cancer Monograph Working Group. A review of human carcinogens–Part E: tobacco, areca nut, alcohol, coal smoke, and salted fish. Lancet Oncol. 2009;10(11):1033–4. https://doi.org/10.1016/s1470-2045(09)70326-2.
23. Shimamoto Y, Ishihara R, Kato Y, Shoji A, Inoue T, Matsueda K, Miyake M, Waki K, Kono M, Fukuda H, Matsuura N, Nagaike K, Aoi K, Yamamoto K, Inoue T, Nakahara M, Nishihara A, Tada T. Real-time assessment of video images for esophageal squamous cell carcinoma invasion depth using artificial intelligence. J Gastroenterol. 2020;55(11):1037–45. https://doi.org/10.1007/s00535-020-01716-5.
24. Shimizu Y, Omori T, Yokoyama A, Yoshida T, Hirota J, Ono Y, Yamamoto J, Kato M, Asaka M. Endoscopic diagnosis of early squamous neoplasia of the esophagus with iodine staining: high-grade intra-epithelial neoplasia turns pink within a few minutes. J Gastroenterol Hepatol. 2008;23(4):546–50. https://doi.org/10.1111/j.1440-1746.2007.04990.x.
25. Slaughter DP, Southwick HW, Smejkal W. Field cancerization in oral stratified squamous epithelium; clinical implications of multicentric origin. Cancer. 1953;6(5):963–8. https://doi.org/10.1002/1097-0142(195309)6:5<963::aid-cncr2820060515>3.0.co;2-q.
26. Takenaka R, Kawahara Y, Okada H, Hori K, Inoue M, Kawano S, Tanioka D, Tsuzuki T, Uemura M, Ohara N, Tominaga S, Onoda T, Yamamoto K. Narrow-band imaging provides reliable screening for esophageal malignancy in patients with head and neck cancers. Am J Gastroenterol. 2009;104(12):2942–8. https://doi.org/10.1038/ajg.2009.426.
27. van Vliet EP, Heijenbrok-Kal MH, Hunink MG, Kuipers EJ, Siersema PD. Staging investigations for oesophageal cancer: a meta-analysis. Br J Cancer. 2008;98(3):547–57. https://doi.org/10.1038/sj.bjc.6604200.
28. Waki K, Ishihara R, Maekawa A, Inoue T, Shoji A, Matsueda K, Miyake M, Fukuda H, Shichijo S, Kanesaka T, Takeuchi Y, Higashino K, Uedo N, Michida T. Endoscopic findings in the soft palatal mucosa are associated with the risk of esophageal squamous cell carcinoma. J Gastroenterol Hepatol. 2021;36(5):1276–85. https://doi.org/10.1111/jgh.15291.
29. Yokoyama A, Mizukami T, Omori T, Yokoyama T, Hirota T, Matsushita S, Higuchi S, Maruyama K, Ishii H, Hibi T. Melanosis and squamous cell neoplasms of the upper aerodigestive tract in Japanese alcoholic men. Cancer Sci. 2006;97(9):905–11. https://doi.org/10.1111/j.1349-7006.2006.00260.x.
30. Yuan XL, Liu W, Lin YX, Deng QY, Gao YP, Wan L, Zhang B, Zhang T, Zhang WH, Bi XG, Yang GD, Zhu BH, Zhang F, Qin XB, Pan F, Zeng XH, Chaudhry H, Pang MY, Yang J, et al. Effect of an artificial intelligence-assisted system on endoscopic diagnosis of superficial oesophageal squamous cell carcinoma and precancerous lesions: a multicentre, tandem, double-blind, randomised controlled trial. Lancet Gastroenterol Hepatol. 2024;9(1):34–44. https://doi.org/10.1016/S2468-1253(23)00276-5.

Japanese Classification and UICC/TNM Classification

5

Shinji Mine

5.1 Introduction

Two major classification systems are widely used for staging esophageal cancer worldwide: the Japanese Classification of Esophageal Cancer by the Japan Esophageal Society (JES) and the TNM Classification by Union for International Cancer Control (UICC) [1]. In September 2022, the 12th edition of the Japanese classification—the most recent version—was published [2, 3], marking the first update in approximately 7 years since the 11th edition [4, 5]. Meanwhile, the ninth edition of the TNM Classification was released in May 2025 [6].

This chapter outlines the historical development of the Japanese classification, the differences between the Japanese and TNM classifications including the major revisions in its 12th edition, and perspectives for the upcoming 13th edition of the Japanese classification.

5.2 History of Both Classifications

5.2.1 History of the Japanese Classification of Esophageal Cancer

In the 1960s, esophageal cancer was recognized as a disease with a poor prognosis and wide variation in treatment outcomes across Japan. This situation highlighted the need for standardized criteria to document and evaluate clinical data—including disease staging, treatment strategies, and outcomes—through interdisciplinary collaboration among surgeons, physicians, radiation oncologists, and pathologists.

S. Mine (✉)
Department of Esophageal and Gastroenterological Surgery, Juntendo University Hospital, Tokyo, Japan
e-mail: s.mine.gv@juntendo.ac.jp

Y. Kitagawa et al. (eds.), *Esophageal Squamous Cell Carcinoma*,
https://doi.org/10.1007/978-981-92-2611-5_5

In response, the Japanese Society for Esophageal Diseases (the predecessor of the JES) published the first edition of the Japanese Classification of Esophageal Cancer in 1969. The goals of this classification were:

- To unify definitions for disease staging and anatomical landmarks, enabling standardized documentation across medical institutions.
- To establish a framework for collecting clinical and pathological data to evaluate treatment strategies and prognostic factors.
- To promote interinstitutional comparisons of treatment outcomes and support research by unifying the recording of clinical, pathological, and statistical data, ultimately aiming to improve patient outcomes.

Although simpler than the current version, the first edition included:

- Anatomical divisions of the esophagus (cervical, thoracic, abdominal).
- Tumor location classification (upper, middle, lower esophagus).
- Staging categories (T, N, M), similar to the current TNM system.
- Histological classification (focused on squamous cell carcinoma).
- Treatment modality classification (surgery, radiation therapy, etc.)
- Clinical findings (c): tumor location and laterality, longitudinal size, histological type, T/N/M status, clinical stage, etc.
- Pathological findings (p): tumor site, lesion size, histological type and grade, depth of invasion, infiltration pattern, vascular/lymphatic invasion, resection margins, multifocality, treatment response, lymph node metastasis, etc.

This first edition was one of Japan's earliest cancer classification systems, alongside those for other gastrointestinal cancers such as gastric cancer (first issued in 1962). It significantly contributed to standardizing care and improving outcomes in esophageal cancer, laying the groundwork for later revisions and national comprehensive registry efforts. It was pioneering in:

- Establishing detailed anatomical subcategories (e.g., subdivisions of the thoracic esophagus, which laid the foundation for subsequent international classifications).
- Emphasizing the relationship between esophagectomy and the extent of lymph node dissection.

In 2003, following organizational restructuring, the Japanese Society for Esophageal Diseases became the Japan Esophageal Society (JES), which continues to oversee the classification's development and revision. The Society regularly updates the classification based on accumulating evidence, compatibility with related guidelines, and alignment with international standards. The 12th edition, released in September 2022, marked the first update in 7 years.

5.2.2 History of the UICC/TNM Classification

In 1933, the International Union Against Cancer—Union Internationale Contre le Cancer (UICC)—was established as a nonprofit and nongovernment organization. Then in the 1940s, the TNM system was developed for the classification of malignant tumors. In 1950, the UICC appointed a Committee on Tumor Nomenclature and Statistics and agreed with general definitions for the local extension of malignant tumors. In 1954, the Research Committee of the UICC set up a special Committee on Clinical Stage Classification and Applied Statistics to extend the general technique of classification to cancer at any site.

Between 1960 and 1967, the Committee published nine pamphlets describing proposals for the classification of 23 sites. In 1968, these pamphlets were combined into a booklet, which was substantially the first edition of the *TNM Classification of Malignant Tumours*.

In 1995, the project started to publish Prognostic Factors in Cancer, a compilation and discussion of the prognostic factors in cancer, both anatomic and nonanatomic, at each of the body sites. The seventh edition of the TNM Classification contained rules of classifications, stage grouping, and prognostic groupings that corresponded with anatomic stage/prognostic groups appearing in the seventh edition of the *American Joint Committee on Cancer (AJCC) Cancer Staging Manual* (2009).

In 2010, the name of the UICC was changed to the Union for International Cancer Control.

In 2017, the eighth edition of the TNM Classification was published at the same time as the eighth edition of the *AJCC Cancer Staging Manual* with the TNM stage and prognostic groups corresponding with AJCC prognostic stage groups.

The ninth edition of the TNM Classification was released in May 2025 as described above.

5.3 Anatomical Subsites—Esophagus and Esophagogastric Junction

5.3.1 The Japanese Classification

The anatomical subsites of the esophagus—tumor location and anatomical esophageal nomenclature—were defined in the first edition (1969). They had almost remained unchanged up to the 11th edition (2015). Esophagus was divided into five parts: cervical esophagus (Ce), upper thoracic esophagus (Ut), middle thoracic esophagus (Mt), lower thoracic esophagus (Lt), and abdominal esophagus (Ae). However, in the latest 12th edition, the definition of the abdominal esophagus (Ae) has been abolished. As a result, the definition of the lower border of the lower thoracic esophagus (Lt) has been defined to 2 cm cephalad from the esophagogastric junction. In addition, the border between Mt. and Lt should be 1 cm distal to the inferior pulmonary vein on computed tomography (CT) in the absence of esophagography. Instead of abdominal esophagus, the zone of the esophagogastric junction (Jz) has been adopted in the latest 12th edition (Fig. 5.1). Jz is defined as the region 2 cm above the esophagogastric junction and 2 cm below the esophagogastric junction. Jz is identical to the esophagogastric junctional area defined by the "Nishi classification."

Definition of the esophagogastric junction (EGJ): In the Japanese classification, the EGJ has been defined comprehensively based on following findings.

Endoscopic findings:

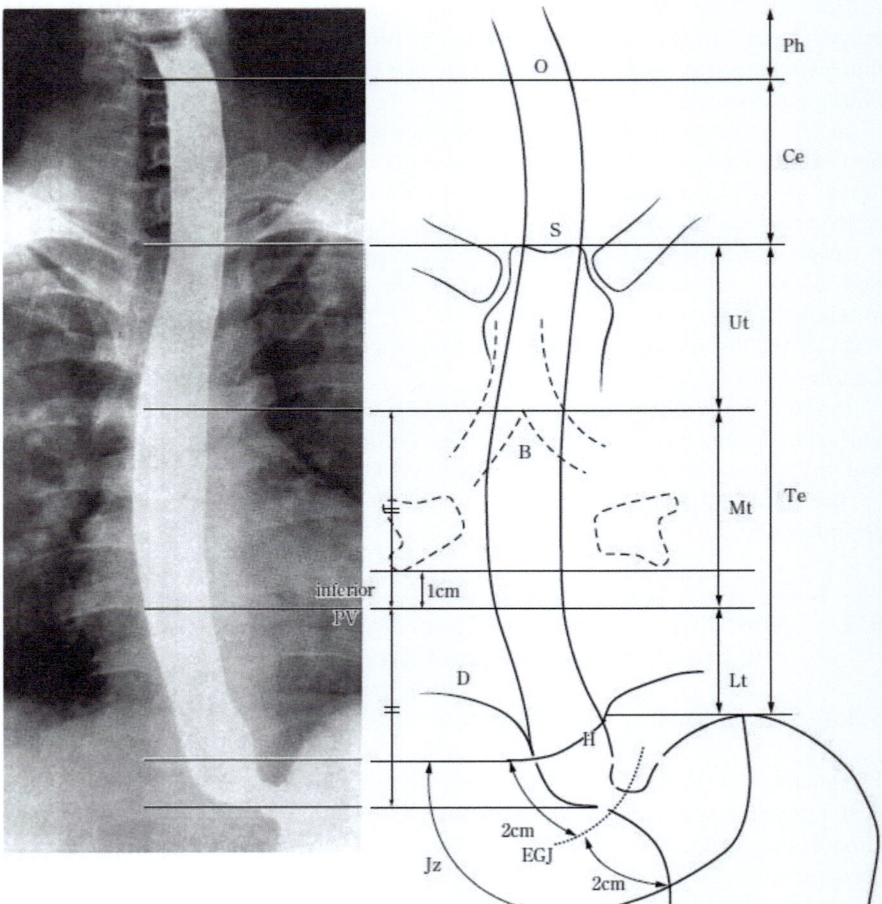

Fig. 5.1 Anatomical subsites (tumor location and anatomical esophageal nomenclature) in the latest 12th edition of the Japanese Classification of Esophageal Cancer [2]. O: esophageal orifice, D: diaphragm, S: superior margin of the sternum, EGJ: esophagogastric junction, B: tracheal bifurcation, H: esophageal hiatus, PV: pulmonary vein. Adapted from Mine et al., *Esophagus, 2024* under CC BY 4.0

- Lower margin of palisading small vessels.
- If the palisading small vessels are unclear, the oral margin of the longitudinal folds of the greater curvature of the stomach is defined as the EGJ.

Upper gastrointestinal imaging (UGI):

- Narrowest locus of the lower esophagus.
- The upper end of the longitudinal folds.

Pathological assessment:

- Macroscopic definition of the surgically resected specimen:
  The EGJ should be defined macroscopically as the point wherein the luminal caliber changes in the area where the tubular esophagus is connected to the vestibular lumen of the stomach.
- Microscopic definition of the surgically or endoscopically resected specimen:
  The EGJ should be defined based on the presence of histological features found in the esophagus (squamous epithelium [including squamous island], proper esophageal glands and their ducts, double-layer muscularis mucosa, or palisading small vessels above muscularis mucosa).

5.3.2 UICC/TNM Classification

Cervical esophagus: This commences at the lower border of the cricoid cartilage and ends at the thoracic inlet (suprasternal notch), approximately 18 cm from the upper incisor teeth.

Intrathoracic esophagus:

- The upper thoracic portion extending from the thoracic inlet to the level of the tracheal bifurcation, approximately 24 cm from the upper incisor teeth.
- The mid-thoracic portion is the proximal half of the esophagus between the tracheal bifurcation and the esophagogastric junction. The lower level is approximately 32 cm from the upper incisor teeth.
- The lower thoracic portion, approximately 8 cm in length (includes the abdominal esophagus), is the distal half of the esophagus between the tracheal bifurcation and the esophagogastric junction. The lower level is approximately 40 cm from the upper incisor teeth.

Esophagogastric junction: Cancers involving the esophagogastric junction (EGJ) whose epicenter is within the proximal 2 cm of the cardia (Siewert types I/II) are to be staged as esophageal cancers. Cancers whose epicenter is more than 2 cm distal from the EGJ will be staged using the Stomach Cancer TNM and Stage even if the EGJ is involved. Please refer to *The Eighth Edition AJCC Cancer Staging Manual*, Chap. 16, Page 188, Figure 16.1 for details [7].

5.4 T Category: Primary Tumor

Generally, the classification of T categories has been almost same between the Japanese and TNM classification except for T1, cT3, cT4 subclassification and metastatic nodes invading other organs.

5.4.1 The Japanese Classification

T0: No evidence of primary tumor.
T1a: Tumor invades mucosa.
  T1a-EP: Carcinoma in situ (Tis).
  T1a-LPM: Tumor invades lamina propria mucosae (LPM).
  T1a-MM: Tumor invades muscularis mucosae (MM).
T1b: Tumor invades submucosa (SM).
  T1b-SM1: Tumor invades the upper third of the submucosal layer.
  T1b-SM2: Tumor invades the middle third of the submucosal layer.
  T1b-SM3: Tumor invades the lower third of the submucosal layer.
T2: Tumor invades muscularis propria (MP).
T3: Tumor invades adventitia (AD).
T4: Tumor invades adjacent structures (AI).

Japanese classification has had a subclassification of T1 depth (Fig. 5.2).

In the latest 12th edition, subdivision of cT3 was introduced and cT4 subclassification was abolished. Due to the challenges of distinguishing cT3 and cT4 lesions by imaging alone, cT3 has been subdivided into "resectable" (cT3r) and "borderline resectable" (cT3br). CT representative images for each were included in the new edition (Fig. 5.3a–c). The cT4a/cT4b subclassification has been eliminated clinically, though it remains in the pathological classification (pT4a/pT4b), and no equivalent subclassification exists for pT3.

When a metastatic lymph node additionally invades a surrounding organ other than the esophagus, it is classified as T4 and recorded as "T4 (metastatic node number invaded organ)," e.g., cT4 (No. 112aoA-Aorta).

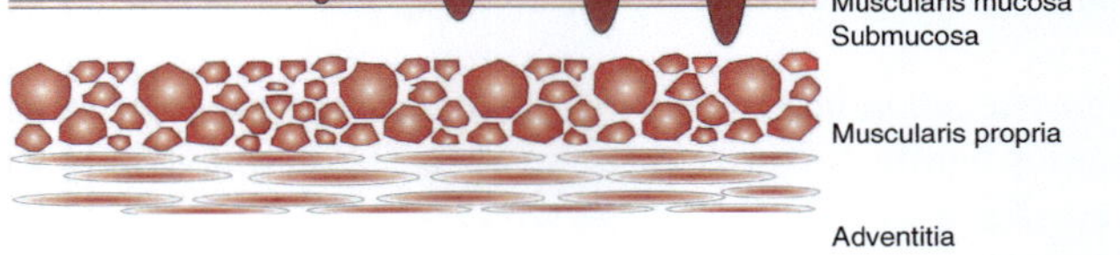

Fig. 5.2 Subclassification of superficial esophageal cancer in the 12th edition of the Japanese Classification of Esophageal Cancer [2]

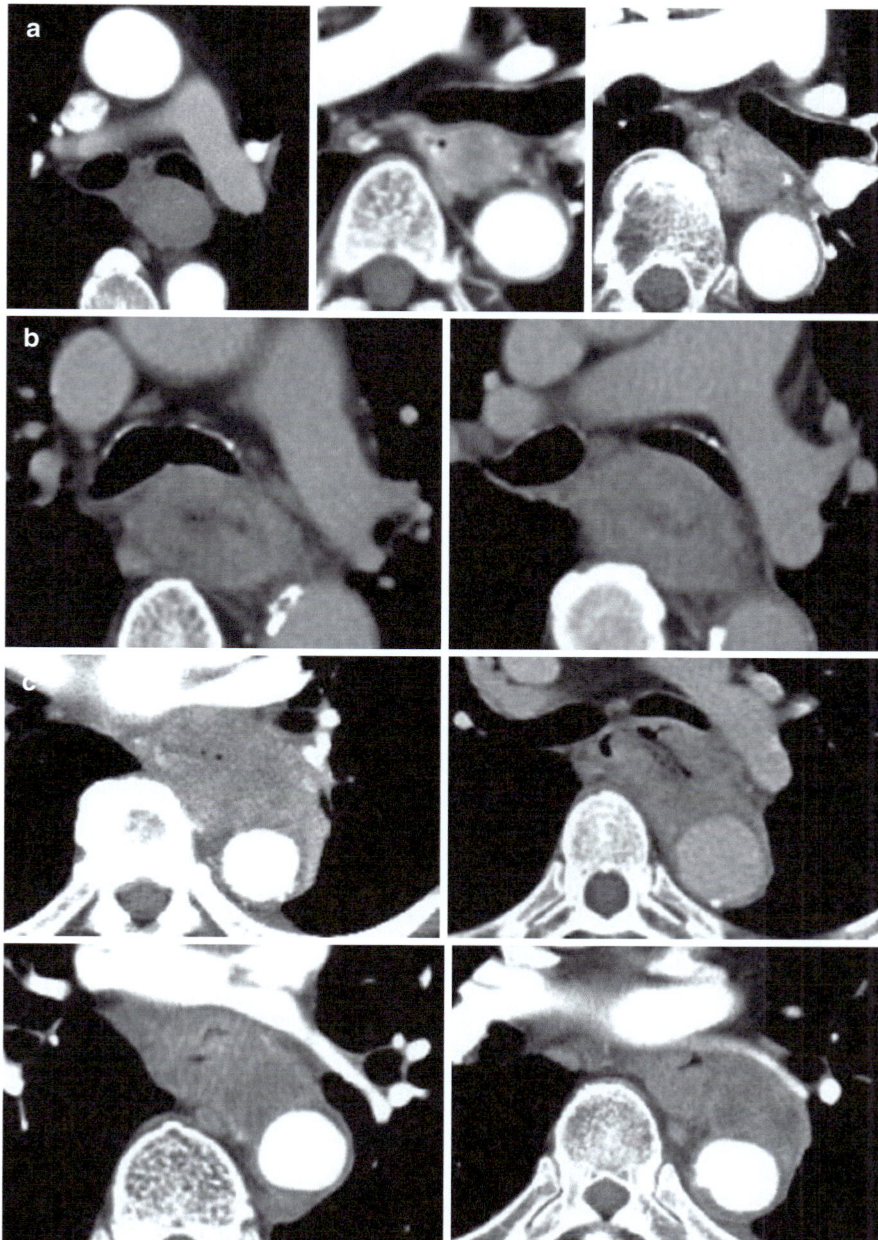

Fig. 5.3 (**a**) Representative CT images of cT3r esophageal cancer [2]. (**b**) Representative CT images of cT3br esophageal cancer [2]. (**c**) Representative CT images of cT4 esophageal cancer [2]

5.4.2 UICC/TNM Classification

Tx: Primary tumor cannot be assessed.
T0: No evidence of primary tumor.
Tis: Carcinoma in site/high-grade dysplasia.
T1: Tumor invades lamina propria, muscularis mucosae, or submucosa.
  T1a: Tumor invades lamina propria or muscularis mucosae.
  T1b: Tumor invades submucosa.
T2: Tumor invades muscularis propria.
T3: Tumor invades adventitia.
T4: Tumor invades adjacent structures.
  T4a: Tumor invades pleura, pericardium, azygos vein, diaphragm, or peritoneum.
  T4b: Tumor invades other adjacent structures such as aorta, vertebral body, or trachea.

In TNM classification, there is no difference between cT and pT status like the Japanese classification.

5.5 N Category: Lymph Node Metastasis

There had been a big difference between the Japanese and TNM classification because the JES had categorized each lymph node into N1, N2, N3, or N4 based on their anatomical location relative to the primary tumor. However, in the latest 12th edition, a numerical system (1–2, 3–6, ≥7 nodes) has been introduced, improving consistency with the TNM classification. Furthermore, supraclavicular lymph nodes (station 104), which have been categorized as M in TNM, are also defined as M1a. This distinction is based on Japanese studies, suggesting survival benefit from prophylactic dissection. Now, a randomized controlled trial (JCOG2013) is ongoing to evaluate this strategy, as it remains a subject of controversy even within Japan.

5.5.1 The Japanese Classification

In the 12th edition, N system based on their anatomical location relative to the primary tumor has been abolished. As a result, regional lymph nodes are the same in patients with thoracic esophageal cancer irrespective of primary tumor locations (e.g., Ut, Mt., or Lt) except for some nodes. The names and numbers of lymph nodes are defined in Table 5.1 and Fig. 5.4. Regional lymph nodes were different in the location of the tumor (Ce, Te, and Jz) as shown in Table 5.2 and Figs. 5.5, 5.6, and 5.7.

Table 5.1 Numbers and naming of regional lymph nodes in the Japanese Classification of Esophageal Cancer in 12th edition [2]

Cervical lymph nodes
100 superficial lymph nodes of the neck
101 cervical paraesophageal lymph nodes
102 deep cervical lymph nodes
103 peripharyngeal lymph nodes
104 supraclavicular lymphnodes
Thoracic lymph nodes
105 upper thoracic paraesophageal lymph nodes
106 thoracic paratracheal lymph nodes
106rec recurrent nerve lymph nodes
106recL left recurrent nerve lymph nodes
106recR right recurrent nerve lymph nodes
106pre pretracheal lymph nodes
106tb tracheobronchial lymph nodes
106tbL left tracheobronchial lymph nodes
106tbR right tracheobronchial lymph nodes
107 subcarinal lymph nodes
108 middle thoracic paraesophageal lymph nodes
109 main bronchus lymph nodes
109 L left mein bronchus lymph nodes
109R right main bronchus lymph nodes
110 lower thoracic paraesophageal lymph nodes
111 supradiaphragmatic lymph nodes
112 posterior mediastinal lymph nodes
112aoA anterio thoracic paraaortic lymph nodes
112aoP posterior thoracic paraaortic lymph nodes
112pul pulmonary ligament lymph nodes
113 ligament arteriosum lymph nodes (Botallo lymph nodes)
114 anterior mediastinal lymph nodes
Abdominal lymph nodes
1 right paracardial lymph nodes
2 left paracardial lymph nodes
3a lesser curvature lymph nodes along the branches of the left gastric artery
3b lesser curvaturte lymph nodes along the second brachches and distal part of the right gastric artery
4 lymph nodes along the greater curvature
4sa lymph nodes along the short gastric artery
4sb lymph nodes along the left gastroepiploic artery
4d lymph nodes along the right gastroepiploic artery
5 suprapyloric lymph nodes
6 Infrapyloric lymph nodes
7 lymph nodes along the left gastric artery
8a lymph nodes along the common hepatic artery (anterosuperior group)
8p lymph nodes along the common hepatic artery (posterior group)
9 lymph nodes along the coeliac artery
10 lymph nodes at the splenic hilum
11 lymph nodes along the splenic artery
11p lymph nodes along the proximal splenic artery
11d lymph nodes along the distal splenic artery
12 lymph nodes in the hepatoduodenal ligament
13 lymph nodes on the posterior surface of the pancreatic head

(continued)

Table 5.1 (continued)

14 lymph nodes along the superior mesenteric vessels
14A lymph nodes along the superior mesenteric artery
14 V lymph nodes along the superior mesenteric vein
15 lymph nodes along the middle colic artery
16 lymph nodes along the abdominal aorta
17 lymph nodes on the anterior surface of the pancreatic head
18 lymph nodes along the inferior margin of the pancreas
19 Infrafdiaphragmatic lymph nodes
20 lymph nodes in the esophageal hiastus of the diaphragm

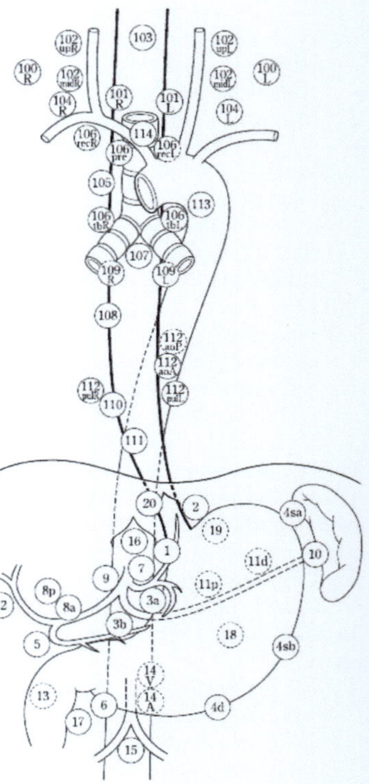

Fig. 5.4 Station numbers of regional lymph nodes in the 12th edition of the Japanese Classification of Esophageal Cancer [2]

Table 5.2 Lymph node groups according to the tumor location in the Japanese Classification of Esophageal Cancer in 12th edition [2]

Tumor location	Regional lymph nodes	M1a	M1b
Cervical (Ce)	Cervical: 100, 101, 102mid, 104	None	Other lymph nodes
	Mediastinal, 105[Note], 106rec[Note]		
Thoracic (Te)	Cervical: 101	104	102
	Mediastinal: 105, 106rec, 106tbL, 107, 108, 109, 110, 111, 112aoA, 112pul		106pre, 106tbR, 112aoP, 16, other lymph nodes
	Abdominal: 1, 2, 3a, 7, 8a, 9, 11p, 19, 20		
Zone of esophagogastric junction (Jz)	Cervical: None	101, 104, 16	Other lymph nodes
	Mediastinal: 105, 106rec, 106tbL, 107, 108, 109, 110, 111, 112aoA, 112pul		
	Abdominal: 1, 2, 3a, 3b, 4sa, 4sb, 4d, 5, 6, 7, 8a, 9, 10, 11p, 11d, 19, 20		

Note: Limited to the area which can be dissected from the cervical incision

5.5.2 UICC/TNM Classification

Coeliac axis nodes and paraesophageal nodes in the neck were defined as the regional lymph nodes, irrespective of the site of the primary tumor. The supraclavicular nodes were excluded from being regional lymph nodes. The N category was classified into four groups as N0 to N3 according to the number of metastasis-positive nodes among the regional lymph nodes, as in *The Eighth Edition AJCC Cancer Staging Manual*, Chapter 16, Page 190, Figure 16.3 for details [7].

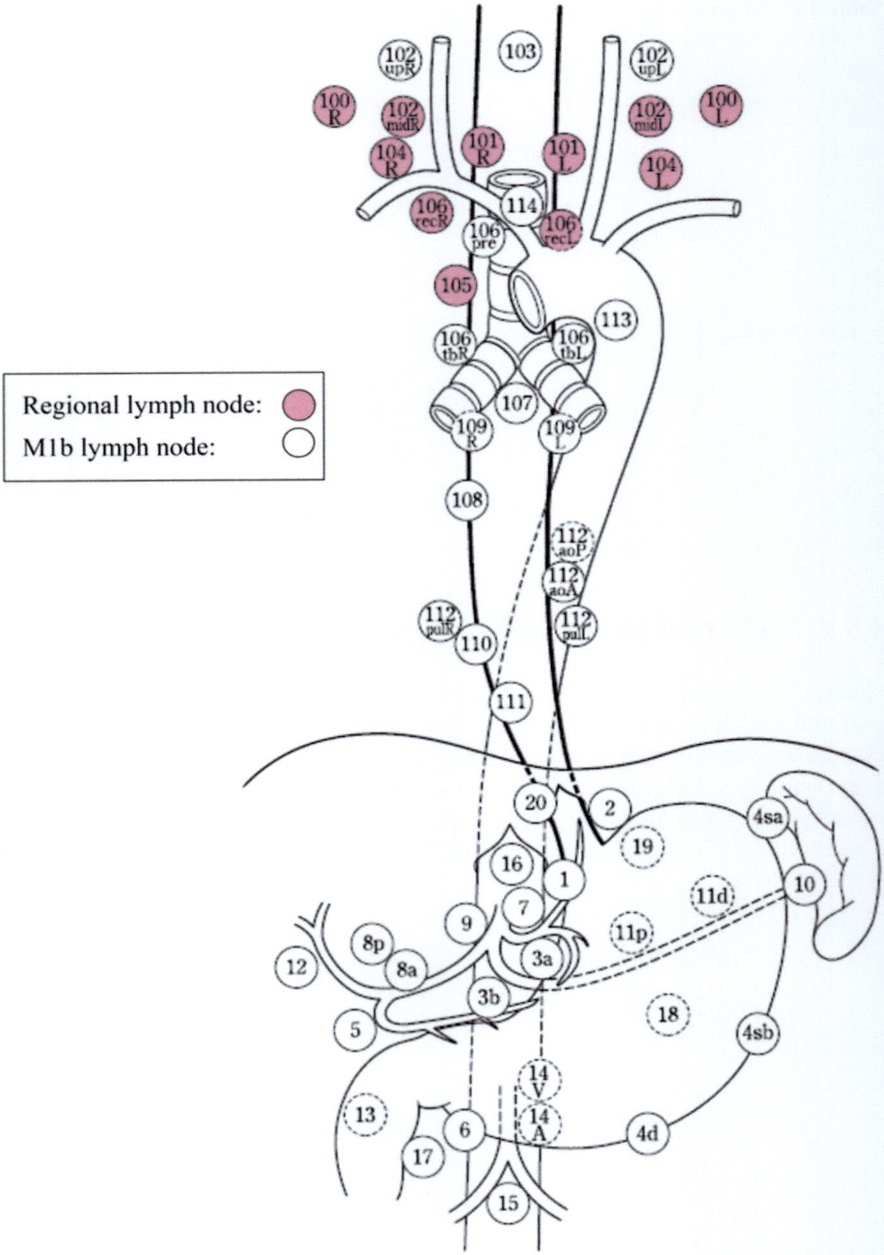

Fig. 5.5 Lymph node maps illustrating the lymph node groups—for cancers in the cervical esophageal cancer (Ce) presented in the 12th edition of Japanese Classification of Esophageal Cancer [2]

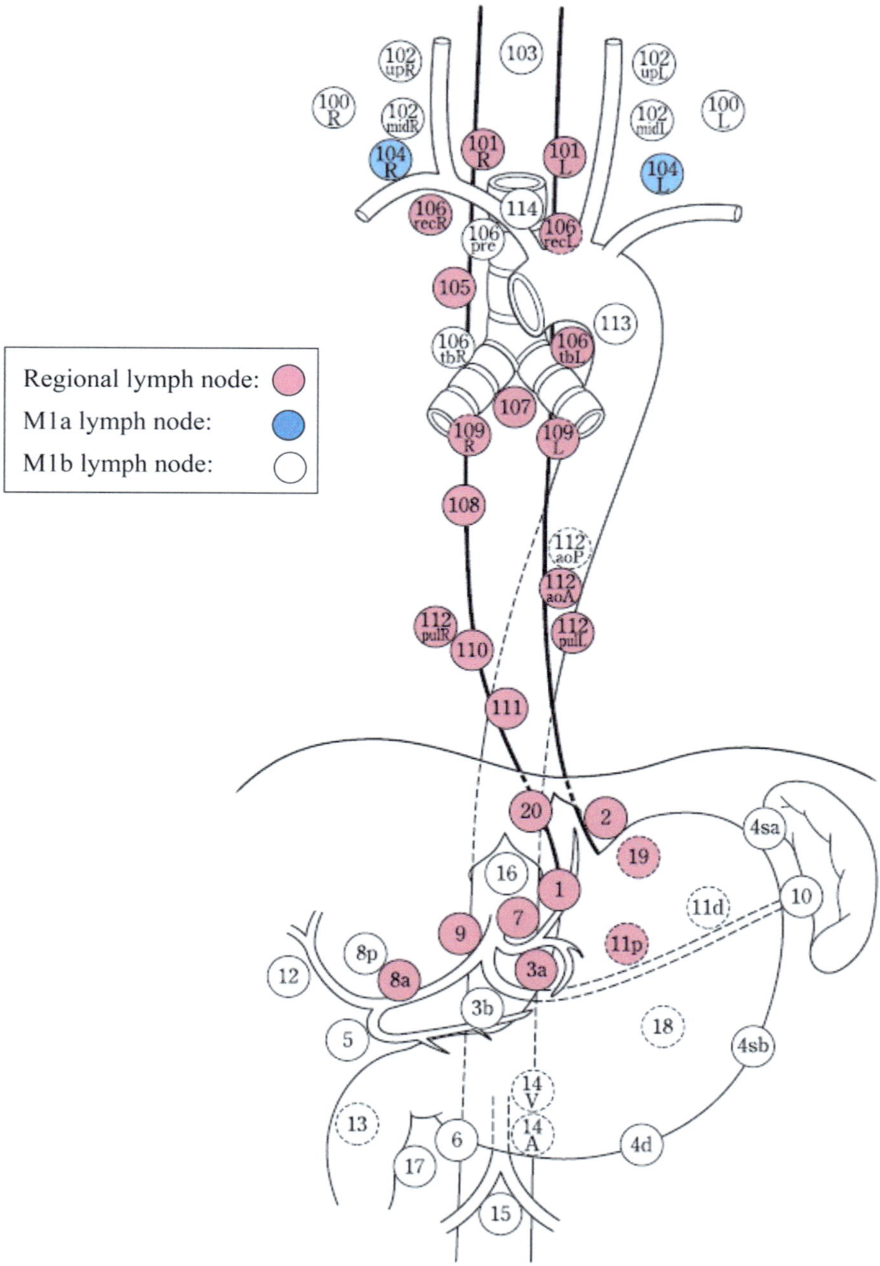

Fig. 5.6 Lymph node maps illustrating the lymph node groups—for cancers in the thoracic esophageal cancer (Te) presented in the 12th edition of Japanese Classification of Esophageal Cancer [2]

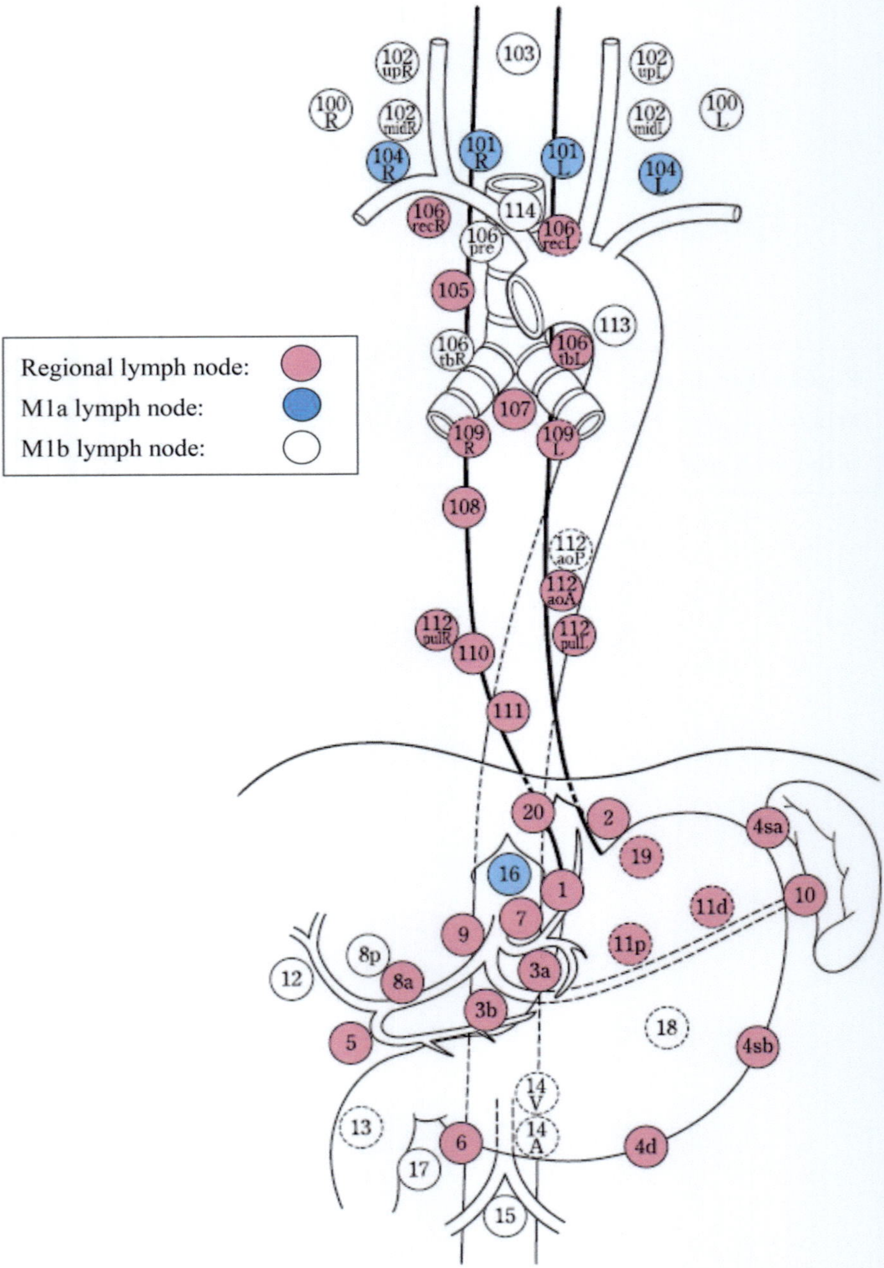

Fig. 5.7 Lymph node maps illustrating the lymph node groups—for cancers in the esophagogastric junction cancer (Jz) presented in the 12th edition of Japanese Classification of Esophageal Cancer [2]

5.6 M Category: Distant Metastasis

5.6.1 Japanese Classification

In the Japanese classification, M1 is divided into M1a and M1b.

M1a: Metastases in lymph nodes that are outside the region but can be expected to have some efficacy in dissection. For instance, #104 for thoracic esophageal cancer and #101, 104, and 16 for the esophagogastric junctional cancer.
M1b: Metastasis to lymph nodes that are neither regional lymph nodes nor M1a or metastasis to distant organs. Intramural metastasis to the stomach was treated as distant metastasis and recorded as M1b (IM1-St).

5.6.2 UICC/TNM Classification

There is no subclassification in M status. Distant organ metastasis and lymph node metastasis other than reginal lymph node are defined as M1.

5.7 Stage Groups

5.7.1 Japanese Classification

In the 12th edition, Japanese Stage grouping has been divided into two stagings: clinical staging and pathological staging as well as UICC/TNM staging (Table 5.3a, b). This staging was based on the data of Japanese comprehensive registry of esophageal cancer [8–10].

5.7.2 UICC/TNM Classification

Apart from clinical and pathological staging, UICC/TNM staging offers pathological prognostic group table (Table 5.4a–c). It contains other factors including histological grading and location.

Table 5.3 Clinical and pathological stage in the Japanese Classification of Esophageal Cancer in 12th edition [2]

(a) Clinical stage				
	N0	N1	N (2–3) M1a	M1b
T0, T1a	0	II	IIIA	IVB
T1b	I	II	IIIA	IVB
T2	II	IIIA	IIIA	IVB
T3r	II	IIIA	IIIA	IVB
T3br	IIIB	IIIB	IIIB	IVB
T4	IVA	IVA	IVA	IVB

(b) Pathological stage					
	N0	N1	N2	N3 M1a	M1b
T0	0	II A	II A	III A	IVB
T1a	0	II A	II B	III A	IVB
T1b	I	II A	III A	III A	IVB
T2	II A	II B	III A	III B	IVB
T3	II B	III A	III B	IVA	IVB
T4a	III B	III B	IVA	IVA	IVB
T4b	IVA	IVA	IVA	IVA	IVB

Table 5.4 Stage in UICC/TNM classification of eighth edition

(a) Clinical stage of esophageal squamous cell carcinoma						
cTNM squamous cell carcinoma						
		N0	N1	N2	N3	M1
Tis	0					
T1		I	I	III	IVA	IVB
T2		II	II	III	IVA	IVB
T3		II	III	III	IVA	IVB
T4a		IVA	IVA	IVA	IVA	IVB
T4b		IVA	IVA	IVA	IVA	IVB

(b) Pathological stage of esophageal squamous cell carcinoma						
pTNM squamous cell carcinoma						
		N0	N1	N2	N3	M1
Tis	0					
T1a		IA	IIB	IIIA	IVA	IVB
T1b		IB	IIB	IIIA	IVA	IVB
T2		IIA	IIIA	IIIB	IVA	IVB
T3		IIB	IIIB	IIIB	IVA	IVB
T4a		IIIB	IIIB	IVA	IVA	IVB
T4b		IVA	IVA	IVA	IVA	IVB

(continued)

Table 5.4 (continued)

(c) Pathological prognostic group of esophageal squamous cell carcinoma								
Pathologic prognostic group								
Squamous cell carcinoma								
			N0					
			L	U/M	N1	N2	N3	M1
	Tis	0						
T1a	G1		IA	IA	IIB	IIIA	IVA	IVB
	G2–3		IB	IB				
	T1b		IB	IIB	IIIA	IVA	IVB	
T2	G1		IB	IB	IIIA	IIIB	IVA	IVB
	G2–3		IIA	IIA				
T3	G1		IIA	IIA	IIIB	IIIB	IVA	IVB
	G2–3		IIA	IIB				
	T4a		IIIB	IIIB	IIIB	IVA	IVA	IVB
	T4b		IVA	IVA	IVA	IVA	IVA	IVB

5.8 Histopathological Grading

5.8.1 Japanese Classification

Histological subtyping must be performed based on the predominant histological features of the tumor: well differentiated, moderately differentiated, and poorly differentiated.

5.8.2 UICC/TNM Classification

The G grading was adopted as a prognostic factor for squamous cell carcinoma of the esophagus since the seventh edition. G grading system has five classifications as follows:

GX: Grade of differentiation cannot be assessed.
G1: Well differentiated.
G2: Moderately differentiated.
G3: Poorly differentiated.
G4: Undifferentiated.

In UICC/TNM classification, if there are different degrees of differentiation in a tumor, one should assign the tumor to the least favorable grade of G1–G4. This is a difference between Japanese and UICC/TNM classifications.

Therefore, when a tumor has a dominant part of well-differentiated squamous cell carcinoma and a less dominant part of poorly differentiated squamous cell carcinoma, it is defined as well differentiated on the Japanese classification and G3 in UICC/TNM classification.

5.9 "Y" Symbol: Post-therapy Classification

In the UICC/TNM classification, the cTNM or pTNM categories were identified by a "y" prefix, in those cases in which classification was performed during or following multimodality therapy:

yc: After multimodality therapy, the y-clinical (yc) classification is assessed based on clinical history, physical examination, and any imaging findings.
yp: After surgery following multimodality therapy, the y-pathological (yp) classification is assessed based on the y-clinical.
TNM classification:post-therapy classificationstage information, operative findings, and pathological evaluation of the resected specimen.

This "y" prefix has not been introduced in the Japanese classification.

5.10 Macroscopic Tumor Type

Macroscopic tumor type is only defined in the Japanese classification. The tumor type classification is decided based on the macroscopic findings: 0-I, 0-II, 0-III, 1, 2, 3, 4, and 5 (Fig. 5.8). Radiological and endoscopic classifications are based on the macroscopic classification.

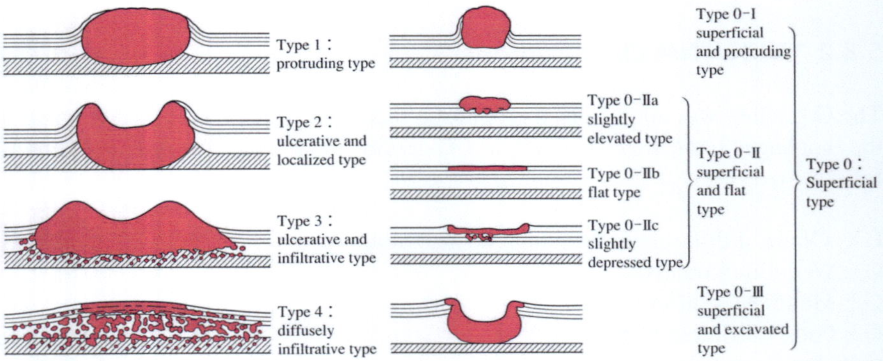

Fig. 5.8 Macroscopic classification (Type 0–4) presented in the 11th edition of the Japanese Classification of Esophageal Cancer [2]

5.11 Extent of Lymph Node Dissection

In the 12th edition of the Japanese classification, two-field and three-field dissection are defined. Then, simply speaking, D2 means two-field dissection and D3 means three-field dissection.

Two-Field Dissection

Mediastinal and abdominal lymph nodes are dissected. The following lymph nodes must be resected: No. 101, 105, 106rec, 106tbl, 107, 108, 109, 110, 111, 112aoA, 112pul, 1, 2, 3, 7, 8a, 9, 11p. (Dissection of No. 106tbl, 111, 8a, and 11p can be omitted.)

Three-Field Dissection:

Cervical, mediastinal, and abdominal lymph nodes are dissected. This is equivalent to two-field dissection plus cervical lymph node dissections.

Based on the location of esophageal cancer, the degree of lymph node dissection is defined as follows:

Cervical esophageal cancer (Ce):

DX: Degree of lymph node dissection cannot be assessed.
D1: Less than D2 lymph node dissection is performed.
D2: Lymph nodes dissection of 100, 101, 102 mid, 104, 105, and 106rec were performed.
D3: Not applicable.

Thoracic esophageal cancer (Te):

DX: Extent of lymph node dissection cannot be assessed.
D1: Incomplete dissection of two-field lymph nodes.
D2: Complete dissection of two-field lymph nodes.
D3: Complete dissection of three-field lymph nodes.

Esophagogastric junctional cancer (Jz):

D1: Lymph node dissection of No. 1, 2, 3a, and 7.
D1+: Lymph node dissection of No. 1, 2, 3a, 7, 8a, 9, and 11p.
D2: Lymph node dissection of No. 1, 2, 3a, 7, 8a, 9, 11p, 19, 20, and 110.
D3: Lymph node dissection of No. 1, 2, 3a, 7, 8a, 9, 11p, 19, 20, 105, 106recL, 106recR, 107, 108, 109 L, 109R, 110, 111, 112aoA, and 112pul.

In the UICC/TNM classification, there is no definition about the extent of lymph node dissection like the Japanese classification.

5.12 Diagnostic Criteria for Depth of Superficial Esophageal Cancer by Magnifying Endoscopy with Narrow-Band Imaging

In the 12th edition of the Japanese classification, a new classification based on narrow-band light-based observation (NBI) and blue laser imaging (BLI) was introduced, which is simple, objective, and useful for differentiating tumors from non-tumors and evaluating tumor depth.

This classification was based on lesions with territoriality that were suspected to be squamous cell carcinomas. Vessels seen in borderline lesions were classified as Type A. Vessels seen in carcinomas were classified as Type B, subclassified as B1, B2, and B3. The subclassification aimed to diagnose the depth of the disease, and the findings in squamous cell carcinomas of T1a-EP and -LPM were classified as Type B1, T1a-MM, and T1b-SM1 as Type B2, and those deeper than T1b-SM2 as Type B3 [11].

5.13 Evaluation of the Primary Tumor Response

Several studies have suggested that preoperative treatment may improve patient survival when it leads to a marked reduction in the primary tumor, even if it does not meet the criteria for a complete response (CR) under RECIST. Accordingly, a new response evaluation system incorporating contrast-enhanced CT and PET-CT has been introduced.

5.13.1 Response Evaluation by CT

5.13.1.1 Measurement by Tumor Short Diameter

Method (Fig. 5.9) [12]

For the primary lesion with ≥20 mm of long diameter in CT (axial), its short diameter is measured on the plane with the longest diameter of the primary lesion.

Reduction rate of primary lesion (ΔTumor short diameter) = [(Short diameter before treatment − Short diameter after treatment)/(Short diameter before treatment)] × 100%.

Response evaluation criteria of the short diameter of the primary lesions by CT:

PR: Reduction rate of the short diameter of the primary lesions ≥30%.
SD: Reduction rate of the short diameter of the primary lesions ≥ − 20%, <30%.
PD: Reduction rate in the short diameter of the primary lesions <−20% (at least 20% increase in short diameter).

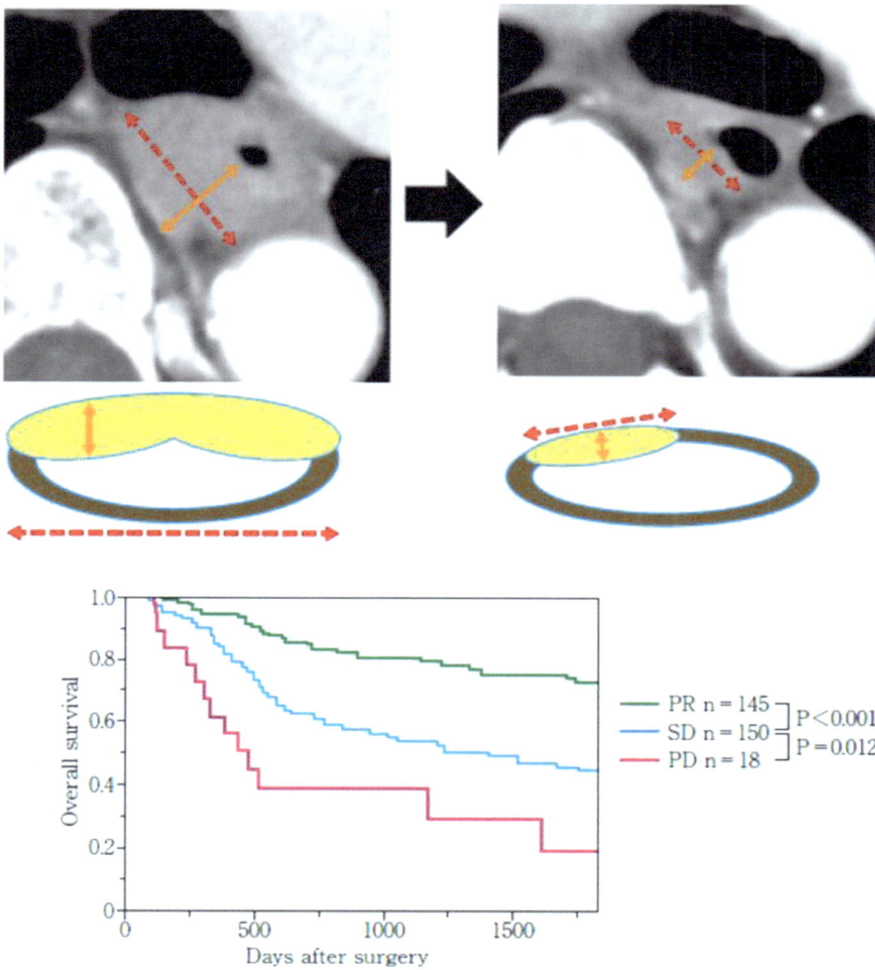

Fig. 5.9 Correlation between the reduction rate of short diameter and survival in patients with esophageal cancer after neoadjuvant treatment in enhanced CT images [12]

5.13.1.2 Measurement by Cross-Section Area of the Esophagus

If it is difficult to evaluate the primary lesion using the method above, the reduction rate of cross-section area of the esophagus can be chosen as an alternative for the primary lesion with ≥20 mm of long diameter in CT (axial) before treatment. This method is not applicable to esophagogastric junction cancer (Jz).

Method (Fig. 5.10) [13]
The cross-sectional area was calculated by multiplying the long esophageal diameter by the short esophageal diameter in the plane with the longest diameter of the primary lesion.

Reduction rate of cross-section area (ΔEsophageal cross-section area) = [(Cross-section area pretreatment − Cross-section area posttreatment)/(Cross-section area pretreatment)] × 100%.

Response evaluation criteria of the cross-section area of the esophagus by CT:

PR: Reduction rate of cross-section area of the esophagus ≥40%.
SD: Reduction rate of the cross-sectional area of the esophagus ≥ − 20%, <40%.
PD: Reduction rate of cross-sectional area of the esophagus <−20% (at least a 20% increase in cross-sectional area).

5.13.2 Response Evaluation by PET-CT

Method [14]
In patients with a primary tumor with cT2–4 and SUVmax ≥3 pretreatment, the reduction rate of SUVmax is calculated.

Reduction rate of SUVmax = [(SUVmax pretreatment − SUVmax posttreatment)/(SUVmax pretreatment)] × 100%.

Response evaluation criteria of SUVmax of the primary lesions by PET-CT:

PR: Reduction rate of SUVmax of the primary lesions ≥50%.
SD: Reduction rate of SUVmax of primary lesions ≥ − 10% and < 50%.
PD: Reduction rate of SUVmax of the primary lesions <−10%.

Perspectives for the 13th Edition of the Japanese Classification
Ongoing efforts for the next revision include:

1. Reclassification of mediastinal lymph nodes:
   Establish standardized criteria for lower mediastinal nodes that can be used consistently across clinical imaging, surgery, and pathology.
2. Review of cT3r/cT3br/cT4 staging:
   Assess the utility and prognostic relevance of the new subclassifications introduced in the 12th edition.
3. Standardization of specimen-based node classification:
   Unify specimen-based lymph node mapping with support materials (videos, diagrams) to improve interinstitutional consistency.

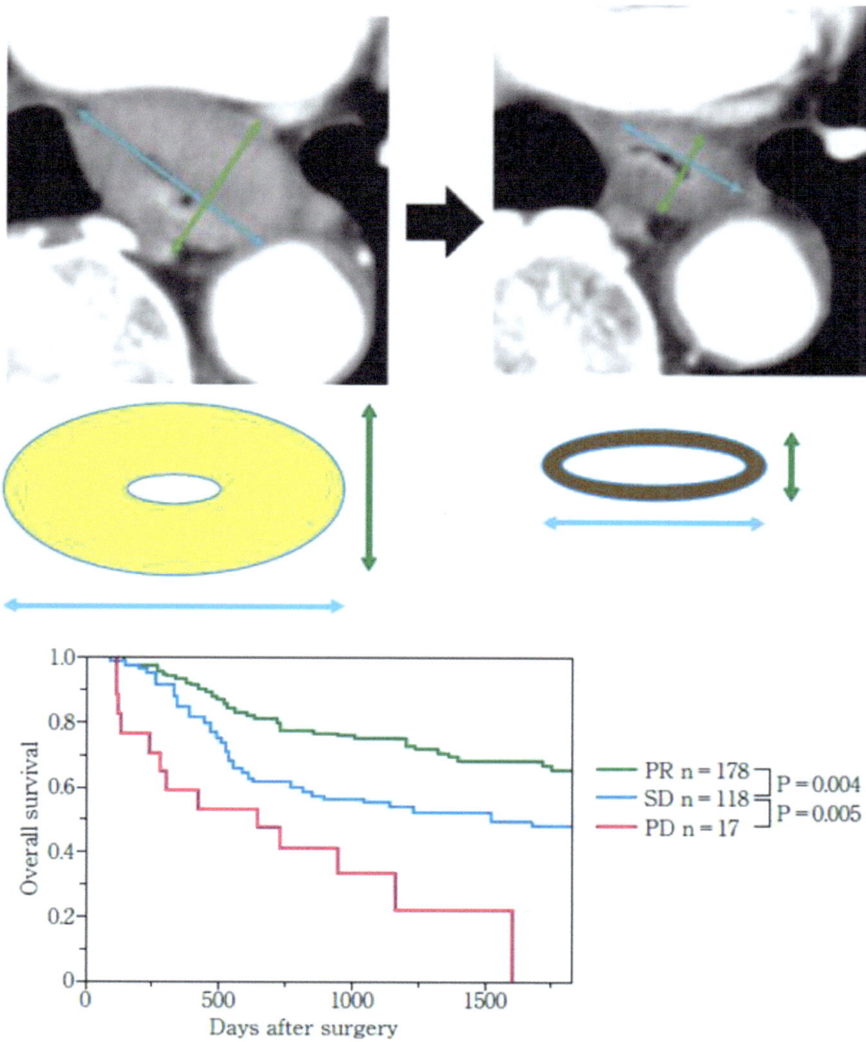

Fig. 5.10 Correlation between reduction rate of the cross-section area and survival in patients with esophageal cancer after neoadjuvant treatment in enhanced CT images [13]

4. MRI-based T4 assessment:

   Develop MRI protocols to support diagnosis of airway or aortic invasion when CT findings are inconclusive [15].
5. Improvement of clinical N status assessment:

   Explore whether the addition of RAD systems [16] or PET-CT improves diagnostic accuracy of lymph node involvement.

The Japanese Esophageal Society remains committed to refining this classification system by collecting and analyzing clinical and pathological data, ultimately aiming to improve the management and outcomes of esophageal cancer patients.

References

1. Brierley JD, Gospodarowicz MK, Wittekind C. TNM classification of malignant tumours. 8th ed. New York: Wiley-Blackwell; 2017.
2. Mine S, et al. Japanese classification of esophageal cancer, 12th Edition: part I. Esophagus. 2024;21(3):179–215.
3. Doki Y, et al. Japanese classification of esophageal cancer, 12th Edition: part II. Esophagus. 2024;21(3):216–69.
4. Japan Esophageal S. Japanese classification of esophageal cancer, 11th Edition: part I. Esophagus. 2017;14(1):1–36.
5. Japan Esophageal S. Japanese classification of esophageal cancer, 11th Edition: part II and III. Esophagus. 2017;14(1):37–65.
6. Brierley JD, Giuliani M, O'Sullivan B, Rous B, Van Eycken E. TNM classification of malignant tumours. 9th ed. Wiley; 2025.
7. Cancer. In: Amin MB, editor. A.J.C.o., AJCC cancer staging manual. 8th ed. Chicago: Springer; 2017.
8. Tachimori Y, et al. Comprehensive registry of esophageal cancer in Japan, 2010. Esophagus. 2017;14(3):189–214.
9. Tachimori Y, et al. Comprehensive registry of esophageal cancer in Japan, 2011. Esophagus. 2018;15(3):127–52.
10. Tachimori Y, et al. Comprehensive registry of esophageal cancer in Japan, 2012. Esophagus. 2019;16(3):221–45.
11. Oyama T, et al. Prediction of the invasion depth of superficial squamous cell carcinoma based on microvessel morphology: magnifying endoscopic classification of the Japan Esophageal society. Esophagus. 2017;14(2):105–12.
12. Taniyama Y, et al. Evaluating the effect of Neoadjuvant chemotherapy for esophageal cancer using the RECIST system with shorter-axis measurements: a retrospective multicenter study. BMC Cancer. 2021;21(1):1008.
13. Yoshida N, et al. Novel criterion using Esophageal major and minor axes is useful to evaluate the therapeutic effect and prognosis after Neoadjuvant chemotherapy followed by surgery in locally advanced Esophageal Cancer. Ann Surg Oncol. 2021;28(13):8474–82.
14. Murakami K, et al. Maximum standardized uptake value change rate before and after neoadjuvant chemotherapy can predict early recurrence in patients with locally advanced esophageal cancer: a multi-institutional cohort study of 220 patients in Japan. Esophagus. 2022;19(2):205–13.
15. Harino T, et al. Impact of MRI on the post-therapeutic diagnosis of T4 esophageal cancer. Esophagus. 2023;20(4):740–8.
16. Elsholtz FHJ, et al. Introducing the node reporting and data system 1.0 (node-RADS): a concept for standardized assessment of lymph nodes in cancer. Eur Radiol. 2021;31(8):6116–24.

Comprehensive Registry in Japan

6

Masayuki Watanabe

6.1 Introduction

Cancer registries are vital for understanding disease incidence, treatment outcomes, and guiding public health initiatives. Globally, many such programs have been established following the lead of initiatives such as the Surveillance, Epidemiology, and End Results (SEER) Program in the United States [1]. In Japan, specific cancer registries for gastric, esophageal, and colorectal cancers were established in 1963 [2], 1976 [3], and 1980 [4], respectively. In this section, we focus on the Comprehensive Registry of Esophageal Cancer in Japan, detailing its historical progression, methodological advancements, its significance for clinical practice, and future perspectives.

6.2 History of the Registry of Esophageal Cancer Cases in Japan

The history of the esophageal cancer registry in Japan is summarized in Table 6.1. The journey of the esophageal cancer registry in Japan began with the establishment of the Japanese Society for Esophageal Diseases (JSDE), the precursor to the Japan Esophageal Society (JES), in October 1965. The Guidelines for Clinical and Pathologic Studies on Carcinoma of the Esophagus, 1st edition, were published in 1969. The guidelines have been renamed the Japanese Classification of Esophageal Cancer and continue to the 12th edition published in 2022. The Registration Committee for Esophageal Cancer was organized in 1976. This committee began registering cases treated in 1976, following guidelines established by the JSDE. The

M. Watanabe (✉)
Cancer Institute Hospital of Japanese Foundation for Cancer Research,
Koto-ku, Tokyo, Japan
e-mail: masayuki.watanabe@jfcr.or.jp

Y. Kitagawa et al. (eds.), *Esophageal Squamous Cell Carcinoma*,
https://doi.org/10.1007/978-981-92-2611-5_6

Table 6.1 History of esophageal cancer registry in Japan

1965	The Japanese Society for Esophageal Diseases (JSDE) was established
1969	Guidelines for clinical and pathologic studies on carcinoma of the esophagus were published
1976	The registration committee was organized
1979	Comprehensive Registry of Esophageal Cancer in Japan, 1976, was published (in Japanese)
1997	Registration software was developed
2003	The project was interrupted to comply with the Act on Protection of Personal Information
2003	The JSDE evolved into the Japan Esophageal Society
2008	The registration project was resumed using the hash function
2010	The National Clinical Database (NCD) was founded
2011	The NCD started data registration
2019	The registration method changed to an internet-based registry using the NCD platform

first issue of the "Comprehensive Registry of Esophageal Cancer in Japan, 1976" was published in 1979. In 1997, registration software was developed, introducing a computer-based system for improved efficiency.

The registry project was interrupted in 2003 due to the implementation of the Act on the Protection of Personal Information, which began enforcement in 2005. This act aimed to protect individual rights and interests in an increasingly information-driven society. In the same year, the JSDE evolved into the JES. To address privacy concerns, a new registration system was developed and completed in 2008. A crucial innovation was the introduction of "anonymity in an unlinkable fashion" using encryption with a "hash function." Patient data were categorized into personal data (e.g., name, date of birth) and disease data (e.g., tumor location, treatment method). Personal data was encrypted into a Hash value, and data packages comprising the encrypted personal data and disease data were sent to a data center. This method enabled the identification of duplicate registrations and the tracking of patient outcomes while maintaining individual privacy. The project, including the use of the hash function, received approval from the Ethics Committee of the JES and the institutional review boards. A trial of the new system involved sending CD-Rs with recording and hash function encryption software to members of the Registration Committee, who then recorded and returned encrypted patient data for cases treated in 2001. This trial confirmed the software's functionality and the feasibility of the data collection process.

In 2010, the National Clinical Database (NCD) in Japan, a large-scale, nationwide, web-based data entry system primarily focused on surgical procedures, was established with significant support from various professional surgical societies in Japan, including the Japan Surgical Society and the Japanese Society of Gastroenterological Surgery [5]. It began collecting data in 2011. The NCD has been actively involved in building organ-specific cancer registration databases in collaboration with several scientific societies. Following this movement, the JES decided to change the registration method from the CD-R submission to an Internet-based registry using the NCD platform. Then, the Comprehensive

Registry of Esophageal Cancer in Japan fully transitioned to the NCD system in 2019, which initially included both retrospective registration for 2013 cases with a 5-year prognosis and prospective registration for 2019 cases with prognosis to be added in 5 years. However, to minimize disruption during the transition period, prospective registration for 2019 cases was temporarily interrupted, and only retrospective registrations continued until 2022. Prospective registration resumed in 2023 and continues to this day. On the occasion of the transition to the NCD, the registry project was approved by the Ethics and Conflict of Interest Committee of the NCD.

Until 2018, data analysis was performed at the data center located in the Department of Medical Physics and Engineering, Osaka University Graduate School of Medicine. After the transition to the NCD, the data center also transitioned to the NCD. Since 2024, two members of the registration committee, endorsed by the JES and certified by the NCD, have analyzed the data.

6.3 Annual Reports

The registration project officially resumed in March 2008 for cases treated in 2001 [3]. After that, the annual registry continues to 2024 for cases in 2016. After completing the data analysis each year, the registration committee sent the "Comprehensive Registry of Esophageal Cancer in Japan" to the participating institutes. An excerpted version was also published in "Esophagus," the official journal of the Japan Esophageal Society, for wider accessibility [6–20].

6.4 Summary of the Comprehensive Registry of Esophageal Cancer in Japan, 2001–2016

6.4.1 Trends in the Number of Cases and Institutions

A total of 103,549 cases had been registered in the registries from 2001 to 2016. The trends of the number of registered cases and participating institutes are shown in Fig. 6.1. The blue bars represent the number of registered cases, while the orange line indicates the number of participating institutions. The number of cases fluctuated in the initial years but showed a general upward trend, reaching over 9000 cases in 2015 and nearly 10,000 in 2016. The number of institutions steadily increased over the years, reaching close to 350 by 2016. The certified esophageal surgeon system, which started certification in 2010, was mandated to participate in the registry. This could have contributed to the increase in the number of participating institutes, particularly the surgical department.

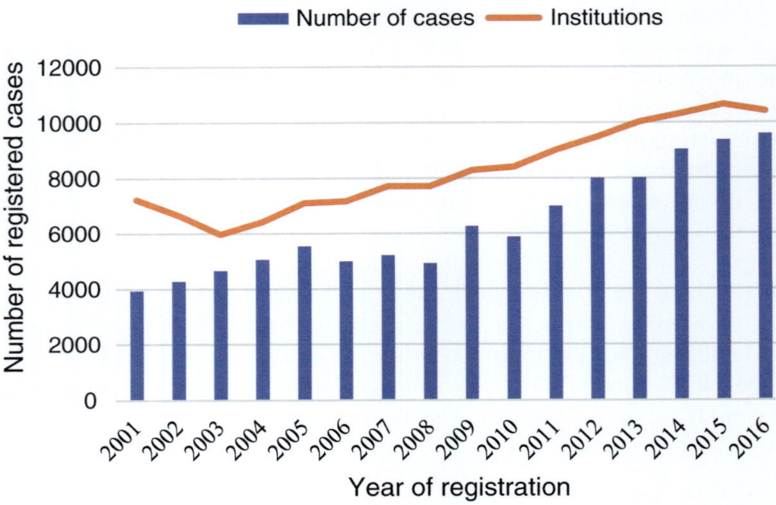

Fig. 6.1 Trend in the number of cases and institutions

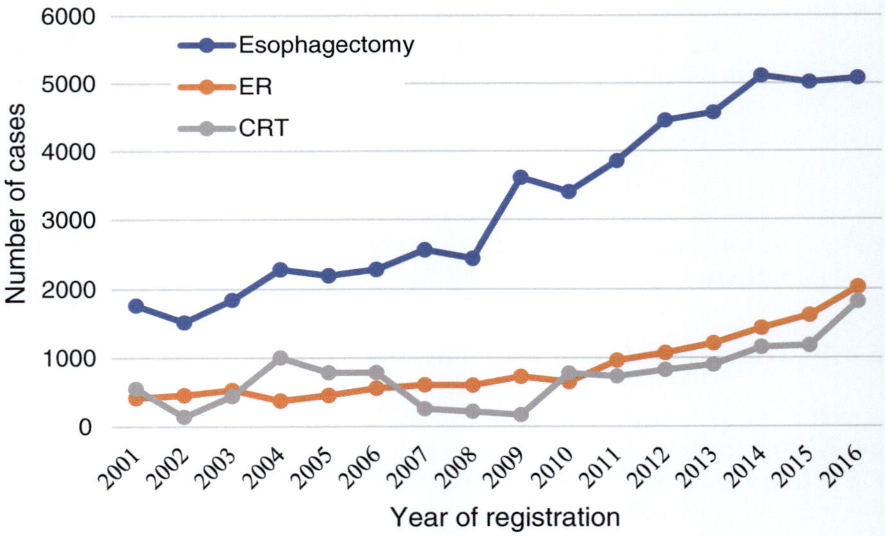

Fig. 6.2 Trends in the number of cases treated with different modalities

6.4.2 Trends of Treatment Modalities

The number of cases treated with different treatment modalities is shown in Fig. 6.2. The number of esophagectomy cases fluctuated in the early 2000s but generally increased over time, surpassing 5000 cases in 2014 and remaining around that level through 2016. Again, the certified esophageal surgeon system may have contributed to the increase in esophagectomy case registrations. The number of cases treated with endoscopic resection (ER) has shown a gradual increase over the years, with a more pronounced rise from approximately 1000 cases in 2011 to over 2000 cases by 2016. However, the number of registered cases appears to be significantly lower than the estimated number of ER cases performed throughout Japan, as the participating institutes of the registry are primarily comprised of surgical departments. The number of chemoradiotherapy (CRT) cases showed a notable increase in the early 2000s, as CRT was attracting attention as a curative treatment option for locally advanced esophageal cancer, replacing surgery during this period. As the standard treatment for locally advanced esophageal cancer has become neoadjuvant chemotherapy followed by esophagectomy, based on the JCOG 9906 [21] and 9907 [22] trials, the number of CRT cases decreased and stabilized for a few years. The CRT cases began a more consistent upward trend from around 2011, reaching close to 2000 cases by 2016. The reasons may include the aging population and the expectation that treatment will maintain quality of life.

6.4.3 Comprehensiveness of Esophagectomy Cases

Comprehensiveness is one of the indicators for evaluating the quality of a registry. After 2011, almost all surgical cases performed in Japan have been registered in the NCD. We compared the number of cases between the Comprehensive Registry of esophageal cancer and the NCD, shown in Fig. 6.3. In 2011, the NCD recorded over 5000 esophagectomy cases, and the trend remained between 6000 and 6500 from 2012 to 2016. The number of JES registered cases remained relatively stable, fluctuating around 3800 to 4500 cases throughout the period, with a slight increase in 2014 and 2016. The coverage rate represents the proportion of JES cases relative to NCD cases, indicated on the right-hand *Y*-axis as a percentage. It dipped slightly in 2012, then steadily increased, reaching over 80% by 2016. The result suggests that the JES registry was capturing a growing proportion of the cases recorded by the NCD over these years. Notably, the increase in coverage after 2013 may indicate the impact of the transition to the NCD registry.

6.4.4 Trends of Minimally Invasive Esophagectomy

The spread of minimally invasive esophagectomy (MIE) is one of the significant topics in esophageal cancer treatment. Figure 6.4 shows the trends of the percentage of minimally invasive esophagectomy procedures recorded by the Comprehensive Registry of Esophageal Cancer in Japan and the NCD. In 2001, MIE accounted for approximately 15% of esophagectomies. The percentage of MIE cases steadily increased over the years, with a noticeable acceleration in the adoption of MIE from around 2009 onward, rising from approximately 30% to over 65% by 2016 in the JES registry. Data for the NCD begins in 2011, where MIE accounted for just over

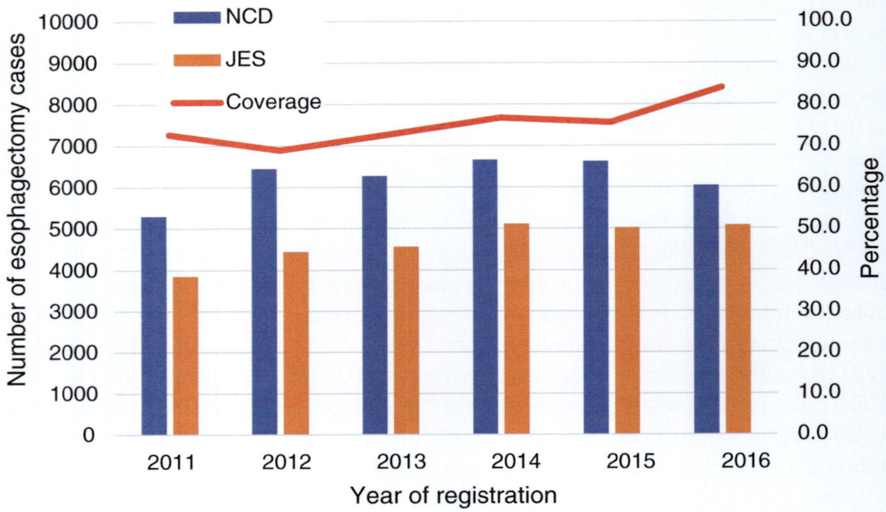

Fig. 6.3 Comparison of the number of esophagectomies between the JES and the NCD and the coverage by the JES registry

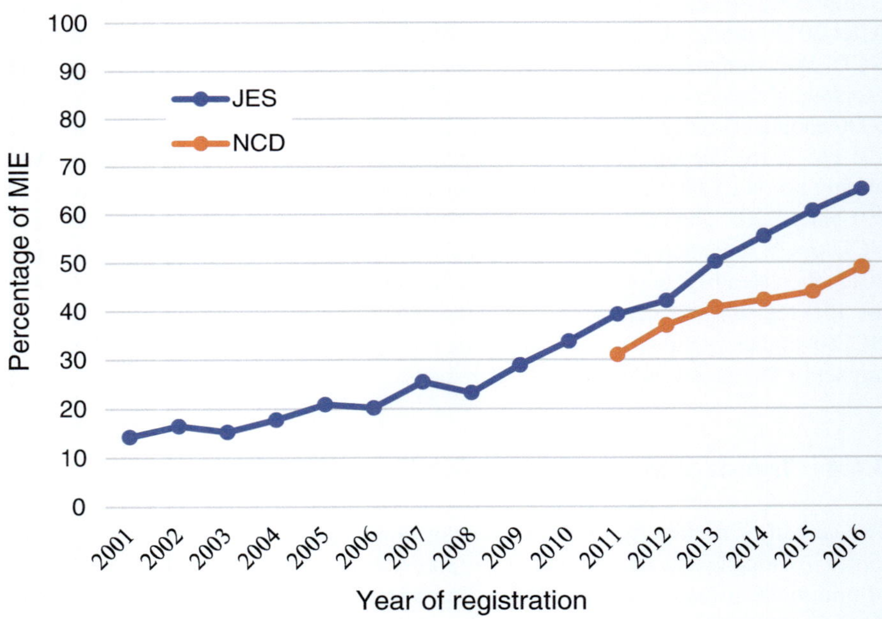

Fig. 6.4 Trends of minimally invasive esophagectomy in the JES registry and the NCD

30% of esophagectomies. The percentage of MIE recorded by the NCD also showed a consistent increase, reaching nearly 50% by 2016. Interestingly, the JES registry showed generally higher percentages of MIE compared to the NCD in the overlapping years. The results suggest that the participating institutes in the JES registry included more advanced facilities, such as high-volume esophageal centers.

6.4.5 Histological Subtypes

Esophageal cancer consisted mainly of two different histologic subtypes, including squamous cell carcinoma (SCC) and adenocarcinoma (ADC). Although ADC is predominant in Europe, North America, and Oceania, SCC exhibits a higher incidence in other regions. Especially, the prevalence of SCC is highest in East Asia. The trend of the percentage of each subtype registered in the registry is shown in Fig. 6.5. SCC is the predominant histological type, consistently accounting for around 90% of registered cases in most years. In contrast, ADC consistently represented a small percentage of registered cases throughout the entire period; however, there is a slight, gradual increase in ADC proportion from 2001 to 2016.

6.4.6 Trends of Clinical Stages

The trend in the number of registered cases, categorized by clinical stage (0/I, II, III, and IV), is shown in Fig. 6.6. Notably, the definition of clinical stage varied substantially among the versions of UICC/TNM. For instance, clinical nodal stage (cN) was categorized by the absence or presence of metastatic nodes until the 6th edition,

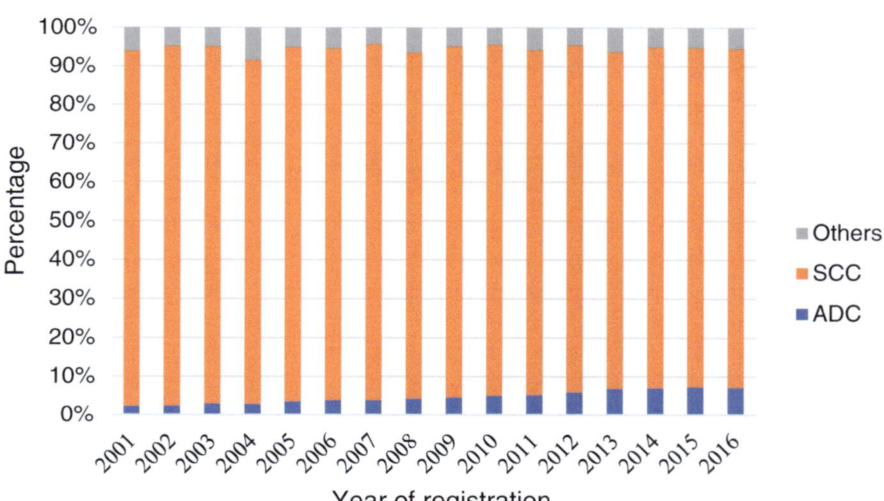

Fig. 6.5 Trends in the histologic subtypes

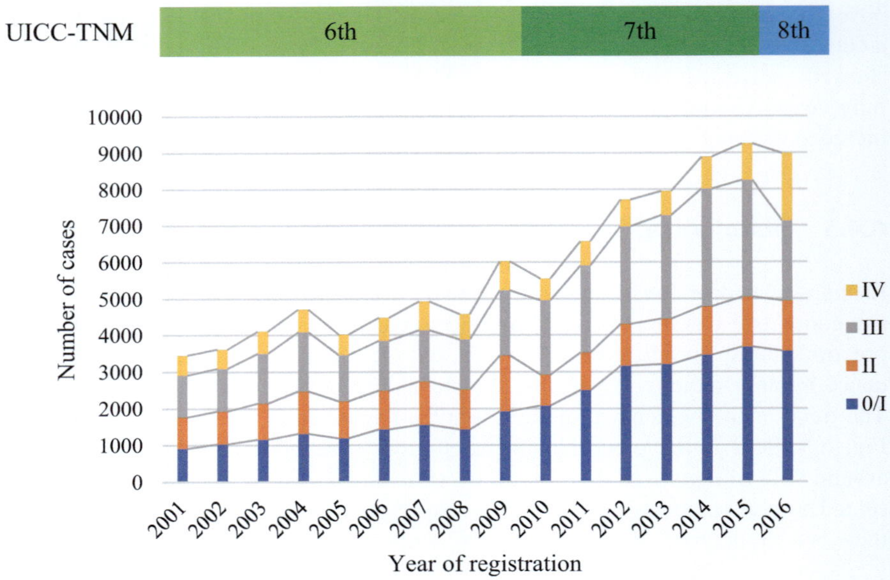

Fig. 6.6 Trends of clinical stages in the registered cases

whereas the number of metastatic nodes categorized it into cN0, cN1, cN2, and cN3 after the 7th edition. cT2N0 changed from cStage II in the 6th edition to cStage IB in the 7th edition, but returned to cStage II in the 8th edition. Additionally, cN3 was categorized as cStage IIIC in the 7th edition, but as cStage IVA in the 8th edition. Although such changes influenced the trends, the number of cases with cStafge 0/I showed a steady increase from approximately 1000 cases in 2001 to over 3500 cases in 2016, suggesting an increase in cases resulting from early cancer detection. In contrast, advanced cases with cStage III or IV have also risen significantly during the period.

6.4.7 Five-Year Survival Rates by Treatment Modality

Figure 6.7 illustrates the 5-year overall survival rates for three different treatment modalities: ER, esophagectomy, and CRT, from the year of registration 2001–2016. ER consistently shows the highest 5-year overall survival rate throughout the period. The survival rate typically ranges from 80% to 90%. There was a slight dip around 2003, but it quickly recovered and remained stable, mostly above 85%, reaching close to 90% by 2016. The 5-year survival rate for esophagectomy has shown a gradual upward trend over the years, increasing from just over 40% in 2001 to nearly 60% in 2016. The 5-year survival rate for CRT began around 20% in 2001 and has shown a general upward trend. By 2016, the survival rate had increased to approximately 35%.

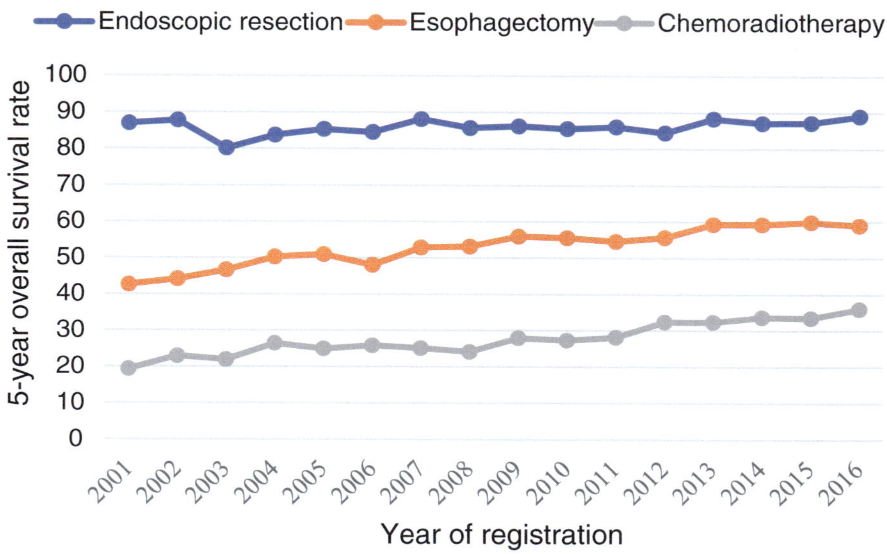

Fig. 6.7 Trends of the 5-year survival rates in patients treated with different modalities

6.5 Research Using the Comprehensive Registry Data

Several studies have been published using data from the Comprehensive Registry of Esophageal Cancer in Japan.

This study evaluated the efficacy of lymph node dissection by node zones based on tumor location for esophageal squamous cell carcinoma. The study analyzed data from 3827 patients in a nationwide registry in Japan who underwent R0 esophagectomy with three-field lymph node dissection for squamous cell carcinoma. The Efficacy Index (EI) was calculated by multiplying the frequency of metastasis to a zone and the 5-year survival rate of patients with metastases to that zone. For upper esophageal tumors, the EI was highest in the supraclavicular and upper mediastinal zones. For middle esophageal tumors, the EI was highest in the upper mediastinal zone, followed by the supraclavicular and perigastric zones. For lower esophageal tumors, the EI was highest in the perigastric zone, followed by the upper and lower mediastinal zones. This study concluded that the extent of lymph node dissection should be determined by lymph node zones and modified by tumor location [23].

This study analyzed the outcomes of patients who underwent radiotherapy alone (RTx) or definitive chemoradiotherapy (CRTx) for thoracic esophageal cancer from the registry of 2009, 2010, and 2011. The median age of patients was significantly higher in the RTx group than in the CRTx group. The 5-year survival rates were 23.2% in the RTx group (41.8%, 18.5%, 9.3%, and 13.9% for cStage 0-I, II, III, and IV, respectively) and 46.6% in the CRTx group (57.8%, 47.8%, 23.4%, and 13.0% for cStage 0-I, II, III, and IV, respectively). This study revealed the real-world status of radiation and chemoradiation therapy for esophageal cancer [24].

This study compared the complete response (CR) rate and 5-year overall survival between radiation doses of 50.4 Gy and 60 Gy in a subgroup of the aforementioned study cohort. The CR rates were comparable between the groups (49.1% and 46.4% in the 50.4 Gy and 60 Gy groups, respectively), and the 5-year overall survival of the 50.4 Gy group was not inferior to that of the 60 Gy group. It was the first study to demonstrate the efficacy of CRT with 50.4 Gy irradiation in Japanese patients with esophageal cancer [25].

This study investigated whether routine thoracic duct (TD) resection improves the prognosis of patients with esophageal cancer after radical esophagectomy, using data from a registry for the period 2007–2012. The 5-year overall survival (57.5% vs. 55.2% in the TD-resected and the TD-preserved groups, respectively) and cause-specific survival (65.6% vs. 63.4% in the TD-resected and the TD-preserved groups, respectively) were comparable between the groups. The TD-resected group had significantly more retrieved mediastinal nodes and significantly fewer lymph node recurrences than the TD-preserved group; however, the number of distant metastatic organs was substantially greater in the TD-resected group. This study concluded that prophylactic TD resection should not be recommended [26].

This study investigated the prognostic significance of TD resection in the subgroup of patients who underwent neoadjuvant CRT followed by esophagectomy from the aforementioned study cohort. Again, TD resection did not improve the 5-year overall and cause-specific survivals compared with the TD-preserved group. Also, the number of retrieved mediastinal lymph nodes was significantly greater in the TD-resected group than in the TD-preserved group, whereas TD resection was associated with metastasis to a greater number of distant organs. This study concluded that indiscriminate TD resection might be avoided in patients undergoing esophagectomy followed by neoadjuvant CRT [27].

6.5.1 Significance of the Registration Project and Future Perspectives

The Comprehensive Registry of Esophageal Cancer in Japan, alongside the "Japanese Classification of Esophageal Cancer" and the "Esophageal Cancer Practice Guidelines," is considered essential for the treatment of esophageal cancer patients in Japan. The project aims to improve all aspects of the diagnosis and treatment of esophageal cancer. Continued efforts are necessary to increase both the quantity and accuracy of registered data, thereby further enhancing the quality of the Comprehensive Registry. The active participation of all doctors involved in managing patients with esophageal cancer is crucial for the ongoing success and importance of this registry.

The Esophageal Surgery Outcomes Database (ESODATA) is a global initiative that aims to collect and analyze standardized data on surgical outcomes for esophageal cancer [28]. The project was initially established by the Esophageal Complications Consensus Group (ECCG) and is currently managed by the International Society for Diseases of the Esophagus (ISDE). The ESODATA project aims to improve clinical outcomes and quality benchmarks by sharing data across high-volume centers, and also to contribute to the development of international guidelines and the improvement of TNM staging. It is necessary to incorporate Japanese data into global guidelines and staging systems by collaborating between the JES registry and the ESODATA project.

References

1. The Surveillance, Epidemiology, and End Results (SEER) Program of the national cancer institute. http://seer.cancer.gov/. Accessed 27 July 2025.
2. Maruyama K, Kaminishi M, Hayashi K, et al. Gastric cancer treated in 1991 in Japan: data analysis of nationwide registry. Gastric Cancer. 2006;9:51–66.
3. Ozawa S, Tachimori Y, Baba H, et al. Comprehensive registry of esophageal cancer in Japan, 2001. Esophagus. 2009;6:95–110.
4. Kotake K, Honjo S, Sugihara K, et al. Changes in colorectal cancer during a 20-year period: an extended report from the multi-institutional registry of large bowel cancer, Japan. Dis Colon Rectum. 2003;46:S32–43.
5. National Clinical Database. https://www.ncd.or.jp/. Accessed 27 July 2025.
6. Ozawa S, Tachimori Y, Baba H, et al. Comprehensive registry of esophageal cancer in Japan, 2002. Esophagus. 2010;7:7–22.
7. Ozawa S, Tachimori Y, Baba H, et al. Comprehensive registry of esophageal cancer in Japan, 2003. Esophagus. 2011;8:9–29.
8. Ozawa S, Tachimori Y, Baba H, et al. Comprehensive registry of esophageal cancer in Japan, 2004. Esophagus. 2012;9:75–98.
9. Tachimori Y, Ozawa S, Fujishiro M, et al. Comprehensive registry of esophageal cancer in Japan, 2005. Esophagus. 2014;11:1–20.
10. Tachimori Y, Ozawa S, Fujishiro M, et al. Comprehensive registry of esophageal cancer in Japan, 2006. Esophagus. 2014;11:21–47.
11. Tachimori Y, Ozawa S, Numasaki H, et al. Comprehensive registry of esophageal cancer in Japan, 2007. Esophagus. 2015;12:101–29.
12. Tachimori Y, Ozawa S, Numasaki H, et al. Comprehensive registry of esophageal cancer in Japan, 2008. Esophagus. 2015;12:130–57.
13. Tachimori Y, Ozawa S, Numasaki H, et al. Comprehensive registry of esophageal cancer in Japan, 2009. Esophagus. 2016;13:110–37.
14. Tachimori Y, Ozawa S, Numasaki H, et al. Comprehensive registry of esophageal cancer in Japan, 2010. Esophagus. 2017;14:189–214.
15. Tachimori Y, Ozawa S, Numasaki H, et al. Comprehensive registry of esophageal cancer in Japan, 2011. Esophagus. 2018;15:127–52.
16. Tachimori Y, Ozawa S, Numasaki H, et al. Comprehensive registry of esophageal cancer in Japan, 2012. Esophagus. 2019;16:221–45.
17. Watanabe M, Tachimori Y, Oyama T, et al. Comprehensive registry of esophageal cancer in Japan, 2013. Esophagus. 2021;18:1–24.
18. Watanabe M, Toh Y, Ishihara R, et al. Comprehensive registry of esophageal cancer in Japan, 2014. Esophagus. 2022;19:1–26.
19. Watanabe M, Toh Y, Ishihara R, et al. Comprehensive registry of esophageal cancer in Japan, 2015. Esophagus. 2023;20:1–28.
20. Kimura Y, Okamura A, Takeuchi M, et al. Comprehensive registry of esophageal cancer in Japan, 2016. Esophagus. 2025;22:475. Published online.
21. Kato K, Muro K, Miinashi K, et al. Phase II study of chemoradiotherapy with 5-fluorouracil and cisplatin for stage II-III esophageal squamous cell carcinoma: JCOG TRIAL (JCOG 9906). Int J Radiat Oncol Biol Phys. 2011;81:684–90.

22. Ando N, Kato H, Igaki H, et al. A randomized trial comparing postoperative adjuvant chemotherapy with cisplatin and 5-fluorouracil versus preoperative chemotherapy for localized advanced squamous cell carcinoma of the thoracic esophagus (JCOG9907). Ann Surg Oncol. 2012;19:68–74.
23. Tachimori Y, Ozawa S, Numasaki H, et al. Efficacy of lymph node dissection by node zones according to tumor location for esophageal squamous cell carcinoma. Esophagus. 2016;13:1–7.
24. Toh Y, Numasaki H, Tachimori Y, et al. Current status of radiotherapy for patients with thoracic esophageal cancer in Japan, based on the Comprehensive Registry of Esophageal Cancer in Japan from 2009 to 2011 by the Japan Esophageal Society. Esophagus. 2020;17:25–32.
25. Nemoto K, Kawashiro S, Toh Y, et al. Comparison of the effect of radiotherapy doses of 50.4 Gy and 60 Gy on outcome of chemoradiotherapy for thoracic esophageal cancer: subgroup analysis based on the comprehensive Registry of Esophageal Cancer in Japan from 2009 to 2011 by the Japan Esophageal Society. Esophagus. 2020;17:122–6.
26. Oshikiri T, Numasaki T, Oguma J, et al. Prognosis of patients with esophageal carcinoma after routine thoracic duct resection. A propensity-matched analysis of 12,237 patients based on the comprehensive registry of Esophageal Cancer in Japan. Ann Surg. 2023;277:e1018–25.
27. Oshikiri T, Numasaki T, Oguma J, et al. Is thoracic duct resection necessary for esophageal squamous cell carcinoma patients treated with neoadjuvant chemoradiotherapy? A propensity-matched analysis based on the Comprehensive Registry of Esophageal Cancer in Japan. Ann Surg Oncol. 2023;30:2691–8.
28. Esodata.org. International Esophageal Database. https://esodata.net/web/. Accessed 27 July 2025.

Esophageal Cancer Practice Guidelines in Japan

7

Eisuke Booka, Hiroya Takeuchi, and Yuko Kitagawa

7.1 Background and Objectives

The Japanese Society of Esophageal Diseases, now the Japan Esophageal Society (JES), has maintained a 5-year revision cycle for its clinical practice guidelines since the first version in 2002. Every cycle has had a slightly different purpose: early editions were mainly to standardize diagnostic and staging procedures; the 2012 edition began to align Japanese descriptions with international TNM; and the 2017 (4th) edition, which we summarized last time, was the first to present the methodology of guideline making together with treatment algorithms and 40-plus Clinical Questions (CQs) [3, 4]. That 2017 text was later translated and published in *Esophagus* (2019) and then reorganized into the ESCC 2nd book as Chap. 8, with us as authors.

The 2022 (5th) edition, published in English in 2023 as "Esophageal cancer practice guidelines 2022 edited by the Japan Esophageal Society: part 1" and "Esophageal cancer practice guidelines 2022 edited by the Japan Esophageal

The contents of this chapter are based on the two publications "Esophageal cancer practice guidelines 2022 edited by the Japan Esophageal Society: part 1" and "Esophageal cancer practice guidelines 2022 edited by the Japan Esophageal Society: part 2" [1, 2]. The latest information that became available since these guidelines were published has been added to provide an update on this topic.

E. Booka · H. Takeuchi (✉)
Department of Surgery, Hamamatsu University School of Medicine, Hamamatsu, Shizuoka, Japan
e-mail: booka@hama-med.ac.jp; takeuchi@hama-med.ac.jp

Y. Kitagawa
Department of Surgery, Keio University School of Medicine, Tokyo, Japan
e-mail: kitagawa.a3@keio.jp

Y. Kitagawa et al. (eds.), *Esophageal Squamous Cell Carcinoma*,
https://doi.org/10.1007/978-981-92-2611-5_7

Society: part 2," is not just another update of drugs or devices; it is a structural reedition [1, 2]. It explicitly adds: (1) participation of nonphysician experts and patients, (2) public comments and external review, (3) a plan to monitor diffusion of recommendations through quality indicator (QI) surveys, (4) a joint statement with the Japanese Gastric Cancer Association (JGCA) on carcinoma of the esophagogastric junction (EGJ), and (5) explicit systemic therapy choices for cStage IVB/recurrent disease, especially regimens containing immune checkpoint inhibitors. These elements were either absent or only alluded to in 2017.

The objective of this chapter is therefore twofold: first, to recreate the readability of our previous chapter—a single, self-contained text that a non-Japanese esophageal surgeon can read without the original articles at hand; second, to incorporate all new 2022 elements without changing the narrative tone. Where the 2022 journal version is intentionally concise (because Esophagus limits space), we will "reinflate" the explanation using the fuller style of the 2017 book and, where appropriate, by recalling background statements from the 2017 guideline so that the logic of the algorithm is transparent. This is consistent with the note in the 2017-based book chapter, which said: "The contents of this chapter are based on … Part 1 and Part 2. The latest information … has been added." We are doing exactly the same, just one cycle later.

Finally, the target readers and target patients are the same as in 2022 Part 1: surgeons, endoscopists, medical oncologists, radiation oncologists, pathologists, and allied professionals who treat adult patients with esophageal squamous cell carcinoma (ESCC), esophageal adenocarcinoma (EAC) of the distal esophagus, and EGJ carcinoma defined by Nishi's classification.

7.2 Method of Guideline Development

In 2017, the JES already introduced GRADE-like processes [3, 4], but in 2022 the method is brought fully in line with the Minds Manual 2017/2020 and documented step by step [1, 2]. This should be described in more detail than last time because it is one of the signature changes. The 2022 committee first defined the scope, then reformulated CQs, then commissioned a systematic review (SR) for each CQ, and finally voted on recommendation strength using a ≥70% agreement threshold. All of this is listed consecutively in the 2023 paper.

1. *Scope formulation.* The committee reconfirmed that the guideline should cover: (1) epidemiology and risk factors; (2) diagnosis and staging; (3) treatment algorithms for cStage 0–I, II–III, IVA, and IVB; (4) surgery, including new approaches; (5) chemotherapy, chemoradiotherapy (CRT), and radiotherapy; (6) follow-up/recurrence; (7) palliation; and (8) Barrett's/EAC and EGJ carcinoma.
2. *Preparation of CQs and literature search.* The 2017 edition had >40 CQs; many of them had become "obvious standards" by 2022 (e.g., endoscopic resection (ER) for T1a-EP/LPM, cisplatin, and 5-fluorouracil (CF) as the basic neoadjuvant regimen). For those, the 2022 committee dropped them from the CQ list and

kept them only in the explanatory text. At the same time, 39 new or revised CQs were drafted for areas where practice had diverged (e.g., post-CRT salvage, immune checkpoint inhibitor (ICI)-containing first-line therapy, and EGJ surgery). A unified SR was then conducted in PubMed, Cochrane, and ICHUSHI, focusing on adult human data, with 2000–2020 as the core period but supplemented by manual 2021–2022 searches for fast-moving areas such as ICIs.

3. *Determination of recommendation strength.* For each CQ, the committee evaluated (1) balance of benefits and harms, (2) quality and directness of evidence, (3) patient preferences and values, and (4) cost/resource use, and then voted. Unlike 2017, every CQ in 2022 reached ≥70% agreement at the first vote; the authors explicitly interpret this as a sign that Japanese esophageal practice has become more uniform. We should keep this observation because it gives authority to the recommendations.
4. *Public hearing and external review.* One innovation of 2022 is to publish the draft on the JES website for a limited period, collect comments from clinicians and patients, and revise the text accordingly. This point is mentioned only briefly in the official guideline publication, but it merits a full paragraph in our chapter because it demonstrates that Japanese guidelines are converging with Western transparency standards. An independent review committee then confirmed consistency, conflict of interest (COI) management, and independence from industry funding.
5. *Plan for dissemination and QI.* Finally, the 2022 guideline states that the society will "improve the convenience for users" and will link the guideline items to nationwide QI surveys—exactly the questionnaire we are now analyzing in another manuscript. This is unique to the Japanese guideline and should be mentioned here to explain why some seemingly "simple" recommendations (e.g., surveillance endoscopy schedule) were retained—they are measurable.

7.3 Major Revisions from the 2017 (4th) to the 2022 (5th) Edition

Readers will want to know "what changed." We therefore list and explain, not just enumerate:

1. *Broader membership and patient participation.* 2022 explicitly lists endoscopists, radiation oncologists, pathologists, and patient representatives as authors (we are also on the list). This means that recommendations on, say, laryngopharyngeal preservation or dysphagia palliation represent consensus across professions, not just surgeons.
2. *Integration with JGCA for EGJ.* In 2017, EGJ carcinoma was mentioned but not operationalized. In 2022, a JES–JGCA joint working group proposes approach and lymph node (LN) dissection according to esophageal invasion length (>2 cm, >4 cm), and this is printed in the guideline with an algorithmic figure.

3. *Update of systemic therapy, especially ICIs*. 2017 could only mention nivolumab/pembrolizumab as emerging agents. 2022 cites KEYNOTE-590 and CheckMate 648 with concrete overall survival (OS) advantages and then incorporates "chemo + ICI" and "ICI + ICI" into the cStage IVB algorithm [5, 6].
4. *Clearer description of salvage/conversion surgery after CRT or induction therapy*. 2017 already acknowledged salvage, but 2022 goes further and quotes long-term outcomes (3-year OS 31–46%) while warning of higher morbidity; it also mentions JCOG1510 as an ongoing randomized control trial (RCT) [7].

7.4 Outline of the 2022 Algorithm

The master algorithm in 2022 has the same skeleton as 2017—diagnose → stage → four stage-specific branches—but the explanatory notes have become more prescriptive. After stating that the Japanese Classification (12th, harmonized with UICC) is to be used [8, 9], the guideline reminds readers that treatment is selected by clinical stage and by patient condition and institutional expertise. This is important because the 2022 edition recognizes minimally invasive/robotic and mediastinoscopic approaches as acceptable surgery, so "institutional expertise" now really affects what is done.

We should describe the four branches in prose:

1. cStage 0–I → ER whenever curative; if not curative, add surgery or CRT.
2. cStage II–III → preoperative therapy (docetaxel, cisplatin, and 5-fluorouracil (DCF) or similar) → esophagectomy with two- or three-field dissection → adjuvant only in selected situations.
3. cStage IVA → definitive CRT or induction therapy followed by conversion/salvage.
4. cStage IVB → systemic therapy as basic treatment, with local therapy for symptoms.

7.5 Treatment of cStage 0–I Disease (Fig. 7.1)

Early ESCC is where Japan has the greatest experience, and the 2022 guideline keeps a very finely stepped algorithm. It starts by noting that the risk of LN metastasis rises sharply once the tumor invades beyond the lamina propria, and therefore "endoscopic resection" is both a therapeutic and staging tool. The text lists three recommendation–explanation pairs: (1) ER is recommended for T1a-epithelium (EP)/lamina propria mucosae (LPM); (2) ER is conditionally recommended for T1a-muscularis mucosae (MM)/T1b-submucosal 1 (SM1) with an obligation to evaluate for additional therapy; (3) surgery or CRT is recommended for T1b-SM2 or deeper.

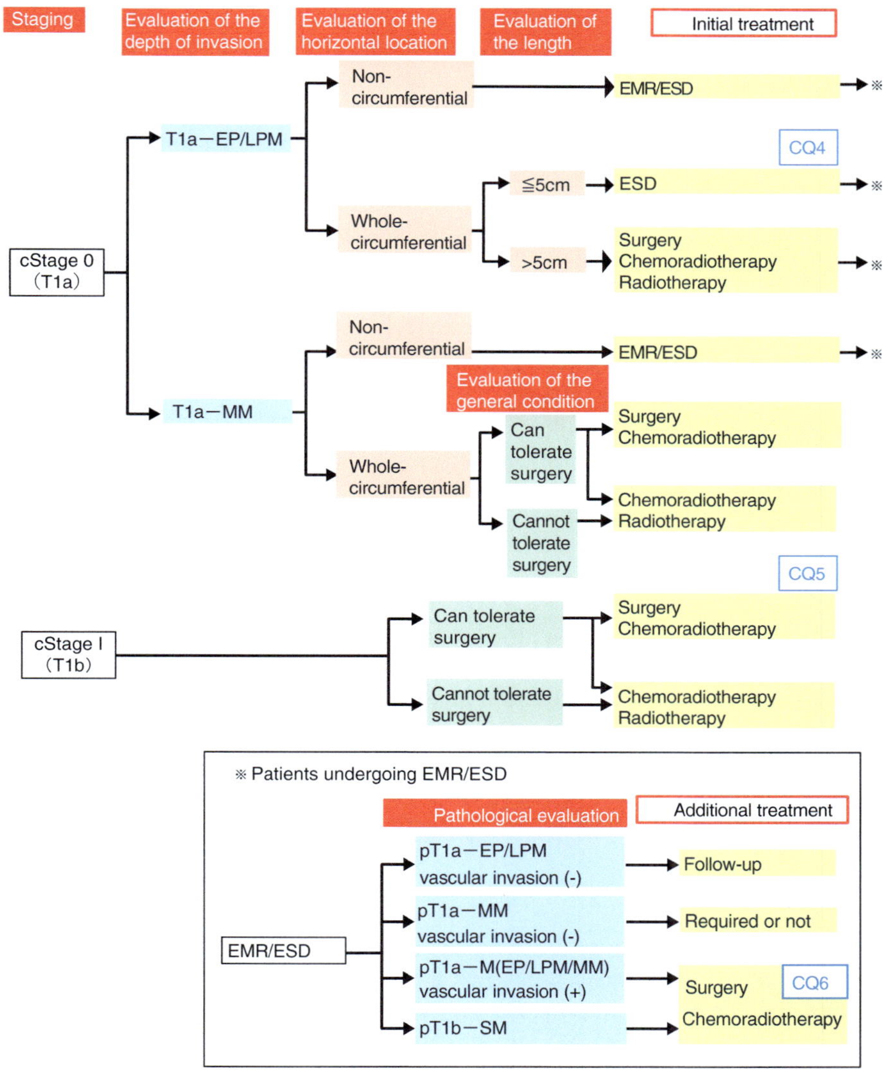

Fig. 7.1 Treatment algorithms for cStage 0, I esophageal cancer

1. Purely mucosal cancers (EP/LPM)

The guideline states that for "cStage 0" lesions (intraepithelial or limited to the lamina propria), ER is strongly recommended because the risk of LN metastasis is "almost negligible." Curative resection is defined pathologically as en bloc resection with negative lateral and vertical margins, well or moderately differentiated squamous cell carcinoma, no lymphovascular (LV) invasion, and depth within LPM. For such cases, no additional treatment or intensified surveillance beyond standard endoscopy is required. In our chapter we should add, as in 2017, that this policy is based on large Japanese series of >1000 ER cases. (This background is in 2017, but it is consistent with 2022.)

2. Muscularis mucosae and superficial submucosa (MM/SM1)

Here the 2022 guideline is more explicit than 2017: it allows ER as initial treatment but immediately states that when any risk factor for LN metastasis is present (LVI, poor differentiation, positive vertical margin, or deeper SM invasion), additional treatment such as esophagectomy with LN dissection or CRT should be considered. This is an important nuance—many Western readers think ER is curative for all T1, but the Japanese guideline stresses the two-step concept. We can keep the sentence: "ER is appropriate for diagnostic and staging purposes; if non-curative, proceed to additional treatment according to the patient's general condition."

3. Submucosal deep invasion (SM2 or deeper)

For these, esophagectomy with regional or extended LN dissection is recommended, or definitive CRT in those unfit for surgery. The 2022 text keeps the same position as 2017, but because it is now part of the stage-based algorithm, we should state clearly that SM2+ disease is not an indication for endoscopic therapy alone.

CQ4 *What would be the recommendation for preventing postoperative stenosis following endoscopic resection of superficial cancer of the esophagus?*

Recommendation statement:

There is evidence to strongly recommend oral prednisolone treatment, submucosal triamcinolone injection, or concurrent oral prednisolone treatment + submucosal triamcinolone injection for preventing stenosis after endoscopic resection. (Rate of consensus: 85.2% [23/27], strength of evidence: C)

CQ5 *Which is recommended, esophagectomy or definitive chemoradiotherapy, in patients with cStage I (T1bN0M0) thoracic esophageal cancer?*

Recommendation statement:

There is weak evidence to recommend esophagectomy in patients with cStage I (T1bN0M0) thoracic esophageal cancer, and there is also weak evidence to recommend definitive chemoradiotherapy with adequate follow-up and salvage therapy in patients with cStage I who desire for esophageal preservation. (Rate of consensus: 92.3% [24/26], strength of evidence: C)

CQ6 Which is recommended as an additional treatment—esophagectomy or chemoradiotherapy—in cases with a pT1a-MM lesion showing positive vascular invasion or a pT1b-SM lesion following endoscopic treatment for superficial esophageal cancer?

Recommendation statement:

There is evidence to recommend esophagectomy or chemoradiotherapy as an additional treatment in patients identified as having a pT1a-MM lesion with positive vascular invasion or a pT1b-SM lesion after endoscopic treatment for superficial esophageal cancer; however, currently there is insufficient evidence to definitively recommend one over the other. (Rate of consensus: 89.3% [25/28]; strength of evidence: C)

7.6 Treatment of cStage II–III (Resectable Advanced) Disease (Fig. 7.2)

Patients with clinically staged II–III thoracic ESCC constitute the largest group of potentially curable cases in Japan, and the 2022 JES guideline, in continuity with the 2017 edition, places this group at the very center of its treatment algorithms. The fundamental policy remains that curative treatment should consist of multimodal therapy with surgery as the principal local treatment, and that preoperative (neoadjuvant) therapy is preferred to postoperative therapy because it improves R0 resection rates and, in Japanese trials, overall survival [10].

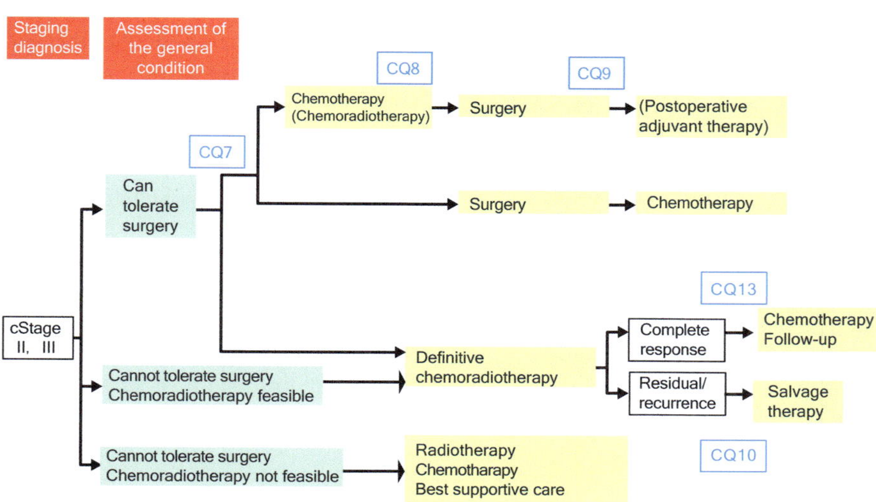

Fig. 7.2 Treatment algorithms for cStage II, III esophageal cancer

The guideline begins by stressing that clinical staging must be accurate and multidisciplinary. Endoscopic ultrasound, contrast-enhanced CT, and where available PET-CT are used to determine T and N, while the Japanese classification of lymph node stations is used to judge the need for cervical or upper mediastinal dissection. Patients are then stratified into: (1) those who are medically fit and whose disease is technically resectable, (2) those who are resectable but have substantial comorbidities or frailty, and (3) those whose disease is technically resectable but locally very advanced (e.g., cT4a with suspected airway involvement), in whom neoadjuvant chemoradiotherapy may be preferable to chemotherapy alone.

For fit patients with standard cStage II–III thoracic ESCC, the current Japanese standard is preoperative triplet chemotherapy with docetaxel, cisplatin, and fluorouracil (DCF), strongly recommended on the basis of JCOG1109 (NExT), which demonstrated superiority of triplet over doublet chemotherapy in this setting [11]. In practice, DCF is administered as three 3-week cycles (docetaxel 70 mg/m^2 day 1, cisplatin 70 mg/m^2 day 1, fluorouracil 750 mg/m^2 days 1–5), followed by restaging and radical esophagectomy with systematic two- or three-field lymphadenectomy. Cisplatin/fluorouracil (CF) remains an alternative when triplet therapy is unsuitable or contraindicated (e.g., advanced age, significant comorbidity, organ dysfunction), recognizing that Japanese protocols explicitly allow de-escalation or even upfront surgery in patients ≥76 years or with substantial comorbidity after multidisciplinary review. Preoperative chemoradiotherapy continues to be positioned as an option for selected cases (e.g., suspected airway involvement, bulky nodal disease), while the routine default in Japan remains chemotherapy-first.

Postoperative therapy is an area where the 2022 guideline introduces an important nuance. For the classic Japanese sequence of neoadjuvant CF followed by R0 esophagectomy, routine adjuvant chemotherapy is not recommended because no survival benefit has been demonstrated and because postoperative morbidity after esophagectomy can compromise the delivery of additional systemic therapy. However, for patients who underwent neoadjuvant chemoradiotherapy followed by surgery and who had residual pathological disease, the guideline newly recommends adjuvant nivolumab for 1 year, in line with the results of the CheckMate 577 trial and subsequent regulatory approvals in Japan [12]. This creates, within the stage II–III pathway, a small but clinically important subgroup in which trimodality therapy is followed by immunotherapy.

For patients who are elderly, frail, or comorbid but still potentially resectable, the guideline allows surgery alone or definitive CRT as weaker recommendations [13]. The reason for preserving these options is pragmatic: in real-world Japanese practice, not all patients can complete neoadjuvant therapy without compromising their condition for surgery, and high-level evidence is limited in such populations. In the same vein, the guideline notes that doublet preoperative chemotherapy other than CF (e.g., oxaliplatin-based) may be used when cisplatin is contraindicated.

CQ7 What should be recommended—primarily surgery, or definitive chemoradiotherapy—in patients with cStage II or III esophageal cancer?

Recommendation statement:

There is weak evidence to recommend primarily surgery for patients with cStage II or III esophageal cancer. (Rate of consensus: 100% [28/28], strength of evidence: C)

CQ8 Which is recommended—preoperative chemotherapy or preoperative chemoradiotherapy—in cStage II or III esophageal cancer patients scheduled to receive surgery as the primary treatment?

Recommendation statement:

In patients with cStage II or III esophageal cancer who are scheduled to receive surgery as the primary treatment, there is strong evidence to recommend preoperative triplet chemotherapy with docetaxel + cisplatin + 5-FU. (Rate of consensus: 84% [21/25], strength of evidence: A)

Q9 Is postoperative adjuvant therapy recommended in patients with cStage II or III esophageal cancer who have undergone preoperative adjuvant therapy plus surgery?

Recommendation statement:

1. In patients with cStage II or III esophageal cancer who failed to show a pathologic complete response after preoperative chemoradiotherapy plus surgery with radical resection, there is strong evidence to recommend postoperative nivolumab therapy, regardless of the histologic type or tumor expression level of programmed death ligand 1 (PD-L1). (Rate of consensus: 81% [21/26], strength of evidence: A)
2. In patients with cStage II or III esophageal cancer who have undergone preoperative chemotherapy plus surgery with radical resection, but failed to achieve a pathologic complete response, there is currently no evidence to recommend postoperative nivolumab therapy. (Rate of consensus: 92% [24/26], strength of evidence: D)

CQ11 Is salvage surgery recommended for residual or recurrent lesions after chemoradiotherapy in patients with untreated resectable esophageal cancer?

Recommendation statement:

There is weak evidence to recommend salvage surgery for residual or recurrent lesions after chemoradiotherapy in patients with untreated resectable esophageal cancer. (Rate of consensus: 96.4% [27/28], strength of evidence: C)

7.7 Treatment of cStage IVA (Locally Advanced, Unresectable or Borderline) (Fig. 7.3)

The 2022 guideline keeps a separate figure (Fig. 7.3) for cStage IVA because these patients sit between clearly resectable II–III and clearly systemic IVB. It begins by stressing accurate staging and assessment of performance status (PS); patients must be discussed by a multidisciplinary team. The guideline then presents two acceptable strategies: (1) definitive CRT and (2) induction chemotherapy/CRT followed by conversion or salvage surgery.

The most "Japanese" part is the description of salvage/conversion surgery. 2022 cites a systematic review showing 3-year OS 31–46.6% after a treatment sequence that included surgery, while acknowledging that this population is highly selected and perioperative mortality is higher than in ordinary cStage II–III surgery. Therefore, the recommendation is weak and accompanied by a caution that careful perioperative management and detailed informed consent are indispensable. We must keep this nuance to avoid overstating the role of salvage surgery.

As the concepts and indications of "conversion" surgery and "salvage" surgery continue to evolve [14], the results of the ongoing JCOG1510 trial are eagerly awaited; this study compares definitive chemoradiotherapy with or without salvage surgery against induction chemotherapy followed—where feasible—by conversion surgery, and is expected to refine patient selection and treatment sequencing.

CQ12 Is chemoradiotherapy recommended for unresectable cStage IVA esophageal cancer?

Recommendation statement:

There is only weak evidence to recommend definitive chemoradiotherapy for the treatment of unresectable cStage IVA esophageal cancer. (Rate of consensus: 100% [28/28]; strength of evidence: C)

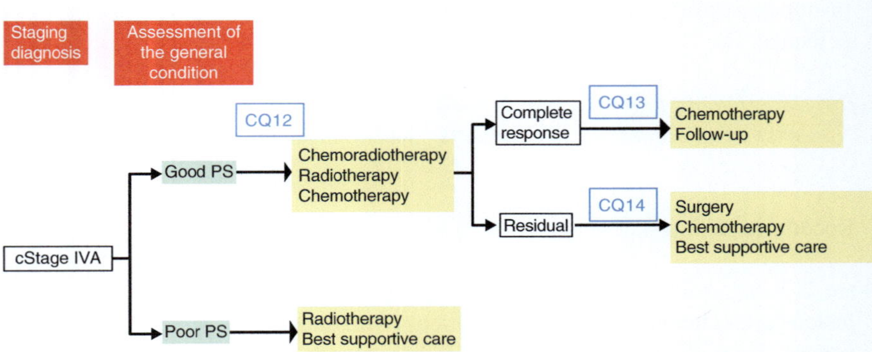

Fig. 7.3 Treatment algorithms for cStage IVA esophageal cancer

CQ13 Is additional chemotherapy recommended for cStage II, III, or IVA esophageal cancer patients who show complete response after definitive chemoradiotherapy?

Recommendation statement:

There is only weak evidence to recommend additional chemotherapy for cStage II, III, or IVA esophageal carcinoma patients who show complete response to definitive chemoradiotherapy. (Rate of consensus: 96.4% [27/28]; evidence level: C)

CQ14 Is surgical resection recommended for patients with unresectable, locally advanced esophageal cancer (cT4 [e.g., aorta, trachea, bronchus] N0-3M0) that becomes resectable after definitive chemoradiotherapy or induction chemotherapy?

Recommendation statement:

There is only weak evidence to recommend surgical resection for patients with unresectable, locally advanced esophageal cancer (cT4 [e.g., aorta, trachea, bronchus] N0-3M0) that becomes resectable after definitive chemoradiotherapy or induction chemotherapy. (Rate of consensus: 89.3% [25/28]; evidence level: C)

7.8 Treatment of cStage IVB and Recurrent Disease (Figs. 7.4 and 7.5)

The 2022 guideline's chapter on cStage IVB and recurrent esophageal cancer represents one of the most visible updates compared with 2017, because it finally aligns the Japanese algorithm with the era of ICI and, at the same time, makes the systemic-therapy-first principle explicit. In 2017, the text said in general terms that

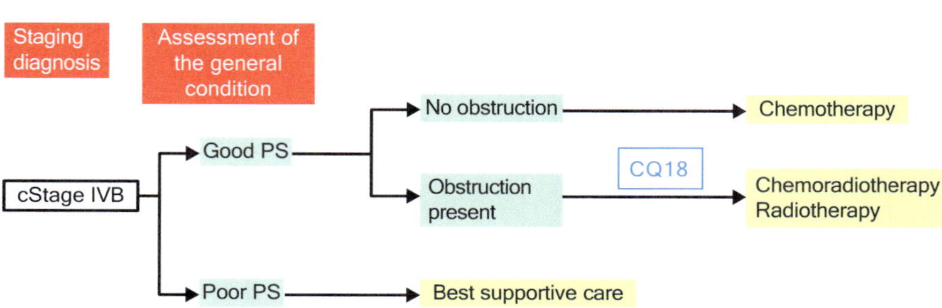

Fig. 7.4 Treatment algorithms for cStage IVB esophageal cancer

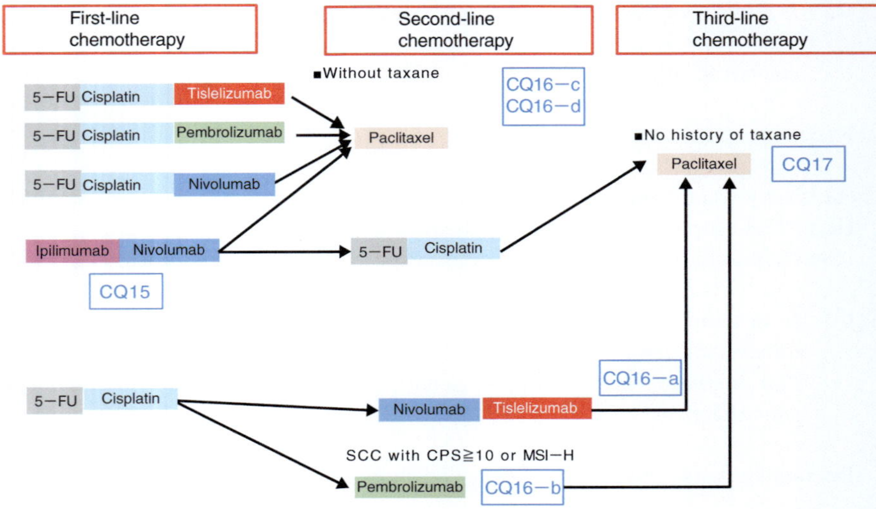

Fig. 7.5 Chemotherapy regimen for cStage IVB esophageal cancer

chemotherapy was the mainstay for stage IVb disease; in 2022, the guideline provides a definite flowchart and lists recommended regimens, including combination regimens with pembrolizumab or nivolumab.

The guideline first underlines that patients with distant metastasis, non-regional lymph node involvement, or disseminated recurrent disease after previous curative treatment should be considered systemic-disease patients. For such patients, purely local treatment—esophagectomy, CRT, or endoluminal therapies—rarely achieves durable disease control and should be reserved for symptom relief (e.g., dysphagia, airway compromise, bleeding). Therefore, systemic therapy is the basic treatment, provided the patient has adequate PS (0–2), preserved organ function, and sufficient oral or enteral intake. The text also contains a distinctly Japanese practical note: if nutrition or hydration is inadequate because of dysphagia or if aspiration pneumonia is present, these problems should be corrected first (by stent, tube feeding, antibiotics, or hydration) before systemic therapy is initiated. This small sentence is important for practitioners outside Japan to understand how Japanese clinicians actually sequence treatments.

With the introduction of ICIs, the first-line systemic therapy menu is now broader. The 2022 guideline lists:

1. Fluoropyrimidine + platinum doublets (CF, FP, FOLFOX) as universal backbones that can be used regardless of PD-L1 status or histologic subtype.
2. Pembrolizumab plus chemotherapy, based largely on the KEYNOTE-590 trial, as a recommended option for unresectable/recurrent ESCC [5]. The trial demonstrated clinically meaningful improvements in overall survival and

progression-free survival, especially in SCC and in tumors with higher PD-L1 expression; the guideline therefore places this regimen in the algorithm rather than only in the text.

3. Nivolumab plus chemotherapy and nivolumab plus ipilimumab, based on the CheckMate 648 trial, as alternative first-line options, again with the caveat that the magnitude of benefit depends on PD-L1 expression and that toxicity profiles differ [6]. In practice, these regimens will be selected according to drug availability, reimbursement, and patient-specific factors (e.g., autoimmune background).
4. Taxane-based second-line therapy (paclitaxel, docetaxel) for patients who fail first-line therapy but remain candidates for further treatment.
5. Nivolumab monotherapy for platinum-refractory ESCC, based on the ATTRACTION-3 trial, showed improved survival over taxanes and a more favorable toxicity profile [15].

In addition to pembrolizumab plus cisplatin and fluorouracil, nivolumab plus cisplatin and fluorouracil, and nivolumab plus ipilimumab, the April 2025 JES rapid update adds tislelizumab plus cisplatin and fluorouracil as a strongly recommended first-line option; PD-L1 expression should be considered when selecting among ICI-based regimens [16]. For patients previously treated with fluoropyrimidine–platinum chemotherapy without prior PD-1 inhibitor exposure, tislelizumab monotherapy is strongly recommended as a second-line option [17].

The guideline emphasizes that treatment choice should consider PD-L1 expression, line of therapy (de novo IVB vs recurrent after surgery/CRT), prior exposure to cisplatin/5-FU, and time to relapse. For example, a patient who recurs early after perioperative CF may go directly to an ICI-containing regimen, while a patient who relapses very late may be retreated with a platinum–fluoropyrimidine doublet.

Another strength of the 2022 text is that it does not ignore local therapy in stage IVB. It specifically mentions that radiotherapy or chemoradiotherapy can be used for symptom control (painful bone metastasis, bleeding, airway invasion, esophageal stenosis) and that esophageal stenting or palliative brachytherapy can be combined with systemic therapy when dysphagia is severe. This hybrid, patient-centered use of local modalities is characteristic of Japanese practice and should be retained in the book chapter, even if Western guidelines would describe such interventions under "palliation" rather than under "systemic therapy."

For patients with poor PS or multiple organ failure, the guideline clearly states that best supportive care (BSC)—including nutrition, swallowing support, pain control, and psychosocial support—should be prioritized over cytotoxic or immunotherapy. By writing this in the same algorithmic section, the committee signals that "doing nothing" is sometimes the most appropriate evidence-based option.

Finally, the 2022 guideline incorporates recurrent disease after prior curative therapy into the same framework as de novo cStage IVB. Recurrence patterns after esophagectomy in Japan often involve distant lymph nodes, lung, liver, or bone. The recommended approach is to treat such patients as stage IVB if the recurrence is disseminated, or to consider local therapy (RT, CRT, surgical resection) if the recurrence is limited and technically controllable. This practical, pattern-of-failure-based approach is consistent with Japanese surgical series and helps clinicians decide quickly even when recurrence does not fit neatly into the TNM framework.

CQ15 *What chemotherapy would be recommended as first-line therapy for patients with unresectable, advanced/recurrent esophageal cancer?*

Recommendation statement:

1. There is strong evidence to recommend pembrolizumab + cisplatin + 5-FU therapy as first-line therapy for the treatment of patients with unresectable, advanced/recurrent esophageal cancer. (Rate of consensus: 92.3% [24/26]; strength of evidence: A)
2. There is strong evidence to recommend nivolumab + cisplatin + 5-FU therapy or nivolumab + ipilimumab therapy as first-line therapy for unresectable, advanced/recurrent esophageal cancer, but the patient's general condition, tumor PD-L1 expression level (tumor proportion score [TPS]), and treatment tolerability should be taken into account. (Rate of consensus: 88.0% [22/25]; strength of evidence: A)

CQ16 *What chemotherapy would be recommended as second-line therapy for patients with unresectable, advanced/recurrent esophageal cancer refractory to first-line chemotherapy, including fluoropyrimidine + platinum therapy?*

Recommendation statement:

(In patients without a history of anti-PD-1 antibody therapy).

1. In patients without a history of anti-PD-1 antibody therapy, there is strong evidence to recommend nivolumab therapy (squamous cell carcinoma). (Rate of consensus: 100% [25/25]; strength of evidence: A)
2. In patients without a history of anti-PD-1 antibody therapy, there is only weak evidence to recommend pembrolizumab therapy (squamous cell carcinoma with a CPS of ≥10 or MSI-H or TMB-H). (Rate of consensus: 96.2% [25/26]; strength of evidence: B)

(In patients without a history of taxane therapy).

3. In patients without a history of anti-PD-1 antibody therapy or taxane therapy, there is only weak evidence to recommend paclitaxel therapy. (Rate of consensus: 96.4% [27/28]; strength of evidence: C)
4. In patients with a history of anti-PD-1 antibody therapy, but no history of taxane therapy, there is only weak evidence to recommend paclitaxel therapy. (Rate of consensus: 100% [28/28]; strength of evidence: C)

CQ17 What would be recommended as third-line therapy for patients with unresectable, advanced/recurrent esophageal cancer who received fluoropyrimidine + platinum combination therapy as first-line therapy and anti-PD-1 antibody therapy as second-line therapy?

Recommendation statement:

In patients without a history of taxane therapy, there is only weak evidence to recommend paclitaxel therapy. (Rate of consensus: 100% [28/28], strength of evidence: C)

CQ18 Is palliative radiotherapy recommended for the treatment of patients with cStage IVB esophageal cancer presenting with obstruction?

Recommendation statement:

There is only weak evidence to recommend palliative radiotherapy for the treatment of patients with cStage IVB esophageal cancer presenting with obstruction. (Rate of consensus: 100% [28/28]; strength of evidence: C)

7.9 Endoscopic Surveillance

Part 2 opens with "Endoscopic surveillance," which means the society now wants this to be visible, not just implied [2]. The rationale is that Japanese patients with ESCC often have multifocal squamous dysplasia related to alcohol-flushing and smoking, so metachronous ESCC is common. Therefore:

1. After ER or CRT, endoscopy of the esophagus, pharynx, and stomach should be done at intervals of 6–12 months;
2. Image-enhanced endoscopy such as NBI is desirable;
3. If Lugol-voiding lesions are found, they should be biopsied or observed closely.

7.10 Surgical Treatment (Including EGJ Carcinoma)

Surgery remains the definitive local therapy for resectable esophageal cancer in Japan. In line with the 2022 guideline, right transthoracic esophagectomy with systematic lymph node dissection is the benchmark, while thoracoscopic, transcervical mediastinoscopic, and robot-assisted techniques are acceptable at experienced centers; the endpoint is consistent oncologic radicality rather than a uniform incision strategy.

1. Choice of approach

For thoracic ESCC, classic right thoracotomy is well established; thoracoscopic esophagectomy is now broadly practiced, and robot assistance is used in selected institutions. Importantly, the multicenter phase III JCOG1409 trial demonstrated non-inferior overall survival for thoracoscopic versus open transthoracic esophagectomy (with reduced blood loss and broadly comparable serious complications apart from a nonsignificant increase in grade ≥3 anastomotic leak), establishing thoracoscopy as a standard option in qualified centers [18]. Subsequently, in November 2025, the JES Guideline Committee issued a rapid update (CQ22) that strongly recommends thoracoscopic esophagectomy for thoracic esophageal cancer (Rate of consensus 95.7% [22/23]; strength of evidence: A), with the proviso that the procedure be performed by a surgeon certified by the Japanese Society for Endoscopic Surgery—or by an equivalently skilled surgeon—or under the direct supervision of an equivalently skilled trainer.

2. Extent of lymph node dissection

Japanese practice continues to emphasize systematic two- or three-field lymphadenectomy depending on tumor location and nodal risk. In JCOG1409, both arms mandated at least D2 dissection, with routine three-field dissection for upper/mid-thoracic disease and centralized intraoperative photo review—reinforcing that nodal clearance quality can be maintained with thoracoscopy at credentialed institutions.

3. Cervical esophageal carcinoma

Laryngopharyngoesophagectomy with vascularized conduit (e.g., free jejunum or gastric tube) remains the standard radical procedure; definitive chemoradiotherapy is a reasonable organ-preserving alternative, with the choice individualized to balance oncologic control and function.

4. Carcinoma of the esophagogastric junction (EGJ)—joint JES–JGCA section (Fig. 7.6).

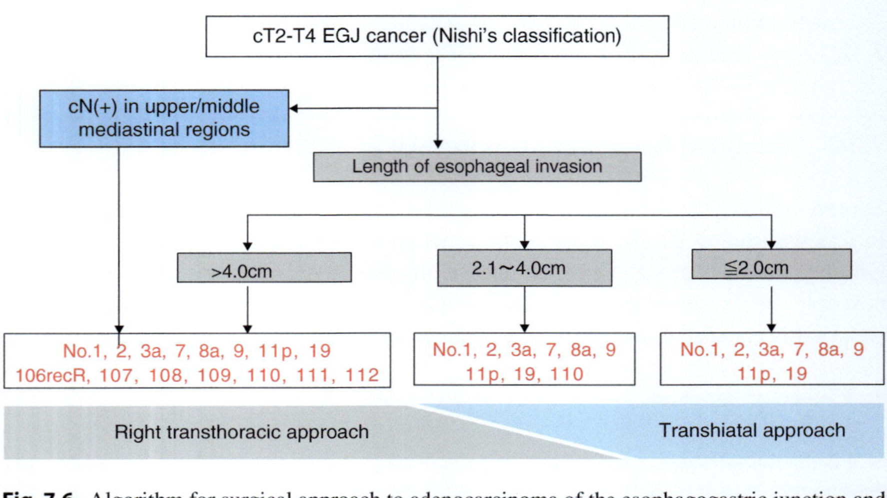

Fig. 7.6 Algorithm for surgical approach to adenocarcinoma of the esophagogastric junction and lymph node dissection

Surgical approach is selected primarily by esophageal invasion length from the EGJ: short invasion (≈≤2 cm) generally permits an abdominal/transhiatal approach with lower mediastinal lymphadenectomy; intermediate invasion (≈2–4 cm) is individualized; and long invasion (>4 cm) or suspected middle/upper mediastinal node involvement favors a right transthoracic approach to secure margins and mediastinal nodal clearance.

5. Reconstruction and perioperative care

A gastric conduit via the posterior mediastinal or retrosternal routes are standards; or subcutaneous route is alternative in selected scenarios. ERAS-type pathways (early enteral/oral feeding, multimodal analgesia, early mobilization) are recommended to optimize recovery; combined with the thoracoscopic approach where appropriate, these measures can reduce perioperative burden without compromising oncologic goals.

7.11 Perioperative Management and Clinical Path

This section is shorter but has to mention ERAS. 2022 guideline says: many Japanese institutions have introduced clinical pathways for perioperative management of esophagectomy, but methods vary and solid evidence of benefit is limited. However, ERAS concepts—short fasting, early oral/enteral nutrition, pain control, and early mobilization—are recommended because international data show reduced complications and shorter hospitalization. It also notes that malnutrition is common in esophageal cancer, so nutritional assessment and (if needed) enteral feeding reduce complications. This links nicely with your current ESPEN work [19].

7.12 Chemotherapy, Chemoradiotherapy, and Adjuvant/Conversion Therapy

Part 2 then deals with systemic and radiation treatments for curative and non-curative settings [2]. We should write this in the same order:

1. Pre- and postoperative therapy

Preoperative triplet chemotherapy with docetaxel, cisplatin, and fluorouracil is the current standard for cStage II–III disease, based on JCOG1109 showing superior survival versus preoperative cisplatin plus fluorouracil (which had been the standard from JCOG9907 and now remains an option when the triplet is unsuitable) [11]. Because preoperative therapy increases toxicity, proactive adverse-event prevention and careful patient selection are required. For postoperative therapy, 1-year nivolumab is recommended only for patients who received neoadjuvant chemoradiotherapy and underwent surgery without achieving pathological complete response; its benefit after preoperative chemotherapy alone is unknown, so use in that setting should be considered cautiously and not routine [12].

2. Definitive chemoradiotherapy

Indications include patients medically inoperable for surgery, those desiring organ preservation (especially cervical esophageal cancer), and cStage IVA disease where multidisciplinary consensus favors nonoperative management or induction therapy. Standard dosing is 50–60 Gy external beam radiotherapy with concurrent cisplatin plus fluorouracil; IMRT is acceptable. Dose escalation can be considered for bulky disease per institutional policy. Careful toxicity prevention is essential because CRT increases acute and late adverse events. Post-CRT assessment must be structured to enable early salvage in non-complete responders.

3. Radiotherapy alone

For very elderly, frail, or poor-performance-status patients, or when chemotherapy is contraindicated, external beam radiotherapy alone may be used for symptom control or selected local control (weak recommendation). Short-course palliative schedules (e.g., 20 Gy/5 fractions or 30 Gy/10 fractions) are reasonable choices for dysphagia, pain, or bleeding, particularly when expected survival is limited.

4. Salvage treatments

After definitive CRT, if local remnant or local recurrence is detected and R0 control seems feasible, endoscopic resection or photodynamic therapy is recommended for superficial/focal disease; salvage esophagectomy is an option for operable localized failure in fit patients, acknowledging higher morbidity than primary surgery and the need for experienced centers. The concepts and indications of "conversion" surgery (after induction therapy) and "salvage" surgery (after CRT) are evolving; the results of JCOG1510 are eagerly awaited and are expected to refine patient selection and sequencing [7].

7.13 Follow-Up After Radical Resection and Treatment of Recurrence

Follow-up aims to detect anastomotic or conduit-site recurrence, regional lymph node recurrence, and metachronous squamous neoplasia (including pharyngeal lesions), while also addressing nutrition, swallowing function, and treatment-related complications. A multimodal strategy is recommended: structured history and physical examination; endoscopic surveillance (with image-enhanced endoscopy when high-risk mucosa is present) to assess the anastomosis/conduit and screen the entire esophagus–pharynx; and contrast-enhanced CT of the neck/chest/abdomen at risk-adapted intervals, with PET-CT selectively for equivocal or oligometastatic disease. Tumor markers are not routine.

Management of recurrence is site-directed. For locoregional failure, consider chemoradiotherapy or re-resection where R0 control is feasible; for superficial/

focal mucosal remnants after CRT, endoscopic resection or photodynamic therapy is appropriate at experienced centers. Distant recurrence is treated with systemic therapy as outlined in Sect. 7.8, with local ablative radiotherapy or surgery for carefully selected oligometastatic lesions and palliation (stent, brachytherapy, short-course external-beam radiotherapy) as needed for symptom control. A uniquely Japanese, practice-oriented point is that endovascular aortic stent grafting may be used for esophago-aortic fistula as an emergency hemostatic measure and bridge to definitive management, acknowledging infection risk and the need for multidisciplinary coordination.

7.14 Palliative Treatment

Palliative care should be integrated into care for all cancers, and every clinician involved in oncology should be competent in its core principles and skills. Because psychological distress—including anxiety and depression—is common, timely screening and referral to mental health professionals are often necessary. In esophageal cancer specifically, dysphagia, malnutrition, and cough from aspiration or aerodigestive fistulae frequently impair quality of life; targeted symptom-relief interventions and nutritional/airway support should be considered from the early stages of treatment to maintain or improve QOL. While the specific palliative modalities used may vary by institutional expertise and resources, practice should be guided by multidisciplinary assessment, with ongoing evaluation and quality improvement to standardize care and outcomes.

7.15 Diagnosis and Treatment of Barrett's Esophagus and Esophageal Adenocarcinoma

In Japan, Barrett's esophagus is an endoscopic diagnosis: columnar epithelium extending into the distal esophagus, with the EGJ defined at the distal end of the palisade vessels; specialized intestinal metaplasia is not required. Western definitions often place the EGJ at the proximal gastric folds and require intestinal metaplasia; segments <1 cm are usually not counted. For consistency with most studies, we use the Western LSBE (≥3 cm maximum length)/SSBE (<3 cm) convention when discussing evidence.

For EAC, management mirrors ESCC by stage: endoscopic resection is appropriate for cT1a lesions, post-resection pT1a-SMM/LPM is generally curative (negative margins, no high-risk features), and even pT1a-DMM may be observed if no lymphovascular invasion or poor differentiation is present. Submucosal invasion, positive margins, or adverse histology warrant additional therapy (esophagectomy with lymphadenectomy or chemoradiotherapy). Surveillance endoscopy of Barrett's mucosa remains essential.

7.16 Future Perspectives

The guideline states plainly that further improvements are planned in public dissemination, in updating when key trial results appear, and in linking practice to QI studies. The biggest challenge will be how to integrate rapidly changing systemic therapies—especially ICIs and combination regimens—into a guideline that is revised every 5 years. The committee notes that when major changes occur (e.g., approval of a new ICI as adjuvant after surgery), they will issue updates on the website.

References

1. Kitagawa Y, Ishihara R, Ishikawa H, et al. Esophageal cancer practice guidelines 2022 edited by the Japan esophageal society: Part 1. Esophagus. 2023;20(3):343–72.
2. Kitagawa Y, Ishihara R, Ishikawa H, et al. Esophageal cancer practice guidelines 2022 edited by the Japan Esophageal Society: Part 2. Esophagus. 2023;20(3):373–89.
3. Kitagawa Y, Uno T, Oyama T, et al. Esophageal cancer practice guidelines 2017 edited by the Japan Esophageal Society: Part 1. Esophagus. 2019;16(1):1–24.
4. Kitagawa Y, Uno T, Oyama T, et al. Esophageal cancer practice guidelines 2017 edited by the Japan esophageal society: Part 2. Esophagus. 2019;16(1):25–43.
5. Sun JM, Shen L, Shah MA, et al. Pembrolizumab plus chemotherapy versus chemotherapy alone for first-line treatment of advanced oesophageal cancer (KEYNOTE-590): a randomised, placebo-controlled, phase 3 study. Lancet. 2021;398(10302):759–71.
6. Doki Y, Ajani JA, Kato K, et al. Nivolumab combination therapy in advanced esophageal squamous-cell carcinoma. N Engl J Med. 2022;386(5):449–62.
7. Terada M, Hara H, Daiko H, et al. Phase III study of tri-modality combination therapy with induction docetaxel plus cisplatin and 5-fluorouracil versus definitive chemoradiotherapy for locally advanced unresectable squamous-cell carcinoma of the thoracic esophagus (JCOG1510: TRIANgLE). Jpn J Clin Oncol. 2019;49(11):1055–60.
8. Mine S, Tanaka K, Kawachi H, et al. Japanese classification of esophageal cancer, 12th edition: Part I. Esophagus. 2024;21(3):179–215.
9. Doki Y, Tanaka K, Kawachi H, et al. Japanese classification of esophageal cancer, 12th edition: Part II. Esophagus. 2024;21(3):216–69.
10. Ando N, Kato H, Igaki H, et al. A randomized trial comparing postoperative adjuvant chemotherapy with cisplatin and 5-fluorouracil versus preoperative chemotherapy for localized advanced squamous cell carcinoma of the thoracic esophagus (JCOG9907). Ann Surg Oncol. 2012;19(1):68–74.
11. Kato K, Machida R, Ito Y, et al. Doublet chemotherapy, triplet chemotherapy, or doublet chemotherapy combined with radiotherapy as neoadjuvant treatment for locally advanced oesophageal cancer (JCOG1109 NExT): a randomised, controlled, open-label, phase 3 trial. Lancet. 2024;404(10447):55–66.
12. Kelly RJ, Ajani JA, Kuzdzal J, et al. Adjuvant nivolumab in resected esophageal or gastroesophageal junction cancer. N Engl J Med. 2021;384(13):1191–203.
13. Takeuchi H, Ito Y, Machida R, et al. A single-arm confirmatory study of definitive chemoradiation therapy including salvage treatment for clinical stage II/III esophageal squamous cell carcinoma (JCOG0909 Study). Int J Radiat Oncol Biol Phys. 2022;114(3):454–62.
14. Booka E, Takeuchi H. Conversion therapy for cT4b and M1 esophageal squamous cell carcinoma: a comprehensive systematic review. Ann Gastroenterol Surg. 2025;
15. Kato K, Cho BC, Takahashi M, et al. Nivolumab versus chemotherapy in patients with advanced oesophageal squamous cell carcinoma refractory or intolerant to previous chemotherapy

(ATTRACTION-3): a multicentre, randomised, open-label, phase 3 trial. Lancet Oncol. 2019;20(11):1506–17.

16. Xu J, Kato K, Raymond E, et al. Tislelizumab plus chemotherapy versus placebo plus chemotherapy as first-line treatment for advanced or metastatic oesophageal squamous cell carcinoma (RATIONALE-306): a global, randomised, placebo-controlled, phase 3 study. Lancet Oncol. 2023;24(5):483–95.
17. Shen L, Kato K, Kim SB, et al. Tislelizumab versus chemotherapy as second-line treatment for advanced or metastatic esophageal squamous cell carcinoma (RATIONALE-302): a randomized phase III study. J Clin Oncol. 2022;40(26):3065–76.
18. Takeuchi H, Machida R, Ando M, et al. Thoracoscopic versus open oesophagectomy for patients with oesophageal cancer (JCOG1409 MONET): a multicentre, open-label, randomised, controlled, phase 3, non-inferiority trial. Lancet Gastroenterol Hepatol. 2025;10(12):1104–16.
19. Weimann A, Bezmarevic M, Braga M, et al. ESPEN guideline on clinical nutrition in surgery – update 2025. Clin Nutr. 2025;53:222–61.

Endoscopic Treatment: EMR and ESD

8

Motohiko Kato, Noriko Matsuura, and Naohisa Yahagi

8.1 Introduction

With recent advancements in therapeutic endoscopy, particularly endoscopic submucosal dissection (ESD), the size limitations for lesions resectable by endoscopy have been effectively eliminated. In the so-called "pre-ESD era," endoscopic mucosal resection (EMR) using an electrocautery snare was the only available technique. However, EMR was limited to small mucosal lesions due to technical constraints. For larger lesions, piecemeal resection was often unavoidable, complicating histological assessment and potentially leading to inaccurate pathological diagnosis [1, 2]. The development of ESD has significantly broadened the indications for endoscopic resection (ER), due to its unique technical advantages. Notably, ESD enables en bloc resection of early gastrointestinal cancers regardless of lesion size or the presence of submucosal fibrosis [3, 4]. This chapter outlines the indications and techniques of both EMR and ESD, as well as the management of procedure-related complications.

8.2 Indication of Endoscopic Resection

According to the Japanese classification of esophageal cancer, superficial carcinoma of the esophagus is defined as a lesion with invasion limited to the submucosal layer [5]. Among these, carcinoma confined to the mucosa, regardless of lymph

M. Kato (✉)
Center for Diagnostic and Therapeutic Endoscopy, Keio University School of Medicine, Shinjuku-ku, Tokyo, Japan
e-mail: motohikokato@keio.jp

N. Matsuura · N. Yahagi
Division of Research and Development for Minimally Invasive Treatment, Cancer Center, Keio University School of Medicine, Shinjuku-ku, Tokyo, Japan

Y. Kitagawa et al. (eds.), *Esophageal Squamous Cell Carcinoma*,
https://doi.org/10.1007/978-981-92-2611-5_8

node metastasis, is referred to as early esophageal cancer. The indication for ER is determined based on the predicted depth of invasion, the risk of lymph node metastasis [5–9], and the circumferential extent of the lesion. If an early cancer invading up to the T1a epithelial or lamina propria mucosae (EP/LPM), where the risk of lymph node metastasis is estimated to be less than 5% [5], is completely resected, curative resection can be expected. The Esophageal Cancer Practice Guidelines 2022 recommend ER for clinically diagnosed T1a-EP/LPM cancers [10].

In contrast, superficial cancers invading the T1a muscularis mucosae (MM) or T1b submucosa to a depth of ≤200 μm (SM1) carry a 10–15% risk of lymph node metastasis [8]. However, alternative treatment options for esophageal squamous cell carcinoma (ESCC), such as chemoradiotherapy (CRT) or surgery, are generally more invasive and associated with a significant risk of major complications. The diagnostic accuracy for clinically diagnosed MM/SM1 cancers has been reported to be relatively low (55.7%) [11]. Therefore, the esophageal ESD/EMR guidelines recommend that the least invasive treatment option, including ER, be selected as the first-line approach for non-circumferential clinical MM/SM1 lesions. Staging with computed tomography (CT) is required prior to treatment for clinically diagnosed MM invasion or deeper, as well as for superficial lesions measuring ≥5 cm.

Mucosal defects involving ≥3/4 of the esophageal circumference after ER have been reported to result in strictures in ≥60% of cases [12]. According to the esophageal ESD/EMR guidelines, local steroid injection is weakly recommended to prevent stricture formation when mucosal defects involve ≥3/4 of the circumference. Even after prophylactic treatment following circumferential resection, stricture rates have been reported to range from 27.3% to 76% [11]. Furthermore, the rate of non-curative resection following ESD for superficial ESCC is reported to be high (17–39%) in circumferential ESCC cases [13–17]. Therefore, the ESD/EMR guidelines weakly recommend ESD for clinically diagnosed T1a-EP/LPM ESCC with a major axis length of ≤50 mm involving the entire esophageal circumference, provided that appropriate preventive measures against stricture are implemented.

8.3 Endoscopic Mucosal Resection (EMR)

Endoscopic mucosal resection (EMR) involves injecting fluid into the submucosa, followed by resection of the mucosa along with a portion of the submucosa using an electrocautery snare. Several technical variations of EMR exist.

EMR with a ligation device (EMR-L) utilizes an O-ring commonly used for esophageal varices ligation (Fig. 8.1) [17]. In this technique, after suctioning the lesion and ligating it with the O-ring to create a pseudo-polyp, endoscopic resection is performed just below the O-ring using a snare. Although submucosal injection before resection is conventionally recommended to prevent unexpected perforation, ER using a ligation device without submucosal injection appears to be acceptable, particularly for early Barrett's neoplasia [18]. In EMR using a cap-fitted endoscope (EMR-C), a transparent hood is attached to the tip of the endoscope [19]. After opening a semilunar snare along the rim of the hood, the lesion, elevated by

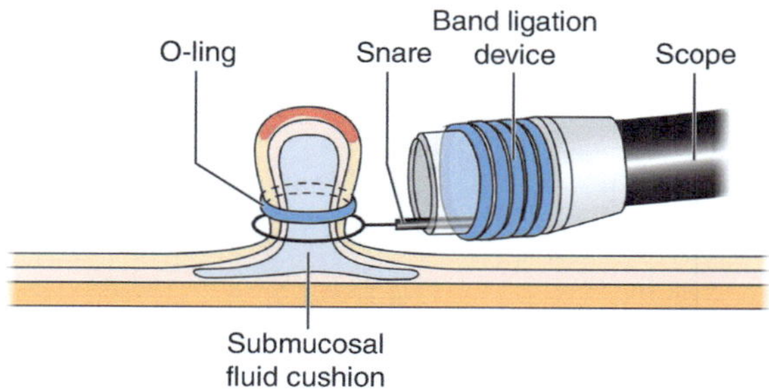

Fig. 8.1 Endoscopic mucosal resection (EMR) with a ligation device (EMR-L). EMR with a ligation device (EMR-L). A lesion is suctioned and ligated with O-ring before resection

submucosal injection, is suctioned into the hood and resected using the snare. In this technique, positioning the snare along the rim of the hood can be difficult and time-consuming, which may occasionally cause operator frustration. In the endoscopic esophageal mucosal resection (EEMR)-tube method, a long transparent silicone overtube is used [20]. After submucosal injection, the lesion is suctioned into the overtube, which is introduced over the endoscope, and then tightened with a snare preliminarily passed through the side channel of the overtube. Resection should be performed only after confirming that the muscularis propria is not involved, as the diameter of the overtube is considerably larger than that of other EMR caps.

The grasping and pulling technique using a two-channel endoscope is known as the two-channel EMR method [21]. A grasping forceps is passed through one working channel and a snare through the other. The lesion, elevated by submucosal injection, is grasped with the forceps and the snare is tightened around the base of the grasped mucosa. As with other methods, resection should be performed only after confirming that the muscularis propria is not involved within the ligated tissue.

Due to the limited size of Snares used in these EMR techniques, the achievable size for en bloc resection is also restricted [3, 4, 22, 23]. The maximum expected size of a single specimen is approximately 2 cm. Furthermore, the resectable size is constrained by the diameter of the O-ring in EMR-L, the hood in EMR-C, and the overtube in the EEMR-tube method. Additionally, severe submucosal fibrosis beneath the lesion often makes resection difficult with these EMR methods, as the snare tends to slip off the target. Therefore, early esophageal cancers measuring 1 cm or less without fibrosis are generally considered suitable candidates for EMR in clinical practice.

8.4 Endoscopic Submucosal Dissection (ESD)

This innovative technique consists of four steps: marking around the lesion after chromoendoscopy, submucosal injection, circumferential mucosal incision, and dissection of the submucosal connective tissue (Fig. 8.2). Because the operator can precisely determine the extent of resection and dissect the submucosal tissue under direct vision, ESD enables reliable en bloc, margin-negative resection regardless of lesion size or the presence of submucosal fibrosis.

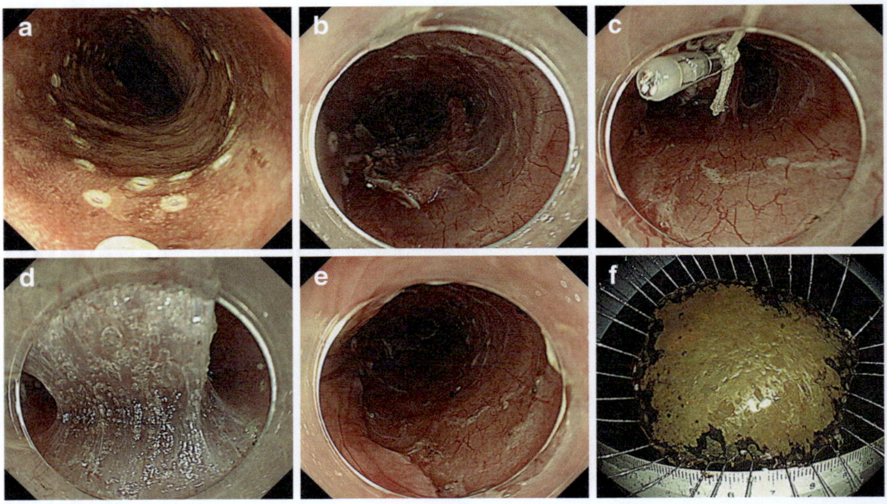

Fig. 8.2 Representative case of esophageal endoscopic submucosal dissection (ESD) using Dualknife J and clip with string traction method. (**a**) Markings are placed around the lesion with an appropriate margin; (**b**) submucosal dissection was started from the opposite side of the gravity force; (**c**) a clip with string was deployed on the proximal side of the lesion; (**d**) good visualization of submucosal layer was obtained by pulling the string; (**e**) resection wound after ESD; (**f**) an en bloc resection enables precise histological assessment (esophageal squamous cell carcinoma, pT1-a, 55 × 40 mm, ly0, v0, pHM0, pVM0)

8.4.1 Details of Practical Skill

Among various electrocautery knives specialized for ESD, pointed tip-type knives are particularly suitable for esophageal ESD due to the narrow lumen and thin wall of the esophagus [24–26]. Moreover, revised types of insulated knives and scissors-type electrocautery knives have also been reported as useful for esophageal ESD [27–29] (Fig. 8.3).

Successful resection requires accurate endoscopic diagnosis of tumor extent. Chromoendoscopy using iodine staining remains the most popular method for delineating lesion boundaries. Recent developments in image-enhanced endoscopy (IEE) have been reported to enable more accurate delineation of tumor margins with IEE-based marking compared to iodine staining [30]. Using the tip of the knife, markings are placed 2–3 mm outside the lesion at intervals of approximately 3 mm.

To create a submucosal cushion, an injection needle is gently advanced into the submucosa outside the markings, and a fluid colored with a small amount of indigo carmine—helpful for visualizing the submucosa—is injected to create sufficient submucosal space for incision and dissection. For submucosal injection, hyaluronic acid solution (MucoUp; Boston Scientific Japan, Tokyo, Japan) or 10% glycerin (Glycerol; Chugai Pharmaceutical Co., Ltd., Tokyo, Japan) is preferred due to its long-lasting cushioning effect. Injection directly into the cancerous area should be avoided to prevent tumor cell implantation into deeper layers.

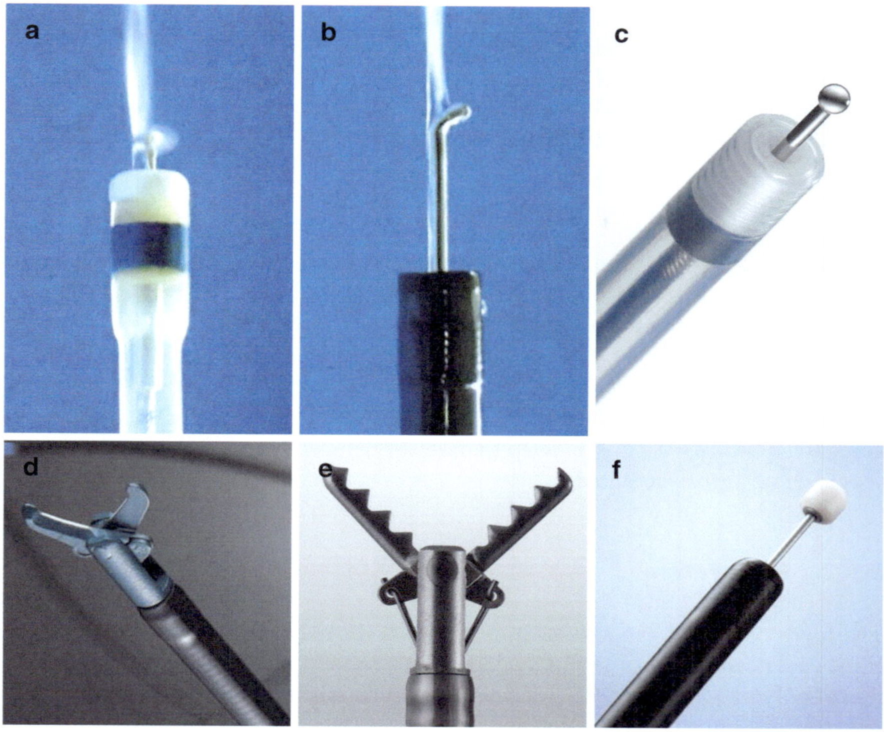

Fig. 8.3 Energy devices for esophageal ESD. (**a**) DualKnifeJ™; (**b**) HookKnifeJ™; (**c**) FlushKnife BT-S; (**d**) SB knife Jr.; (**e**) ClutchCutter (**f**) ITknife nano

The mucosa 1–2 mm outside the markings is typically incised using a cutting current with a specialized knife. Immediately after the partial mucosal incision, initial submucosal dissection should be performed along the incision line using coagulation current. To ensure precise identification of the endpoint of submucosal dissection, it is preferable to first dissect the anal side of the lesion, followed by continuation of the procedure from the oral side.

It is essential to perform submucosal dissection under direct vision using a transparent hood. For large lesions, the tunneling technique or traction devices, such as a clip with a line, are useful for achieving adequate submucosal exposure (Fig. 8.2). During submucosal dissection, the knife should be moved parallel to the muscular layer to avoid muscular injury or perforation. Submucosal injection, mucosal incision, and submucosal dissection should be repeated stepwise until the procedure is complete. In recent years, the use of traction methods, such as clip-with-line techniques, has been reported to shorten the procedure time [31, 32]. Red dichromatic imaging (RDI) is an endoscopic technique that provides better visualization of the deep submucosal blood vessels. RDI has been reported to reduce the incidence of bleeding and hematoma formation during submucosal injection in esophageal ESD

[33]. The resected specimen is pinned onto a board, fixed in formalin, and subsequently subjected to histological evaluation.

8.5 Management of Complications

8.5.1 Bleeding

In cases of minor bleeding during ESD, initial hemostasis should be attempted using the retracted tip of the knife. If bleeding is difficult to control or becomes profuse, hemostatic forceps should be utilized. Following specimen retrieval, the resection ulcer must be carefully inspected for any visible vessels. All exposed, thick vessels should be coagulated with caution to avoid excessive thermal injury. Unlike gastric ESD, the incidence of postoperative bleeding after esophageal ESD is relatively low (0–0.7%) [34–40]. In cases of delayed bleeding, immediate endoscopic hemostasis is required.

8.5.2 Perforation

The reported rate of intraoperative perforation ranges from 0% to 6.9% [34–41]. Most cases can be successfully managed with endoscopic clipping or the application of polyglycolic acid (PGA) sheets in combination with fibrin glue. Injury to the muscular layer may result in delayed perforation, potentially leading to fatal mediastinitis. Therefore, close postoperative monitoring is essential, particularly after intraoperative perforation, muscular injury, or significant thermal damage. The incidence of delayed perforation is relatively low, ranging from 0% to 0.1% [34–41]. Endoscopists should collaborate with surgeons to determine the most appropriate management strategy. In cases with mild inflammatory signs and symptoms, conservative treatment—such as fasting, antibiotic therapy, and mediastinal drainage—may be sufficient. However, in cases of severe inflammation, invasive interventions such as subtotal esophagectomy, pleural drainage, or temporary stent placement may be required [42].

8.5.3 Mediastinal Emphysema

Given the absence of a serosal layer in the esophagus, exposure of the muscularis propria during ESD can result in mediastinal emphysema [43, 44]. Although mediastinal emphysema is often difficult to detect on chest X-ray (CXR), CT has revealed its presence in approximately half of patients following esophageal ESD. However, the majority of these cases are subclinical and do not require any therapeutic intervention [44]. Most cases of mediastinal emphysema detected on chest CT are minor and have little impact on the clinical course. To reduce the risk of severe mediastinal emphysema, esophageal ESD should be performed using carbon dioxide (CO_2), which is rapidly absorbed by tissues, rather than room air. Insufflation with air may lead to serious complications, even when only the muscularis propria is exposed [45].

8.5.4 Postoperative Stricture

The risk of postoperative stricture exceeds 60% in esophageal ESD defects involving more than three-fourths of the circumference and reaches 100% in circumferential defects without any preventive measures (Fig. 8.4) [12–16, 46]. The efficacy of various preventive strategies, including endoscopic balloon dilation (EBD), local steroid injection, oral steroid administration, PGA sheets, cultured oral mucosal epithelial cell sheets, and stent placement, has been reported [47–52]. Triamcinolone acetonide (TAC), a corticosteroid, is used for locoregional injection as a slurry. Several studies have demonstrated the significant superiority of locoregional TAC injection compared to historical controls in preventing post-ESD esophageal stricture formation [47, 52]. In the JCOG1217 study, which evaluated the superiority of oral steroid administration over local steroid injection for preventing strictures after ESD for superficial ESCC involving more than half—but not the entire—circumference, oral steroid administration did not show superiority in stricture-free survival [53]. This study established local steroid injection therapy as the standard treatment for stricture prevention following esophageal ESD. The Japanese ESD/EMR guideline states: "Local injection of triamcinolone is weakly recommended when mucosal defects affecting ≥3/4 of the esophageal circumference occur after ER for superficial ESCC."

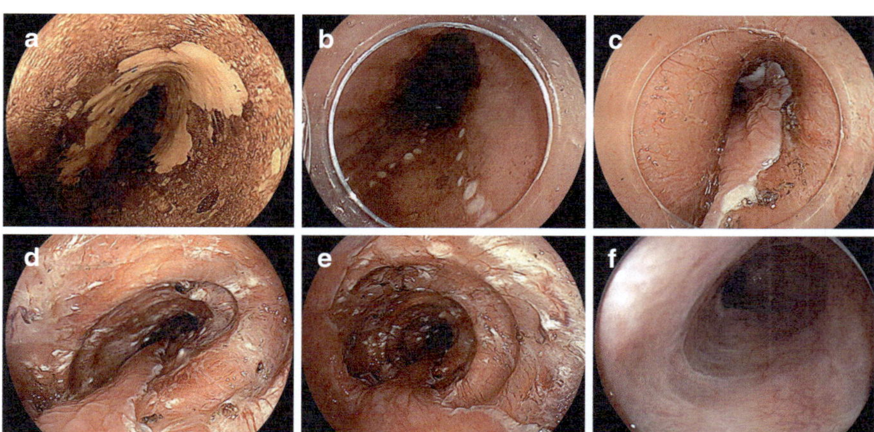

Fig. 8.4 Prevention of stricture following extensive resection. (**a**) Superficial cancer involving three-quarters of the esophageal circumference; (**b**) placement of marking dots; (**c**) the resection wound becomes semi-circumferential; (**d**) steroid solution is injected into the remaining submucosa to prevent severe stricture; (**e**) ulcer after ESD; (**f**) endoscopic image at 3 months after the initial ESD. The mucosal defect has completely healed without significant stricture

Incidental injection of TAC into the muscularis propria can cause mural necrosis [54]; therefore, it is essential to administer steroids into the submucosal layer of the esophagus. Circumferential mucosal defects following esophageal ESD are known to be more prone to stricture formation and require a longer time for stricture resolution compared to non-circumferential defects. Oral steroid administration is another option that may prevent strictures after circumferential ESD [13–16]; however, concerns remain regarding adverse events such as infection and diabetes. Furthermore, preclinical trials investigating novel approaches, including adipose tissue-derived stem cell transplantation [55], cultured cell sheet transplantation [56, 57], and small interfering RNA with anti-fibrotic properties [58], are underway, but no definitive method has yet been established. Further research is necessary to overcome this challenge.

8.5.5 Postoperative Pneumonia

Pneumonia may result from the aspiration of saliva or gastric reflux during treatment. The incidence of postoperative pneumonia following esophageal ESD has been reported to range from 1.6% to 2.6% [34–40]. While post-procedural pneumonia following esophageal ESD is commonly evaluated using CXR, a previous study reported CT detected pneumonia in 21% of patients on the day after the procedure [59]. Patients with underlying conditions such as emphysema are at increased risk of developing severe pneumonia; therefore, any post-operative fever or hypoxemia should prompt evaluation for possible pneumonia. Performing ESD under general anesthesia may reduce the risk of aspiration pneumonia and should be considered, especially for procedures involving the cervical esophagus.

8.6 Curability and Additional Treatment After ER

The curability of ER is determined based on the histopathological findings of the resected specimens. For pathological EP or LPM cancers without vascular invasion and with negative resection margins, the risk of lymph node metastasis is extremely low, and such cases are considered curatively resected. In a follow-up cohort of patients with pathological MM cancer without vascular invasion and with negative vertical margins, the lymph node metastasis rate was reported to be 5.6% [11]. According to the ESD/EMR guidelines, it is weakly recommended to avoid additional surgical resection or CRT for pathological MM cancers, given concerns about reduced quality of life (QOL), delayed adverse events, and treatment-related mortality [11]. However, if the pathological findings indicate submucosal invasion (≥SM1) or positive vascular invasion, additional treatment, including surgical resection or CRT, is recommended. In patients with non-curative ER for ESCC, long-term outcomes following additional treatment were comparable between surgical resection and CRT [60].

8.7 Outcomes of ESD for Esophageal Squamous Cell Carcinoma

8.7.1 Short-Term Outcomes

Favorable treatment outcomes have been reported from high-volume centers, particularly in Japan [35–39]. Regarding the short-term outcomes and technical feasibility of esophageal ESD, recent studies have reported en bloc and complete resection rates ranging from 96.7% to 100% and 84.5% to 94.5%, respectively. The incidence of major complications, such as delayed bleeding or perforation, remains below 1% at high-volume centers [35–39]. Even when complications occur, they can usually be managed conservatively and rarely become life-threatening. Given the potential severity of postoperative complications, ESD remains a considerably less invasive resection method compared to surgery.

8.7.2 Long-Term Outcomes

Long-term outcomes of ESD are also favorable. The 5-year disease-specific survival rate for pathological T1a esophageal cancer has been reported to be 99.1% [61], indicating that endoscopic local resection is sufficient for curative treatment of esophageal SCC with negligible risk of lymph node metastasis. Following ER for ESCC, endoscopic surveillance is recommended for early detection of metachronous esophageal cancers. The presence of multiple iodine-unstained lesions is a known risk factor for the development of metachronous ESCC after ER. Metachronous cancer occurs annually in more than 10% of patients with multiple iodine-unstained lesions [62]. The Japanese ESD/EMR guidelines recommend endoscopic surveillance every 6–12 months after ER. In cases of pathological T1a-MM or T1b-SM1, both CT scanning and endoscopy every 6–12 months are strongly recommended if additional treatments (surgery or CRT) are declined after complete local resection.

8.8 Summary

Compared to other treatment options, endoscopic treatment is the least invasive approach for patients with esophageal cancer who have a negligible risk of lymph node metastasis. Successful endoscopic treatment requires accurate preoperative diagnosis of the lesion, precise endoscopic manipulation, and comprehensive knowledge of potential complications. ESD is superior to EMR because it enables reliable, margin-negative en bloc resection regardless of lesion size or the presence of submucosal fibrosis. Therefore, although technically demanding, ESD can preserve gastrointestinal function and provide patients with a better QOL.

References

1. Ishihara R, Iishi H, Takeuchi Y, et al. Local recurrence of large squamous-cell carcinoma of the esophagus after endoscopic resection. Gastrointest Endosc. 2008;67:799–804.
2. Ishihara R, Iishi H, Uedo N, et al. Comparison of EMR and endoscopic submucosal dissection for en bloc resection of early esophageal cancers in Japan. Gastrointest Endosc. 2008;68:1066–72.
3. Takahashi H, Arimura Y, Masao H, et al. Endoscopic submucosal dissection is superior to conventional endoscopic resection as a curative treatment for early squamous cell carcinoma of the esophagus (with video). Gastrointest Endosc. 2010;72:255–64.
4. Teoh AY, Chiu PW, Yu Ngo DK, et al. Outcomes of endoscopic submucosal dissection versus endoscopic mucosal resection in management of superficial squamous esophageal neoplasms outside Japan. J Clin Gastroenterol. 2010;44:e190–4.
5. Japan Esophageal Society. Japanese classification of esophageal cancer, 12th edition: Part I. Esophagus. 2024;21:179–215.
6. Shimada H, Nabeya Y, Matsubara H, et al. Prediction of lymph node status in patients with superficial esophageal carcinoma: analysis of 160 surgically resected cancers. Am J Surg. 2006;191:250–4.
7. Eguchi T, Nakanishi Y, Shimoda T, et al. Histopathological criteria for additional treatment after endoscopic mucosal resection for esophageal cancer: analysis of 464 surgically resected cases. Mod Pathol. 2006;19:475–80.
8. Katada C, Muto M, Momma K, et al. Clinical outcome after endoscopic mucosal resection for esophageal squamous cell carcinoma invading the muscularis mucosae – a multicenter retrospective cohort study. Endoscopy. 2007;39:779–83.
9. Griffin SM, Burt AD, Jennings NA. Lymph node metastasis in early esophageal adenocarcinoma. Ann Surg. 2011;254:731–6.
10. Kitagawa Y, Ishihara R, Ishikawa H, et al. Esophageal cancer practice guidelines 2022 edited by the Japan esophageal society: Part 1. Esophagus. 2023;20:343–72.
11. Ishihara R, Arima M, Iizuka T, et al. Endoscopic submucosal dissection/endoscopic mucosal resection guidelines for esophageal cancer. Dig Endosc. 2020;32:452–93.
12. Ono S, Fujishiro M, Niimi K, et al. Predictors of postoperative stricture after esophageal endoscopic submucosal dissection for superficial squamous cell neoplasms. Endoscopy. 2009;41:661–5.
13. Sato H, Inoue H, Kobayashi Y, et al. Control of severe strictures after circumferential endoscopic submucosal dissection for esophageal carcinoma: oral steroid therapy with balloon dilation or balloon dilation alone. Gastrointest Endosc. 2013;78:250–7.
14. Kadota T, Yoda Y, Hori K, et al. Prophylactic steroid administration against strictures is not enough for mucosal defects involving the entire circumference of the esophageal lumen after esophageal endoscopic submucosal dissection (ESD). Esophagus. 2020;17:440–7.
15. Miwata T, Oka S, Tanaka S, et al. Risk factors for esophageal stenosis after entire circumferential endoscopic submucosal dissection for superficial esophageal squamous cell carcinoma. Surg Endosc. 2016;30:4049–56.
16. Kadota T, Ishihara R, Hatta W, et al. Multi-institutional questionnaire on treatment strategies for superficial entire circumferential esophageal squamous cell carcinoma. DEN Open. 2023;3:e206.
17. Suzuki H. Endoscopic mucosal resection using ligating device for early gastric cancer. Gastrointest Endosc Clin N Am. 2001;11:511–8.
18. Pouw RE, van Vilsteren FG, Peters FP, et al. Randomized trial on endoscopic resection-cap versus multiband mucosectomy for piecemeal endoscopic resection of early Barrett's neoplasia. Gastrointest Endosc. 2011;74:35–43.
19. Inoue H, Endo M, Takeshita K, et al. A new simplified technique of endoscopic esophageal mucosal resection using a cap-fitted panendoscope (EMRC). Surg Endosc. 1992;6:264–5.

20. Makuuchi H. Endoscopic mucosal resection for early esophageal cancer – indication and techniques. Dig Endosc. 1996;8:175–9.
21. Shimizu Y, Takahashi M, Yoshida T, et al. Endoscopic resection (endoscopic mucosal resection/endoscopic submucosal dissection) for superficial esophageal squamous cell carcinoma: current status of various techniques. Dig Endosc. 2013;25(Suppl. 1):13–9.
22. Yamashita T, Zeniya A, Ishii H, et al. Endoscopic mucosal resection using a cap-fitted panendoscope and endoscopic submucosal dissection as optimal endoscopic procedures for superficial esophageal carcinoma. Surg Endosc. 2011;25:2541–6.
23. Urabe Y, Hiyama T, Tanaka S, et al. Advantages of endoscopic submucosal dissection versus endoscopic oblique aspiration mucosectomy for superficial esophageal tumors. J Gastroenterol Hepatol. 2011;26:275–80.
24. Yahagi N, Uraoka T, Ida Y, et al. Endoscopic submucosal dissection using the Flex and the Dual knives. Tech Gastrointest Endosc. 2011;13:74–8.
25. Fukami N, Ryu CB, Said S, et al. Prospective, randomized study of conventional versus HybridKnife endoscopic submucosal dissection methods for the esophagus: an animal study. Gastrointest Endosc. 2011;73:1246–53.
26. Ishii N, Horiki N, Itoh T, et al. Endoscopic submucosal dissection with a combination of small-caliber-tip transparent hood and flex knife is a safe and effective treatment for superficial esophageal neoplasias. Surg Endosc. 2010;24:335–42.
27. Akahoshi K, Minoda Y, Komori K, et al. Endoscopic submucosal dissection using the "Clutch Cutter" for early esophageal squamous cell carcinoma. Endoscopy. 2013;45:1035–8.
28. Kuwai T, Yamaguchi T, Imagawa H, et al. Endoscopic submucosal dissection for early esophageal neoplasms using the stag beetle knife. World J Gastroenterol. 2018;24:1632–40.
29. Kitagawa Y, Suzuki T, Hara T, et al. Safety and efficacy of endoscopic submucosal dissection using IT knife nano with clip traction method for early esophageal squamous cell carcinoma. Surg Endosc. 2018;32:450–5.
30. Kono M, Kanesaka T, Ishihara R, et al. Delineating the extent of esophageal squamous cell carcinoma. Esophagus. 2021;18:790–6.
31. Koike Y, Hirasawa D, Fujita N, et al. Usefulness of the thread-traction method in esophageal endoscopic submucosal dissection: randomized controlled trial. Dig Endosc. 2015;27:303–9.
32. Yoshida M, Takizawa K, Nonaka S, et al. Conventional versus traction-assisted endoscopic submucosal dissection for large esophageal cancers: a multicenter, randomized controlled trial (with video). Gastrointest Endosc. 2020;91(55–65):e2.
33. Miyazaki K, Kato M, Sasaki M, et al. Red dichromatic imaging reduces bleeding and hematoma during submucosal injection in esophageal endoscopic submucosal dissection. Surg Endosc. 2022;36:8076–85.
34. Repici A, Hassan C, Carlino A, et al. Endoscopic submucosal dissection in patients with early esophageal squamous cell carcinoma: results from a prospective Western series. Gastrointest Endosc. 2010;71:715–21.
35. Ono S, Fujishiro M, Niimi K, et al. Long-term outcomes of endoscopic submucosal dissection for superficial esophageal squamous cell neoplasms. Gastrointest Endosc. 2009;70:860–6.
36. Yamashina T, Ishihara R, Uedo N, et al. Safety and curative ability of endoscopic submucosal dissection for superficial esophageal cancers at least 50 mm in diameter. Dig Endosc. 2012;24:220–5.
37. Higuchi K, Tanabe S, Azuma M, et al. A phase II study of endoscopic submucosal dissection for superficial esophageal neoplasms (KDOG 0901). Gastrointest Endosc. 2013;78:704–10.
38. Tsujii Y, Nishida T, Nishiyama O, et al. Clinical outcomes of endoscopic submucosal dissection for superficial esophageal neoplasms: a multicenter retrospective cohort study. Endoscopy. 2015;47:775–83.
39. Ishihara R, Oyama T, Takeuchi M, et al. Multicenter retrospective analysis of complications and risk factors in endoscopic resection for esophageal cancer across Japan. Esophagus. 2024;21:430–7.
40. Okubo Y, Ishihara R. Endoscopic submucosal dissection for esophageal cancer: current and future. Life (Basel). 2023;13:892.

41. Seehawong U, Morita Y, Nakano Y, et al. Successful treatment of an esophageal perforation that occurred during endoscopic submucosal dissection for esophageal cancer using polyglycolic acid sheets and fibrin glue. Clin J Gastroenterol. 2019;12:29–33.
42. Omae M, Konradsson M, Baldaque-Silva F. Delayed perforation after endoscopic submucosal dissection treated successfully by temporary stent placement. Clin J Gastroenterol. 2018;11:118–22.
43. Maeda Y, Hirasawa D, Fujita N, et al. Mediastinal emphysema after esophageal endoscopic submucosal dissection: its prevalence and clinical significance. Dig Endosc. 2011;23:221–6.
44. Maeda Y, Hirasawa D, Fujita N, et al. A pilot study to assess mediastinal emphysema after esophageal endoscopic submucosal dissection with carbon dioxide insufflation. Endoscopy. 2012;44:565–71.
45. Nonaka S, Saito Y, Takisawa H, et al. Safety of carbon dioxide insufflation for upper gastrointestinal tract endoscopic treatment of patients under deep sedation. Surg Endosc. 2010;24:1638–45.
46. Nonaka K, Miyazawa M, Ban S, et al. Different healing process of esophageal large mucosal defects by endoscopic mucosal dissection between with and without steroid injection in an animal model. BMC Gastroenterol. 2013;13:72.
47. Hashimoto S, Kobayashi M, Takeuchi M, et al. The efficacy of endoscopic triamcinolone injection for the prevention of esophageal stricture after endoscopic submucosal dissection. Gastrointest Endosc. 2011;74:1389–93.
48. Mizutani T, Tadauchi A, Arinobe M, et al. Novel strategy for prevention of esophageal stricture after endoscopic surgery. Hepato-Gastroenterology. 2010;57:1150–6.
49. Yano T, Yoda Y, Nomura S, et al. Prospective trial of biodegradable stents for refractory benign esophageal strictures after curative treatment of esophageal cancer. Gastrointest Endosc. 2017;86:492–9.
50. Takagi R, Murakami D, Kondo M, et al. Fabrication of human oral mucosal epithelial cell sheets for treatment of esophageal ulceration by endoscopic submucosal dissection. Gastrointest Endosc. 2010;72:1253–9.
51. Isomoto H, Yamaguchi N, Nakayama T, et al. Management of esophageal stricture after complete circular endoscopic submucosal dissection for superficial esophageal squamous cell carcinoma. BMC Gastroenterol. 2011;11:46.
52. Hanaoka N, Ishihara R, Takeuchi Y, et al. Intralesional steroid injection to prevent stricture after endoscopic submucosal dissection for esophageal cancer: a controlled prospective study. Endoscopy. 2012;44:1007–11.
53. Tanaka M, Ono H, Takizawa K, et al. Gastrointestinal endoscopy study group of the japan clinical oncology group. A randomized controlled phase 3 trial of oral prednisolone administration versus local triamcinolone injection therapy for esophageal stricture prevention after extensive endoscopic submucosal dissection (JCOG1217). Dig Endosc. 2026;38:e70195.
54. Yamashita S, Kato M, Fujimoto A, et al. Inadequate steroid injection after esophageal ESD might cause mural necrosis. Endosc Int Open. 2019;7:E115–21.
55. Honda M, Hori Y, Nakada A, et al. Use of adipose tissue-derived stromal cells for prevention of esophageal stricture after circumferential EMR in a canine model. Gastrointest Endosc. 2011;73:777–84.
56. Ohki T, Yamato M, Murakami D, et al. Treatment of oesophageal ulcerations using endoscopic transplantation of tissue-engineered autologous oral mucosal epithelial cell sheets in a canine model. Gut. 2006;55:1704–10.
57. Ohki T, Yamato M, Ota M, et al. Prevention of esophageal stricture after endoscopic submucosal dissection using tissue-engineered cell sheets. Gastroenterology. 2012;143:582–8.
58. Sato H, Sagara S, Nakajima N, Akimoto T, Suzuki K, Yoneyama H, Terai S, Yahagi N. Prevention of esophageal stricture after endoscopic submucosal dissection using RNA-based silencing of carbohydrate sulfotransferase 15 in a porcine model. Endoscopy. 2017;49:491–7.
59. Mizutani M, Minesaki D, Morioka K, et al. Prospective cross-organ analysis for the causes of fever and increased inflammatory response after endoscopic resection. Dig Endosc. 2024;36:918–26.

60. Yamamoto Y, Ishihara R, Kawakubo H, et al. Comparison of outcomes between surgery and chemoradiotherapy after endoscopic resection for pT1a-MM with lymphovascular invasion or pT1b esophageal squamous cell carcinoma: Japanese multicenter propensity score-matched study. J Gastroenterol. 2025;60:43–54.
61. Oda I, Shimizu Y, Yoshio T, et al. Long-term outcome of endoscopic resection for intramucosal esophageal squamous cell cancer: a secondary analysis of the Japan Esophageal Cohort study. Endoscopy. 2020;52:967–75.
62. Katada C, Yokoyama T, Yano T, et al. Alcohol consumption and multiple dysplastic lesions increase risk of squamous cell carcinoma in the esophagus, head, and neck. Gastroenterology. 2016;151:860–9.e7.

Surgery: Transthoracic Esophagectomy

9

Hirofumi Kawakubo

9.1 Introduction

Many therapeutic options including endoscopic therapy, surgical resection, chemotherapy, and radiotherapy are used for treatment of esophageal cancer. A multimodality treatment combining surgical resection, radiotherapy, and chemotherapy is necessary for advanced esophageal carcinoma [1, 2]. Among these options, surgical resection has been most frequently used to obtain locoregional control and has consistently played a central role in management of esophageal cancer [3].

The histopathological profile of esophageal cancer differs markedly between Western countries and East Asia. In Western countries, adenocarcinoma (ADC), arising from Barrett's esophagus, is predominant, whereas in East Asian countries such as Japan, China, and Korea, squamous cell carcinoma (SCC) is more common [4, 5]. ADC and SCC also tend to differ in tumor location and metastatic lymphatic spread patterns. SCC most frequently arises in the middle thoracic esophagus and is often associated with lymph node metastases involving all three fields, including the cervical and upper mediastinal regions. In contrast, most ADCs are located in the lower esophagus and at the esophagogastric junction, and are a higher incidence of metastases to the middle and lower mediastinal as well as abdominal lymph nodes [6]. The distribution of lymph node metastases according to the location of the primary lesion in thoracic esophageal SCC, as reported by Ando et al., is shown in Fig. 9.1 [7]. As illustrated, thoracic esophageal SCC frequently presents with extensive lymph node metastases extending from the neck to the upper abdomen. In upper thoracic esophageal cancer, cervical and upper mediastinal nodes are most commonly involved, whereas in lower thoracic esophageal cancer, metastases predominantly affect the lower mediastinal and peri-gastric nodes. Middle thoracic

H. Kawakubo (✉)
Japanese Foundation for Cancer Research, Cancer Institute Hospital, Tokyo, Japan
e-mail: hkawakubo@keio.jp

Y. Kitagawa et al. (eds.), *Esophageal Squamous Cell Carcinoma*,
https://doi.org/10.1007/978-981-92-2611-5_9

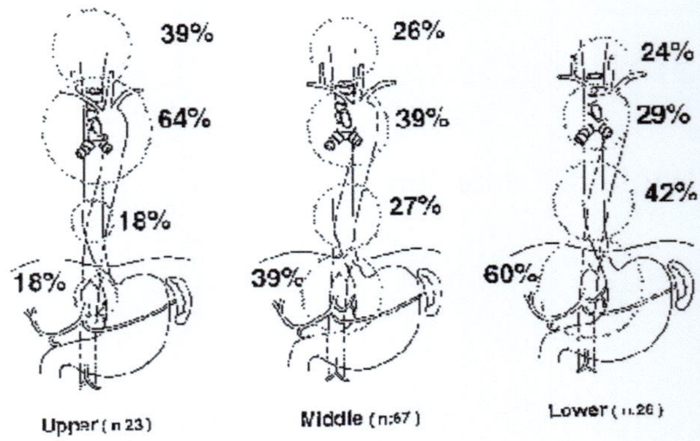

Fig. 9.1 The status of lymph node metastases according to the location of the primary tumor as reported by Ando et al.

esophageal cancer is particularly characterized by a high incidence of widespread nodal involvement from the cervical to the abdominal regions.

In Japan, where the majority of esophageal cancers are SCC, the concept of three-field lymphadenectomy was developed in the 1980s for resectable cancers. This approach includes systematic dissection of cervical, mediastinal, and abdominal lymph nodes [6]. Although the oncological benefit of extended three-field lymphadenectomy for esophageal cancer has not yet been definitively established in large randomized prospective trials [8, 9], numerous reports from Japan and several high-volume centers in other countries have emphasized the importance of esophagectomy with three-field lymph node dissection [3, 6–13].

In this chapter, we describe the standard transthoracic esophagectomy with three-field lymphadenectomy for thoracic esophageal SCC, focusing on the operative technique used in Japanese routine clinical practice.

9.2 Surgery for SCC of Thoracic Esophagus

9.2.1 Esophagectomy

Curative resection of the primary lesion includes resection of the gross tumor as well as potential microscopic spread of esophageal carcinoma. Because adequate mediastinal lymphadenectomy is essential, a right transthoracic approach with systematic lymph node dissection and total extirpation of the thoracoabdominal esophagus is generally performed.

9.2.2 Regional Extent of Lymphadenectomy

The distribution and incidence of lymph node metastasis vary according to the location, size, and depth of tumor invasion. Therefore, preoperative evaluation using computed tomography, ultrasonography, magnetic resonance imaging, and positron

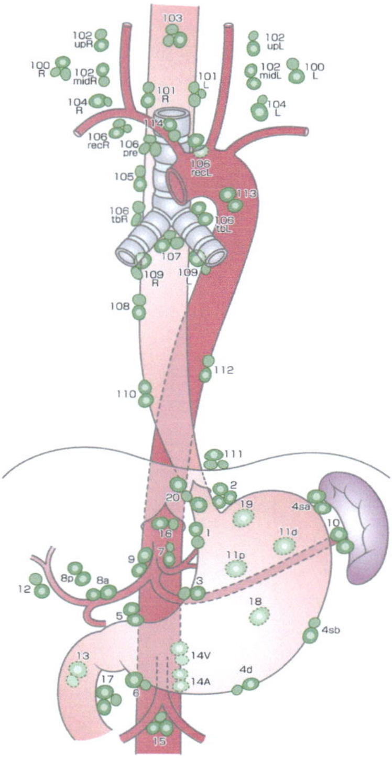

1) Cervical lymph nodes
No. 101 Cervical paraesophageal lymp nodes
No. 104 Superclavicular lymph nodes

2) Thoracic lymph nodes
No. 105 Upper thoracic paraesophageal lymph nodes
No. 106 Thoracic paratracheal lymph nodes
No. 106rec Recurrent nerve lymph nodes
No. 106pre Pretracheal lymph nodes
No. 106tb Trancheobronchial lymph nodes
No. 107 Subcarinal lymph nodes
No. 108 Middle thoracic paraesophageal lymph nodes
No. 109 Main bronchus lymph nodes
No. 110 Lower thoracic paraesophageal lymph nodes
No. 111 Superadiaphragmatic lymph nodes
No. 112 Posterior mediastinal lymph nodes

3) Abdominal lymph nodes
No. 1 Right cardiac lymph nodes
No. 2 Left cardiac lymph nodes
No. 3 Lymph nodes along the lesser curvature
No. 7 Lymph nodes along the left gastric artery
No. 8 Lymph nodes along the common hepatic artery
No. 9 Lymph nodes along the celiac artery

Fig. 9.2 The naming and numbers of lymph nodes defined according to the location of the nodes

emission tomography is important for determining the appropriate extent of lymph node dissection in each patient. The naming and numbers of lymph nodes defined according to the location of lymph nodes [14] are shown in Fig. 9.2.

9.2.2.1 Upper Thoracic Esophageal Carcinoma

In cases of upper thoracic esophageal carcinoma, lymph node metastasis occurs mainly in the cervical and upper mediastinal region. Although metastasis to lower mediastinal or abdominal lymph nodes is less frequent, lymphadenectomy usually covers all three regions in potentially curable cases.

9.2.2.2 Middle Thoracic Esophageal Carcinoma

In middle thoracic esophageal carcinoma, lymph node metastases are frequently found in the cervical, upper, middle, and lower mediastinal, and abdominal regions. In addition to thoracic and abdominal approaches, a cervical approach is necessary to achieve secure dissection of cervical lymph nodes, including those in the supraclavicular region.

9.2.2.3 Lower Thoracic Esophageal Carcinoma

In lower thoracic esophageal carcinoma, lymph node metastases occur mainly in the mediastinal and abdominal regions, but cervical lymph node metastases may also occur at a lower frequency. The optimal extent of dissection in this setting is controversial: some surgeons advocate inclusion of cervical lymphadenectomy, whereas others regard mediastinal and abdominal lymphadenectomy as sufficient.

9.3 Surgical Procedure

9.3.1 Surgical Approach

Open approaches used for esophageal resection include the transhiatal approach, right transthoracic approach, and left transthoracic approach, including the left thoracoabdominal approach. The choice of approach depends on various factors, such as the location of the tumor, the general condition of the patient, and the choice of conduit for esophageal reconstruction.

Because adequate mediastinal lymph node dissection is critical for oncological control in SCC of the thoracic esophagus, the standard approach is right thoracotomy with mediastinal lymph node dissection and total extirpation of the thoracoabdominal esophagus.

Two main transthoracic procedures are widely used:

- *McKeown esophagectomy:*

This operation is typically performed with the patient initially in the left lateral decubitus position. The procedure begins with the thoracic phase, including mobilization of the esophagus and mediastinal lymphadenectomy, followed by the abdominal phase with gastric mobilization and abdominal lymphadenectomy. Finally, a cervical esophagogastrostomy is performed through a left cervical incision. This approach is appropriate for tumors located in the middle to upper thoracic esophagus.

- *Ivor Lewis esophagectomy:*

This procedure is initiated with the patient in the supine position. The abdominal phase is performed first, including gastric mobilization and abdominal lymphadenectomy, followed by the thoracic phase, during which the esophagus is mobilized, mid-to-lower mediastinal lymphadenectomy is completed, and an intrathoracic esophagogastric anastomosis is performed. The Ivor Lewis esophagectomy is particularly suitable for tumors of the lower thoracic esophagus and esophagogastric junction.

9.3.2 Upper Mediastinal Procedure

After the azygous arch is divided, the posterior side of the right-upper mediastinal pleura is incised along the posterior edge of the esophagus up to the right subclavian artery. For open esophagectomy, the right bronchial artery is carefully isolated and preserved. The dorsal and left sides of the upper esophagus are dissected from the left pleura.

Next, the anterior side of the right-upper mediastinal pleura is incised along the right vagal nerve up to the right subclavian artery. The right recurrent laryngeal nerve (RLN) is identified at the caudal end of the right subclavian artery, and the lymph nodes around the right RLN are carefully dissected to prevent nerve injury (Fig. 9.3). The anterior part of the upper esophagus is circumferentially dissected together with surrounding lymphatic tissue.

By retracting the taped esophagus posteriorly and the trachea anteriorly, the left anterior aspect of the trachea can be approached. Lymph nodes along the left RLN are dissected from the aortic arch to the cervical region. The left subclavian artery is exposed to facilitate dissection of left RLN nodes. During dissection of left tracheobronchial lymph nodes, the left RLN and left bronchial artery are preserved on the surface of the trunk of the left pulmonary artery between the aortic arch and the left main bronchus (Fig. 9.4).

9.3.3 Middle and Lower Mediastinal Procedure

The pleura of the middle and lower mediastinum is incised along the anterior aspect of the vertebral bodies down to the hiatus. The posterior side of the middle-to-lower esophagus is dissected to expose the aortic arch and descending aorta (Fig. 9.5). The thoracic duct is ligated and divided behind the lower esophagus and is resected combined with the esophagus.

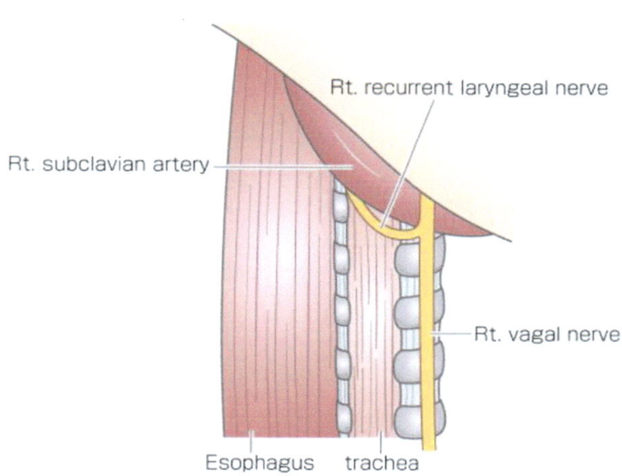

Fig. 9.3 The right recurrent laryngeal nerve was identified at the caudal end of the right subclavian artery, and lymph nodes around the right recurrent laryngeal nerve were dissected

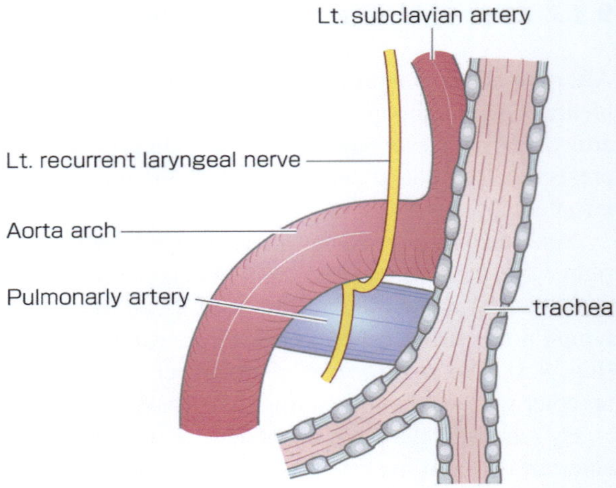

Fig. 9.4 The left subclavian artery was exposed to dissect the left recurrent laryngeal lymph nodes. The trunk of the left pulmonary artery between the aortic arch and the left main bronchus was exposed to dissect the left tracheobronchial lymph nodes

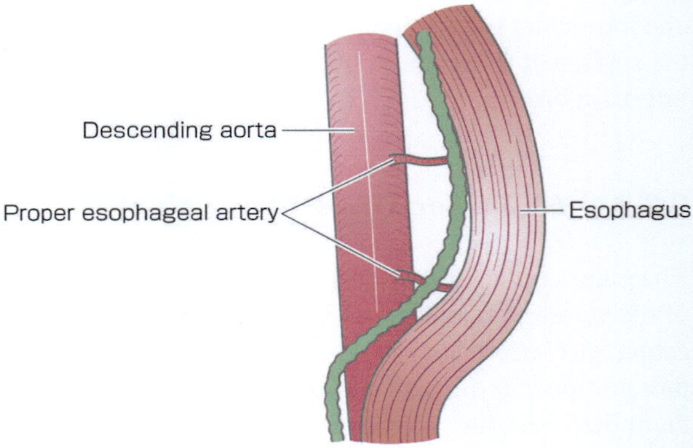

Fig. 9.5 The posterior side of the middle to lower esophagus was dissected to expose the descending aorta. The thoracic duct was ligated and divided behind the lower esophagus and resected together with the esophagus

The esophagus is divided with a linear stapler above the primary tumor, and the proximal stump of the esophagus, together with surrounding mediastinal tissue, is dissected down to the hiatus. Subcarinal lymph nodes are separately resected (Fig. 9.6). Esophageal mobilization and mediastinal lymphadenectomy are then complete.

The view after esophagectomy and mediastinal lymph node dissection is shown in Fig. 9.7a–e. The bilateral RLNs, bilateral subclavian arteries, trachea, main bronchi, aorta, left pulmonary artery and vein, left pleura, pericardium, and hiatus are all skeletonized.

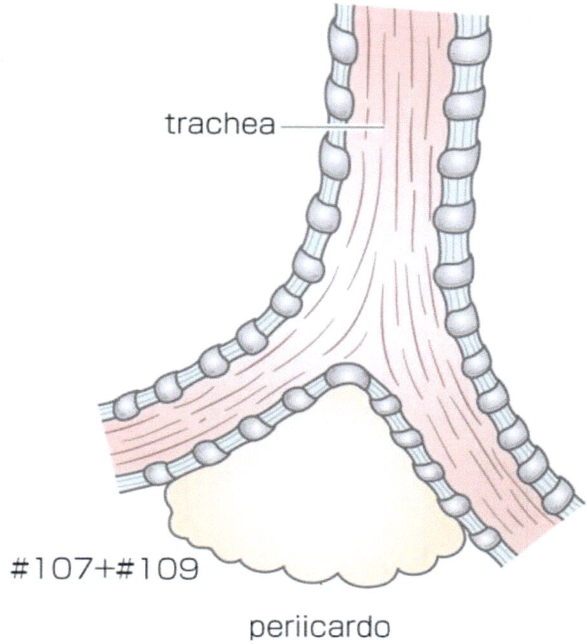

Fig. 9.6 The subcarinal nodes were separately dissected

9.3.4 Abdominal Procedures

The greater omentum is divided 4–5 cm from the arcade of the gastroepiploic vessels. The left gastroepiploic and short gastric vessels are divided along the splenic hilum. The lesser omentum is opened, and the right gastric vessels are preserved. The distal esophagus is dissected and mobilized.

The greater omentum is divided 4–5 cm from the arcade of the gastroepiploic vessels. The left gastroepiploic and short gastric vessels are divided along the splenic hilum. The lesser omentum is opened, and the right gastric vessels are preserved. The distal esophagus is dissected and mobilized.

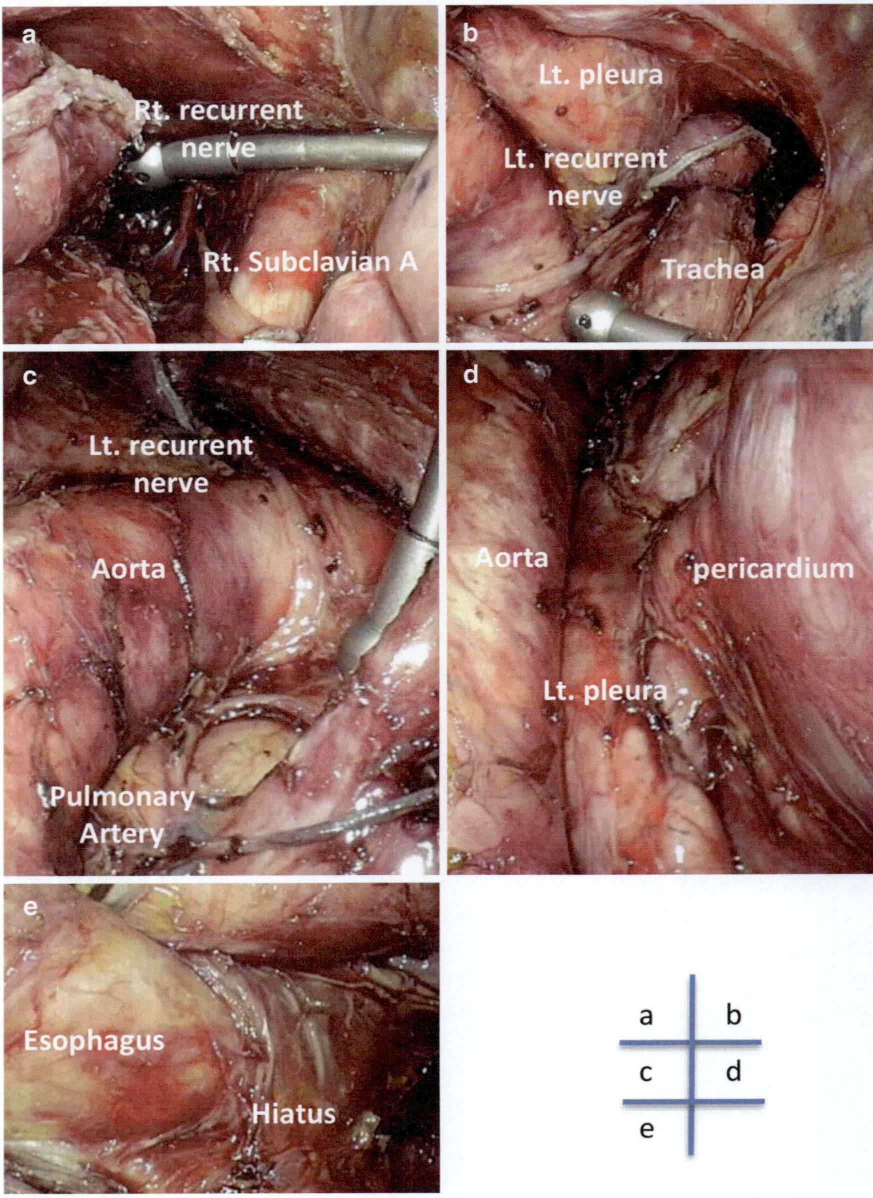

Fig. 9.7 View after esophagectomy and mediastinal lymph node dissection. (**a**) View after dissection of the right recurrent laryngeal nerve lymph node. The right recurrent laryngeal nerve and the right subclavian artery were exposed. (**b**) View after dissection of the left recurrent laryngeal nerve lymph node. The left recurrent laryngeal nerve, the left pleura, and the aortic arch were exposed. (**c**) View after dissection of the left tracheobronchial lymph nodes. Recurrent site of the left recurrent laryngeal nerve under the aortic arch and pulmonary artery were exposed and left bronchial artery was preserved. (**d**) View after procedure of mid to lower mediastinum. The descending aorta, the left pleura, and pericardium were exposed. (**e**) View after dissection of the supradiaphragmatic lymph nodes

9.4 Mortality and Morbidity After Esophagectomy

Transthoracic esophagectomy is one of the most invasive procedures in thoracic and gastrointestinal surgery. Patients undergoing this procedure are at risk of respiratory, cardiovascular, and other systemic complications. Despite substantial advances in preoperative risk evaluation, surgical technique, and perioperative care, the risks of morbidity and mortality after esophagectomy remain significant.

Takeuchi et al. analyzed 5354 patients who underwent esophagectomy in 713 institutions across Japan using data from the National Clinical Database (NCD) in 2011 [15]. The 30-day mortality rate in this cohort was 1.25%, and the operative mortality rate was 3.4%. The overall morbidity rate was 41.9%. The most common postoperative complications included pneumonia (15.4%), anastomotic leakage (13.3%), and septic shock (1.8%).

9.4.1 Mortality

Postoperative mortality after esophagectomy has been clearly linked to institutional and surgeon case volume. Metzger et al. conducted a meta-analysis of 13 studies evaluating the impact of surgical volume on mortality after esophagectomy [16]. They demonstrated a significant reduction in postoperative mortality with increasing annual case volume. The most plausible explanation for this association is that high-volume centers have lower complication rates and greater expertise in managing complications. They concluded that an annual experience of more than 20 esophagectomies per center is required to achieve a significant reduction in mortality, which decreased to approximately 4.9%, and that esophagectomy for esophageal carcinoma should preferably be concentrated in high-volume hospitals.

Rodgers et al. identified surgical volume as a significant predictor of mortality in a retrospective review of the Nationwide Inpatient Sample database, which included 3243 esophagectomies [17]. Independent risk factors for mortality included comorbidities, age ≥65 years, female sex, race, and lower surgical volume.

In Japan, mortality rates after esophagectomy have decreased over time. According to the comprehensive registry of esophageal cancer in Japan, the 30-day mortality rate was 6.8% during 1979–1982, 3.0% during 1988–1994, and 1.0% in 2006 [18–20]. These mortality rates are lower than those reported in many contemporary Western series. Fujita et al. demonstrated that 30-day and in-hospital mortality rates in low-volume hospitals (fewer than five esophagectomies per year) were approximately three times higher than those in high-volume hospitals (more than 40 esophagectomies per year), based on data from 31,380 esophagectomies performed at 709 institutions in Japan between 2001 and 2006 [21]. These findings strongly support centralization of esophagectomy to high-volume centers.

9.4.2 Morbidity

9.4.2.1 Pulmonary Complications

Pulmonary complications are the most frequent complications after esophagectomy and are implicated in nearly two-thirds of postoperative deaths [22]. The incidence of pneumonia has been directly linked to technical aspects of the surgical procedure and perioperative management [23]. The incidence of pneumonia has been reported to be higher after transthoracic esophagectomy than after transhiatal esophagectomy (THE) [24] and higher than after minimally invasive esophagectomy (MIE) [25].

9.4.2.2 Cardiovascular Complications

Atrial fibrillation is a common cardiovascular complication after esophagectomy. In a retrospective review of 379 patients, Atkins et al. reported a 13.7% incidence of arrhythmia after esophagectomy [22]. Several studies have demonstrated associations between atrial fibrillation and other perioperative complications, such as anastomotic leakage and pulmonary complications, as well as increased perioperative mortality.

Murthy et al. reviewed 921 patients who underwent esophagectomy and found a 22% incidence of atrial fibrillation [26]. Patients who developed atrial fibrillation had significantly higher rates of pulmonary complications and renal failure, a six-fold increase in anastomotic leak rates, and a 3.7-fold increase in mortality compared with those without atrial fibrillation. Myocardial infarction has been reported in 1.1–3.8% of patients after esophagectomy [22, 27, 28].

9.4.2.3 Recurrent Laryngeal Nerve Injury

Injury to the recurrent laryngeal nerves is more frequent in procedures that include cervical anastomoses and three-field lymph node dissection. The incidence of RLN injury has been reported to range from 2% to 20% [29]. RLN palsy is associated with an increased incidence of aspiration and perioperative pulmonary complications [30, 31]. Injury can occur due to traction or thermal damage during extensive dissection of RLN lymph nodes (No. 106-recL and 106-recR). Approximately half of cases of vocal cord dysfunction after esophagectomy resolve spontaneously over time [32].

9.4.2.4 Chylothorax

Injury to the thoracic duct during esophagectomy can result in clinically significant chyle leakage, sometimes exceeding 2–4 L per day into the thoracic cavity. Diagnosis is based on increased drainage from the chest tube after enteral feeding and a change in the character of the fluid to a milky appearance. High-volume chyle leaks increase the risk of pulmonary and systemic complications due to loss of fluid, lymphocytes, and protein, leading to immunosuppression and malnutrition.

Initial management of chylothorax includes cessation of enteral feeding and the initiation of total parenteral nutrition (TPN). Lymphangiography and thoracic duct embolization can be effective, but their success is highly dependent on the experience of the interventional radiologist. Early surgical intervention is recommended by many surgeons in cases of high-output leaks or after failure of conservative management. The site of leakage can be identified by administering a high-fat liquid, such as milk or cream, via a nasogastric or jejunostomy tube at least 1 h before surgery. Some studies have demonstrated the utility of ICG fluorescence imaging, which enabled real-time visualization of lymphatic flow and precise localization of chyle leakage sites [33–35]. When the leak site is identified, the duct is ligated both proximally and distally. If the precise site of leakage cannot be identified, mass ligation of all tissue between the spine and the aorta around the esophageal hiatus is performed.

9.5 Discussion

9.5.1 Open Transthoracic Esophagectomy

Thoracoscopy-assisted esophagectomy and robot-assisted esophagectomy have been reported as promising surgical procedures, in view of their minimal invasiveness, superior cosmetics outcomes, reduced postoperative pain, lower incidence of postoperative respiratory complications, adequate oncological radicality, and favorable long-term outcomes. Various other novel procedures such as mediastinoscopy-assisted esophagectomy have also been reported as minimal invasive esophagectomy techniques. Previous reports have suggested that these endoscopy-assisted esophagectomy allow preservation of the vasculature and nerves while providing detailed visualization of the microanatomy and improving the accuracy of lymph node dissection through higher-magnification imaging.

Three large-scale randomized controlled trials have been reported comparing open esophagectomy with thoracoscopic esophagectomy. The TIME trial was a multicenter, open label randomized controlled trial comparing totally minimally invasive esophagectomy (thoracoscopic and laparoscopic approach) with conventional open esophagectomy in patients with resectable esophageal cancer [36]. The study demonstrated a significantly lower incidence of postoperative pulmonary complications in the minimally invasive group compared with the open surgery group (9% vs. 29%, $p = 0.005$). Short-term mortality and oncological outcomes were comparable between the two approaches. This trial provided the first high-level evidence that minimally invasive esophagectomy reduces respiratory morbidity without compromising early oncological safety.

The MIRO trial was a multicenter randomized phase III study comparing hybrid minimally invasive esophagectomy (laparoscopic abdominal phase combined with open thoracic esophagectomy) with conventional open esophagectomy for esophageal cancer [37]. The hybrid approach significantly reduced the rate of major postoperative complications, particularly pulmonary complications, compared with open surgery (36% vs. 64%). Long-term oncological outcomes, including overall survival, were comparable between the two groups. The MIRO trial established hybrid minimally invasive esophagectomy as a safer alternative to open esophagectomy with equivalent oncological efficacy.

JCOG1409 (MONET trial) was a multicenter randomized phase III non-inferiority trial conducted in Japan to compare thoracoscopic esophagectomy with open esophagectomy for thoracic esophageal squamous cell carcinoma. The primary endpoint was overall survival [38]. Thoracoscopic esophagectomy was demonstrated to be non-inferior to open esophagectomy with respect to long-term survival. In addition, thoracoscopic surgery was associated with improved perioperative outcomes, particularly a reduction in pulmonary complications. This trial confirmed that thoracoscopic esophagectomy is an oncologically sound and less invasive alternative to open esophagectomy in high-volume centers.

There have also been reports from the Netherlands comparing open esophagectomy with robotic-assisted esophagectomy. The robot-assisted minimally invasive esophagectomy (RAMIE) trial was a multicenter randomized controlled study comparing RAMIE with conventional open transthoracic esophagectomy in patients with resectable esophageal cancer [39]. A total of 112 patients were randomly assigned to either RAMIE or open surgery. The primary endpoint was the incidence of postoperative complications of Clavien–Dindo grade II or higher. RAMIE was associated with a significantly lower overall complication rate, particularly a reduction in pulmonary complications, compared with open esophagectomy. Perioperative mortality, R0 resection rate, and the number of retrieved lymph nodes were comparable between the two groups, indicating that RAMIE provided improved short-term outcomes without compromising oncological safety. The long-term follow-up of the RAMIE trial evaluated oncological outcomes after robot-assisted minimally invasive esophagectomy compared with open transthoracic esophagectomy [40]. The study demonstrated no significant differences between the two groups in overall survival, disease-free survival, or patterns of recurrence at 5 years. These findings confirmed that RAMIE achieves long-term oncological outcomes comparable to open surgery while maintaining the advantages of reduced postoperative morbidity observed in the initial randomized trial.

Based on these recent studies, minimally invasive surgery (MIS) has demonstrated its usefulness in patients with stage I–III esophageal cancer. However, with recent advances in neoadjuvant chemotherapy and radiotherapy, the number of patients undergoing conversion surgery for initially unresectable locally advanced esophageal cancer, as well as salvage surgery after definitive chemoradiotherapy, has been increasing. In such complex cases, the safety of MIS has not yet been fully established, and open esophagectomy remains the first-line surgical approach at many institutions.

9.5.2 The Three-Field Lymphadenectomy

The concept of three-field dissection was developed in Japan in the 1980s. In Japan, three-field lymph node dissection, including dissection of the cervical, mediastinal, and abdominal lymph nodes, is the standard procedure for surgically curable esophageal cancer located in the middle or upper thoracic esophagus. Although the effectiveness of extended lymphadenectomy for esophageal cancer has not yet been proven by randomized prospective studies, better survival outcomes have been reported with three-field lymph node dissection than with two-field lymph node dissection in Japan.

The largest study demonstrating the benefits of the three-field lymph node dissection from a single institution was reported by Akiyama et al. in 1994 [6]. The authors performed 393 cases of esophagectomy with a two-field lymph node dissection between 1973 and 1984 and 324 cases of esophagectomy with a three-field lymph node dissection between 1984 and 1993. In both node-negative and node-positive patients, the survival of patients after extensive three-field dissection was significantly better than that after the less extensive two-field dissection. The authors speculated that the differences might be attributable to the removal of occult metastatic lymph nodes in the cervical and other regions, which may have been present and omitted from dissection and analysis in the group with less extensive dissections, but were removed by extensive dissection. The 5-year survival rate of patients with all depth of cancer invasion after extensive three-field and the less extensive two-field dissection were 53.3% and 37.5%, respectively. Although this study was a non-randomized, historical control study, the 5-year survival rate of 53.3% after three-field dissection was remarkable high.

Tsurumaru et al. studied the patterns of lymph node metastasis in cases with only a single node metastasis [10]. A single node metastasis in patients with thoracic esophageal cancer was located in the cervical (14.1%), mediastinal (upper, 31.0%; middle, 11.3%; and lower, 8.5%), and abdominal areas (35.2%). They also studied the state of lymph node metastasis in 5-year survivors of these cases and showed that 14.2% had a single node metastasis in the cervical area, 49.3% had a single node in the mediastinum (upper, 19.4%; middle, 22.4%; and lower 7.5%), and 37.3% had a single node in the abdomen. Even in the presence of cervical or abdominal lymph node metastasis, many patients achieved long-term survival following extended lymphadenectomy.

These results suggested that lymph nodes in the cervical and abdominal areas were regional lymph nodes of the thoracic esophagus. However, these studies were retrospective in nature and subject to significant bias. Nevertheless, only two prospective studies have been published from Japan. One was a prospective randomized trial comparing three-field with two-field lymph node dissection published by Nishihira et al. [8]. They demonstrated a survival benefit for three-field over two-field lymph node dissection (65% vs. 48%); however, the study was limited by a small sample size at a single institution, and the difference did not reach statistically significance. Another prospective study was published from the National Cancer Center in Tokyo [9]. This non-randomized, case-matched trial demonstrated that the 5-year survival rate was significantly higher after three-field dissection than after two- field dissection (48% vs. 33%; $p = 0.03$). The 5-year survival rate among patients with cervical lymph node metastasis was as high as 30%. These findings suggested both a survival benefit of three-field lymphadenectomy and that cervical and abdominal lymph nodes are regional lymph nodes for thoracic esophageal squamous cell carcinoma.

Recent large-scale randomized trials from China indicate that while three-field lymphadenectomy improves nodal staging, it does not confer a survival advantage over two-field lymphadenectomy in middle and lower thoracic esophageal cancer. Li and colleagues conducted a large, multicenter randomized controlled trial comparing three-field lymphadenectomy with two-field lymphadenectomy in patients with middle and lower thoracic esophageal cancer, predominantly squamous cell carcinoma [41]. A total of 400 patients were randomly assigned to undergo either three-field lymphadenectomy or two-field lymphadenectomy. With a median follow-up of approximately 55 months, there was no significant difference in overall survival (OS) between the two groups, with a 5-year OS of 63% in both groups (hazard ratio [HR] 1.019, 95% CI 0.727–1.428; $p = 0.912$). Similarly, disease-free survival (DFS) did not differ significantly (5-year DFS: 59% in the three-field lymphadenectomy group vs. 53% in the two-field lymphadenectomy group; HR 0.868, 95% CI 0.636–1.184; $p = 0.371$). Although three-field lymphadenectomy resulted in a greater number of the retrieved lymph nodes and more frequent detection of cervical lymph node metastases, this did not translate into a survival benefit. The authors concluded that, for middle and lower thoracic esophageal cancer, routine three-field lymphadenectomy does not provide a clear survival advantage over two-field dissection for middle and lower thoracic esophageal cancer.

Mao and colleagues conducted a recent multicenter randomized trial in China (NST-1503) to evaluate whether two-field lymphadenectomy is non-inferior to three-field lymphadenectomy in patients with thoracic esophageal squamous cell carcinoma without clinical right recurrent laryngeal nerve lymph node involvement [42]. This study was designed as a non-inferiority trial, focusing on overall and disease-free survival as primary endpoints. Interim analyses demonstrated that in patients without suspected right recurrent laryngeal nerve lymph node metastasis, two-field lymphadenectomy was non-inferior to three-field lymphadenectomy in terms of both OS and DFS, while reducing the extent of surgery. These findings support a more individualized strategy for lymphadenectomy rather than routine three-field dissection, in selected patients with thoracic esophageal squamous cell carcinoma.

Role of three-field lymph node dissection for adenocarcinoma of the distal third of the esophagus remains unclear. In cases of lower thoracic esophageal carcinoma, lymph node metastasis occurs primarily in the mediastinal and abdominal regions, but metastasis to cervical lymph nodes can also occur at a lower frequency. The prognosis of a patient with cervical lymph node metastases from lower thoracic esophageal carcinoma is extremely poor [1]. Therefore, mediastinal and abdominal lymphadenectomy may be adequate for lower thoracic esophageal carcinoma.

Although the incidence of esophageal cancer is increasing, the number of candidates for curative resection remains limited. Consequently, large-scale prospective randomized trials are difficult to complete within a reasonable timeframe, and the establishment of multi-institutional high-volume randomized studies poses significant challenges.

In summary, the cervical lymph nodes are at a risk of being involved by cancer metastasis from either upper or middle thoracic esophageal cancers. Therefore, three-field lymphadenectomy, including bilateral cervical, mediastinal, and abdominal lymphadenectomy, is recommended. In contrast, for lower thoracic esophageal cancer, the appropriate extent of regional lymphadenectomy may be limited to the mediastinal and abdominal fields.

9.6 Conclusion

There have been many criticisms of the extension of transthoracic esophagectomy. The most common negative reason against extended lymph node dissection was the increase in mortality and morbidity. The effect on postoperative quality of life has been apparent because of the invasiveness of this procedure. Based on recent studies, minimally invasive surgery (MIS) has demonstrated its usefulness in patients with stage I–III esophageal cancer. However, with recent advances in systemic chemotherapy and radiotherapy, the number of patients undergoing conversion surgery for initially unresectable locally advanced esophageal cancer, as well as salvage surgery after definitive chemoradiotherapy, has been increasing. In such complex cases, the safety of MIS has not yet been fully established, and open esophagectomy remains the first-line surgical approach at many institutions.

References

1. Bedenne L, Michel P, Bouche O, et al. Chemoradiation followed by surgery compared with chemoradiation alone in squamous cancer of the esophagus: FFCD 9102. J Clin Oncol. 2007;25:1160–8.
2. Suntharalingam M. Definitive chemoradiation in the management of locally advanced esophageal cancer. Semin Radiat Oncol. 2007;17:22–8.
3. Udagawa H, Akiyama H, et al. Surgical treatment of esophageal cancer: Tokyo experience of the three-field technique. Dis Esophagus. 2001;14:110–4.
4. Vizcaino AP, Moreno V, Lambert R, et al. Time trends incidence of both major histologic types of esophageal carcinoma in selected countries, 1973–1995. Int J Cancer. 2002;99:860–8.
5. Jamal A, Bray F, Center MM, et al. Global cancer statistics. CA Cancer J Clin. 2011;61:69–90.
6. Akiyama H, Tsurumaru M, Udagawa H, et al. Radical lymph node dissection for cancer of the thoracic esophagus. Ann Surg. 1994;220:364–73.
7. Ando N, Ozawa S, Kitagawa Y, et al. Improvement in the results of surgical treatment of advanced squamous esophageal carcinoma during 15 consecutive years. Ann Surg. 2000;232:225–32.
8. Nishihira T, Hirayama K, Mori S. A prospective randomized control trial of extended cervical and superior mediastinal lymphadenectomy for carcinoma of the thoracic esophagus. Am J Surg. 1998;175:47–51.
9. Kato H, Watanabe H, Tachimori Y, et al. Evaluation of the neck lymph node dissection for thoracic esophageal carcinoma. Ann Thorac Surg. 1991;51:931–5.
10. Tsurumaru M, Kajiyama Y, Udagawa H, et al. Outcomes of extended lymph node dissection for squamous cell carcinoma of the thoracic esophagus. Ann Thorac Cardiovas Surg. 2001;7:325–9.

11. Fujita H, Kakegawa T, Yamana H, et al. Mortality and morbidity rates, postoperative course, quality of life, and prognosis after extended radical lymphadenectomy for oesophageal cancer. Comparison of three-field lymphadenectomy with two- field lymphadenectomy. Ann Surg. 1995;222:654–62.
12. Altorki N, Kent M, Ferrara RN, et al. Three-field lymph node dissection for squamous cell and adenocarcinoma of the esophagus. Ann Surg. 2002;236:177–83.
13. Lerut T, Nafteux P, Moons J, et al. Three-field lymphadenectomy for carcinoma of the esophagus and gastroesophageal junction in 174 R0 resections: impact on staging, disease-free survival, and outcome: a plea for adaptation of TNM classification in upper-half esophageal carcinoma. Ann Surg. 2004;240:962–72.
14. Japanese Society for Esophageal Diseases. Japanese classification of esophageal cancer, tenth edition: part I. Esophagus. 2009;6:1–25.
15. Takeuchi H, Miyata H, Gotoh M, et al. A risk model for esophagectomy using data of 5354 patients included in Japanese nationwide web-based database. Ann Surg. 2014;260(2):259–66.
16. Metzer R, Bollschweiler E, Vallbohmer D, et al. High volume centers for esophagectomy: what is the number needed to achieve low postoperative mortality? Dis Esophagus. 2004;17(4):310–4.
17. Rodgers M, Jobe BA, O'Rourke RW, et al. Case volume as a predictor of inpatient mortality after esophagectomy. Arch Durg. 2007;142(9):829–39.
18. Japanese Research Society for Esophageal Diseases. The report of treatment results of esophageal carcinoma in Japan (1979, 1980, 1982, 1982) (in Japanese). 10th ed. Tokyo: National Cancer Center; 2000.
19. Japanese Research Society for Esophageal Diseases. Comprehensive registry of esophageal cancer in Japan (1988~1994). 1st ed. Chiba: Japanese Society for Esophageal Diseases; 2000.
20. Tachimori Y, Ozawa S, Fujishiro M, et al. Comprehensive registry of esophageal cancer in Japan, 2006. Esophagus. 2010;23(2):145–52.
21. Fujita H, Ozawa S, Kuwano H, et al. Esophagectomy for cancer: clinical concerns support centralizing operations within the larger hospitals. Dis Esophagus. 2014;11:21–47.
22. Atkins BZ, Shah AS, Hutcheson KA, et al. Reducing hospital morbidity and mortality following esophagectomy. Ann Thorac Surg. 2004;78(5):1783–9.
23. Ferri LE, Law S, Wong KH, et al. The influence of technical complications on postoperative outcome and survival after esophagectomy. Ann Surg Oncol. 2006;13:557–64.
24. Hulscher JB, van Sandick JW, de Boer AG, et al. Extended transthoracic resection compared with limited transhiatal resection for adenocarcinoma of the esophagus. N Engl J Med. 2002;347:1662–9.
25. Biere SS, van Berg Henegouwen MI, Maas KW, et al. Minimally invasive versus open oesophagectomy for patients with oesophageal cancer; a multicenter, open-label, randomized controlled trial. Lancet. 2012;379:1887–92.
26. Murthy SC, Law S, Whooley BP, et al. Atrial fibrillation after esophagectomy is a marker for postoperative morbidity and mortality. J Thorac Cardiovas Surg. 2003;126:1162–7.
27. Bailey SH, Bull DA, Harpole DH, et al. Outcomes after esophagectomy: a ten-year prospective cohort. Ann Thorac Surg. 2003;75(1):217–22.
28. Martin RE, Letsos P, Taves DH. Oropharyngeal dysphagia in esophageal cancer before and after transhiatal esophagectomy. Dysphagia. 2001;16(1):23–31.
29. Raymond D. Complication of esophagectomy. Sug Clin North Am. 2012;92:1299–313.
30. Berry MF, Atkins BZ, Tong BC, et al. A comprehensive evaluation for aspiration after esophagectomy reduces the incidence of postoperative pneumonia. J Thorac Cardiovas Surg. 2010;140:1266–71.
31. Dumont P, Wihlm JM, Hentz JG, et al. Respiratory complications after surgical treatment of esophageal cancer. A study of 309 patients according to the type of resection. Eur J Cardiothorac Surg. 1995;9:539–43.
32. Baba M, Natsugoe S, Shimada M, et al. Dose hoarseness of voice from recurrent nerve paralysis after esophagectomy for carcinoma influence patient quality of life? J Am Coll Surg. 1999;188:231–6.

33. Kamiya S, Nishiwaki N, Hachimaru A, et al. Indocyanine green fluorescent lymphography for detection of thoracic duct leakage after esophagectomy. Ann Thorac Surg. 2009;88:1345–8.
34. Kaburagi T, Takeuchi H, Kawakubo H, et al. Intraoperative identification of thoracic duct with indocyanine green fluorescence imaging in esophageal cancer surgery. Ann Surg Oncol. 2013;20:640–5.
35. Matsutani T, Hagiwara N, Yokoyama Y, et al. Fluorescent lymphography using indocyanine green to identify chyle leakage during surgery for postoperative chylothorax after esophagectomy. Surg Endosc. 2014;28:3314–9.
36. Biere SSAY, van Berge Henegouwen MI, Maas KW, et al. Minimally invasive versus open oesophagectomy for patients with oesophageal cancer: a multicentre, open-label, randomised controlled trial (TIME trial). Lancet. 2012;379:1887–92.
37. Mariette C, Markar SR, Dabakuyo-Yonli TS, et al. Hybrid minimally invasive esophagectomy for esophageal cancer (MIRO trial). N Engl J Med. 2019;380:152–62.
38. Takeuchi H, Kataoka K, Mizusawa J, et al. Thoracoscopic versus open esophagectomy for patients with resectable thoracic esophageal cancer: a randomized phase III non-inferiority trial (JCOG1409, MONET trial). Lancet Gastroenterol Hepatol. 2025;10(12):1104–16.
39. van der Sluis PC, van der Horst S, May AM, et al. Robot-assisted minimally invasive thoraco-laparoscopic esophagectomy versus open transthoracic esophagectomy for resectable esophageal cancer: a randomized controlled trial (RAMIE trial). Ann Surg. 2019;269:621–30.
40. de Groot EM, van der Sluis PC, Ruurda JP, et al. Long-term oncologic outcomes of robot-assisted minimally invasive esophagectomy versus open transthoracic esophagectomy. Ann Surg. 2021;274:569–76.
41. Li B, Zhang Y, Miao L, et al. Esophagectomy with three-field versus two-field lymphadenectomy for middle and lower thoracic esophageal cancer: long-term outcomes of a randomized clinical trial. J Thorac Oncol. 2021;16:310–7.
42. Mao Y, Chen Y, Zhou J, et al. Three-field versus two-field lymphadenectomy in thoracic esophageal squamous cell carcinoma: a multicenter randomized non-inferiority trial (NST-1503). J Natl Cancer Cent. 2025;5(2):203–11.

Surgery: Minimally Invasive Esophagectomy and Robot Assisted Esophagectomy

10

Kazuo Koyanagi

10.1 Introduction

Multimodal treatment modalities have led to improved oncologic outcomes in patients with esophageal squamous cell carcinoma (ESCC) [1, 2]. The usefulness of chemoradiotherapy and perioperative adjuvant chemotherapy has been demonstrated; however, esophagectomy remains the mainstay as curative treatment for patients with localized ESCC. Transthoracic esophagectomy with radical lymph node dissection is established and adopted as the standard surgical procedure and was reported to improve disease control and survival for ESCC [3–5].

Although there have been remarkable advances in perioperative management, esophagectomy is a complex and highly invasive operative procedure among the gastrointestinal surgeries; consequently, the operative morbidity and mortality associated with esophagectomy have been major concerns [6]. A long thoracotomy incision and one-lung ventilation during esophagectomy are thought to be partly responsible for the high surgical invasiveness of this procedure and subsequent respiratory complications.

Since 1990s, thoracoscopic and/or laparoscopic surgery has been attracting attention as a less invasive approach for the treatment of ESCC [7, 8]. Cuschieri et al. first reported a thoracoscopic minimally invasive esophagectomy (MIE) in 1992 [9], then many surgeons have been interested in performing the procedure, because MIE has the potential to lower the morbidity associated with the resection and to enable a quicker return to normal function. Also, this increase in MIE can be attributable to technical advances in endoscopic equipment for thoracoscopic surgery, including dissectors, ultrasonic coagulating shears, and vessel-sealing

K. Koyanagi (✉)
Department of Gastroenterological Surgery, Tokai University School of Medicine, Isehara, Kanagawa, Japan
e-mail: kkoyanagi@tokai.ac.jp

Y. Kitagawa et al. (eds.), *Esophageal Squamous Cell Carcinoma*,
https://doi.org/10.1007/978-981-92-2611-5_10

systems, which are now available for thoracoscopic esophagus resection with extended mediastinal lymphadenectomy.

Moreover, with the recent introduction of robot-assisted minimally invasive esophagectomy (RAMIE), it is expected that esophagectomy with fewer complications will be performed [10]. The potential advantages of this technological innovation are thought to allow surgeons to carry out minimally invasive procedures more precisely and ergonomically, compared with MIE. Robotic techniques may be most suitable for esophagectomy, because the esophagus is located in the mediastinum adjacent to vital organs, requiring extremely precise and delicate manipulation.

In this chapter, the establishment of MIE and the current trend toward RAMIE in esophageal cancer surgery will be described.

10.2 Overview of MIE and RAMIE

10.2.1 Terminology

To date, several thoracoscopic and laparoscopic approaches for resection of thoracic esophageal cancer have been defined as MIE, based on tumor location, clinical stage, and patient demographics [11]. Although total thoracoscopic and laparoscopic esophagectomy represent (total) MIE in a narrow sense, thoracoscopic procedures, mini-thoracotomy procedures, and laparoscopic procedures are all included in the scope of MIE. Hybrid MIE is defined as esophagectomy using either a thoracoscopic or laparoscopic approach. Transhiatal esophagectomy under mediastinoscopy was developed primarily for resection of esophageal or esophagogastric junction adenocarcinoma arising from Barrett's esophagus [12]. For esophagogastric anastomosis after thoracoscopic esophagectomy, cervical anastomosis or intrathoracic anastomosis with the Ivor Lewis procedure was applied in clinical practice. Recently, some surgical robot systems have been developed by several companies and are being clinically applied at MIE [13]. More recently, non-transthoracic radical esophagectomy both with transcervical and transhiatal approaches using surgical robot system was developed with feasible surgical outcomes. Esophagectomy using robot surgical systems are collectively referred to as RAMIE. This chapter focuses on explaining MIE and RAMIE using a transthoracic approach.

10.2.2 History

Since the first report of thoracoscopic esophagectomy by Cuschieri et al. in 1992 where the prone position was adopted, MIE has become increasingly popular and was performed widely. In 1993, the first mediastinoscope-assisted blunt dissection of the esophagus was reported [14]. Meanwhile, in Japan, Sadanaga et al. reported the first laparoscopic transhiatal esophagectomy in 1994 [15]. Akaishi et al. reported the first use of thoracoscopic total esophagectomy with en bloc mediastinal lymphadenectomy in 1996 [16]. In 1999, Kawahara et al. provided the details of thoracoscopic esophagectomy with extended lymphadenectomy [17], and Osugi et al. described the long-term survival of 77 patients with ESCC in 2003 [18].

The first robotic system became available in 1998 [19], and the da Vinci Surgical System (Intuitive Surgical, Inc., Sunnyvale, CA, USA) was approved by the United States Food and Drug Administration in 2000 [20]. The first case of robot-assisted esophagectomy for esophageal carcinoma reported in the literature was carried out by Horgan et al. in 2001 [21], in which their procedure was a transhiatal esophagectomy. Robot-assisted thoracoscopic esophagectomy was first reported in 2004 by Kernstine et al. [22], whereas, in Japan, robot-assisted transthoracic esophagectomy was introduced by Uyama et al. in 2009 [23]. Since its inclusion in the insurance coverage in 2018, the number of robot-assisted esophagectomy cases in Japan has been increasing rapidly.

10.2.3 Indication

The surgical indications for MIE and RAMIE are almost the same. They are currently used for locally advanced esophageal cancer, even after neoadjuvant or definitive chemoradiotherapy as reported in several studies. In general, contraindications for the MIE and RAMIE procedure may include severe pleural adhesion, bulky or locally infiltrative tumors (especially those in close proximity with the tracheabronchial tree, pulmonary vein, and aorta) [11]. Recently, MIE and RAMIE have become increasingly applicable to conversion surgery performed when organ invasion is resolved by induction therapy.

10.2.4 Patient Position

To date, two patient positions were used for MIE: the left lateral decubitus position (LLDP), similar to that adopted for right transthoracic open esophagectomy (OE) and the prone position. The differences between the two positions in MIE were discussed in the literature [11].

The most significant advantage of the prone position is that it provides a good surgical field: The view of the posterior mediastinum, including the esophagus, can be obtained without any retraction of the right lung using a retractor or sutures, and blood pooling does not obscure the surgical field. The middle mediastinal organs and right lung naturally fall away because of the gravity and the additional carbon dioxide insufflation of the thoracic cavity in the prone position [24]. The LLDP, on the other hand, requires skillful retraction of the right lung by assistants to obtain the appropriate surgical field. In addition, prone position was considered to have several theoretical physiological and ergonomic advantages for both the patient and the surgeon. The prone position is well known to be beneficial for arterial oxygenation [25]. Furthermore, since the surgeon can operate in a plane parallel to the camera and the ports used by the operator are located at the elbow level of the surgeon, the ergonomics and fatigue experienced by the surgeon may be improved in the prone position.

However, the prone position is still considered problematic in terms of safety, since it is technically difficult to perform urgent conversion to right thoracotomy in emergency situations such as sudden massive bleeding. To resolve this issue, the left semi-prone position was utilized [26]. This position enables safe and precise extended lymphadenectomy in the optimal position (e.g., LLDP or prone position) by rotating the operating table.

Robotic esophagectomy can also take either position. When robot surgical systems were first introduced, each institute that performed MIE in the LLDP also adopted the same position for RAMIE in consideration of safety. However, as surgeons became more accustomed to operating robots, the prone position came to be adopted more frequently. This is mainly because operating a robotic arm is considered more suitable in the prone position, and because the number of robotic arms available has increased, making it possible to perform solo-surgery without the need for an assistant.

10.2.5 LN Dissection

Since lymph node (LN) metastases occur primarily from the cervical to the abdominal field, especially in ESCC, importance of extended LN dissection includes the dissection of upper mediastinal nodes along bilateral recurrent laryngeal nerves (RLNs) has been emphasized in Japan. In the 1980s, the three-field LN dissection during transthoracic esophagectomy, a procedure for cervico-thoraco-abdominal LN dissection, was established. Currently, this procedure is widely accepted worldwide [27]. This upper mediastinal lymphadenectomy along bilateral RLNs is also feasible, even with MIE and RAMIE [28]. MIE and RAMIE can offer magnified surgical view and precise surgical techniques, which are expected to improve the accuracy of mediastinal LN dissection compared to OE.

10.2.6 Reconstruction Procedure

In general, a gastric conduit is used as reconstructed organ after MIE and RAMIE as well as OE. Reconstruction after esophagectomy must be technically safe and easy to perform. In that regard, intrathoracic esophagogastric anastomosis is considered superior to cervical esophagogastric anastomosis, associated with a lower incidence of anastomotic leakage and a better cosmetic effect in patients undergoing OE with two-field lymphadenectomy. However, during reconstruction after MIE and RAMIE, esophagogastric anastomosis is preferred in the cervical portion, since intrathoracic esophagogastric anastomoses are technically difficult during minimally invasive procedures with circular or linear staplers. Several research groups, including ours, have developed an easy and secure minimally invasive intrathoracic esophagogastric anastomosis procedure [29]. These anastomosis procedures use a circular stapler with transoral placement of the anvil or linear staplers and can be applied after Ivor Lewis MIE and RAMIE.

10.2.7 Advantage and Disadvantage of RAMIE

The da Vinci Surgical System is the most widely used as robot surgical system in the world and its features are described below.

The functional advantages of the da Vinci system include improved stereoscopic visibility through high-resolution 3D imaging, multi-joint functionality, hand tremor prevention, and motion scaling (Fig. 10.1). Transthoracic surgery using thoracoscope differs from abdominal surgery in that the bony thoracic cage, including the ribs and vertebrae, makes it difficult to obtain a wide surgical field, and further limits the surgeon's forceps manipulation. In esophageal cancer surgery, injury to vital organs can lead to severe complications, but with robot surgical system, improved surgical instrument maneuverability enables precise procedures, and a reduction in intraoperative and postoperative complications is expected.

LN dissection around the recurrent laryngeal nerve is extremely important from the perspective of curative treatment, but on the other hand, postoperative recurrent laryngeal nerve palsy carries the risk of significantly impairing quality of life in daily life. High-resolution 3D images are useful for understanding local anatomy during lymph node dissection. Additionally, the multi-joint function can overcome the difficulty sometimes encountered when using linear forceps in MIE. While delicate manipulation is required around nerves, the tremor reduction function and motion scale function are considered effective.

The advantages of robot surgical system are also recognized in middle and lower mediastinal procedures. In particular, the multi-joint functionality is a useful feature for left-sided esophageal dissection. Suturing and ligation procedures are also much smoother than in MIE, and improvements in surgeon ergonomics are expected. MIE

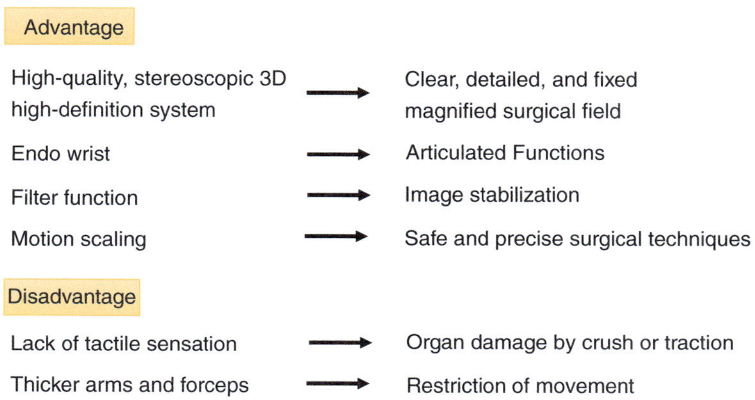

Fig. 10.1 Advantages and disadvantages of surgical robot system

is considered a patient-friendly procedure due to its small incisions, whereas RAMIE is expected to be a surgeon-friendly procedure as well, due to its high level of ergonomics.

On the other hand, one of the disadvantages is that robotic forceps lack tactile sensation. It is necessary to pay close attention to organ damage caused by crushing or excessive traction due to the grip of robotic forceps. In addition, the robot arms and forceps are thicker than conventional ones, and this can cause interference between them outside or inside the patient's body, leading to movement restrictions. This interference can cause unexpected movements of the robotic forceps and may lead to organ injury. Careful consideration must be given to port placement and arm settings. The arm closest to the patient's head is likely to come into contact with the patient's right arm, in which case this arm may not be operable during lower mediastinal procedures.

10.3 Our Procedure of MIE and RAMIE

10.3.1 Preceding Anterior Approach

Considering the possibility of emergency thoracotomy, the patient is first fixed in a left semi-lateral decubitus position and then turned into a prone position using bed rotation (Fig. 10.2). In RAMIE, rather than placing the patient in a completely prone position, slightly raising the right chest improves the operability of the robot arm and facilitates management of the endotracheal tube by the anesthesiologist (Fig. 10.3).

As we have previously proposed, based on the theory that the prone position maximizes the effects of gravity, MIE and RAMIE employ a preceding anterior approach, which involves prior processing of the ventral side of the esophagus. Also, because thorough LN dissection around bilateral recurrent laryngeal nerves could contribute to a favorable prognosis, we perform upper mediastinal LN dissection prior to middle and lower mediastinal dissection. Therefore, mediastinal

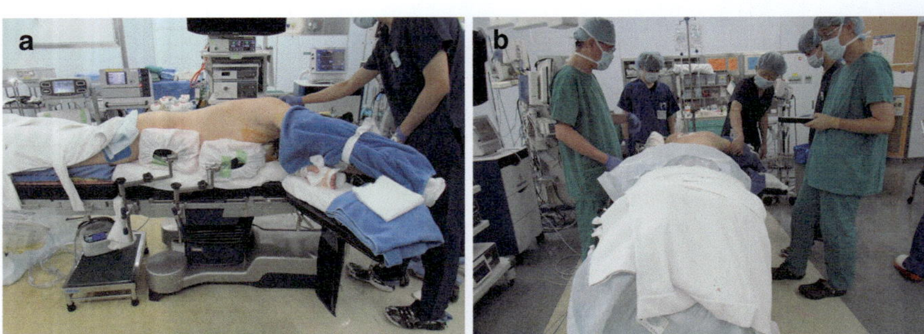

Fig. 10.2 Patient position. (**a**) Left semi-lateral decubitus position; (**b**) turn into a prone position using bed rotation

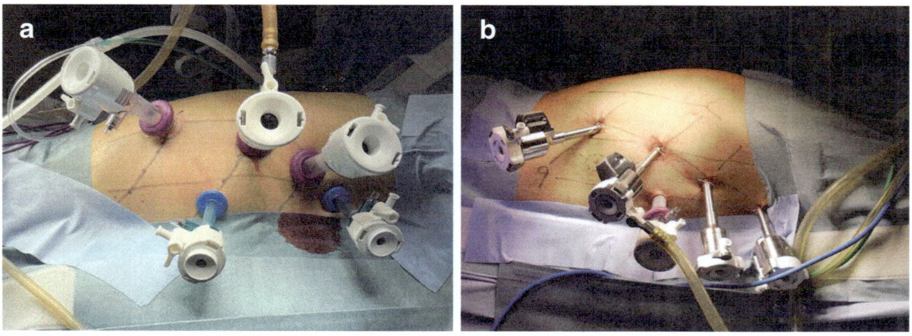

Fig. 10.3 Port placement. (**a**) MIE: 9th intercostal space (ICS) on the inferior scapular angle line, 7th ICS on the posterior axially line, 7th ICS on the middle axially line, 5th ICS on the posterior axially line, 3rd ICS on the middle axially line; (**b**) RAMIE: it is almost the same as MIE, but an assistant port is inserted at the 6th ICS on middle axillary line

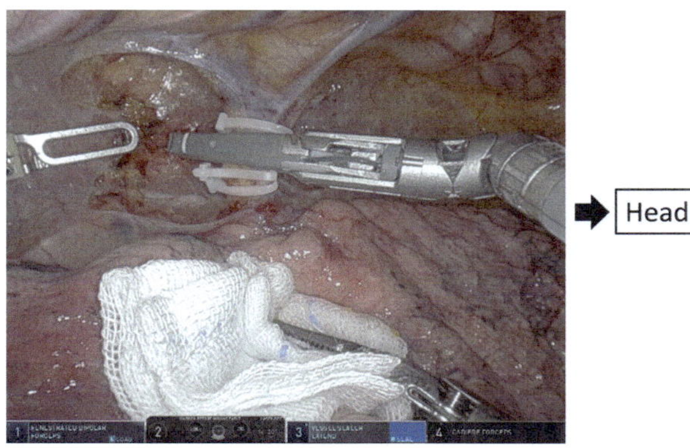

Fig. 10.4 Resection of azygous vein

procedures are performed in the following order: (1) ventral upper mediastinum esophagus, (2) dorsal upper mediastinum esophagus, (3) ventral middle and lower mediastinum esophagus, and (4) dorsal middle and lower mediastinum esophagus. In the case of RAMIE, the azygos vein is first dissected (Fig. 10.4). Subsequently, by dissecting around the right bronchial artery, the ventral side of the esophagus in the mediastinum is exposed, making it easier to obtain the gravity effect of the prone position.

10.3.2 LN Dissection Along the Right Recurrent Nerve

We identify the right vagus nerve running across the right bronchial artery, incise the mediastinal pleura on the ventral side of the upper mediastinal esophagus, and confirm the right vagus nerve cephalad to the right subclavian artery. Then, we incise the pleura over the right subclavian artery and expose the arterial wall. By performing dissection between the upper esophagus and tracheobronchial region in

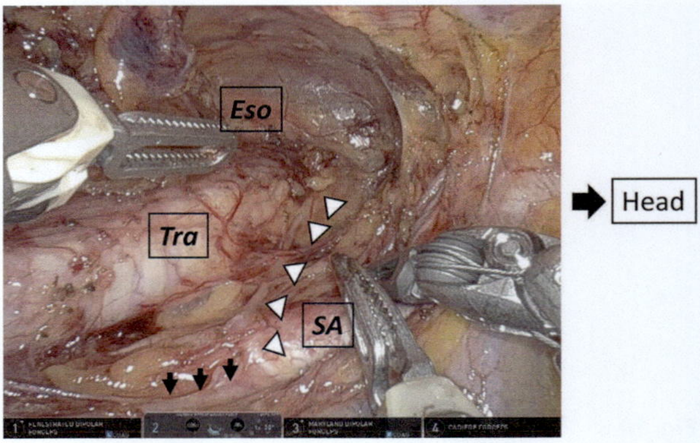

Fig. 10.5 LN dissection along right recurrent laryngeal nerve: arrows, right vagal nerve; arrow heads, right recurrent laryngeal nerve; Eso esophagus, Tra trachea, SA subclavian artery

the direction of the cervical portion, it is possible to mesenterize the fat tissue containing the right recurrent laryngeal nerve and surrounding LNs. Next, we expose the right recurrent laryngeal nerve while retracting the fatty tissue and performing LN dissection. At this point, it is necessary to carefully handle small blood vessels from the neck to avoid unnecessary bleeding. RAMIE provides a very clear and magnified surgical field, so care must be taken to sharply dissect the tissue surrounding the nerves and avoid excessive traction or damage to the right recurrent laryngeal nerve. If there are no anatomical or oncological difficulties, it is usually possible to perform a radical resection from the thoracic cavity to the right neck (Fig. 10.5).

10.3.3 LN Dissection Along the Left Recurrent Nerve

Incising the pleura on the dorsal side of the upper esophagus, the upper esophagus is pulled toward the right thoracic cavity, and dissection is continued until the aortic arch and left subclavian artery are visible. The thoracic duct is preserved if there is no tumor infiltration around the thoracic duct. After sufficiently dissecting the upper esophagus from the posterior mediastinum, we pull up the upper esophagus toward the patient's back. Dissecting the left side of the tracheobronchial tree as much as possible will make it easier to retract the esophagus. Using double taping technique to pull the esophagus and a robotic arm to compress the tracheobronchial tree, it is possible to spread the fat tissue containing the left recurrent laryngeal nerve and surrounding LNs widely between the esophagus and trachea (Fig. 10.6a). In RAMIE, the lymphatic tissue between the left recurrent laryngeal nerve and the trachea is usually dissected as a lymphatic chain. The left recurrent laryngeal nerve is identified and traced to the aortic arch to confirm. After LN dissection, we sharply dissect the esophageal branch of the recurrent laryngeal nerve,

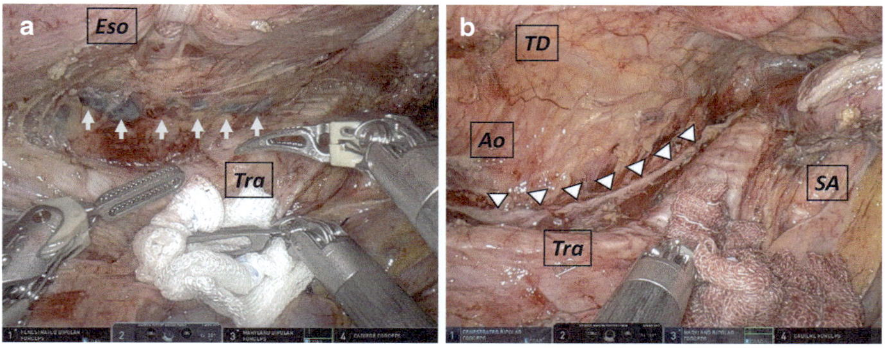

Fig. 10.6 LN dissection along left recurrent laryngeal nerve. (**a**) Double taping technique and mesenterization between esophagus and trachea: arrows, lymphatic chain along left recurrent laryngeal nerve. (**b**) Completion LN dissection along left recurrent laryngeal nerve: arrow heads, left recurrent laryngeal nerve; Tra trachea, SA subclavian artery, Ao aortic arch, TD thoracic duct

then transect the upper esophagus, and complete the upper mediastinal procedure (Fig. 10.6b).

10.3.4 LN Dissection of the Ventral Side of the Middle and Lower Mediastinal Esophagus

By dissecting the esophageal branch of the right vagus nerve, it becomes easier to perform procedures on the ventral side of the middle and lower mediastinum. After dissecting the pleura on the ventral side of the middle and lower mediastinal esophagus, we perform the dissection between the esophagus and pericardium until the contralateral pleura is visible. LN dissection around the esophageal hiatus is performed, and then the tracheal bifurcation and left and right main bronchia LN dissection are performed (Fig. 10.7).

10.3.5 LN Dissection of the Dorsal Side of the Middle and Lower Mediastinal Esophagus

By dissecting the pleura on the dorsal side of the esophagus in the middle and lower mediastinum, the esophagus can be pulled into the right thoracic cavity. The esophageal artery should be carefully handled to fully expose the descending aorta. While having an assistant pull on the esophageal anal end as needed, we resect the esophageal branch of the left vagus nerve, expose the left pleura, and perform LN dissection up to the diaphragm.

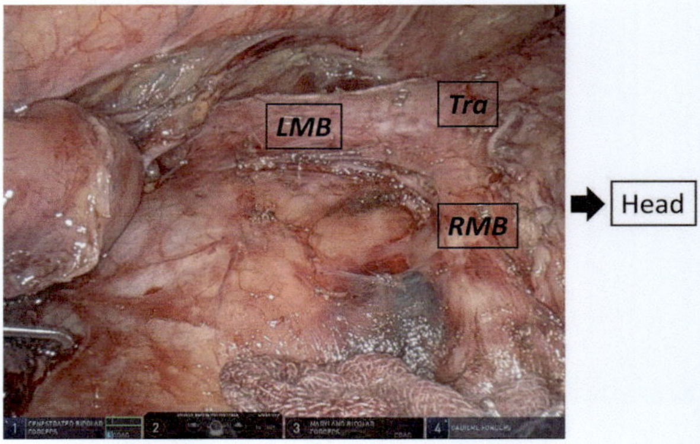

Fig. 10.7 Tracheal bifurcation and left and right main bronchia LN dissection: Tra trachea, LMB left main bronchus, RMB right main bronchus

10.4 Surgical Outcome of MIE

10.4.1 MIE

A study group in Europe reported the results of the first multicenter randomized control trial (RCT), the TIME trial, that compared MIE with OE [30]. The primary outcome of the TIME trial was the incidence of pulmonary infections within the first 2 weeks after surgery and during the entire hospital stay. The RCT randomly assigned 56 patients to the OE group and 59 patients to the MIE group. MIE was performed by right thoracoscopy with the patient in the prone position using single-lumen tracheal intubation, upper abdominal laparoscopy, and cervical incision. To maintain partial collapse of the right lung during thoracoscopy, the thoracic cavity was insufflated with 8 mmHg carbon dioxide. The MIE and OE procedures included two-field esophagectomy with gastric conduit formation followed by cervical or intrathoracic anastomosis. The incidence of pulmonary infection was considerably lower in the MIE group than the OE group, both within the first 2 weeks after surgery and during the entire hospital stay. MIE was also beneficial with lower operative blood loss, better postoperative quality of life, and shorter hospital stay; however, the 30-day and the in-hospital mortality rates did not differ significantly between the groups. Pathological parameters such as the number of retrieved LNs did not differ markedly between the two groups. These findings provided evidence for the short-term benefits of MIE in patients with esophageal cancer. Regarding long-term survival, subsequent reports showed no significant differences in disease-free and overall 3-year survival rates between MIE and OE [31].

Regarding the number of retrieved mediastinal and/or total LNs, most studies demonstrated that MIE was almost equivalent to OE [32], whereas a meta-analysis emphasized that the number of retrieved LNs was significantly higher with MIE compared with OE [33].

Several studies have compared the short-term outcomes in MIE with those of OE using nationwide or prospective data (Table 10.2) [34–36]. These studies reported that although MIE was associated with lower rates of respiratory complications than

OE, the overall rate of surgical complications was higher with MIE compared to OE. In institutions with limited experience using MIE, the rate of surgical complications may be especially higher for MIE than for OE. MIE is commonly categorized as a high-skilled operation and should especially be performed by skilled surgeons.

Recently, Japan Clinical Oncology Group conducted the multicenter randomized phase III trial that compared surgical outcomes between MIE and OE [37]. Eligible patients were cStage I–III, excluding T4, thoracic ESCC, and the primary endpoint was overall survival, with secondary endpoints including relapse-free survival, the proportion of R0 resection, adverse events, postoperative respiratory dysfunction and quality of life score. A total of 300 patients were randomly assigned into MIE and OE. They demonstrated non-inferiority of MIE to OE regarding overall survival and also better 3-year relapse-free survival in MIE compared to OE [38]. R0 resection proportions were higher in MIE, and perioperative morbidities were equivalent between two arms. The proportion of respiratory dysfunction at 3 months after surgery was lower in MIE than in OE. Although skillful esophageal surgeons in Japan were involved in the study and therefore there might be a potential difference from clinical practice in real world, MIE has been shown to enable more precise surgical techniques and offer advantages in terms of postoperative recovery for patients; therefore, MIE should be expected to become more widely used as the standard surgical procedure for ESCC.

10.4.2 RAMIE

As RAMIE became more popular, surgical outcomes have improved compared to when it was first introduced. Operative time and blood loss have been reduced, and the number of harvested lymph nodes has increased. Postoperative complications, such as pulmonary complications, anastomotic leakage, and recurrent laryngeal nerve paralysis, were feasible [39–42] (Table 10.1). Indications for RAMIE are similar to those for MIE, and recent papers report that robotic esophagectomy is feasible for patients with a high body mass index [43], the elderly [44], and patients undergoing neoadjuvant chemoradiotherapy [45]. Regarding the learning curve, significant reduction in total operative time was identified after the initial 20 or 30 cases [46, 47].

The first RCT to validate the efficacy of RAMIE was conducted in Europe. The ROBOT trial compared RAMIE to OE regarding postoperative morbidity, mortality, and survival [48]. A total of 112 patients were randomized. The primary endpoint was the percentage of overall surgery-related postoperative complications. The overall complication rate was significantly lower in the RAMIE group, which was likely attributable to significantly lower rates of pulmonary complications and cardiac complications. Furthermore, RAMIE was associated with less intraoperative blood loss, lower postoperative pain scores, faster functional recovery, and better quality of life when compared to OE. Regarding long-term survival, subsequent reports showed that overall survival did not differ between the groups, indicating

Table 10.1 Surgical outcomes of RAMIE at a single institute after standardization of the procedure

Author	No. of cases	Operation time (min)	Blood loss (mL)	Hospital stay (days)	No. of retrieved LN	Respiratory complications (%)	Anastomotic leakage (%)	Recurrent laryngeal nerve paralysis (%)
Boone et al. [39]	47	450	625	18	29	45	21	19
Puntambekar et al. [40]	83	205	87	10	18	1	4	2
Cerfolio et al. [41]	85	360	35	8	22	7	4	NA
Park et al. [42]	114	420	309	16	44	10	15	26

RAMIE robot-assisted minimally invasive esophagectomy, *LN* lymph node, *NA* not available that RAMIE offers short-term benefits while maintaining the high oncological standards of an open esophagectomy [49].

The RAMIE trial was designed as a prospective, multicenter, randomized, controlled clinical trial that compares the efficacy and safety of RAMIE and MIE in the treatment of resectable ESCC [50]. Early results demonstrate that both RAMIE and MIE are safe and feasible for the treatment of ESCC. This trial showed RAMIE can achieve shorter operative duration and better LN dissection in patients who received neoadjuvant therapy. Long-term results are pending for further follow-up investigations.

The REVATE trial was performed to compare the efficacy and safety of RAMIE versus MIE in patients with ESCC [51]. The primary endpoint was the success rate of left recurrent laryngeal nerve LN dissection. Success was defined as the removal of at least one LN without causing nerve damage lasting longer than 6 months. Secondary endpoints were perioperative and oncological outcomes. In the trial, MIE leads to more successful left recurrent laryngeal nerve LN dissection than MIE, including a lower rate of short- and long-term recurrent laryngeal nerve injury. Postoperative complication rates were comparable between the two groups and there were no in-hospital deaths.

In Japan, insurance coverage for RAMIE started in 2018, and then the number of RAMIE cases has been increasing. Using the Japanese National Clinical Database, registered as esophageal malignant tumors between October 2018 and December 2019, the propensity score matching study was conducted to compare the RAMIE and MIE [52]. The primary outcome measure was postoperative complications. The RAMIE group had a significantly longer operation time and greater blood loss than the MIE group. Furthermore, the R0 resection rate was lower in the RAMIE group than in the MIE. However, RAMIE and MIE demonstrated comparable morbidity rates when performed by skilled board-certified endoscopic surgeons. This study demonstrated that RAMIE was safely introduced in Japan after insurance coverage.

10.5 Future Prospects

MIE has been shown to be useful from RCTs in terms of minimally invasiveness, reduction of postoperative complications, and maintenance of quality of life (QOL), and is recognized as the standard surgery for ESCC. RAMIE has some advantages that complement the motion restriction of conventional MIE, and it is expected that the number of procedures will increase in the future from the perspective of improving surgeon ergonomics and shortening the learning curve. However, RAMIE is still in its infancy, and there are several issues that need to be clarified.

First, there is still no clear statistical significance when compared to MIE, especially in terms of long-term prognosis. Second, it is necessary to establish an educational system for the widespread use of RAMIE. Third, there is a need to improve surgical procedures by further reducing the diameter of the robotic arm and forceps. Fourth, high costs are a major problem in hospital management, and improvements in profitability are required. Finally, we hope that these challenges will be overcome and that remote surgery using RAMIE will become a reality.

References

1. Higuchi T, Shoji Y, Koyanagi K, et al. Multimodal treatment strategies to improve the prognosis of locally advanced thoracic esophageal squamous cell carcinoma: a narrative review. Cancers. 2023;15:10.
2. Booka E, Takeuchi H, Suda K, et al. Meta-analysis of the impact of postoperative complications on survival after oesophagectomy for cancer. BJS Open. 2018;2:276–84.
3. Ando N, Ozawa S, Kitagawa Y, et al. Improvement in the results of surgical treatment of advanced squamous esophageal carcinoma during 15 consecutive years. Ann Surg. 2000;232:225–32.
4. Akiyama H, Tsurumaru M, Udagawa H, et al. Radical lymph node dissection for cancer of the thoracic esophagus. Ann Surg. 1994;220:364–72.
5. Isono K, Sato H, Nakayama K. Results of a nationwide study on the three-field lymph node dissection of esophageal cancer. Oncology. 1991;48:411–20.
6. Booka E, Takeuchi H, Nishi T, et al. The impact of postoperative complications on survivals after esophagectomy for esophageal cancer. Medicine (Baltimore). 2015;94:e1369.
7. Koyanagi K, Tabuchi S, Kato T, et al. Stapled resection for bronchogenic cyst of the esophagus performing using video-assisted thoracic surgery. Esophagus. 2011;8:191–5.
8. Koyanagi K, Nakagawa M, Ozawa S, et al. Thoracoscopic enucleation for small-sized gastrointestinal stromal tumor of the esophagus: report of two cases. Esophagus. 2010;7:219–24.
9. Cuschieri A, Shimi S, Banting S. Endoscopic oesophagectomy through a right thoracoscopic approach. J R Coll Surg. 1992;37:7–11.
10. Seto Y, Mori K, Aikou S. Robotic surgery for esophageal cancer: merits and demerits. Ann Gastroenterol Surg. 2017;1:193–8.
11. Koyanagi K, Ozawa S, Tachimori Y. Minimally invasive esophagectomy performed with the patient in a prone position: a systematic review. Surg Today. 2016;46:275–84.
12. Shoji Y, Kanamori K, Koyanagi K, et al. Conversion surgery for esophageal and esophagogastric junction cancer. Int J Clin Oncol. 2024;29:1777–84.
13. Nakauchi M, Uyama I, Suda K, et al. Robotic surgery for the upper gastrointestinal tract: current status and future perspectives. Asian J Endosc Surg. 2017;10:354–63.
14. Bumm R, Holscher AH, Feussner H, et al. Endodissection of the thoracic esophagus. Technique and clinical results in transhiatal esophagectomy. Ann Surg. 1993;218:97–104.
15. Sadanaga N, Kuwano H, Watanabe M, et al. Laparoscopy-assisted surgery: a new technique for transhiatal esophageal dissection. Am J Surg. 1994;168:355–7.
16. Akaishi T, Kaneda I, Higuchi N, et al. Thoracoscopic en bloc total esophagectomy with radical mediastinal lymphadenectomy. J Thorac Cardiovasc Surg. 1996;112:1533–40.
17. Kawahara K, Maekawa T, Okabayashi K, et al. Video-assisted thoracoscopic esophagectomy for esophageal cancer. Surg Endosc. 1999;13:218–23.
18. Osugi H, Takemura M, Higashino M, et al. A comparison of video-assisted thoracoscopic oesophagectomy and radical lymph node dissection for squamous cell cancer of the oesophagus with open operation. Br J Surg. 2003;90:108–13.
19. Broeders IA, Ruurda JP. Robotics in laparoscopic surgery: current status and future perspectives. Scand J Gastroenterol. 2002;37(236):76–80.
20. Watson TJ. Robotic esophagectomy: is it an advance and what is the future? Ann Thorac Surg. 2008;85:S757–9.
21. Horgan S, Berger RA, Elli EF, et al. Robotic-assisted minimally invasive transhiatal esophagectomy. Am Surg. 2003;69:624–6.

22. Kernstine KH, DeArmond DT, Karimi M, et al. The robotic, 2-stage, 3-field esophagolymphadenectomy. J Thorac Cardiovasc Surg. 2004;127:1847–9.
23. Suda K, Nakauchi M, Inaba K, et al. Robotic surgery for upper gastrointestinal cancer: current status and future perspectives. Dig Endosc. 2016;28:701–13.
24. Palanivelu C, Prakash A, Senthilkumar R, et al. Minimally invasive esophagectomy: thoracoscopic mobilization of the esophagus and mediastinal lymphadenectomy in prone position–experience of 130 patients. J Am Coll Surg. 2006;203:7–16.
25. Yatabe T, Kitagawa H, Yamashita K, et al. Better postoperative oxygenation in thoracoscopic esophagectomy in prone positioning. J Anesth. 2010;24:803–6.
26. Takeuchi H, Oyama T, Saikawa Y, et al. Novel thoracoscopic intrathoracic esophagogastric anastomosis technique for patients with esophageal cancer. J Laparoendosc Adv Surg Tech A. 2012;22:88–92.
27. Matsuda S, Takeuchi H, Kawakubo H, et al. Three-field lymph node dissection in esophageal cancer surgery. J Thorac Dis. 2017;9:731–40.
28. Ozawa S, Ito E, Kazuno A, et al. Thoracoscopic esophagectomy while in a prone position for esophageal cancer: a preceding anterior approach method. Surg Endosc. 2013;27:40–7.
29. Shoji Y, Nakashima R, Tajima K, et al. Near-infrared fluorescence clip guided robot-assisted minimally invasive esophagectomy for esophagogastric junction cancer: a case report. Discov Med. 2024;1:31.
30. Biere SS, van Berge Henegouwen MI, Maas KW, et al. Minimally invasive versus open oesophagectomy for patients with oesophageal cancer: a multicentre, open-label, randomised controlled trial. Lancet. 2012;379:1887–92.
31. Straatman J, van der Wielen N, Cuesta MA, et al. Minimally invasive versus open esophageal resection: three-year follow-up of the previously reported randomized controlled trial: the TIME trial. Ann Surg. 2017;266:232–6.
32. Koyanagi K, Igaki H, Iwabu J, et al. Recurrent laryngeal nerve paralysis after esophagectomy: respiratory complications and role of nerve reconstruction. Tohoku J Exp Med. 2015;237:1–8.
33. Dantoc M, Cox MR, Eslick GD. Evidence to support the use of minimally invasive esophagectomy for esophageal cancer: a meta-analysis. Arch Surg. 2012;147:768–76.
34. Seesing MFJ, Gisbertz SS, Goense L, et al. A propensity score matched analysis of open versus minimally invasive transthoracic esophagectomy in The Netherlands. Ann Surg. 2017;266:839–46.
35. Mamidanna R, Bottle A, Aylin P, et al. Short-term outcomes following open versus minimally invasive esophagectomy for cancer in England: a population-based national study. Ann Surg. 2012;255:197–203.
36. Nozaki I, Mizusawa J, Kato K, et al. Impact of laparoscopy on the prevention of pulmonary complications after thoracoscopic esophagectomy using data from JCOG0502: a prospective multicenter study. Surg Endosc. 2018;32:651–9.
37. Kataoka K, Takeuchi H, Mizusawa J, et al. A randomized phase III trial of thoracoscopic versus open esophagectomy for thoracic esophageal cancer: Japan clinical oncology group study JCOG1409. Jpn J Clin Oncol. 2016;46:174–7.
38. Takeuchi H, Ando M, Tsubosa Y, et al. Survival outcomes of thoracoscopic vs open oesophagectomy for oesophageal cancer: a multicentre, open-label, randomised, controlled, phase 3 trial (JCOG1409 MONET). Lancet Gastroenterol Hepatol. 2025;10(12):1104–16.
39. Boone J, Schipper ME, Moojen WA, et al. Robot-assisted thoracoscopic oesophagectomy for cancer. Br J Surg. 2009;96:878–86.
40. Puntambekar S, Kenawadekar R, Kumar S, et al. Robotic transthoracic esophagectomy. BMC Surg. 2015;23:47.
41. Cerfolio RJ, Wei B, Hawn MT, et al. Robotic esophagectomy for cancer: early results and lessons learned. Semin Thorac Cardiovasc Surg. 2016;28:160–9.
42. Park SY, Kim DJ, Yu WS, et al. Robot-assisted thoracoscopic esophagectomy with extensive mediastinal lymphadenectomy: experience with 114 consecutive patients with intrathoracic esophageal cancer. Dis Esophagus. 2016;29:326–32.

43. Salem AI, Thau MR, Strom TJ, et al. Effect of body mass index on operative outcome after robotic-assisted Ivor-Lewis esophagectomy: retrospective analysis of 129 cases at a single high-volume tertiary care center. Dis Esophagus. 2017;30:1–7.
44. Abbott A, Shridhar R, Hoffe S, et al. Robotic assisted Ivor Lewis esophagectomy in the elderly patient. J Gastrointest Oncol. 2015;6:31–8.
45. Shridhar R, Abbott AM, Doepker M, et al. Perioperative outcomes associated with robotic Ivor Lewis esophagectomy in patient's undergoing neoadjuvant chemoradiotherapy. J Gastrointest Oncol. 2016;7:206–12.
46. Hernandez JM, Dimou F, Weber J, et al. Defining the learning curve for robotic assisted esophagogastrectomy. J Gastrointest Surg. 2013;17:1346–51.
47. Sarkaria IS, Rizk NP, Grosser R, et al. Attaining proficiency in robotic-assisted minimally invasive esophagectomy while maximizing safety during procedure development. Innovations. 2016;11:268–73.
48. van der Sluis PC, van der Horst S, May AM, et al. Robot-assisted minimally invasive thoraco-laparoscopic esophagectomy versus open transthoracic esophagectomy for resectable esophageal cancer: a randomized controlled trial. Ann Surg. 2019;269:621–30.
49. de Groot EM, van der Horst S, Kingma BF, et al. Robot-assisted minimally invasive thoraco-laparoscopic esophagectomy versus open esophagectomy: long term follow-up of a randomized clinical trial. Dis Esophagus. 2020;33(Supplement_2):doaa079.
50. Yang Y, Li B, Yi J, Hua R, et al. Robot-assisted versus conventional minimally invasive esophagectomy for resectable esophageal squamous cell carcinoma: early results of a multicenter randomized controlled trial: the RAMIE trial. Ann Surg. 2022;275:646–53.
51. Chao YK, Li Z, Jiang H, et al. Multicentre randomized clinical trial on robot-assisted versus video-assisted thoracoscopic oesophagectomy (REVATE trial). Br J Surg. 2024;111(7):znae143.
52. Nishigori T, Kumamaru H, Obama K, et al. Short-term outcomes of robot-assisted versus conventional minimally invasive esophagectomy: a propensity score-matched study via a nationwide database. Ann Gastroenterol Surg. 2025;9:109–18.

Reconstruction 11

Akihiko Okamura and Masayuki Watanabe

11.1 Introduction

Esophagectomy is the mainstay of curative treatment for esophageal cancer, and it is one of the most invasive surgeries with high rates of morbidity and mortality, despite advances in operative procedures and perioperative management [1, 2]. Anastomotic leakage is a significant complication after esophagectomy, and it is well known that leakage is associated with prolonged hospital stay and increased costs and may adversely affect long-term outcomes. Recent nationwide studies in Japan reported the incidence of leakage remains high, with reported incidences of more than 10% [3, 4]. Therefore, every effort should be made to decrease the incidence.

Sufficient conduit length is required for esophageal reconstruction due to the considerably long defect along the digestive tract. There are several variations in reconstructive organs, routes, anastomotic locations, and techniques [5]. Reconstruction should be performed according to the situation, with a thorough understanding of the characteristics and suitability of the various options.

11.2 Reconstructive Organs

The stomach has been the most frequently used substitute [6], with a reported rate of about 90% in a recent Japanese comprehensive registry of esophageal cancer. Meanwhile, for patients in whom a gastric tube is not available because of previous gastrectomy or synchronous gastric cancer, the jejunum and colon graft are choices for reconstruction [7].

A. Okamura (✉) · M. Watanabe
Division of Esophageal Surgery, Department of Gastroenterological Surgery, Cancer Institute Hospital of Japanese Foundation for Cancer Research, Tokyo, Japan
e-mail: akihiko.okamura@jfcr.or.jp; masayuki.watanabe@jfcr.or.jp

Y. Kitagawa et al. (eds.), *Esophageal Squamous Cell Carcinoma*,
https://doi.org/10.1007/978-981-92-2611-5_11

11.2.1 Stomach

The stomach has an abundant intramural microvascular network, making reconstruction using the stomach straightforward. Therefore, the stomach is generally the first choice for esophageal reconstruction after esophagectomy. In clinical practice, there are two major types of gastric conduits with different widths, including the whole (including subtotal) stomach and the narrow gastric tube.

In the canine model, comparative studies of gastric tubes of different widths reported that maximum blood flow at the proposed anastomosis site was obtained with the 3 cm wide gastric tube [8]. In contrast, another study evaluating gastric tube perfusion using indocyanine green angiography in the setting of clinical esophagectomy found that creating a wide conduit of more than 5 cm is a significant factor in improving gastric tube perfusion [9]. Several clinical studies comparing outcomes between whole stomach and narrow gastric tube conduits have consistently shown that the clinical outcomes are similar between the two types of conduits, although reflux may be more frequent in the whole stomach than in the narrow gastric tube [10–14]. In general, the whole stomach can preserve the microvascular network of the gastric wall, but it is not as long as the narrow gastric tube. In contrast, the narrow gastric tube has an advantage in terms of length, but it lacks sufficient blood supply at the tip. Considering these characteristics, we should select an appropriate type of conduit depending on various situations.

In addition, several reconstruction methods using the stomach have been proposed with some modifications, including microvascular anastomosis (MVA; supercharge and/or superdrainage), which would be helpful in troublesome situations where there is an insufficient length or poor blood perfusion (Fig. 11.1). The

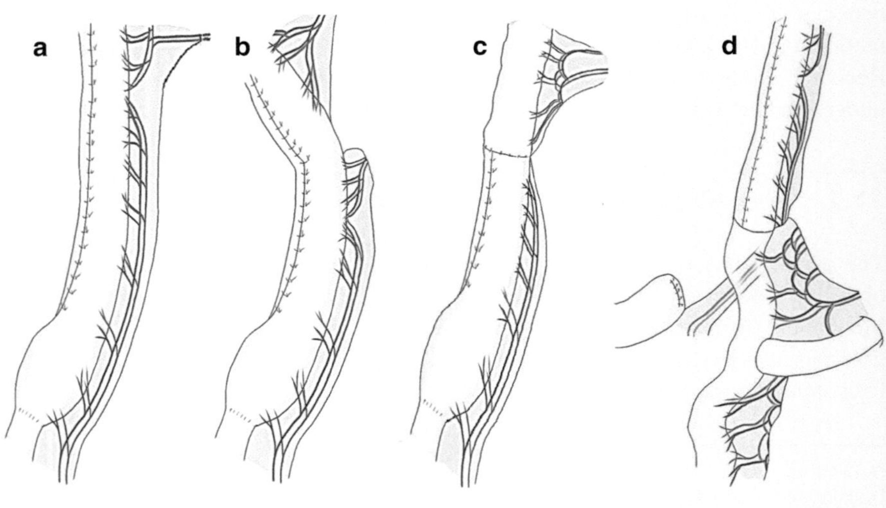

Fig. 11.1 Reconstructive modifications using the stomach. (**a**): Gastric tube with additional MVA, (**b**): elongated gastric tube with MVA, (**c**): gastric tube combined with free jejunal transfer, (**d**): pedicled gastric tube with Roux-en-Y anastomosis. (Modified from Okamura et al. [16])

modifications include additional MVA between short gastric or left gastroepiploic vessels and appropriate cervical vessels (Fig. 11.1a), elongated gastric conduit creation with preservation of the left gastric vessels that are anastomosed with the appropriate cervical vessels (Fig. 11.1b), a gastric conduit combined with free jejunal transfer with MVA (Fig. 11.1c), and a pedicled gastric conduit with Roux-en-Y anastomosis where the gastric antrum is resected with preservation of the right gastroepiploic vessel and the distal end of the conduit is reconstructed with the pedicled jejunum using the Roux-en-Y method (Fig. 11.1d) [15, 16].

11.2.2 Colon

The colon can provide a sufficiently long graft for esophageal reconstruction, although the procedure is complicated. Meanwhile, postoperative diarrhea symptoms are relatively common. In addition, polyps and malignancies are frequently observed, and endoscopic evaluation before and after surgery is strongly recommended.

There are three candidate colon grafts used for esophageal reconstruction, including the right colon graft, the left colon graft, and the ileocolon graft [7]. The right colon graft is created using the middle colic vessels as a pedicle (Fig. 11.2a). Transection of the right colic and ileocolic vessels is typically required, and a segment from the terminal ileum to the ascending colon is placed for isoperistaltic interposition. A left colon graft is created using the ascending branch of the left colic artery and the inferior mesenteric vein as a pedicle (Fig. 11.2b). The middle colic vessels are transected, preserving the communication between the right and left branches of these vessels. A segment from the transverse colon to the splenic flexure is used for isoperistaltic interposition. As a modified alternative to the right colon graft, the ileocolon graft is created using the ileocolic vessels as a pedicle (Fig. 11.2c) [17].

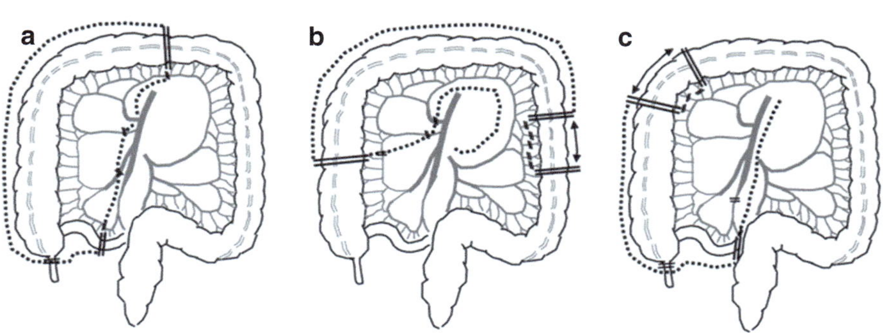

Fig. 11.2 Colon grafts for esophageal reconstruction. (**a**): Right colon graft using middle colic vessels as a pedicle. (**b**): left colon graft using left colic artery and inferior mesenteric vein as a pedicle. (**c**): ileocolon graft using ileocolic vessels as a pedicle. (Modified from Watanabe et al. [7])

The right colon can prevent postoperative regurgitation and reflux esophagitis due to the presence of the Bauhin valve. It also has a reservoir-like capacity due to the large caliber of the cecum, and the anastomosis between the terminal ileum and the cervical esophagus is easy because their diameters are similar. In contrast, there are many vascular variations in the ileocecal region, and discontinuity in the marginal vessels is occasionally observed. In this case, additional MVA is required to maintain the blood supply to the ileum. Meanwhile, the ileocolic graft has a more abundant blood supply than the right colon graft; however, the graft length is limited by the length of the ileocolic mesentery, and a relatively long segment of the terminal ileum is required.

Regarding the left colon graft, there are few variations in the vessels around the middle and left colic regions, allowing us to use a long segment graft from the root of the left colic vessels to the territory of the middle colic vessels. However, the inferior mesenteric artery is sometimes affected by atherosclerosis in the elderly, which may cause graft ischemia. In addition, regurgitation is more common than the right colon graft due to the lack of an antireflux valve.

11.2.3 Jejunum

The jejunum exhibits vigorous peristalsis, which facilitates the comfortable passage of food and prevents regurgitation, although it lacks a reservoir function. Malignancy of the jejunum is rare, and postoperative diarrhea is uncommon. Depending on the extent of esophagectomy, pedicled jejunal grafts of different lengths are created. However, the length of the jejunal graft is limited by the mesenteric arcade. In a long-segment jejunal graft, supercharge or superdrainage is occasionally required due to impaired blood perfusion.

For reconstruction after lower esophagectomy, it is sufficient to create a pedicled jejunum in the same manner as after gastrectomy (Fig. 11.3a). Meanwhile, after subtotal esophagectomy, an intrathoracic or cervical anastomosis is performed between the remnant esophagus and the elongated jejunal graft (Fig. 11.3b, c) [18, 19]. Generally, transection of the second and third jejunal vessels is required to achieve a long graft. However, supercharging and superdraining with MVA is often necessary when pulling up the pedicled jejunal flap. Meanwhile, it has been reported that the improved pedicled jejunal flap, in which the first jejunal vascular arcade is preserved and up to the second jejunal vessels are transected, can reduce the need for MVA in cervical anastomosis [19].

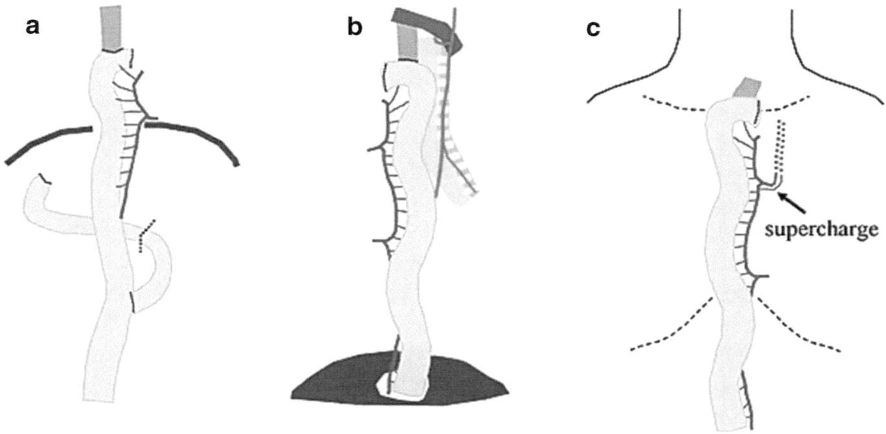

Fig. 11.3 Esophageal reconstruction using a pedicled jejunal flap. (**a**): Roux-en-Y reconstruction with anastomosis between the middle esophagus and pedicled jejunum. (**b**): intrathoracic anastomosis with upper esophagus and elongated pedicled jejunum. (**c**): cervical anastomosis using supercharged jejunal pedicle. (Modified from Watanabe et al. [7])

11.3 Reconstruction Route

The substitute organs can be pulled up through the subcutaneous, retrosternal, or posterior mediastinal route. Although most esophageal surgeons believe that the posterior mediastinal route is the shortest, debates persist regarding which route is the shortest [20–25]. Recently, Yasuda et al. compared the length of each reconstruction route using measurements obtained during surgery and showed that the retrosternal route is the shortest for esophageal reconstruction in Japanese patients [25].

In general, the subcutaneous route has a higher risk of anastomotic leakage, may cause food stasis in the bending conduit, and may be detrimental to the patient's appearance. However, it is easy and safe to manage anastomotic problems. The posterior mediastinal route is the most physiological route without cosmetic disadvantages, but it carries the risk of serious complications such as intrathoracic infection and gastrotracheal fistula. Also, regurgitation is relatively common after reconstruction through this route. Meanwhile, the retrosternal route is not physiological, and the substitute organ can press against the heart. The advantage of this route is that it is easy and safe to manage graft or anastomotic problems compared to the posterior mediastinal route.

Previous meta-analyses of randomized controlled trials comparing outcomes between the retrosternal and posterior mediastinal routes showed no significant difference in anastomotic leakage, cardiopulmonary complications, and mortality between the two routes [26, 27]. In contrast, a recent nationwide Japanese study showed that the incidence of anastomotic leakage and surgical site infection was significantly lower in the posterior mediastinal route than in the retrosternal route, while the incidence of pneumonia was significantly higher in the posterior mediastinal route [28].

Recently, it has been suggested that the frequency of paraconduit hiatal herniation after esophagectomy has increased significantly as a result of the widespread use of a minimally invasive approach, in which intra-abdominal adhesions occur less frequently compared to open surgery [29, 30]. Therefore, the frequency of retrosternal route reconstruction has gradually increased, rather than the posterior mediastinal route in Japan. Since paraconduit hiatal hernia is a challenging complication that can occur as an early to a late complication after esophagectomy, preventive measures need to be taken, such as hiatoplasty with omentum fixation [31], when using the posterior mediastinal route.

11.4 Anastomosis

11.4.1 Anastomotic Location

The anastomotic location can be selected based on the location and the extent of the tumor. There are two main types of esophagectomy, including McKeown esophagectomy (cervical anastomosis) and Ivor Lewis esophagectomy (intrathoracic anastomosis). McKeown esophagectomy is often indicated for patients with esophageal squamous cell carcinoma because it is often located in the upper to middle esophagus. In contrast, Ivor Lewis esophagectomy is the preferred procedure for patients with esophageal or esophagogastric adenocarcinoma because it is typically located in the lower third of the esophagus. Therefore, Ivor Lewis esophagectomy is often selected in Western countries, while McKeown is more commonly used in Asian countries.

The optimal location of the anastomosis has been debated to reduce the risk of anastomotic leakage. A previous retrospective study and a randomized clinical trial from the Netherlands consistently showed that Ivor Lewis esophagectomy was significantly associated with a lower incidence of anastomotic leakage than McKeown esophagectomy [32, 33]. However, the incidence of anastomotic leakage after minimally invasive McKeown esophagectomy in a Japanese nationwide study is much lower than in the studies [3]. Therefore, further validation is needed to determine whether the results from Western countries can be applied to Asian countries.

Meanwhile, in the above trial, Ivor Lewis esophagectomy showed a higher incidence of reoperation among patients with anastomotic leakage than McKeown esophagectomy [33], which may indicate that cervical anastomotic leakage is easier to manage than thoracic anastomotic leakage.

11.4.2 Anastomotic Technique

There are many kinds of anastomotic techniques, including hand-sewn (HS), circular stapling (CS), and linear stapling (LS). HS anastomosis is performed in an end-to-end or end-to-side fashion with an interrupted or running suture in all single layers, such as Gambee, or through double layers, including layer-to-layer and Albert-Lembert. In the CS, an anvil head is inserted and secured in the remnant esophagus, and then the body of the stapler is inserted from the conduit tip. After anastomosis is made by CS in an end-to-side fashion, the entry hole is closed with a linear stapler. LS anastomosis can be made in an end-to-end or side-to-side fashion. Triangulating stapling is commonly used for end-to-end LS anastomosis, which has been utilized traditionally for colonic surgery but has also been implemented in esophageal surgery [34–36]. Of the side-to-side technique, Collard anastomosis is widely used, which is ordinally a linear stapled cervical semi-mechanical side-to-side anastomosis technique, but it has now adapted to design a totally mechanical anastomosis technique [37, 38]. Many meta-analyses have been performed to compare different types of anastomotic techniques. Overall, anastomoses using LS appear to be advantageous in reducing anastomosis-related complications, including anastomotic leakage and stricture [39–43].

Our standard procedure for cervical esophagogastric anastomosis (McKeown esophagectomy) is LS with triangulating stapling, while that for intrathoracic anastomosis (Ivor Lewis esophagectomy) is semi-mechanical LS anastomosis. In conventional triangulating stapling, the posterior one-third wall is stapled in an inverted fashion, while the other two-thirds are stapled in an everted fashion. Meanwhile, we have introduced total everted triangulating stapling, in which all three walls are stapled in an everted fashion (Fig. 11.4), which may reduce the incidence of anastomotic stricture compared to conventional stapling [44].

For the intrathoracic anastomosis, the LS anastomosis is performed with the intracorporeal overlap technique, and the common entry hole is closed with interrupted or running HS sutures (Fig. 11.5) [45, 46]. However, it requires considerable technical skill in the minimally invasive approach, as it must be performed with a straight instrument in the limited intercostal space. Recently, robotic surgery has been increasingly implemented, and it was suggested that the articulating function of the robotic forceps may improve anastomotic manipulation and reduce postoperative anastomotic leakage [47].

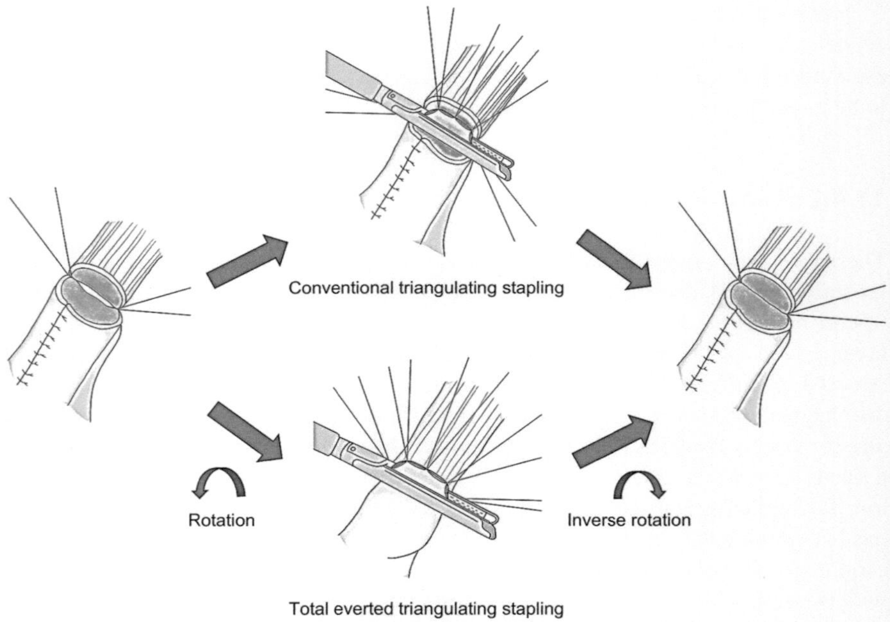

Fig. 11.4 Triangulating stapling technique for cervical esophagogastric anastomosis using three linear staplers. In conventional triangulating stapling, the posterior one-third wall is stapled in an inverted fashion. In the total everted triangulating stapling, the anastomotic region is half-turned and the posterior wall is anastomosed in an everted fashion. After that the anastomotic region is half-turned inversely. In both techniques, the other two-thirds are stapled in an everted fashion. (Modified from Takahashi et al. [44])

Fig. 11.5 Semi-mechanical linear-stapled anastomosis with the intracorporeal overlap technique. Linear stapling anastomosis is performed with the intracorporeal overlap technique and the common entry hole is closed with interrupted or running hand-sewn suture

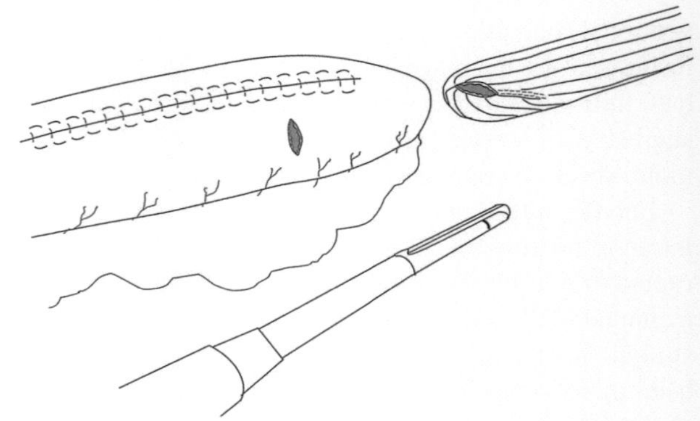

11.5 Reconstruction in Specific Situations

11.5.1 Reconstruction Following Cervical Esophagectomy

In patients with tumors confined to the cervical esophagus, a free jejunal transfer is usually chosen. However, there have been few reports of the outcomes of cervical esophagectomy because cervical esophageal carcinoma is rare. From a recent nationwide study in Japan, the incidence of anastomotic leakage after free jejunum transfer in cervical esophagectomy was 6.8% [48]. Also, reoperation is required in 10.2% of cases, and patients should be carefully monitored postoperatively, with particular attention to the possibility of graft failure [48]. Reconstruction from the neck is possible as long as the distal end is limited to the upper edge of the aortic arch.

A 30–40-cm-long segment of jejunum is harvested using the second or third jejunal vessels as donor vessels. The jejunum is placed in the isoperistal direction. It is then trimmed to the appropriate length and stretched as straight as possible. The distal jejuno-esophageal anastomosis is created in an end-to-end fashion whether using HS or CS techniques. Subsequently, the jejunum is anastomosed to the pharynx as an end-to-end HS anastomosis. The MVA is then made between the donor vessels and the appropriate cervical vessels. The transverse cervical artery is the first choice for the recipient artery. Other cervical vessels, including the facial artery, lingual artery, and superior thyroid artery, may be used if necessary.

11.5.2 Reconstruction Following Pharyngolaryngectomy with Total Esophagectomy

Pharyngolaryngectomy with total esophagectomy is sometimes indicated in patients with synchronous head and neck cancer and thoracic esophageal cancer or in those with either tumor that extends to the other. In this situation, the defect of the digestive tract is so long that a long conduit is required for reconstruction, making reconstructive surgery challenging. However, as mentioned above, several modifications may be helpful when using the stomach as a reconstructive organ [16]. A recent Japanese nationwide study suggested that a gastric conduit combined with free jejunal transfer is significantly associated with reduced rates of anastomotic leakage or necrosis in the gastric tube. However, given that it did not reduce the overall and severe complications associated with digestive reconstruction, we should be aware that additional digestive anastomosis and MVA may cause other complications [49].

11.5.3 Reconstruction Following Esophagectomy in Patients with a History of Total Pharyngolaryngectomy

In patients with a history of total pharyngolaryngectomy for head and neck cancer, two procedures are available for metachronous esophageal cancer: total esophagectomy with cervical anastomosis (Fig. 11.6a, McKeown esophagectomy) and subtotal esophagectomy with intrathoracic anastomosis (Fig. 11.6b, Ivor Lewis esophagectomy). Prior surgery or postoperative irradiation to the neck may cause severe fibrotic changes and dense adhesions, which carry the risk of injury to the replaced free jejunal graft, anastomosed vessels, and trachea. In addition, severe fibrotic changes in the thoracic inlet may compromise the blood supply to the conduit in the McKeown esophagectomy. However, Ivor Lewis esophagectomy may avoid such risks when oncologically and technically feasible. Reportedly, no patient has experienced necrosis of the remnant esophagus following Ivor Lewis esophagectomy. Ivor Lewis esophagectomy is preferred to reduce anastomotic leakage when oncologically and technically feasible [50–52].

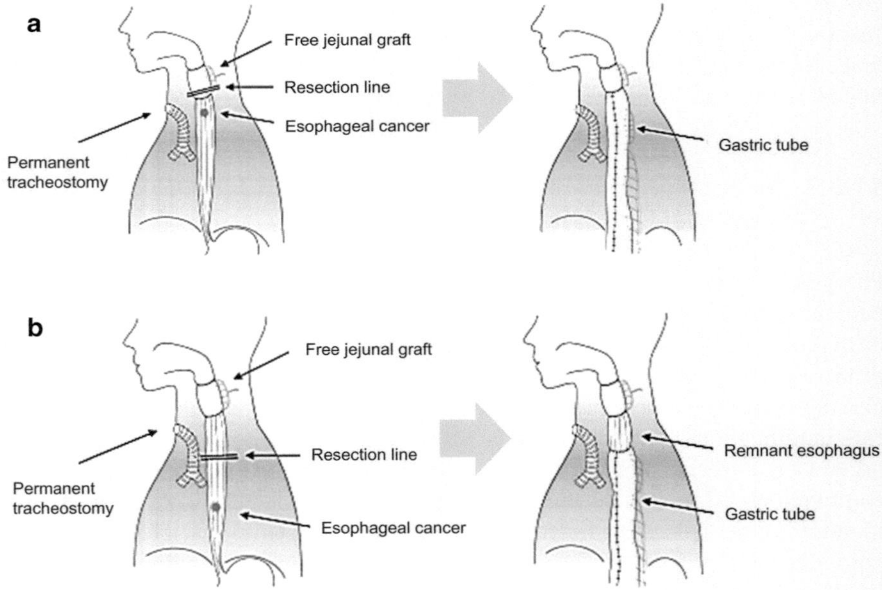

Fig. 11.6 Surgical procedure and reconstruction in patients with a history of total pharyngolaryngectomy. (**a**): McKeown esophagectomy, (**b**): Ivor Lewis esophagectomy. (Modified from Kuriyama et al. [51])

References

1. Watanabe M, Okamura A, Toihata T, Yamashita K, Yuda M, Hayami M, Fukudome I, Imamura Y, Mine S. Recent progress in perioperative management of patients undergoing esophagectomy for esophageal cancer. Esophagus. 2018;15:160–4.
2. Watanabe M, Otake R, Kozuki R, Toihata T, Takahashi K, Okamura A, Imamura Y. Recent progress in multidisciplinary treatment for patients with esophageal cancer. Surg Today. 2020;50:12–20.
3. Okamura A, Endo H, Watanabe M, Yamamoto H, Kikuchi H, Kanaji S, Toh Y, Kakeji Y, Doki Y, Kitagawa Y. Influence of patient position in thoracoscopic esophagectomy on postoperative pneumonia: a comparative analysis from the National Clinical Database in Japan. Esophagus. 2023;20:48–54.
4. Okamura A, Yamamoto H, Watanabe M, Miyata H, Kanaji S, Kamiya K, Kakeji Y, Doki Y, Kitagawa Y. Association between preoperative HbA1c levels and complications after esophagectomy: analysis of 15,801 esophagectomies from the national clinical database in Japan. Ann Surg. 2022;276:e393–9.
5. Booka E, Takeuchi H, Morita Y, Hiramatsu Y, Kikuchi H. What is the best reconstruction procedure after esophagectomy? A meta-analysis comparing posterior mediastinal and retrosternal approaches. Ann Gastroenterol Surg. 2023;7:553–64.
6. Watanabe M, Takahashi N, Tamura M, Terayama M, Kuriyama K, Okamura A, Kanamori J, Imamura Y. Gastric conduit reconstruction after esophagectomy. Dis Esophagus. 2024;37:doae045.
7. Watanabe M, Mine S, Nishida K, Kurogochi T, Okamura A, Imamura Y. Reconstruction after esophagectomy for esophageal cancer patients with a history of gastrectomy. Gen Thorac Cardiovasc Surg. 2016;64:457–63.
8. Sugimachi K, Ikeda M, Kai H, Ueo H, Okudaira Y, Inokuchi K. Assessment of the blood flow in various gastric tubes for esophageal substitutes. J Surg Res. 1982;33:463–8.
9. Ishikawa Y, Chang AC, Lin J, Orringer MB, Lynch WR, Lagisetty KH, Wakeam E, Reddy RM. Wider gastric conduit morphology is associated with improved blood flow during esophagectomy. J Gastrointest Surg. 2023;27:845–54.
10. Tabira Y, Sakaguchi T, Kuhara H, Teshima K, Tanaka M, Kawasuji M. The width of a gastric tube has no impact on outcome after esophagectomy. Am J Surg. 2004;187:417–21.
11. Zhang C, Wu QC, Hou PY, Zhang M, Li Q, Jiang YJ, Chen D. Impact of the method of reconstruction after oncologic oesophagectomy on quality of life–a prospective, randomised study. Eur J Cardiothorac Surg. 2011;39:109–14.
12. Shu YS, Sun C, Shi WP, Shi HC, Lu SC, Wang K. Tubular stomach or whole stomach for esophagectomy through cervico-thoraco-abdominal approach: a comparative clinical study on anastomotic leakage. Ir J Med Sci. 2013;182:477–80.
13. Zhang W, Yu D, Peng J, Xu J, Wei Y. Gastric-tube versus whole-stomach esophagectomy for esophageal cancer: a systematic review and meta-analysis. PLoS One. 2017;12:e0173416.
14. Sasaki K, Tsuruda Y, Shimonosono M, Noda M, Uchikado Y, Omoto I, Setoyama T, Matsushita D, Arigami T, Baba K, et al. Comparison of the subtotal and narrow gastric conduit for cervical esophagogastrostomy after esophagectomy in esophageal cancer patients: a propensity score-matched analysis. Esophagus. 2024;21:41–50.
15. Kosumi K, Baba Y, Watanabe M, Ida S, Nagai Y, Baba H. Pedunculated gastric conduit interposition with duodenal transection after salvage esophagectomy: an option for increasing the flexibility of the gastric conduit. J Am Coll Surg. 2012;214:e31–3.
16. Okamura A, Watanabe M, Kanamori J, Imamura Y, Takahashi K, Ushida Y, Kamiyama R, Seto A, Shimbashi W, Sasaki T, et al. Digestive reconstruction after pharyngolaryngectomy with total esophagectomy. Ann Surg Oncol. 2021;28:695–701.
17. Kawano T, Nishikage T, Kawada K, Nakajima Y, Kojima K, Nagai K. Subcutaneous reconstruction using ileocolon with preserved ileocolic vessels following esophagectomy or in esophageal bypass operation. Dig Surg. 2009;26:200–4.

18. Ninomiya I, Okamoto K, Oyama K, Hayashi H, Miyashita T, Tajima H, Kitagawa H, Fushida S, Fujimura T, Ohta T. Feasibility of esophageal reconstruction using a pedicled jejunum with intrathoracic esophagojejunostomy in the upper mediastinum for esophageal cancer. Gen Thorac Cardiovasc Surg. 2014;62:627–34.
19. Shirakawa Y, Noma K, Koujima T, Maeda N, Tanabe S, Ohara T, Sakurama K, Fujiwara T. Operative technique of antethoracic esophageal reconstruction with pedicled jejunal flap. Esophagus. 2014;12:57–64.
20. Ngan SY, Wong J. Lengths of different routes for esophageal replacement. J Thorac Cardiovasc Surg. 1986;91:790–2.
21. Coral RP, Constant-Neto M, Silva IS, Kalil AN, Boose R, Beduschi T, Gemelle TF. Comparative anatomical study of the anterior and posterior mediastinum as access routes after esophagectomy. Dis Esophagus. 2003;16:236–8.
22. Chen H, Lu JJ, Zhou J, Zhou X, Luo X, Liu Q, Tam J. Anterior versus posterior routes of reconstruction after esophagectomy: a comparative anatomic study. Ann Thorac Surg. 2009;87:400–4.
23. Hu H, Ye T, Tan D, Li H, Chen H. Is anterior mediastinum route a shorter choice for esophageal reconstruction? A comparative anatomic study. Eur J Cardiothorac Surg. 2011;40:1466–9.
24. Yang J, Xu C, Lian D, Ye S, Zeng Z, Liu D, Zhuang C. Esophageal reconstruction: posterior mediastinal or retrosternal route. J Surg Res. 2016;201:364–9.
25. Yasuda T, Shiraishi O, Kato H, Hiraki Y, Momose K, Yasuda A, Shinkai M, Kimura Y, Imano M. A comparative study of the lengths of different reconstruction routes used after thoracic esophagectomy. Esophagus. 2021;18:468–74.
26. Yan D, Zheng H, Wang P, Yin Y, Zhang Q, Zhang L, Liang H, Shi D, Hu L, Fan H, et al. Surgical outcomes of two different reconstruction routes for esophagectomy in esophageal cancer patients: a meta-analysis. Dis Esophagus. 2022;35:doab070.
27. Yoshida S, Fujii Y, Hoshino N, Tokoro Y, Tsunoda S, Obama K, Watanabe N. Anterior versus posterior mediastinal reconstruction after esophagectomy in esophageal cancer patients: a systematic review and meta-analysis. Langenbeck's Arch Surg. 2024;409:88.
28. Kikuchi H, Endo H, Yamamoto H, Ozawa S, Miyata H, Kakeji Y, Matsubara H, Doki Y, Kitagawa Y, Takeuchi H. Impact of reconstruction route on postoperative morbidity after esophagectomy: analysis of esophagectomies in the japanese national clinical database. Ann Gastroenterol Surg. 2022;6:46–53.
29. Murad H, Huang B, Ndegwa N, Rouvelas I, Klevebro F. Postoperative hiatal herniation after open vs. minimally invasive esophagectomy; a systematic review and meta-analysis. Int J Surg. 2021;93:106046.
30. Kuvendjiska J, Jasinski R, Hipp J, Fink M, Fichtner-Feigl S, Diener MK, Hoeppner J. Postoperative hiatal hernia after Ivor Lewis esophagectomy-a growing problem in the age of minimally invasive surgery. J Clin Med. 2023;12:5724.
31. Holscher AH, Fetzner UK. Paraconduit hiatal hernia after esophagectomy. Prevention-indication for surgery-surgical technique. Dis Esophagus. 2021;34:doab025.
32. van Workum F, Slaman AE, van Berge Henegouwen MI, Gisbertz SS, Kouwenhoven EA, van Det MJ, van den Wildenberg FJH, Polat F, Luyer MDP, Nieuwenhuijzen GAP, Rosman C. Propensity score-matched analysis comparing minimally invasive Ivor Lewis versus minimally invasive Mckeown esophagectomy. Ann Surg. 2020;271:128–33.
33. van Workum F, Verstegen MHP, Klarenbeek BR, Bouwense SAW, van Berge Henegouwen MI, Daams F, Gisbertz SS, Hannink G, Haveman JW, Heisterkamp J, et al. Intrathoracic vs cervical anastomosis after totally or hybrid minimally invasive esophagectomy for esophageal cancer: a randomized clinical trial. JAMA Surg. 2021;156:601–10.
34. Venkatesh KS, Morrison N, Larson DM, Ramanujam P. Triangulating stapling technique: an alternative approach to colorectal anastomosis. Dis Colon Rectum. 1993;36:73–6.
35. Furukawa Y, Hanyu N, Hirai K, Ushigome T, Kawasaki N, Toyama Y, Nakayoshi T, Yanaga K. Usefulness of automatic triangular anastomosis for esophageal cancer surgery using a linear stapler (TA-30). Ann Thorac Cardiovasc Surg. 2005;11:80–6.

36. Toh Y, Sakaguchi Y, Ikeda O, Adachi E, Ohgaki K, Yamashita Y, Oki E, Minami K, Okamura T. The triangulating stapling technique for cervical esophagogastric anastomosis after esophagectomy. Surg Today. 2009;39:201–6.
37. Collard JM, Romagnoli R, Goncette L, Otte JB, Kestens PJ. Terminalized semimechanical side-to-side suture technique for cervical esophagogastrostomy. Ann Thorac Surg. 1998;65:814–7.
38. De Giacomo T, Francioni F, Venuta F, Trentino P, Moretti M, Rendina EA, Coloni GF. Complete mechanical cervical anastomosis using a narrow gastric tube after esophagectomy for cancer. Eur J Cardiothorac Surg. 2004;26:881–4.
39. Honda M, Kuriyama A, Noma H, Nunobe S, Furukawa TA. Hand-sewn versus mechanical esophagogastric anastomosis after esophagectomy: a systematic review and meta-analysis. Ann Surg. 2013;257:238–48.
40. Deng XF, Liu QX, Zhou D, Min JX, Dai JG. Hand-sewn vs linearly stapled esophagogastric anastomosis for esophageal cancer: a meta-analysis. World J Gastroenterol. 2015;21:4757–64.
41. Zhou D, Liu QX, Deng XF, Min JX, Dai JG. Comparison of two different mechanical esophagogastric anastomosis in esophageal cancer patients: a meta-analysis. J Cardiothorac Surg. 2015;10:67.
42. Kamarajah SK, Bundred JR, Singh P, Pasquali S, Griffiths EA. Anastomotic techniques for oesophagectomy for malignancy: systematic review and network meta-analysis. BJS Open. 2020;4:563–76.
43. Chen B, Xia P, Tang W, Huang S. Which anastomotic techniques is the best choice for cervical esophagogastric anastomosis in esophagectomy? A Bayesian network meta-analysis. J Gastrointest Surg. 2023;27:422–32.
44. Takahashi K, Watanabe M, Ushida Y, Kanie Y, Kozuki R, Toihata T, Otake R, Kanamori J, Okamura A, Imamura Y, Mine S. Comparison of the outcomes between total eversion and conventional triangulating stapling technique in cervical esophagogastric anastomosis after esophagectomy: a propensity score-matched analysis. Esophagus. 2021;18:475–81.
45. Irino T, Tsai JA, Ericson J, Nilsson M, Lundell L, Rouvelas I. Thoracoscopic side-to-side esophagogastrostomy by use of linear stapler-a simplified technique facilitating a minimally invasive Ivor-Lewis operation. Langenbeck's Arch Surg. 2016;401:315–22.
46. Kanamori J, Watanabe M, Kozuki R, Toihata T, Otake R, Takahashi K, Okamura A, Imamura Y, Mine S. Successful transition from open to minimally invasive approach in Ivor Lewis esophagectomy: a single-center experience in Japan. Langenbeck's Arch Surg. 2021;406:1407–14.
47. Kanamori J, Watanabe M, Maruyama S, Kanie Y, Kuriyama K, Terayama M, Takahashi N, Tamura M, Okamura A, Imamura Y. Fully robotic side-to-side stapled anastomosis provides less anastomotic leakage than conventional minimally invasive approach in Ivor Lewis esophagectomy. Asian J Endosc Surg. 2024;17:e13340.
48. Nakajima Y, Tachimori H, Miyawaki Y, Fujiwara N, Kawada K, Sato H, Miyata H, Sakuramoto S, Shimada H, Watanabe M, et al. A survey of the clinical outcomes of cervical esophageal carcinoma surgery focusing on the presence or absence of laryngectomy using the national clinical database in Japan. Esophagus. 2022;19:569–75.
49. Okamura A, Watanabe M, Mukoyama N, Ota Y, Shiraishi O, Shimbashi W, Baba Y, Matsui H, Shinomiya H, Sugimura K, et al. A nationwide survey on digestive reconstruction following pharyngolaryngectomy with total esophagectomy: a multicenter retrospective study in Japan. Ann Gastroenterol Surg. 2022;6:54–62.
50. Takahashi K, Mine S, Kozuki R, Toihata T, Okamura A, Imamura Y, Watanabe M. Ivor-Lewis esophagectomy for patients with squamous cell carcinoma of the thoracic esophagus with a history of total pharyngolaryngectomy. Esophagus. 2019;16:382–5.
51. Kuriyama K, Okamura A, Kanie Y, Maruyama S, Sakamoto K, Kanamori J, Imamura Y, Watanabe M. McKeown versus Ivor-Lewis esophagectomy for patients with a history of total pharyngolaryngectomy: a comparison study. World J Surg. 2023;47:2479–87.
52. Okamura A, Watanabe M, Okui J, Kuriyama K, Shiraishi O, Kurogochi T, Abe T, Sato H, Miyata H, Kawaguchi Y, et al. Esophagectomy for esophageal cancer in patients with a history of total pharyngolaryngectomy: a Japanese nationwide retrospective cohort study. Esophagus. 2024;21:438–46.

Salvage/Conversion Esophagectomy for T4b ESCC

12

Shigeto Nakai, Tomoki Makino, and Yuichiro Doki

12.1 Introduction

Esophageal squamous cell carcinoma (ESCC) exhibits an aggressive behavior due to the lack of a serosal layer, facilitating direct invasion into adjacent structures. The Union for International Cancer Control/American Joint Committee on Cancer (UICC/AJCC) 8th edition classifies tumors with definitive invasion into the aorta, trachea, bronchus, vertebral body, or other mediastinal structures as stage cT4b [1]. These patients are conventionally treated with definitive chemoradiotherapy (dCRT) or systemic chemotherapy; however, complete response (CR) rates range from 0% to 39%, local failure exceeds 30%, and fistula formation occurs in up to 15% of cases [1–3]. Consequently, long-term survival remains poor, with 5-year overall survival (OS) rates below 20%.

Two induction-based paradigms are recognized: salvage esophagectomy (a rescue resection performed after definitive chemoradiotherapy ≥50 Gy for residual or recurrent disease) and conversion esophagectomy (resection after a tumor initially deemed unresectable becomes resectable following induction therapy) [4]. When T4 invasion is downstaged, conversion surgery becomes feasible; historical CRT (40–60 Gy) has enabled curative resection in 32–60% of cT4b cases with favorable prognosis. Although induction chemotherapy alone offers inferior local control compared with CRT, intensive triplet regimens such as DCF (docetaxel, cisplatin, and 5-fluorouracil) can achieve outcomes comparable to induction CRT [5, 6]. The advent of immune checkpoint inhibitors (ICI) targeting PD-1/PD-L1 further expanded induction options and growing series now report successful conversion surgery after ICI-chemotherapy [7, 8]. However,

S. Nakai · T. Makino (✉) · Y. Doki
Department of Gastroenterological Surgery, Osaka University Graduate School of Medicine, Osaka, Japan
e-mail: snakai@gesurg.med.osaka-u.ac.jp; tmakino@gesurg.med.osaka-u.ac.jp; ydoki@gesurg.med.osaka-u.ac.jp

Y. Kitagawa et al. (eds.), *Esophageal Squamous Cell Carcinoma*,
https://doi.org/10.1007/978-981-92-2611-5_12

conversion surgery—particularly salvage esophagectomy—is technically demanding because prior radiotherapy induces dense fibrosis and tissue edema, obscuring anatomic planes and necessitating complex dissection to identify safe resection margins. Postoperatively, it carries a high risk of serious complications including airway ischemia/necrosis, anastomotic leakage, and gastric conduit necrosis, thus being classified as a high-risk surgery.

This review integrates systematic and contemporary data to evaluate patient selection criteria, induction regimens, surgical techniques, perioperative management, and long-term outcomes for cT4b ESCC.

12.2 Recommended Treatments for cT4b Esophageal Cancer by Guidelines

According to the NCCN Clinical Practice Guidelines in Oncology for Esophageal and Esophagogastric Junction Cancers (Version 3.2025), dCRT is the recommended standard treatment for patients with clinical T4b ESCC, as these tumors are considered unresectable at presentation [9]. In patients who are not candidates for dCRT, palliative chemotherapy or radiation therapy should be offered according to performance status and comorbidity profiles. If sufficient tumor downstaging is achieved following CRT, salvage surgery may be considered as a treatment option.

Salvage esophagectomy for esophageal cancer refers to a rescue surgical procedure performed after definitive (chemo)radiotherapy of ≥50 Gy, targeting residual or recurrent tumor foci. According to Esophageal Cancer Practice Guidelines 2022 edited by the Japan esophageal society, there is weak evidence to recommend salvage surgery for residual or recurrent lesions after chemoradiotherapy in patients with untreated resectable esophageal cancer (*evidence level: C*) [10]. On the other hand, conversion esophagectomy involves planned resection after induction therapy in tumors initially staged as unresectable. According to Esophageal Cancer Practice Guidelines 2022 edited by the Japan esophageal society, there is only weak evidence to recommend surgical resection for patients with unresectable, locally advanced esophageal cancer (cT4 [e.g., aorta, trachea, bronchus] N0-3M0) that becomes NCCN resectable after definitive chemoradiotherapy or induction chemotherapy (*evidence level: C*) [10].

12.3 Induction Treatments Followed by Surgery for cT4b Esophageal Cancer

As shown in Tables 12.1 and 12.2, 25 studies (22 retrospective trials and 3 phase II trials) have analyzed the outcome of patients with T4 esophageal cancer that underwent conversion/salvage surgery following induction treatments of induction chemoradiotherapy (ICRT) or induction chemotherapy (ICT) (6.11–34). In ICRT, the combination of CF with concurrent 36–60 Gy irradiation was the most common

Table 12.1 Summary of conversion/salvage surgery for patients with clinical T4 esophageal cancer

Authors	Design	Year	*N*	Conversion or salvage	Histology (SCC/AC/other)	Total radiation dose/chemotherapy regimen	1/3/5 year overall survival rate (%)
Ikeda et al. [11]	P2	2001	37	Salvage	37/0/0	60 Gy/CF	45/23/23
Yokota et al. [12] (COSMOS)	P2	2016	48[a]	Conversion or salvage	47/0/1	DCF ($n = 18$) DCF + 30–60 Gy/CF ($n = 2$)	67/47/NA
Sugimura et al. [6]	P2	2021	99	Conversion or salvage	99/0/0	50.4 Gy/CF or DCF	NA/35.5/NA
Van Raemdonck et al. [13]	Retro	1997	18	Conversion	15/3/0	36–50 Gy/CF or MF	62/43/NA
Yano et al. [14]	Retro	1999	45	Conversion	45/0/0	40 Gy/CF	48/35/25
Noguchi et al. [15]	Retro	2003	41	Conversion	41/0/0	40 Gy/CF	24/5/0
Fujita et al. [16]	Cohort	2005	53	Conversion	53/0/0	36 Gy(+24 Gy[b])/CF	73/28/17
Seto et al. [17]	Retro	2007	88	Conversion	88/0/0	40 Gy/CF	68/38/20
Manzoni et al. [18]	Retro	2007	51	Salvage	51/0/0	50–60 Gy/CF	NA/9/6
Miyoshi et al. [19]	Retro	2009	42	Conversion	42/0/0	40 Gy/CF or ACF	66/45/38
Miyata et al. [20]	Retro	2012	169	Conversion or salvage	169/0/0	40–60 Gy/CF ($n = 41$) FAP or DCF ($n = 41$) Both ($n = 16$)	NA/48/40
Shimoji et al. [21]	Cohort	2013	43	Conversion or salvage	42/1/0	40–60 Gy/FN ($n = 17$) FAN ($n = 26$)	52/35/35
Pimiento et al. [22]	Retro	2013	45	Conversion	6/36/3	NA/platinum-based	75/50/35
Akutsu et al. [23]	Retro	2014	40	Conversion or salvage	40/0/0	40 Gy/CF 53 Gy/CF	74/48/26 72/36/37
Ohira et al. [24]	Retro	2015	91	Conversion or salvage	91	40–60 Gy/CF or FN	NA/NA/51
Yamaguchi et al. [25]	Retro	2018	13	Conversion	13/0/0	30–40 Gy/CF	62/NA/26
Takeuchi et al. [26]	Retro	2019	87	Conversion or salvage	87/0/0	50–60 Gy/CF or DCF	NA/NA/NA
Booka et al. [27]	Retro	2020	18	Salvage	18/0/0	60 Gy/CF	89/NA/52
Sugawara et al. [28]	Retro	2020	31	Conversion or salvage	31/0/0	50–60 Gy + CF or SN or FN	NA/59/NA
Defize et al. [29]	Retro	2021	24	Salvage	23/1/0	50.4 Gy/CBDCA + PTX	83/NA/NA

(continued)

Table 12.1 (continued)

Authors	Design	Year	*N*	Conversion or salvage	Histology (SCC/AC/other)	Total radiation dose/chemotherapy regimen	1/3/5 year overall survival rate (%)
Abe et al. [30]	Retro	2021	36	Conversion	36/0/0	DCF	NA/61/54
Teranishi et al. [31]	Retro	2023	200	Conversion or salvage	200/0/0	40–60 Gy/DCF FP or DCF	81/63 (2-year)
Makino et al. [32]	Retro	2025	90	Conversion or salvage	89/0/1	40–60 Gy/DCF or FP	NA/41 (2-year)/NA
Xu et al. [33]	Retro	2024	64	Conversion	64/0/0	nab-PTX + CDDP or nab-PTX + CDDP + ICI	98 (PC + ICI)/84 (PC) (2-year)
Huang et al. [34]	Retro	2024	150	Conversion	150/0/0	CF/DF or CF/DF + ICI	NA/NA/NA

SCC squamous cell carcinoma, *AC* adenocarcinoma, *P2* phase II study, *retro*, retrospective study, cohort, *cohort* Study, *CF/FP* 5-fluorouracil and cisplatin, *DCF* docetaxel, cisplatin, and 5-fluorouracil, *MF* mitomycin C and 5-fluorouracil, *ACF* adriamycin, cisplatin, and 5-fluorouracil, *FAP* 5-fluorouracil, adriamycin, and cisplatin, *FN* 5-fluorouracil and nedaplatin, *FAN* 5-fluorouracil, adriamycin, and nedaplatin, *SN* S-1 and nedaplatin, *PTX* paclitaxel, *CBDCA* carboplatin, nab-PTX albumin-bound paclitaxel, *CDDP* cisplatin, *DF* docetaxel and 5-fluorouracil, *ICI* immune checkpoint inhibitor, NA data not available

[a] Patients with clinical T4 disease and/or unresectable supraclavicular lymph node metastasis

[b] Postoperative dose

regimen used as primary treatment. In ICT, some more recent studies applied triplet chemotherapy regimens, including DCF, adriamycin, cisplation, and 5-FU (ACF), and the combination of 5-FU, adriamycin, and nedaplatin (FAN). JCOG1510 (TRIANgLE) is a multicenter, randomized Phase III trial initiated in February 2018, evaluating the efficacy and safety of induction chemotherapy with DCF, followed by surgical conversion or definitive CRT in patients with locally advanced, unresectable intrapleural squamous cell carcinoma of the esophagus, compared to CRT monotherapy, to determine whether it improves overall survival. The results are eagerly awaited. Recently, there have been increasing reports on conversion surgery performed after combination therapy with immune checkpoint inhibitors and chemotherapy, despite limited evidence. Existing reports have used regimens such as ICI plus paclitaxel and cisplatin (ICI–PC), ICI plus cisplatin and 5-FU (ICI–CF), and ICI plus docetaxel and 5-FU (ICI–DF).

Table 12.2 Summary of outcomes in conversion/salvage surgery

Author	year	*N*	Interval[a] (week)	Combined resection rate (%)	Postoperative complications (%)	Mortality (%)	Resection rate[b] (%)	Curative resection rate[b] (%)	Clinical response rate (%)	pCR rate (%)		1/3/5 year overall survival rate (%)	
										Main	All	Grade 3	Grade 0–2
Ikeda et al.	2001	37	NA	0	NA	0	35	32	76	8	8	NA	NA
Yokota et al. (COSMOS)	2016	20	Within 8	0	38 (recurrent nerve palsy) 24 (pleural effusion) 14 (lung infection)	0	42	40	NA	20	20	NA	NA
Sugimura et al.	2021	99	NA	6	Total 56 27 (pneumonia) 11 (anastomic leakage) 15 (recurrent nerve palsy)	0	82	94	0	28	19	NA	NA
Van Raemdonck et al.	1997	18	4–8	0	11 (recurrent nerve palsy) 11 (surgical site infection)	0	100	83	50	17	17	100/100/NA	53/32/NA
Yano et al.	1999	45	4	NA	Total 62 43 (respiratory) 25 (delirium) 21 (recurrent nerve palsy)	0	62	44	64	29	25	86/86/86	65/35/20
Noguchi et al.	2003	41	4–6	0	Total 29 17 (anastomotic leak)	21	59	NA	59	17	17	100/75/25	20/0/0

(continued)

Table 12.2 (continued)

Author	year	N	Interval[a] (week)	Combined resection rate (%)	Postoperative complications (%)	Mortality (%)	Resection rate[b] (%)	Curative resection rate[b] (%)	Clinical response rate (%)	pCR rate (%)		1/3/5 year overall survival rate (%)	
										Main	All	Grade 3	Grade 0–2
Fujita et al.	2005	30	4–6	0	Total 87 50 (recurrent nerve palsy) 35 (respiratory) 23 (tracheal ischemia) 23 (pyothorax)	7	57	34	63	15	7	NA	NA
Seto et al.	2007	59	NA	17 (respiratory tract) 10 (lung) 10 (pericardium)	NA	5	NA	NA	68	14	7	NA	NA
Manzoni et al.	2007	51	NA	NA	NA	10	78	39	20	NA	13	NA	NA
Miyoshi et al.	2009	42	4	NA	NA	NA	NA	NA	83	21	21	90/78/78	58/30/30
Miyata et al.	2012	98	3–4	NA	NA	NA	58	47	78	16	16	NA	NA
Shimoji et al.	2013	43	4 (chemo) 6 (CRT)	0	63	13	70	61	54	14	14	NA	NA
Pimiento et al.	2013	45	NA	0	Total 52 22 (respiratory) 17 (DGE)	4	NA	96	NA	42	42	85/61/53	NA

Akutsu et al.	2014	40	3–4	NA	NA	8	26	NA	100	22	NA	NA	NA
Ohira et al.	2015	40	NA	0	NA	NA	45	40	67	NA	NA	NA	NA
Yamaguchi et al.	2018	13	NA	NA	NA	NA	NA	NA	NA	NA	NA	NA	NA
Takeuchi et al.	2019	87	NA	0	Total 23 5 (pneumonia) 8 (anastomic leakage) 6 (recurrent nerve palsy)	0	46	72	NA	2	2	NA	NA
Booka et al.	2020	18	19	NA	6 (pneumonia) 39 (anastomic leakage) 42 (recurrent nerve palsy)	0	NA	78	NA	28	28	96/NA/83	NA
Sugawara et al.	2020	31	NA	0	Toal 51	10	39	71	0	39	39	NA	NA
Defize et al.	2021	24	NA	NA	46 (pneumonia) 25 (anastomic leakage) 25 (recurrent nerve palsy)	0	47	92	NA	54	46	NA	NA
Abe et al.	2021	36	NA	0	17 (pneumonia) 3 (anastomic leakage) 19 (recurrent nerve palsy)	0	65	81	4	17	17	NA	NA

(continued)

Table 12.2 (continued)

Author	year	N	Interval[a] (week)	Combined resection rate (%)	Postoperative complications (%)	Mortality (%)	Resection rate[b] (%)	Curative resection rate[b] (%)	Clinical response rate (%)	pCR rate (%)		1/3/5 year overall survival rate (%)	
										Main	All	Grade 3	Grade 0–2
Teranishi et al.	2023	200	NA	16	Total 36 14 (pneumonia) 5 (anastomic leakage) 4 (recurrent nerve palsy)	0	NA	NA	3	19	14	NA	NA
Makino et al.	2025	90	8	70 (trachea/bronchus) 22 (large vessel) 5 (both)	Total 54 14 (pneumonia) 4 (anastomic leakage) 7 (recurrent nerve palsy	2	100	NA	9	9	9	NA/75/55 (grade 2–3)	NA/27/21 (grade 0–1)
Xu et al.	2024	64	NA	NA	17 (pneumonia) 5 (anastomic leakage)	1	71	87	8	13	13	NA	NA
Huang et al.	2024	150	NA	NA	12 (pneumonia) 12 (anastomic leakage)	1	67	90	NA	16	0	NA	NA

pCR pathological complete response, *NA* data not available, *CR* complete response, [a]Interval from the completion of chemoradiotherapy to the operation, [b]Calculated with intention to treat analysis; *chemo* chemotherapy, *CRT* chemoradiotherapy, *DGE* delayed gastric emptying

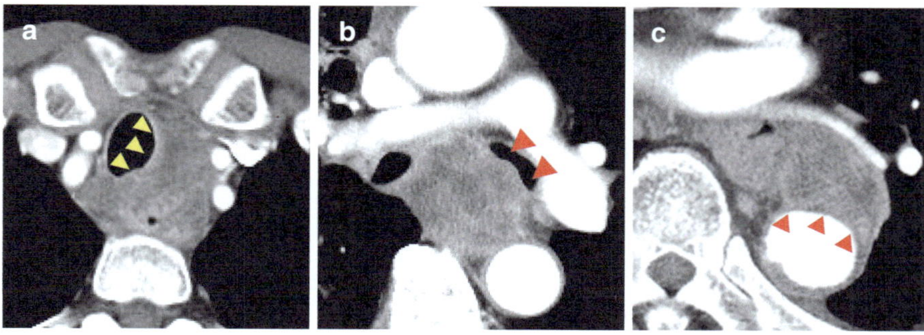

Fig. 12.1 Representative computed tomography images of cT4 esophageal cancer: (**a**) trachea, (**b**) left main bronchus, (**c**) large vessel

12.4 Indications and Preoperative Considerations for Conversion/Salvage Surgery for cT4 Esophageal Cancer

Surgical candidates are those with sufficient operative fitness and downstaging of T4 disease after induction therapy. Tracheobronchial invasion is diagnosed when the layered interface with the airway is lost and the airway is compressed, deviated, or narrowed; bronchoscopy complements CT. Aortic invasion is diagnosed when the aorta–tumor interface is obscured and the contact (Picus) angle is ≥110° over ≥10 mm craniocaudally, or 90–110° over ≥20 mm, or when tumor contour collapse with aortic contact/encasement is present (Fig. 12.1) [10]. cT4 assessment integrates contrast-enhanced CT with upper endoscopy and esophagography (considering dominant wall and gross type), with MRI, PET-CT, or EUS as needed. If these abnormalities resolve after induction therapy, the cT4 designation is considered reversed and conversion surgery considered. It is essential to ensure proper patient positioning that allows immediate conversion to thoracotomy in the left lateral decubitus position in case of intraoperative emergencies such as major organ injury or massive bleeding. Close coordination with anesthesiologists, medical engineers, and nursing staff is crucial.

12.5 Summary of Outcomes in Conversion/Salvage Surgery

Table 12.2 shows summary of outcomes in conversion/salvage surgery. First, the Phase II trial is described in detail. In a Japanese, multicenter, Phase II study evaluating the efficacy of induction chemotherapy (three cycles of cisplatin +5-FU + docetaxel) followed by radical resection (COSMOS trial) (Fig. 12.2) [12] based on evaluation of the effect of induction chemotherapy, resectable patients underwent surgery, while unresectable patients received definitive chemoradiotherapy, and if the cancer became resectable after irradiation at 40–60 Gy, conversion

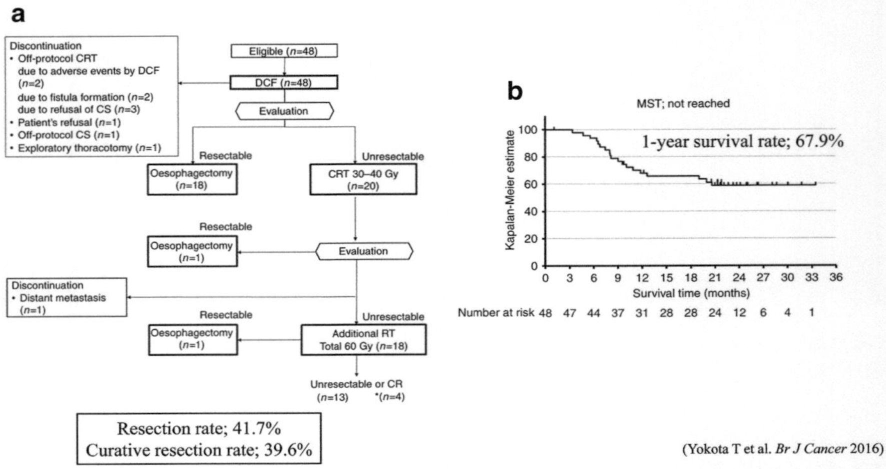

Fig. 12.2 COSMOS trial: (**a**) CONSORT flow diagram, (**b**) Kaplan–Meier plot showing overall survival MST; median survival time

surgery was undertaken. Of the 48 patients enrolled, 42% (20 patients) underwent surgery, corresponding to an R0 resection rate of 95.0% (19/20 cases). In the enrolled patient population overall, the 1- and 3-year overall survival rates were 66.7%, 46.6%, respectively, and the 1- and 3-year progression-free survival rates were 50.6% and 39.6%, respectively. In the 19 patients with R0 resection, the 1- and 3-year overall survival rates were 100.0% and 71.4%, respectively, and the 1- and 3-year progression-free survival rates were 83.6% and 61.3%, respectively. There were no intraoperative complications such as organ injury, and the Grade 3 postoperative complications according to the CTCAE were recurrent laryngeal nerve paralysis, respiratory infection, wound infection, pulmonary fistula, and dysphagia, in 4.8% of the patients each; there were no ≥Grade 4 serious complications or postoperative in hospital deaths.

Sugimura et al. conducted a multicenter randomized Phase II trial (Fig. 12.3) [6] to evaluate the efficacy and safety of two induction treatment strategies—CRT and DCF—prior to conversion/salvage surgery in patients with cT4b ESCC. A total of 99 patients were randomly assigned to either upfront CRT ($n = 49$) or upfront DCF chemotherapy ($n = 50$). Conversion surgery was ultimately performed in 84% of patients in both groups. However, a significantly higher proportion of patients in the CRT group underwent surgery after initial treatment (69% vs. 50%, $p = 0.049$). The R0 resection rate was comparable between groups (78% in CRT vs. 76% in DCF). Notably, the CRT group achieved a significantly higher pathological complete response rate (40% vs. 17%, $p = 0.028$). Postoperative complications occurred in 55% of patients in the CRT group and 59% in the DCF group ($p = 0.824$), showing no significant difference. Common complications included pneumonia (18% in CRT vs. 37% in DCF), recurrent laryngeal nerve palsy (18% vs. 12%), and anastomotic leakage (13% vs. 10%). Although the

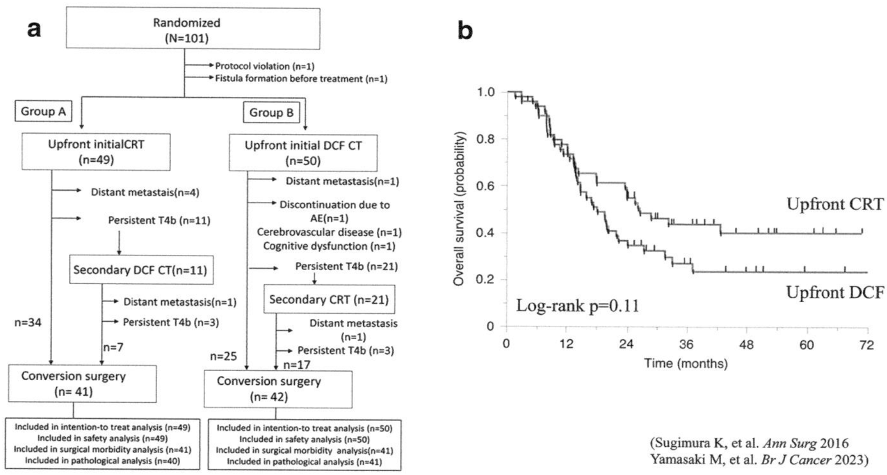

Fig. 12.3 A multicenter randomized Phase II trial by Sugimura et al.: (**a**) CONSORT diagram, (**b**) Kaplan–Meier curves. Overall survival in the intention-to-treat population by initial induction treatment. CRT group ($n = 49$), CT group ($n = 50$)

incidence of pneumonia tended to be higher in the DCF group, the difference did not reach statistical significance ($p = 0.080$). No in-hospital deaths were reported in either group. Although neither difference reached statistical significance, CRT was associated with higher 2-year overall survival (55.1% vs. 34.7%; $p = 0.11$) and showed a trend toward improved 2-year progression-free survival (40.8% vs. 24.0%; $p = 0.12$) compared with CT alone. Local and regional lymph node recurrence in patients undergoing R0 resection was significantly higher in the CT group compared to the CRT group (local: 30% vs. 8%, respectively, $p = 0.03$; regional: 37% vs. 8%, respectively, $p = 0.002$).

Summarizing the results of the retrospective study, the interval between the completion of ICT or ICRT and CS was 3–8 weeks. The resection rates ranged from 26% to 100%, with R0 resection rates of 32% to 96% across studies. Perioperative morbidity in patients undergoing conversion/salvage surgery has varied widely (29–87%, see table for details), with mortality rates of 0–21% across series. Clinical response rates ranged from 20% to 100%, but true pathological complete response (pCR) was achieved in only 8–42% of primary tumors and 7–42% of all involved lesions. Regarding prognosis, 1-, 3-, and 5-year overall survival (OS) rates after CS varied widely at 24–100%, 5–50%, and 0–51%, respectively. When stratified by pathological response, grade 3 responders enjoyed markedly better outcomes (1-, 3-, 5-year OS of 85–100%, 61–100%, and 25–86%) than grade 0–2 patients (1-, 3-, 5-year OS of 20–65%, 0–35%, and 0–30%). Combined resection of involved adjacent organs is also a crucial surgical strategy in conversion surgery for cT4b esophageal cancer. Makino et al. evaluated 90 cT4 patients undergoing conversion surgery and reported combined resections of trachea/bronchus in 63 (70.0%), large vessel in 22 (24.4%), and both 5 (5.6%). Representative intraoperative photographs are shown in (Fig. 12.4).

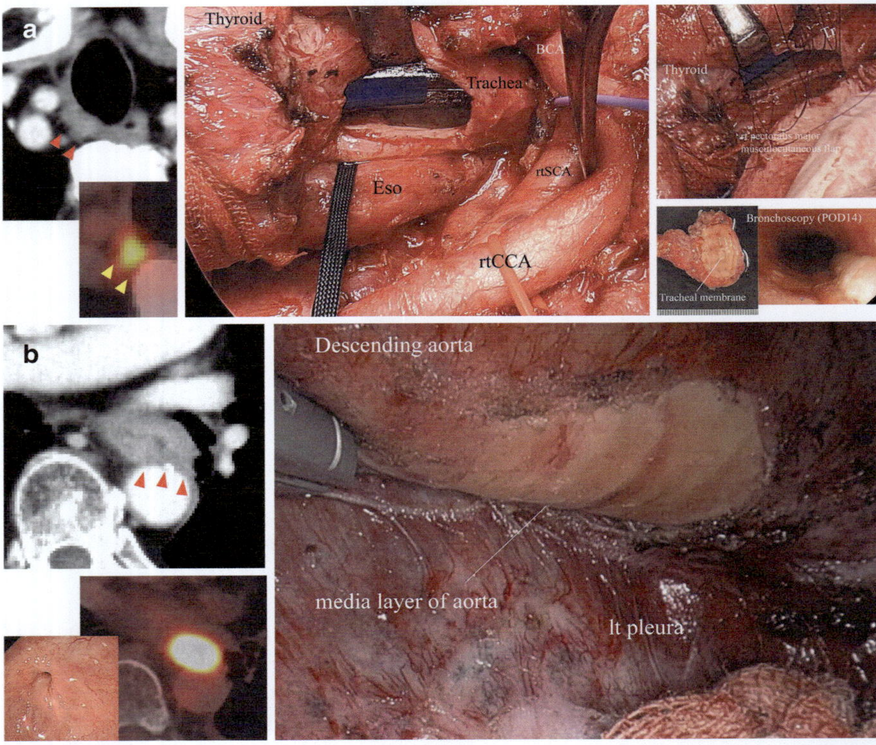

Fig. 12.4 A representative case with all-layer resection of the trachea (**a**), resection of aortic adventitia layer via a robotic approach (**b**). Red and yellow arrow indicate recurrent tumor. BCA brachiocephalic artery, Eso esophagus, rtSCA right subclavian artery, rtCCA right common carotid artery, POD postoperative, Ao aorta, SCA subclavian artery, CCA common carotid artery

Immune checkpoint inhibitors combined with chemotherapy have been evaluated as induction therapy to convert initially unresectable locally advanced esophageal squamous cell carcinoma (including cT4b) to resectable disease. In a retrospective single-center series of cT4b ESCC, PD-1 inhibitor plus chemotherapy yielded higher conversion (81.3% vs. 66.7%), R0 resection (94.2% vs. 82.2%), pathologic complete response (23.1% vs. 6.7%), and 2-year event-free survival (76.4% vs. 42.4%) than chemotherapy alone without increased grade ≥3 toxicity [33]. A multicenter retrospective cohort similarly demonstrated that induction immunochemotherapy produced superior surgical conversion (84.7% vs. 49.7%), pCR (22.0% vs. 5.1%), and overall survival (HR 0.215) compared with induction chemotherapy [35]. The real-world RICE-retro study confirmed feasibility and safety, reporting a 74.8% conversion rate, 94% R0 resection, 22.4% pCR, acceptable high-grade adverse events, and lower anastomotic leak relative to traditional chemotherapy [34]. Mechanistically, chemotherapy may induce immunogenic cell death and remodel the tumor microenvironment to enhance T-cell infiltration, synergizing with ICIs. These data support immunochemotherapy as a preferred induction strategy to improve resectability and survival in unresectable/cT4 ESCC; careful perioperative coordination and management of immune-related adverse events are essential.

12.6 Surgical Strategies: Open to Minimally Invasive Esophagectomy (MIE) or Robot-Assisted Minimally Invasive Esophagectomy (RAMIE)

Historically, open transthoracic esophagectomy provides excellent exposure for radical resection of esophageal tumors but at the cost of greater surgical trauma, higher blood loss, longer intensive care and hospital stays, and increased pulmonary and wound-related complications. With the advent of minimally invasive esophagectomy (MIE) using conventional thoracoscopy, these morbidities were significantly reduced: thoracoscopic MIE yields lower postoperative pain, improved respiratory function, and shorter recovery compared with open surgery.

Robot-assisted esophagectomy is a modern evolution of MIE that addresses some limitations of conventional thoracoscopy. In RAMIE, surgeons use a robotic platform (e.g., DaVinci system) to control a 3D high-definition camera and wristed instruments from a console. This provides a stable, magnified 3D view of the operative field and enhanced dexterity for precise dissection. These features are especially advantageous in cT4b ESCC, where tumors adhere to vital structures. The articulating instruments allow surgeons to approach an invaded area from multiple angles, enabling meticulous dissection along tissue planes that would be difficult with straight laparoscopic tools. For example, around the descending aorta (a common site of T4b invasion), conventional thoracoscopic instruments often must come at a perpendicular angle, whereas the robotic instruments can work parallel to the aorta, markedly improving operative freedom. The robotic system also filters tremors and provides motion scaling, which is beneficial when operating near delicate structures like major vessels or the tracheobronchial tree. Surgeons have reported that the robot's strength in retraction is useful for managing dense fibrosis after chemoradiation, allowing strong but controlled traction on scar tissue during salvage T4b resections.

Crucially, emerging evidence suggests that RAMIE can achieve at least equivalent, if not superior, oncological and perioperative outcomes compared to conventional approaches. A meta-analysis indicated that compared to standard thoracoscopic MIE, RAMIE is associated with significantly lower estimated blood loss and tends to have lower rates of morbidity, recurrent laryngeal nerve (RLN) palsy, and pneumonia. In other words, the robotic approach may better preserve the recurrent laryngeal nerves and reduce pulmonary complications, likely owing to the improved visualization and precision. Recent comparative studies focused on locally advanced tumors support these advantages: Fujita et al. reported that RAMIE yielded a lower incomplete resection (R1/R2) rate (9.0% vs. 16.6%) compared to conventional MIE for borderline cT3/cT4b tumors and a slightly higher

3-year survival rate [36]. Another propensity-matched study by Daiko et al. found that although total operative time was longer with RAMIE, the thoracic phase was shorter and patients in the RAMIE group had signs of faster recovery—such as a lower peak CRP on postoperative day 3, fewer surgical site infections, and shorter ICU stays for cT3 or T4 advanced esophageal cancer [37]. These findings highlight that RAMIE can facilitate gentle tissue handling and meticulous lymphadenectomy (yielding a similar number of lymph nodes as thoracoscopy) without compromising oncological efficacy.

12.7 Points to Note During Salvage Surgery and Postoperative Complications

In conversion (i.e., salvage) esophagectomy following definitive chemoradiotherapy (CRT), fatal postoperative complications—most notably tracheal ischemia and necrosis—have been reported. Therefore, it is imperative during dissection to identify and preserve, under endoscopic visualization, the bronchial arteries, branches of the inferior thyroid arteries supplying the trachea, and the lateral longitudinal anastomotic vessels that interconnect these arterial networks. One characteristic complication after posterior mediastinal reconstruction with a gastric conduit is a gastric conduit–tracheal fistula. Although its incidence is rare, once it occurs, digestive fluid enters the airway through the fistula, leading to severe aspiration pneumonia, making treatment difficult and potentially fatal. Therefore, in salvage surgery, reconstruction is generally performed via the subcutaneous or retrosternal route, except in cases where supporting tissue is required on the dorsal side of the trachea, such as when the membranous portion of the trachea is deeply shaved during tumor dissection. If posterior mediastinal reconstruction with a gastric conduit is chosen, it is important to bury the stapler line of the gastric division or anastomosis securely to reduce the risk of gastric conduit–tracheal fistula. In addition, salvage surgery has been reported to have a relatively high rate of anastomotic leakage. If the radiation field includes the gastric cardia, it is advisable to avoid performing the anastomosis in the irradiated area as much as possible. Furthermore, when a moderate or greater amount of pericardial effusion due to radiation is observed at the time of surgery, pericardiotomy should be considered intraoperatively for long-term postoperative management. Reported in-hospital mortality rates for salvage esophagectomy was 5% [38], and although more recent series suggest a downward trend, mortality remains unacceptably high. To minimize surgical invasiveness and reduce perioperative risk, strategies such as limiting the extent of resection, staging the operation, or placing a feeding jejunostomy tube for postoperative nutritional support should be considered on a case-by-case basis. These procedures should ideally be conducted in high-volume centers with multidisciplinary teams capable of providing comprehensive perioperative management and postoperative care.

12.8 Summary and Perspectives

Conversion and salvage esophagectomy have emerged as potentially curative strategies for patients with initially unresectable cT4b esophageal squamous cell carcinoma (ESCC), particularly in the era of multimodal induction therapy. Accumulating evidence indicates that both induction chemotherapy (ICT) and induction chemoradiotherapy (ICRT) can downstage tumors and enable R0 resection in selected cases, with pathological complete response (pCR) rates reaching up to 40% in some series. Moreover, the integration of immune checkpoint inhibitors (ICIs) into induction regimens has markedly improved response rates, resectability, and survival without significantly increasing perioperative risks.

From a surgical standpoint, salvage esophagectomy for cT4b cases remains technically demanding due to tumor invasion into adjacent vital structures, tissue fibrosis after radiation, and the risk of fatal complications such as tracheal necrosis. To mitigate these risks, meticulous intraoperative dissection with preservation of critical vascular supply to the airway is imperative. It is also essential to have a thorough understanding of the indications and perioperative management considerations. The use of robot-assisted minimally invasive esophagectomy (RAMIE) has been increasingly adopted in high-volume centers, offering superior visualization, tremor filtration, and articulation that enhance precision during complex resections. Comparative studies suggest that RAMIE may reduce intraoperative blood loss, pulmonary complications, and recurrent laryngeal nerve injury, while achieving comparable oncologic outcomes to conventional approaches.

Looking forward, standardization of patient selection criteria, refinement of induction protocols, and multidisciplinary perioperative management are essential to optimize outcomes. The role of RAMIE in conversion and salvage settings warrants further validation through prospective studies. Importantly, ongoing trials such as JCOG1510 (TRIANgLE) and emerging data from immunochemotherapy cohorts will help define optimal therapeutic algorithms. In parallel, artificial intelligence (AI) and augmented reality (AR) can broaden indications and enhance safety via AR overlays for patient-specific 3D navigation, AI-assisted interpretation of intraoperative signals, and perioperative AI for risk prediction and early complication detection. With advancing connectivity and robotics, telesurgery may become feasible in selected cases, enabling safer R0 resections and improved outcomes in cT4b ESCC.

References

1. Makino T, Miyata H, Yano M, et al. Conversion surgery for cT4 esophageal squamous cell carcinoma: a systematic review. Ann Gastroenterol Surg. 2019;3(1):21–30.
2. Kaneko K, Ito H, Konishi K, et al. Definitive chemoradiotherapy for patients with malignant stricture due to T3 or T4 squamous cell car cinoma of the oesophagus. Br J Cancer. 2003;88:18–24.
3. Itoh Y, Fuwa N, Matsumoto A, et al. Outcomes of radiotherapy for inoperable locally advanced (T4) esophageal cancer- retrospective analysis. Radiat Med. 2001;19:231–5.

4. Mine S, et al. Japanese classification of esophageal cancer, 12th edition: part I. Esophagus. 2024;21(3):179–215.
5. Makino T, Yamasaki M, Miyazaki Y, et al. Utility of initial induction chemotherapy with 5-fluorouracil, cisplatin, and docetaxel (DCF) for T4 esophageal cancer: a propensity score-matched analysis. Dis Esophagus. 2018;31. https://doi.org/10.1093/dote/dox130.
6. Sugimura K, Miyata H, Tanaka K, et al. Multicenter randomized phase 2 trial comparing chemoradiotherapy and docetaxel plus 5-fluorouracil and cisplatin chemotherapy as initial induction therapy for subsequent conversion surgery in patients with clinical T4b esophageal cancer: short-term results. Ann Surg. 2021;274:e465–72.
7. KEYNOTE 590 Investigators. Pembrolizumab plus chemotherapy versus chemotherapy alone for first line treatment of advanced esophageal carcinoma: results from the KEYNOTE 590 trial. J Clin Oncol. 2020;38(23):WCH 590.
8. Doki Y, Ajani JA, Kato K, et al. Nivolumab combination therapy in advanced esophageal squamous-cell carcinoma. N Engl J Med. 2022;386:449–62.
9. National Comprehensive Cancer Network. NCCN clinical practice guidelines in oncology: esophageal and esophagogastric junction cancers. Version 2.2025. Fort Washington: National Comprehensive Cancer Network; 2025.
10. Kitagawa Y, Ishihara R, Ishikawa H, et al. Esophageal cancer practice guidelines 2022 edited by the Japan Esophageal Society: part 1. Esophagus. 2023;20(3):343–72.
11. Ikeda K, Ishida K, Sato N, et al. Chemoradiotherapy followed by surgery for thoracic esophageal cancer potentially or actually involving adjacent organs. Dis Esophagus. 2001;14:197–201.
12. Yokota T, Kato K, Hamamoto Y, et al. Phase II study of chemo selection with docetaxel plus cisplatin and 5- fluorouracil in duction chemotherapy and subsequent conversion surgery for locally advanced unresectable oesophageal cancer. Br J Cancer. 2016;115:1328–34.
13. Chiarion-Sileni V, Corti L, Ruol A, et al. Phase II trial of docetaxel, cisplatin and fluorouracil followed by carboplatin and radio therapy in locally advanced oesophageal cancer. Br J Cancer. 2007;96:432–8.
14. Yano M, Tsujinaka T, Shiozaki H, et al. Concurrent chemotherapy (5- fluorouracil and cisplatin) and radiation therapy followed by surgery for T4 squamous cell carcinoma of the esophagus. J Surg Oncol. 1999;70:25–32.
15. Noguchi T, Moriyama H, Wada S, et al. Resection surgery with neo adjuvant chemoradiotherapy improves outcomes of patients with T4 esophageal carcinoma. Dis Esophagus. 2003;16:94–8.
16. Fujita H, Sueyoshi S, Tanaka T, et al. Esophagectomy: is it necessary after chemoradiotherapy for a locally advanced T4 esophageal cancer? Prospective nonrandomized trial comparing chemoradiotherapy with surgery versus without surgery. World J Surg. 2005;29:25–30.
17. Seto Y, Chin K, Gomi K, et al. Treatment of thoracic esophageal car cinoma invading adjacent structures. Cancer Sci. 2007;98:937–42.
18. de Manzoni G, Pedrazzani C, Pasini F, et al. Chemoradiotherapy followed by surgery for squamous cell carcinoma of the thoracic esophagus with clinical evidence of adjacent organ invasion. J Surg Oncol. 2007;95:261–6.
19. Miyoshi N, Yano M, Takachi K, et al. Myelotoxicity of preoperative chemoradiotherapy is a significant determinant of poor prognosis in patients with T4 esophageal cancer. J Surg Oncol. 2009;99:302–6.
20. Miyata H, Yamasaki M, Kurokawa Y, et al. Clinical relevance of in duction triplet chemotherapy for esophageal cancer invading adjacent organs. J Surg Oncol. 2012;106:441–7.
21. Shimoji H, Karimata H, Nagahama M, Nishimaki T. Induction chemotherapy or chemoradiotherapy followed by radical esophagectomy for T4 esophageal cancer: results of a prospective cohort study. World J Surg. 2013;37:2180–8.
22. Pimiento JM, Weber J, Hoffe SE, et al. Outcomes associated with surgery for T4 esophageal cancer. Ann Surg Oncol. 2013;20:2706–12.

23. Akutsu Y, Kono T, Uesato M, et al. Is the outcome of a salvage surgery for T4 thoracic esophageal squamous cell carcinoma really poor? World J Surg. 2014;38:2891–7.
24. Van Raemdonck D, Van Cutsem E, Menten J, et al. Induction therapy for clinical T4 oesophageal carcinoma; a plea for continued surgical exploration. Eur J Cardiothorac Surg. 1997;11:828–37.
25. Yamaguchi S, Morita M, Yamamoto M, et al. Long-term outcome of definitive chemoradiotherapy and induction chemoradiotherapy followed by surgery for T4 esophageal cancer with tracheobronchial invasion. Ann Surg Oncol. 2018;25:3280–7.
26. Takeuchi M, Kawakubo H, Mayanagi S, et al. The benefits of docetaxel plus cisplatin and 5-fluorouracil induction therapy in conversion to curative treatment for locally advanced esophageal squamous cell carcinoma. World J Surg. 2019;43:2006–15.
27. Booka E, Haneda R, Ishii K, et al. Appropriate candidates for salvage esophagectomy of initially unresectable locally advanced T4 esophageal squamous cell carcinoma. Ann Surg Oncol. 2020;27:3163–70.
28. Sugawara K, Yagi K, Okumura Y, et al. Long-term outcomes of multimodal therapy combining definitive chemoradiotherapy and salvage surgery for T4 esophageal squamous cell carcinoma. Int J Clin Oncol. 2020;25:552–60.
29. Defize IL, Van Der Horst S, Bulbul M, et al. Salvage robot-assisted minimally invasive esophagectomy (RAMIE) for T4b esophageal cancer after definitive chemoradiotherapy. Ann Surg Oncol. 2021;28:2730–8.
30. Abe T, Higaki E, Hosoi T, et al. Long-term outcome of patients with locally advanced clinically unresectable esophageal cancer undergoing conversion surgery after induction chemotherapy with docetaxel plus cisplatin and 5-fluorouracil. Ann Surg Oncol. 2021;28:712–21.
31. Teranishi R, Makino T, Tanaka K, Yamashita K, Saito T, Yamamoto K, et al. Long-term survival and prognostic factors associated with curative conversion surgery for ct4b esophageal squamous cell carcinoma: analysis of 200 consecutive cases. Surgery. 2023;174(3):558–66. https://doi.org/10.1016/j.surg.2023.05.040.
32. Makino T, Yamasaki M, Nakai S, et al. Surgical and longterm outcomes of combined organ resection for esophageal cancer invading adjacent organs: experience of 90 consecutive cases. J Thorac Cardiovasc Surg. 2025;S0022–5223(25):00088–1.
33. Xu Z, You Z, Chen M, et al. Comparison of immunochemotherapy and chemotherapy alone in conversion therapy for locally advanced unresectable esophageal squamous cell carcinoma. Front Oncol. 2024;14:1370353.
34. Huang S, Wu H, Cheng C, et al. Conversion surgery following immunochemotherapy in initially unresectable locally advanced esophageal squamous cell carcinoma-a real world multicenter study (RICE-retro). Front Immunol. 2022;13:935374.
35. Huang S, Wang S, Gao Z, et al. Induction immunochemotherapy yields a higher conversion rate and better overall survival than chemotherapy in initially unresectable esophageal squamous cell carcinoma. Ann Surg Oncol. 2024;31(10):6635–44.
36. Fujita T, Sato K, Kajiyama D, et al. Short and middle term outcomes of robot assisted minimally invasive esophagectomy for highly locally advanced esophageal cancer with stage cT3 borderline and cT4b at initial diagnosis. Surg Endosc. 2025;39:2994–3005.
37. Daiko H, Oguma J, Ishiyama K, et al. Technical feasibility and oncological outcomes of robotic esophagectomy compared with conventional thoracoscopic esophagectomy for clinical T3 or T4 locally advanced esophageal cancer: a propensity-matched analysis. Surg Endosc. 2024;38:3590–601.
38. Petric J, Handshin S, Bright T, Watson DI. Planned oesophagectomy after chemoradiotherapy versus salvage oesophagectomy following definitive chemoradiotherapy: a systematic review and meta-analysis. ANZ J Surg. 2023;93(4):829–39.

Mediastinoscopic Esophagectomy

13

Hitoshi Fujiwara, Hirotaka Konishi, and Atsushi Shiozaki

13.1 Introduction

Transthoracic esophagectomy (TTE) with total mediastinal lymphadenectomy has been recognized as a standard procedure for esophageal squamous cell carcinoma (ESCC) [1], in which the upper mediastinum along the bilateral recurrent laryngeal nerves (RLN) is the most important region for radical surgery for ESCC [2, 3]. With advances of endoscopic surgery, thoracoscopic TTE, or thoracoscopic esophagectomy (TE), is now performed widely as a minimally invasive esophagectomy (MIE) [4]. Mediastinoscopic esophagectomy (ME) is another MIE, which is originated from transhiatal esophagectomy (THE). THE, first reported as "esophagectomy without thoracotomy" by Orringer et al. in 1978, is characterized by blunt dissection of the esophagus in a blind manner with fingers [5]. THE has been accepted as a standard procedure for esophageal cancer in Western countries, mostly for distal esophageal and junction tumors or those with a histology of adenocarcinoma. THE is regarded as less invasive than open TTE since it avoids thoracotomy [6]. However, THE has been a limited option for ESCC due to lymphadenectomy limited to the lower mediastinum [7]. In the 1990s, mediastinoscopy was introduced into THE to improve the safety and curability of THE [8–10]. However, although it enabled esophageal mobilization and lymph node sampling under direct vision through the scope, it was unsuitable for lymphadenectomy as it only provides narrow surgical view around the scope tip.

In the last decade, with the introduction of single-port mediastinoscopy or robotic surgery, novel approach with equivalent lymphadenectomy to TTE has been developed [11]. In this chapter, we review conventional and novel approaches in ME mainly focusing on published studies and introduce our surgical procedure.

H. Fujiwara (✉) · H. Konishi · A. Shiozaki
Division of Digestive Surgery, Department of Surgery, Kyoto Prefectural University of Medicine, Kyoto, Japan
e-mail: hfuji@koto.kpu-m.ac.jp; shiozaki@koto.kpu-m.ac.jp

Y. Kitagawa et al. (eds.), *Esophageal Squamous Cell Carcinoma*,
https://doi.org/10.1007/978-981-92-2611-5_13

13.2 Different Approaches in ME

13.2.1 Conventional Approach (Fig. 13.1, Left)

Since clinical introduction, dedicated rigid endoscope has been used as mediastinoscopy [8–10]. However, due to the limitation of surgical view and handling for lymphadenectomy, mediastinoscopy-assisted THE, often abbreviated as MATHE, has been indicated mostly for clinical T1–2 tumors without lymph node metastasis, or Stage I–II tumors, in ESCC patients who are unsuitable for thoracotomy or one lung ventilation because of severe pleural adhesion or poor pulmonary function due to previous thoracic surgery or disease as a limited surgery in Asia [10, 12–18]. Although transcervical approach using a pneumomediastinum or single-port technique is reported, it was only used for esophageal dissection, not lymphadenectomy [19, 20].

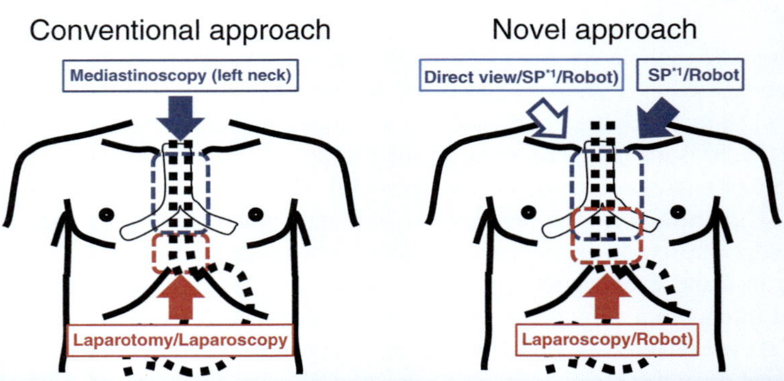

	Conventional approach	Novel approach
Mediastinoscopy	· Dedicated rigid scope without PM*2	· SP*1with PM*2
Transcervical procedure	· Left side alone	· Bilateral sides
Upper and middle mediastinal LND*3	· Sampling (limited surgery)	· Equivalent to TTE(radical surgery)
Surgical indication (patient risk)	· Limited to high-risk patients*4	· Expanded to low-risk patients
Surgical indication (tumor stage)	· Limited to T1-2N0, Stage I-II	· Expanded to T3N(+), Stage III

*1 SP, Single-port mediastinoscopy; *2 PM, Pneumomediastinum; *3 LND, Lymph node dissection

*4 Those with a difficulty in thoracotomy due to poor pulmonary function, severe pleural adhesion

Fig. 13.1 ME types (conventional and novel)

13.2.2 Novel Approach (Fig. 13.1, Right)

Since 2010s, novel minimally invasive techniques were introduced into transhiatal or transcervical procedure to establish novel radical esophagectomy without thoracotomy for ESCC. Robot-assisted transhiatal procedure for the middle and lower mediastinal lymphadenectomy was first reported by Mori et al. as a case report in 2013 [21], followed by a case series with a comparison of short-term outcomes with open TTE [22], and then, the left transcervical procedure for the upper mediastinal lymphadenectomy using a single-port mediastinoscopy was reported by Fujiwara et al. [23, 24]. These procedures contributed greatly to safe and reliable mediastinal lymphadenectomy, especially in the deep mediastinum, or subcarinal and subaortic arch region, farthest from both the neck and abdomen. Since then, different approaches from different countries have been reported, mainly from Japan [25–34] (Table 13.1).

Novel approach, which allows complete mediastinal lymphadenectomy, can be applied to a wide range of ESCC cases, including advanced diseases or those suitable for thoracotomy. In Japan, it was approved for national insurance coverage in 2018 based on the short-term outcomes and is now recognized, along with TTE, as a standard procedure for ESCC.

Reports on novel approach are increasing, but its name is not yet standardized. In Japan, it was first reported as "non-transthoracic esophagectomy (NTTE)" [22] and "single-port mediastinoscope-assisted THE" [26]. In China, it has been reported under names such as esophagectomy with "single-port inflatable mediastinoscopy" or "pneumatic mediastinoscopy" [30, 35]. At present, in Japan, the term "transmediastinal radical esophagectomy (TME)" is used more often to equally emphasize both transcervical and transhiatal lymphadenectomies [11]. In Western countries, the abbreviation TME is regarded unsuitable because it is identical to the concept of lymphadenectomy in rectal cancer. In addition, to clearly distinguish from THE, the term MICE (minimally invasive transcervical esophagectomy) is now proposed [33]. For robot-assisted surgery, terms such as "robot-assisted transmediastinal esophagectomy (RATME)" [36] and "robot-assisted transcervical esophagectomy (RACE)" have been reported [34].

Table 13.1 TME: first clinical reports from different countries (except for a case report)

Author	Country	Year	Case	Minimally invasive technique		Novel finding	Reference
				Transcervical	Transhiatal		
Fujiwara	Japan	2015	*n* = 12	SP (LN)	Laparoscopy	First SP approach	[23]
Mori	Japan	2016	*n* = 22	Non-SP (LN)	Robot	First robotic approach	[22]
Tokairin	Japan	2019	*n* = 10	SP (BN)	Laparoscopy	SP approach from RN	[28]
Nakauchi	Japan	2019	*n* = 6	Robot (LN)	Robot	Robotic approach from neck	[29]
Wang	China	2019	*n* = 80	SP (LN)	Laparoscopy	First SP approach in China	[30]
Daiko	Japan	2021	*n* = 16	SP (BN)	Laparoscopy	Simultaneous SP approaches from BN	[31]
Klarenbeek	The Netherlands	2023	*n* = 3	SP (LN)	Laparoscopy	First SP approach in the Netherland	[33]
Fujita	Japan	2024	*n* = 10	Robot (BN)	Robot	Totally robotic approach	[34]

SP single-port mediastinoscopy, *LN* left neck, *RN* right neck, *BN* bilateral neck

13.3 Our Surgical Procedure

At our institution (KPUM), TME is a standard procedure for ESCC. In principle, all cases judged to be resectable either before surgery or following neoadjuvant chemotherapy are considered candidates for TME. For bulky tumors with suspected invasion to the tracheobronchi or aorta, open TTE alone or in combination with transmediastinal approach is considered.

13.3.1 Overview

TME was performed according to previously reported procedures [23–25] with a modification. In brief, the patient was placed in the supine position with both upper limbs secured to the trunk and the lower limbs abducted. First, following placement of a single-port instrument through the left cervical incision, a transcervical procedure was performed using the single-port mediastinoscopy technique with forced pneumomediastinum initiated at 6 mmHg, then increased to 8 mmHg, and finally to 10 mmHg, depending on the expansion of the dissected space. During esophageal mobilization, upper mediastinal lymphadenectomy, including dissection of lymph nodes along the left RLN, was performed. This was followed by the right cervical procedure under direct vision for lymphadenectomy along the right RLN. Subsequently, transhiatal esophageal mobilization with middle and lower mediastinal lymphadenectomy was performed using either a hand-assisted or totally laparoscopic technique with a pneumomediastinum of 10 mmHg. Subcarinal lymphadenectomy (dissection of the carinal and bilateral main bronchial lymph nodes) was performed mainly through the left transcervical approach and supplemented by the transhiatal procedure if necessary. Finally, after cervical transection of the esophagus and extraction through the abdominal incision (Fig. 13.2), reconstruction was performed with a gastric conduit via the retrosternal route. The procedure for total mediastinal lymphadenectomy is shown in Table 13.2.

13.3.2 Technical Tips and Key Considerations in Lymphadenectomy

During the left transcervical procedure, the esophagus is separated from the trachea, together with the left RLN and lymph nodes, and finally, the nerve is dissected free to allow en bloc dissection (Fig. 13.3). Separating the nerve from the trachea can minimize the left RLN palsy risk associated with lymphadenectomy of the right upper mediastinum and subcarinal region from the left neck.

13.3.2.1 Lymphadenectomy Along the Left RLN

With solo surgery by the operator, lymphadenectomy along the left RLN can be performed sufficiently under good surgical view until subaortic arch region, without the need to avoid the trachea or esophagus. However, in the long and narrow

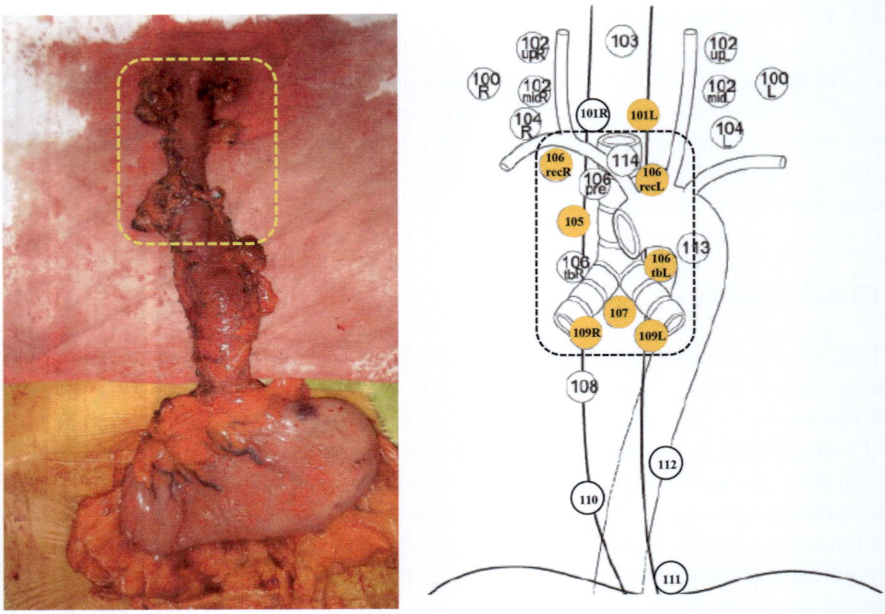

Fig. 13.2 Intraoperative finding of the esophagus and stomach extracted through the abdominal incision. Dotted square indicates the dissection range by the left transcervical procedure

Table 13.2 Our standardized procedure for TME

Approach	Procedure	LN dissection
1. Left neck (direct vision)	Single-port placement	No. 101L
2. Mediastinoscopy	Esophageal dissection (left side and posterior plane)	No. 106recL-106tbL (left side dissection)
	Esophageal dissection (anterior plane)	No. 106recL-106tbL (right side dissection)
	Esophageal dissection (right side)	No. 105-106recR
	Subcarinal dissection (right side)	No. 107-109R
	Left RLN isolation	No. 106recL-106tbL (complete dissection)
	Subcarinal dissection (left side)	No. 109L
3. Right neck (direct vision)	Right RLN isolation	No. 101R/No. 106recR (addition)
4. Laparoscopy	Esophageal dissection (anterior and posterior planes)	No. 109L (addition)
	Esophageal dissection (left and right sides)	No. 112/No. 108–110

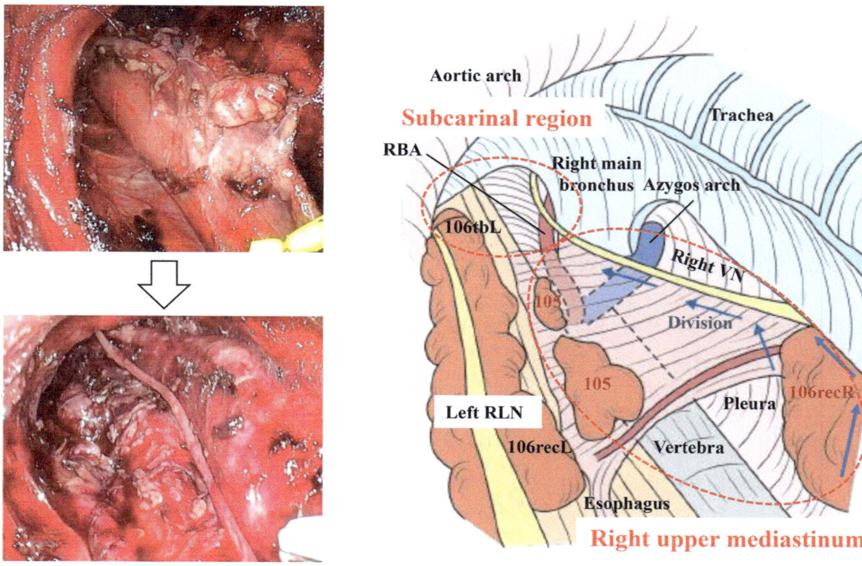

Fig. 13.3 Left transcervical procedure: concept and rationale

mediastinum, careful procedure is required to avoid RLN palsy due to device handling always close to the nerve. Exposure of the nerve at the aortic arch early during esophageal dissection is helpful as a good landmark to predict the nerve course. Keeping the nerve as straight as possible while dividing the branches one by one is also important to reduce the risk of RLN palsy on lymphadenectomy.

13.3.2.2 Lymphadenectomy Along the Right RLN

The right RLN lymph nodes can generally be dissected from the right neck, but surgical view over the right subclavian artery is limited, which may lead to insufficient dissection. Depending on mediastinal anatomy, the view from the left neck using mediastinoscopy may be clearer. Therefore, for complete dissection, it is important to combine both approaches, rather than relying on either single approach. During dissection from the left neck, care is needed to avoid the right RLN palsy due to traction. When bulky nodes are present, dissection from the right neck is often performed first.

13.3.2.3 Subcarinal Lymphadenectomy

Subcarinal lymphadenectomy is most difficult as it is the deepest procedure both from the neck and abdomen, and is generally performed via the left cervical approach, which offers better access and avoids cardiac compression seen in the transhiatal approach, thus preventing arrhythmia or circulation instability. However, careful handling of bronchial arteries and lymph node traction is required, with attention to the left RLN injury. Depending on mediastinal anatomy, a combined cervical and transhiatal approaches may be necessary [37]. In particular, the left main bronchial nodes are often difficult to remove from the left neck due to the aortic arch and RLN, but can be more easily dissected by the transhiatal approach.

13.3.3 Perioperative Tools to Reduce Morbidity

13.3.3.1 Preoperative 3D-CT Evaluation

Preoperative 3D-CT evaluation is performed for all cases scheduled for TME to better understand transmediastinal anatomy (Fig. 13.4). The bronchial arteries show considerable variation, and assessing their relationship to the esophagus on 3D-CT is useful for safe esophageal dissection and lymphadenectomy [38]. Observing sequential axial images from the neck to the deep mediastinum visualizes the esophagus, surrounding organs, and bronchial arteries through a cervical approach, and allows appropriate handling of the arteries to reduce the risk of bleeding or RLN injury (Fig. 13.5). In addition, sagittal images enable quantitative assessment of mediastinal shape or narrowness, helping to predict the difficulty of lymphadenectomy in the deep mediastinum [37].

13.3.3.2 Continuous Intraoperative Nerve Monitoring (CIONM)

The cervical single-port approach carries a high risk of the left RLN palsy due to device insertion and manipulation along the nerve in the narrow mediastinum. Injury may result not only from heat, traction, or compression by the devices at the visible area around scope tip but also from traction or compression in blind areas

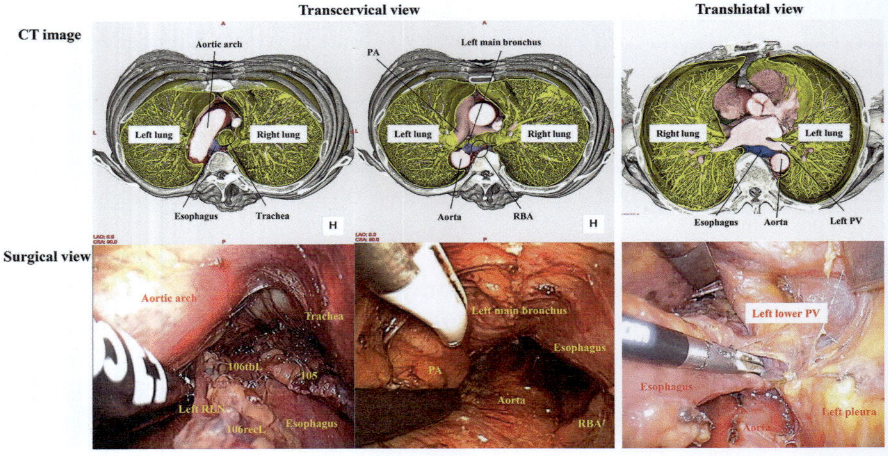

Fig. 13.4 Preoperative 3D-CT simulation

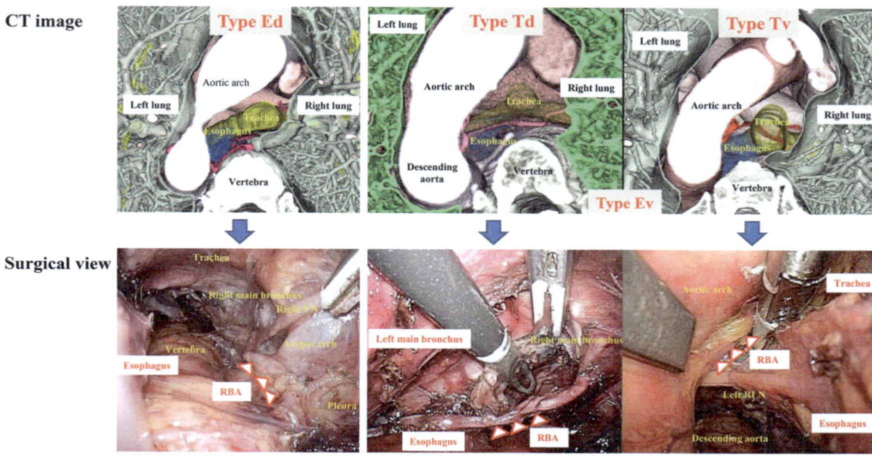

Fig. 13.5 Transcervical view of RBA. RBA right bronchial arteries

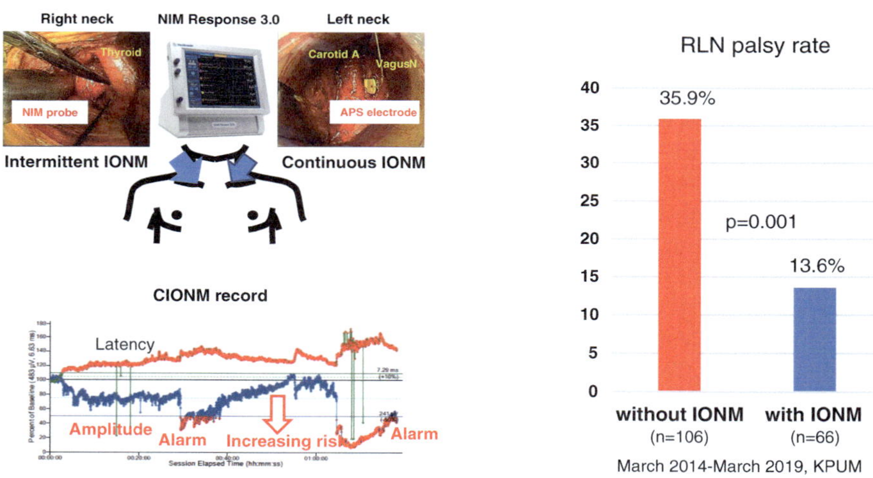

Fig. 13.6 IONM

proximal to the device tip. To reduce the risk, we are employing continuous intraoperative nerve monitoring (CIONM) with periodic electric stimulation of the vagus nerve during the left cervical single-port approach, in addition to intermittent RLN stimulation by the probe during bilateral cervical dissection (Fig. 13.6). CIONM enables real-time detection and subsequent cessation of the risk procedure to avoid RLN injury during surgery, and learning of the risk events after surgery helps improve surgical procedure or technique. Since the risk varies by case, CIONM is considered essential to minimize RLN palsy. Our initial outcome is also shown in Fig. 13.6.

13.4 Surgical Outcomes and Comparison with TTE

A recent meta-analysis from China showed that, compared with TE, ME results in shorter operation time, less blood loss, fewer pneumonias but more RLN palsy, and fewer dissected lymph nodes, while survival is similar [39]. The difference in lymph node yield reflects the fact that ME is generally applied as a limited surgery, with different indications from TE. Similarly, recent reports from Japan compared TE and single-port ME in a single institutional study, where ME was preferentially indicated for high-risk cases, and concluded that ME may be feasible in terms of short-term outcomes and survival when compared with TE [40, 41].

On the other hand, no studies have compared ME and TE as standard procedures for ESCC. Ogawa et al. reported favorable short-term outcomes of TME, including reduced pulmonary complications, when compared with open TTE, and that surgical approach (TME) is an independent factor for reducing pulmonary complications in multivariate analysis [42]. Yagi et al. compared open TTE with robot-assisted TME, and demonstrated for the first time that, after propensity score matching, TME had significantly better OS and RFS than open TTE [36].

ME has fewer pulmonary complications but more RLN palsy than TTE. IONM is useful for reducing RLN palsy, but most evidence comes from intermittent probe stimulation in TE [43], while reports on CIONM are limited [44–47]. A recent report showed that combining intermittent and continuous monitoring reduces RLN palsy and increases lymph node yield along RLNs in TTE [46]. Similarly, a significant reduction in RLN palsy with CIONM is reported in TME [47]. More evidence is needed to confirm its value in ME.

A recent nationwide survey in Japan reported short-term outcomes of esophagectomy by surgical approach [48]. Compared with TE, ME showed more RLN palsy but a similar rate of pneumonia. The number of cases was much smaller in ME and differences in surgical indications and surgeon skills should be considered for fair evaluation. Multicenter studies are needed to clarify the true value of ME in short- and long-term outcomes. Our short-term outcomes after IONM introduction are shown in Table 13.3.

Table 13.3 Short-term outcomes after IONM induction at KPUM (n=246, Aug 2017-Sep 2023)

Operation time (median)	332 min
Blood loss (median)	120 mL
No. of resected med + abd LNs (median)	36
R0 resection	224 (91.1%)
Pneumonia (≥CD II)	15 (6.1%)
Vocal cord palsy (≥CD I)	
Clinical symptom (hoarseness)	44 (17.9%)
Laryngoscopy on POD7	69 (28.0%)
Tracheotomy/tracheostomy	4 (1.7%)
Anastomotic leak (≥CD II)	35 (14.2%)
Unplanned conversion to thoracotomy	4 (1.6%)
Tracheobronchial injury	2 (0.8%)
Mediastinal bleeding	2 (0.8%)
Chyle leak	1 (0.4%)

13.5 Future Perspectives

The cervical single-port approach has improved the safety of ME, but have not necessarily expanded its indications. In Japan, some centers use ME as the standard for ESCC, while others apply it only as a limited option for selected cases, maintaining TE as the standard. Because of anatomical differences from TTE and technical challenges of the cervical single-port approach, its use is mostly limited to high-volume centers. More than 100 cases are reported to be needed to overcome the learning curve [49]. For safe dissemination of ME, standardization of surgical procedures is essential. Robotic approach may be promising to perform deep mediastinal procedures safely and reliably [34, 50]. CIONM, which is well suited to the cervical single-port approach, will likely be indispensable in overcoming RLN palsy, while improving the accuracy of lymphadenectomy along RLNs. Furthermore, if surgical difficulty could be predicted based on individual patient characteristics and tumor factors as well as mediastinal shape or narrowness, it would facilitate appropriate case selection according to the surgeon's level of proficiency in ME.

References

1. Watanabe M, Toh Y, Ishihara R, et al. Comprehensive registry of esophageal cancer in Japan, 2015. Esophagus. 2023;20:1–28.
2. Tachimori Y, Ozawa S, Numasaki H, et al. Efficacy of lymph node dissection by node zones according to tumor location for esophageal squamous cell carcinoma. Esophagus. 2016;13:1–7.
3. Udagawa H, Ueno M, Shinohara H, et al. The importance of grouping of lymph node stations and rationale of three-field lymphadenectomy for thoracic esophageal cancer. J Surg Oncol. 2012;106:742–7.
4. Marubashi S, Takahashi A, Kakeji Y, et al. Surgical outcomes in gastroenterological surgery in Japan: report of the national clinical database 2011–2019. Ann Gastroenterol Surg. 2021;5:639–58.
5. Orringer MB, Sloan H. Esophagectomy without thoracotomy. J Thorac Cardiovasc Surg. 1978;76:643–54.
6. Boshier PR, Anderson O, Hanna GB. Transthoracic versus transhiatal esophagectomy for the treatment of esophagogastric cancer: a meta-analysis. Ann Surg. 2011;254:894–906.
7. Akiyama H, Hiyama M, Miyazono H. Total esophageal reconstruction after extraction of the esophagus. Ann Surg. 1975;182:547–52.
8. Buess G, Kaiser J, Manncke K, et al. Endoscopic microsurgical dissection of the esophagus (EMDE). Int Surg. 1997;82:109–12.
9. Bumm R, Hölscher AH, Feussner H, et al. Endodissection of the thoracic esophagus. Technique and clinical results in transhiatal esophagectomy. Ann Surg. 1993;218:97–104.
10. Tangoku A, Yoshino S, Abe T, et al. Mediastinoscope-assisted transhiatal esophagectomy for esophageal cancer. Surg Endosc. 2004;18:383–9.
11. Fujiwara H, Shiozaki A, Konishi H, et al. Transmediastinal approach for esophageal cancer: a new trend toward radical surgery. Asian J Endosc Surg. 2019;12:30–6.
12. Okumura H, Uchikado Y, Matsumoto M, et al. Clinical significance of mediastinoscope-assisted transhiatal esophagectomy in patients with esophageal cancer. Langenbeck's Arch Surg. 2015;400:699–706.
13. Wu B, Qiu M, Zheng X, et al. Video-assisted mediastinoscopic transhiatal esophagectomy combined with laparoscopy for esophageal cancer. J Cardiothorac Surg. 2010;5:132–6.

14. Feng MX, Wang H, Zhang Y, Tan LJ, Xu ZL, Qun W. Minimally invasive esophagectomy for esophageal squamous cell carcinoma: a case-control study of thoracoscope versus mediastinoscope assistance. Surg Endosc. 2012;26:1573–8.
15. Koide N, Takeuchi D, Suzuki A, et al. Mediastinoscopy-assisted esophagectomy for esophageal cancer in patients with serious comorbidities. Surg Today. 2012;42:127–34.
16. Wang QY, Tan LJ, Feng MX, et al. Video-assisted mediastinoscopic resection compared with video-assisted thoracoscopic surgery in patients with esophageal cancer. J Thorac Dis. 2014;6:663–7.
17. Wang QY, Li JP, Zhang L, et al. Mediastinoscopic esophagectomy for patients with early esophageal cancer. J Thorac Dis. 2015;7:1235–40.
18. Wang J, Wei N, Lu Y, et al. Mediastinoscopy-assisted esophagectomy for T2 middle and lower thoracic esophageal squamous cell carcinoma patients. World J Surg Oncol. 2018;16:58.
19. Ikeda Y, Niimi M, Kan S, et al. Mediastinoscopic esophagectomy using carbon dioxide insufflation via the neck approach. Surgery. 2001;129:504–6.
20. Parker M, Bowers SP, Goldberg RF, et al. Transcervical videoscopic esophageal dissection during two-field minimally invasive esophagectomy: early patient experience. Surg Endosc. 2011;25:3865–9.
21. Mori K, Yamagata Y, Wada I, et al. Robotic-assisted totally transhiatal lymphadenectomy in the middle mediastinum for esophageal cancer. J Robot Surg. 2013;7:385–7.
22. Mori K, Yamagata Y, Aikou S, et al. Short-term outcomes of robotic radical esophagectomy for esophageal cancer by a nontransthoracic approach compared with conventional transthoracic surgery. Dis Esophagus. 2016;29:429–34.
23. Fujiwara H, Shiozaki A, Konishi H, et al. Single-port mediastinoscopic lymphadenectomy along the left recurrent laryngeal nerve. Ann Thorac Surg. 2015;100:1115–7.
24. Fujiwara H, Shiozaki A, Konishi H, Otsuji E. Mediastinoscope and laparoscope-assisted esophagectomy. J Vis Surg. 2016;2:125.
25. Fujiwara H, Shiozaki A, Konishi H, et al. Perioperative outcomes of single-port mediastinoscope-assisted transhiatal esophagectomy for thoracic esophageal cancer. Dis Esophagus. 2017;30:1–8.
26. Mori K, Aikou S, Yagi K, et al. Technical details of video-assisted transcervical mediastinal dissection for esophageal cancer and its perioperative outcome. Ann Gastroenterol Surg. 2017;1:232–7.
27. Tokairin Y, Nakajima Y, Kawada K, et al. A feasibility study of mediastinoscopic radical esophagectomy for thoracic esophageal cancer from the viewpoint of the dissected mediastinal lymph nodes validated with thoracoscopic procedure: a prospective clinical trial. Esophagus. 2019;16:214–9.
28. Tokairin Y, Nakajima Y, Kawada K, et al. The usefulness of a bilateral trans-cervical pneumomediastinal approach for mediastinoscopic radical esophagectomy: a right transcervical approach is an available option. Gen Thorac Cardiovasc Surg. 2019;67:884–90.
29. Nakauchi M, Uyama I, Suda K, et al. Robot-assisted mediastinoscopic esophagectomy for esophageal cancer: the first clinical series. Esophagus. 2019;16:85–92.
30. Wang X, Li X, Cheng H, et al. Single-port inflatable mediastinoscopy combined with laparoscopic-assisted small incision surgery for radical esophagectomy is an effective and safe treatment for esophageal cancer. J Gastrointest Surg. 2019;23:1533–40.
31. Daiko H, Oguma J, Fujiwara H, et al. Novel universally applicable technique for performing bilateral transcervical mediastinoscopic-assisted transhiatal laparoscopic esophagectomy: a truly minimally invasive procedure. Surg Endosc. 2021;35:5186–92.
32. Hu W, Yuan P, Yuan Y, et al. Learning curve for inflatable mediastinoscopic and laparoscopic-assisted esophagectomy. Surg Endosc. 2023;37:4486–94.
33. Klarenbeek BR, Fujiwara H, Scholte M, et al. Introduction of Minimally Invasive trans Cervical oEsophagectomy (MICE) according to the IDEAL framework. Br J Surg. 2023;110:1096–9.
34. Fujita T, Sato K, Fujiwara N, et al. Robot-assisted transcervical esophagectomy with a bilateral cervical approach for thoracic esophagectomy. Surg Endosc. 2024;38:1617–25.

35. Jin Y, Lu X, Xue L, et al. Retrospective comparison of two minimally invasive esophagectomy in the treatment of esophageal cancer: pneumatic medastinoscopy versus thoracoscopy. Adv Surg Tech A. 2019;29:638–42.
36. Yagi K, Aikou S, Yajima S, et al. Survival outcomes of robot-assisted transmediastinal esophagectomy in patients with esophageal squamous cell carcinoma. Dis Esophagus. 2025;38:1–11.
37. Furuke H, Konishi H, Fujiwara H, et al. Predictors of the difficulty of transcervical subcarinal lymph node dissection for esophageal cancer. Esophagus. 2023;20:420–6.
38. Maeda T, Fujiwara H, Konishi H, et al. Preoperative 3D-CT evaluation of the bronchial arteries in transmediastinal radical esophagectomy for esophageal cancer. Esophagus. 2022;19:77–84.
39. Fang P, Zhou J, Liu Y, et al. Substitute or coexistence? Mediastinoscopy-assisted versus thoracoscope-assisted esophagectomy in esophageal cancer: a meta-analysis of perioperative outcomes and long-term survival. Int J Surg. 2024;110:5802–17.
40. Daiko H, Ishiyama K, Kurita D, et al. Bilateral transcervical mediastinoscopic-assisted transhiatal laparoscopic esophagectomy compared with thoracolaparoscopic esophagectomy for esophageal cancer: a propensity score-matched analysis. Surg Endosc. 2024;38:5746–55.
41. Sasaki K, Tsuruda Y, Shimonosono M, et al. A comparison of the surgical invasiveness and short-term outcomes between thoracoscopic and pneumatic mediastinoscopic esophagectomy for esophageal cancer. Surg Today. 2022;52:1759–65.
42. Ogawa K, Akashi Y, Hisakura K, et al. Clinical advantage of transmediastinal esophagectomy in terms of postoperative respiratory complications. Int J Clin Oncol. 2023;28:748–55.
43. Peyser Cardoso R, Agarwal L, Cardoso SA, et al. Impact of intraoperative recurrent laryngeal nerve monitoring on minimally invasive esophagectomy outcomes for esophageal cancer: a meta-analysis of case-control studies. Dis Esophagus. 2025;38:doae116.
44. Tsang RK, Law S. Adaptation of continuous intraoperative vagus nerve stimulation for monitoring of recurrent laryngeal nerve during minimally invasive esophagectomy. World J Surg. 2016;40:137–41.
45. Wong I, Tong DKH, Tsang RKY, et al. Continuous intraoperative vagus nerve stimulation for monitoring of recurrent laryngeal nerve during minimally invasive esophagectomy. J Vis Surg. 2017;3:9.
46. Wong IYH, Zhang RQ, Tsang RKY, et al. Improving outcome of superior mediastinal lymph node dissection during esophagectomy: a novel approach combining continuous and intermittent recurrent laryngeal nerve monitoring. Ann Surg. 2021;274:736–42.
47. Komatsu S, Konishi T, Matsubara D, et al. Continuous recurrent laryngeal nerve monitoring during single-port mediastinoscopic radical esophagectomy for esophageal cancer. J Gastrointest Surg. 2022;26:2444–50.
48. Committee for Scientific Affairs, The Japanese Association for Thoracic Surgery, Minatoya K, Sato Y, Toh Y, et al. Thoracic and cardiovascular surgeries in Japan during 2019: annual report by the Japanese Association for Thoracic Surgery. Gen Thorac Cardiovasc Surg. 2023;71:595–628.
49. Li W, Gan X, Lv L, et al. The learning curve for laparoscopic-assisted single-port mediastinoscopic esophagectomy: an analysis of proficiency. BMC Surg. 2025;25:29.
50. Hadzijusufovic E, Lozanovski VJ, Griemert EV, et al. Single-Port da Vinci robot-assisted cervical esophagectomy: how to do it. Thorac Cardiovasc Surg. 2024;72:654–8.

Perioperative Management

14

Shuhei Mayanagi

14.1 Introduction

Among gastrointestinal (GI) surgeries, esophagectomy for esophageal cancer is one of the most invasive procedures and is associated with high morbidity due to postoperative complications. Recently, video-assisted thoracoscopic esophagectomy was shown to reduce the incidence of pulmonary complications compared with conventional open surgery [1], and furthermore, robot-assisted esophagectomy was reported to have an even lower incidence of pneumonia than thoracoscopic surgery [2]. However, in a real-world big data analysis from the Japanese National Clinical Database of 5354 patients who underwent esophagectomy in 2011, overall morbidity was significantly higher in the minimally invasive esophagectomy group than in the open esophagectomy group (44.3% vs. 40.8%, respectively) [3]. In 2020, when minimally invasive esophagectomy will account for more than 70% of all esophagectomies, the proportion of patients aged 80 years or older will be 8.2%, and the frequency of serious postoperative complications of Clavien–Dindo classification grade IIIa or higher will be higher at 23.0%, with a slight increase over time [4]. In parallel with advances in surgical techniques, various perioperative management methods have been introduced to reduce the risk of postoperative complications. The accurate assessment of the tolerability of esophageal surgery and appropriate perioperative management based on adequate risk management are critical.

S. Mayanagi (✉)
Division of Esophageal Surgery, Shizuoka Cancer Center Hospital, Shizuoka, Japan
e-mail: s.mayanagi@scchr.jp

Y. Kitagawa et al. (eds.), *Esophageal Squamous Cell Carcinoma*,
https://doi.org/10.1007/978-981-92-2611-5_14

14.2 Enhanced Recovery After Surgery (ERAS)

The perioperative management of esophageal cancer surgery evolved from nutritional and transfusional support to the application of the Enhanced Recovery After Surgery (ERAS) program. The ERAS program, also known as fast-track surgery, was initiated by Henrik Kehlet in the 1990s [5–7]. This program aims to minimize surgical stress, reduce surgery-related complications, and accelerate postoperative recovery during the perioperative period. The ERAS program has been successfully implemented in various surgically treated diseases, especially colorectal surgeries [8]. The ERAS guidelines for esophagectomy were developed relatively late because esophagectomy is a particularly complex surgical procedure owing to the documented high levels of perioperative morbidity and mortality. However, in the introduction to the guidelines for perioperative care in esophagectomy [9], the ERAS Society indicated that the high morbidity and mortality after esophagectomy accentuate the need for providing an ERAS program, a standardized format for esophagectomy that can be routinely applied and audited to improve international outcomes. Initially, over 60 potential sections for inclusion into the ERAS guidelines were proposed. After two Delphi surveys, 39 sections were identified for inclusion in the esophagectomy ERAS project. The ERAS sections were divided into procedure- and non-procedure-specific components. As shown in Table 14.1, the procedure-specific components were further divided into preoperative, operative,

Table 14.1 Elements, levels of evidence, and recommendation grade of ERAS recommendations for esophagectomy

Elements	Level of evidence	Recommendation grade
Procedure-specific components		
Preoperative issues (5 sections)		
Preoperative nutritional assessment and treatment	C	A
Preoperative nutritional intervention	C	A
Preoperative oral pharmaconutrition	B	A
Multidisciplinary tumor board	B	A
Prehabilitation programs	C	B
Operative issues (14 sections)		
Timing of surgery following neoadjuvant therapy	B	B
Access: Minimally invasive or open	B	B
Choice of conduit (gastric conduit/tubulized stomach)	C/B[a]	A
Role of pyloroplasty (no strong evidence of effect)	C	A
Lymphadenectomy	B	A
Perianastomatic drains	B	B
NG tube/gastric decompression	B	A
Chest drain management following esophagectomy	C	B
Routine use of enteric feeding tubes	B	B
Esophagectomy: Perioperative fluid management	A/B[a]	A/B/C[a]
Anesthetic management	B	A

(continued)

Table 14.1 (continued)

Elements	Level of evidence	Recommendation grade
Anesthetic maintenance	A/B[a]	A
Two-lung ventilation	A/B[a]	A
One-lung ventilation	A/B/C[a]	A/B[a]
Post- and perioperative issues (6 sections)		
Intensive care unit utilization	B	A
Perioperative pain control for esophagectomy	B/C[a]	A/C[a]
Postoperative early nutrition: Oral vs. jejunostomy	B	A
Early mobilization	B	A
The role of multidisciplinary standardized clinical pathways	C	A
Audit (continuous institutional audit of outcomes)	B	A
Non-procedure-specific components (14 sections)		
Preoperative counseling patient/family	C	A
Smoking–alcohol cessation	B	A
Cardiopulmonary assessment	C	B
Bowel preparation (taking into account issues regarding colonic reconstruction)	B	A
Preoperative fasting (avoidance of fasting)	A	A
Preanesthetic analgesics and anxiolytics	B	C
Postoperative nausea and vomiting	C	A
Beta-blockade	B	A
Prophylaxis of atrial dysrhythmia	B	B
Antithrombotic prophylaxis	A	A
Hypothermia (avoidance of intraoperative hypothermia)	A	A
Postoperative glycemic control	B	A
Bowel stimulation	C	C
Foley catheter management (expeditious removal of urinary catheter)	A	A

Adapted from Low et al. [9]
Level of evidence; High: A, Moderate: B, Low: C
Recommendation grade; Strong: A, Moderate: B, Weak: C
[a]Depending on the subdivided recommendations

and post- and perioperative sections. The clinical impact of guideline-based ERAS program implementation for esophageal surgery have also been evaluated by randomized clinical trials (RCTs), and have been shown to reduce the overall complication rate, pulmonary complications, length of hospital stay, and time to flatus following esophagectomy [10–15]. The ERAS guidelines for esophagectomy are comprehensive and comparable to the entire textbook on esophageal cancer surgery. Several components are outlined in the following sections.

14.3 Preoperative Nutritional Assessment

Preoperative nutritional status is highly correlated with the incidence of postoperative complications [16–20]. Furthermore, the nutritional status directly influenced the prognosis after esophagectomy [20–26]. Approximately 50–80% of patients with esophageal cancer are malnourished at the time of diagnosis [17, 18, 27, 28]. Therefore, nutritional management is an essential key strategy to improve both short-term and long-term results in patients with esophageal cancer. Several nutritional indicators have been proposed for the initial prediction of the incidence of complications after esophagectomy. Some of these indicators also affect oncologic prognosis. Regardless of the indicator selected, the most important goal is to improve of nutritional status through appropriate management before and after esophageal cancer surgery.

14.3.1 Global Leadership Initiative on Malnutrition

The leading clinical nutrition societies of the world have collaborated to propose new adult undernutrition diagnostic criteria, the Global Leadership Initiative on Malnutrition (GLIM) (Fig. 14.1) [29]. Malnutrition diagnosis using the GLIM criteria initially identifies the "at-risk" status by the use of any validated screening tool, e.g., the Nutritional Risk Screening (NRS)-2002 scores, established as part of the European Society for Clinical Nutrition and Metabolism (ESPEN) guideline for nutrition screening [30] (Table 14.2). Patients identified as "at-risk" subsequently undergo a comprehensive assessment to establish the diagnosis of malnutrition and grade its severity. The diagnosis of malnutrition is based on three phenotypic

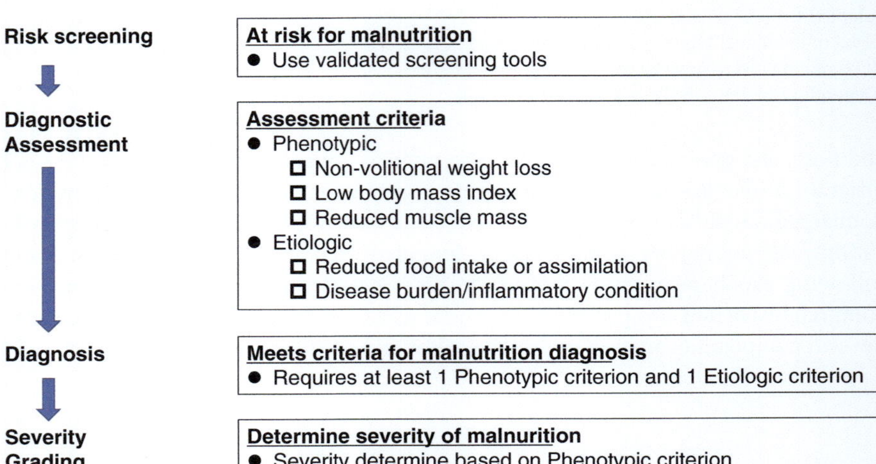

Fig. 14.1 The Global Leadership Initiative on Malnutrition (GLIM) diagnostic schema for screening, assessment, and grading of malnutrition. (Adapted from Cederholm et al. [29])

Table 14.2 Nutritional Risk Screening (NRS)-2002

Impaired nutritional status		Severity of disease	
Absent (score 0)	Normal nutritional status	Absent (score 0)	Normal nutritional requirements
Mild (score 1)	Weight loss >5% in 3 months or food intake below 50–75% of normal requirements	Mild (score 1)	Hip fracture, chronic patients in particular with acute complications; cirrhosis, COPD, chronic hemodialysis, diabetes, and oncology
Moderate (score 2)	Weight loss >5% in 2 months or BMI <18.5–20.5 + impaired general condition or food intake below 25–60% of normal requirements in preceding week	Moderate (score 2)	Major abdominal surgery, stroke, severe pneumonia, hematological malignancy
Severe (score 3)	Weight loss >5% in 1 months (>15% in 3 months) or BMI <18.5 + impaired general condition or food intake 0–25% of normal requirements in preceding week	Severe (score 3)	Head injury, bone marrow transplantation, intensive care patients (APACHE >10)
Total score	Add scores		
Age	If ≥70 years: Add 1 to total score above		

Score ≥3: the patient is nutritionally at-risk and a nutritional care plan is initiated
Score <3: weekly rescreening of the patient. If the patient, e.g., is scheduled for a major operation, a preventive nutritional care plan is considered to avoid the associated risk status
Adapted from Kondrup et al. [29]

criteria (non-volitional weight loss, low body mass index, and reduced muscle mass) and two etiologic criteria (reduced food intake or assimilation, and inflammation or disease burden). In addition, phenotypic metrics for grading severity as Stage 1 (moderate) and Stage 2 (severe) malnutrition are proposed. A systematic review indicated that malnutrition diagnosed using the GLIM criteria was associated with poorer postoperative complications, length of hospital stay, survival, and possibly hospital readmission in patients with cancer [31]. In patients with esophageal cancer, severe malnutrition based on the GLIM criteria was not only predictive of overall complications (odds ratio, 8.75; $p < 0.001$), major complications (odds ratio, 15.6; $p < 0.001$), and delayed hospital discharge (odds ratio, 7.38; $p = 0.001$) but was also associated with poor overall and disease-free survival (respectively: hazard ratio, 3.75; $p = 0.015$; and hazard ratio, 4.18; $p = 0.028$) [32]. Notably, patients with severe malnutrition were more clinically impaired than those with moderate malnutrition.

14.3.2 Controlling Nutritional Status Score

The Controlling Nutritional Status score (CONUT), was first validated and reported by Ignacio de Ulíbarri et al. [27] is a screening tool for the early detection and continuous control of hospital undernutrition. The formula for calculating CONUT,

Serum albumin g/dl	Score
≧3.5	0
3.0-3.4	2
2.5-2.9	4
< 2.5	6

Total lymphocyte count /μl	Score
≧1600	0
1200-1599	1
800-1199	2
< 800	3

Total cholesterol mg/dl	Score
≧180	0
140-179	1
100-139	2
< 100	3

Total score	Undernutrition degree
0-1	A Normal
2-4	B Mild
5-8	C Moderate
≧9	D Severe

Fig. 14.2 Assessments of undernutrition degrees by the CONUT (Controlling Nutritional Status)

including serum albumin and cholesterol levels, as well as total lymphocyte count, is shown in Fig. 14.2. A retrospective study of 352 patients who underwent elective esophagectomy for esophageal cancer reported that 58% of patients had normal nutrition, 36% had light malnutrition, and 6% had moderate or severe malnutrition according to CONUT assessed before surgery [33]. The length of hospital stay was significantly longer in patients with moderate or severe malnutrition than in the other patients. Logistic regression analysis revealed that moderate or severe malnutrition was an independent risk factor for any and severe morbidity [33]. The authors subsequently reported that patients with moderate or severe malnutrition, as determined by the preoperative CONUT, had a significantly poorer prognosis, in both overall survival and cancer-specific survival [26]. The meta-analysis found a significant association of the CONUT with overall survival (hazard ratio = 2.51, $p < 0.001$), cancer-specific survival (hazard ratio = 2.60, $p < 0.001$), and recurrence-free survival (hazard ratio = 2.08, $p < 0.001$) [34].

14.3.3 Geriatric Nutritional Risk Index

The Geriatric Nutritional Risk Index (GNRI), originally developed to examine the nutritional status of elderly hospitalized patients, consists of three objective nutritional variables: height, body weight, and serum albumin concentration (Fig. 14.3)

Fig. 14.3 GNRI (Geriatric Nutritional Risk Index) formula and assessment of nutrition-related risk

GNRI = [1.489 x albumin (g/L)] + [41.7 x (real weight / ideal weight)]

Ideal weight was calculated from the Lorentz equations (WLo) as follows:
For men: WLo = *Hight (cm)* - 100 - [(*Hight* - 150)/4]
For women: WLo = *Hight (cm)* - 100 - [(*Hight* -150)/2.5]

GNRI	Nutrition-related risk
82>	major risk
82-91	moderate risk
92-98	low risk
98<	no risk

[16]. A retrospective study examining GNRI and postoperative outcomes in 373 patients with esophageal cancer who underwent esophagectomy after neoadjuvant chemotherapy showed that the low-GNRI group had a higher rate of postoperative complications compared with the high-GNRI group (odds ratio 2.023) [35]. Several studies have investigated the impact of the GNRI on long-term outcomes in patients with esophageal squamous cell carcinoma who undergo esophagectomy [20, 22, 24]. The preoperative GNRI score was identified as an independent predictor of overall survival in the multivariate analysis. In one of these studies, multivariate analysis also revealed that severe and moderate nutritional risk (GNRI: <92) (hazard ratio 0.50; $p = 0.002$), T factor (≥T2) (hazard ratio 0.52; $p = 0.026$), and N positive factor (hazard ratio 0.47; $p = 0.004$) were independent prognostic factors [20]. Another study showed that the GNRI was significantly associated with tumor depth ($p = 0.001$), level of carcinoembryonic antigen ($p = 0.009$), and C-reactive protein level ($p = 0.028$) [24]. The meta-analysis also showed that lower GNRI had a negative impact on overall survival (hazard ratio: 1.75, 95%, $p < 0.01$) and cancer-specific survival (hazard ratio: 1.77, $p < 0.01$) [36].

14.3.4 Prognostic Nutritional Index

Onodera's Prognostic Nutritional Index (PNI) was calculated using the serum albumin concentration and total lymphocyte counts in peripheral blood (Fig. 14.4). The PNI was originally defined as a predictor of postoperative complications in patients with GI cancer. A subsequent study demonstrated the usefulness of preoperative PNI for predicting the occurrence of complications and length of hospital stay following esophagectomy in patients with esophageal cancer [23]. The study further demonstrated a positive correlation between PNI at 6 months post-surgery and overall survival. The preoperative PNI is also an independent predictor of long-term postoperative survival in patients with various cancers [37–41], including esophageal squamous cell carcinoma [21, 25]. Preoperative PNI was also shown to be an independent prognostic factor for overall survival among patients undergoing salvage esophagectomy [42].

Fig. 14.4 PNI (Prognostic Nutritional Index) formula and a definition of malnutrition

PNI = 10 × serum albumin (g/dl) + 0.005 × total lymphocyte count (/mm^3)

PNI < 45 is defined as moderate to severe malnutrition [19, 20]

14.4 Preoperative Nutritional Intervention

Moderate to severe dysphagic patients may experience prolonged periods of near fasting, which can not only result in malnutrition but also damage the intestinal mucosal and immune barrier, upset the balance of the intestinal microbiota, and contribute to postoperative gastrointestinal dysfunction. Therefore, nutritional interventions are recommended for patients with esophageal cancer and malnutrition based on nutritional assessment such as the GLIM criteria [29, 43]. In patients with gastrointestinal cancer, counseling and nutritional support can improve postoperative outcome [44, 45]. For esophageal cancer, adequate protein and energy supplement was achieved through intensive dietary counseling by surgical oncology specialized dieticians, which contributed to maintaining and increasing preoperative weight, and to reducing severe postoperative complications [46]. Furthermore, patients with severe esophageal stenosis should receive enteral support with tube feeding. Although this was a small RCT, for patients with esophageal cancer with an NRS-2002 score ≥3 and apparent difficulty swallowing, preoperative enteral nutrition using tube feeding can shorten the recovery time of gastrointestinal function, reduce the incidence of gastrointestinal complications, and accelerate postoperative recovery when compared with parenteral nutrition [47].

14.4.1 Preoperative Oral Pharmaconutrition, Immunonutrition

Immunonutrition refers to the oral or enteral administration of a formula containing one or more added nutrients, such as omega-3 fatty acids (FAs), nucleic acid, arginine, glutamine, or antioxidants; these formulas are called immuno-enhanced or immuno-modulating diets. In a recent meta-analysis, including many RCTs, of 48 studies of 4825 patients with gastrointestinal and head and neck cancers, immunonutritional therapy reduced postoperative complications (relative risk ratio: 0.78; 95% CI, 0.66–0.93) and infectious complications (relative risk ratio 0.71; 95% CI, 0.61–0.82) [48]. However, with a focus on esophageal cancer, no consensus has been reached on the benefits of immunonutrition on outcomes. The results of a multicenter RCT to determine the impact of preoperative and postoperative immunonutrition versus standard nutrition in patients with esophageal cancer were published in 2018 [49]. This comparatively large trial, which including 276 patients from 11 Australian sites, did not reveal any positive effects of immunonutrition. The incidence of infective complications was similar between all groups (37% in the perioperative standard nutrition group, 51% in the perioperative immunonutrition group, 34% in the preoperative immunonutrition group, and 40% in the postoperative immunonutrition group). There were no significant differences in any other clinical or quality of life outcomes. In addition, the results of a multicenter, double-blind, RCT on immunonutrition in patients with esophagogastric cancer undergoing neoadjuvant therapy were reported in 2025 [50]. Approximately 1000 kcal of additional immunonutrition, a complete nutritional formula rich in fish oil and supplemented with arginine and nucleotides, was administered orally or via tube feeding at least 1 week before the start of neoadjuvant therapy. A total of 300 patients were randomly assigned to this RCT. As a result, no significant differences were observed between groups in the primary outcome, patients' health-related quality of life, or 30-day postoperative complications. In meta-analyses of esophageal cancer by Mingliang et al. [51] reported that immunonutrition did not improve postoperative outcomes. According to the latest ESPEN recommendations peri- or at least postoperative administration of immunonutrition is only recommended for malnourished patients [43]. At present, there is no evidence base to strongly recommend the routine immunonutrition use during neoadjuvant therapy. It may be more important for clinicians to introduce early enteral nutrition using any type of enteral feeding products than the use of an immunonutrition formula.

14.5 Sarcopenia

Patients with advanced esophageal cancer frequently present with sarcopenia, defined as the loss of muscle mass and function, upon cancer diagnosis. Dysphagia and weight loss often result from malignant esophageal stenosis. Skeletal muscle loss related to cancer is the outcome of a negative energy and protein balance driven by a variable combination of reduced food intake and abnormal metabolism [52]. At the Asian Working Group for Sarcopenia 2019, sarcopenia was diagnosed and evaluated using three indices: muscle strength, muscle function, and muscle volume [53]. To investigate the impact of preoperative sarcopenia on postoperative complications or survival in patients undergoing esophagectomy, skeletal muscle mass was assessed using preoperative computed tomographic scans by measuring the cross-sectional muscle area at the third lumbar vertebral level, which was defined as the skeletal muscle index. In several meta-analyses, it was shown not only to increase the risk of postoperative complications, including pulmonary complications and anastomotic leakage, but also to adversely affect survival [54–56]. Sarcopenic dysphagia, defined as dysphagia associated with whole-body sarcopenia, has recently attracted attention in various fields, and a large proportion of patients with esophageal cancer are expected to develop sarcopenic dysphagia. A systematic review suggested that preoperative sarcopenia in swallowing-related muscles, such as the geniohyoid muscle and tongue, might be associated with postoperative pneumonia or dysphagia after esophagectomy [57].

14.5.1 Prehabilitation Program

A key determinant of the success of ERAS program is the rapid return to an acceptable level of functional activity after highly invasive surgery. Since functional capacity has been shown to be an important issue associated with postoperative complications, it seems logical that efforts to optimize and improve a patient's physiological reserve before surgery would improve outcomes. Several randomized controlled trials have investigated the use of exercise training alone as a preoperative intervention in esophagectomy [58–60]. Although the results of these clinical trials showed improvement in perioperative functional capacity (e.g., cardiopulmonary fitness (peak VO2), maximum inspiratory pressure, inspiratory muscle endurance, 6-min walk distance), the reduction in postoperative complications was limited. "Prehabilitation" generally refers to a multimodal approach that incorporates not only a structured and goal-directed exercise program combining aerobic and strengthening activities but also nutritional intervention, medical optimization (e.g., glycemic control, blood pressure control, smoking cessation, alcohol reduction), and psychological intervention. Colorectal cancer patients undergoing the 4-week in-hospital supervised multimodal prehabilitation program that consisted of a high-intensity exercise program, nutritional intervention, psychological support, and a smoking cessation program when needed experienced fewer severe complications and medical complications (e.g., cardiovascular or respiratory) [61]. The value of multimodal prehabilitation in improving outcomes in patients undergoing esophageal surgery requires further research.

14.6 Postoperative Early Enteral Nutrition

Early enteral nutrition in the critical care setting is defined as standard nutritional support initiated within 24 h after intensive care admission based on evidence that intestinal barrier changes can be observed within 24 h, including intestinal ischemia, increased permeability, bacterial translocation, and dysbiosis. In more critically ill patients, early enteral nutrition may attenuate these changes through various "non-nutritional benefits" and improve outcomes compared with delayed enteral nutrition [62]. Since the latter half of the 1990s, postoperative early enteral nutrition has been widely used to improve nutritional status and potentially decrease the incidence of postoperative complications and length of hospital stay in comparison with parenteral nutrition. At present, early enteral nutrition within 24 h shall be initiated in patients undergoing gastrointestinal cancer surgery in the ESPEN practical guidelines [43]. A meta-analysis of 10 RCTs from Japan and China concluded that postoperative early enteral nutrition after esophagectomy could decrease the morbidity of severe complications, such as pulmonary complications and anastomotic leakage, and maintain patients at a better nutritional status compared with parenteral nutrition support [63]. Studies on the effects of postoperative early enteral nutrition have used various protocols for enteral nutrition beginning from within 24 h to within 72 h or more after surgery. Two studies investigated the ideal period of initiating enteral nutrition after surgery for esophageal cancer. In one study, 42 patients were retrospectively divided into two groups. Group D1 started enteral nutrition within 24 h after surgery, whereas Groups D2–3 started enteral nutrition within 24–72 h after surgery [64]. There were no significant differences between the groups in clinical factors, including days to first fecal passage, dose of postoperative albumin infusion, difference in serum albumin levels between pre- and post-operation, incidence of postoperative infection, and use of total parenteral nutrition. In the other study, a total of 208 patients were divided into three groups (Groups 1, 2, and 3) based on whether they received enteral nutrition within 48 h, 48–72 h, or more than 72 h, respectively [65]. Group 1 had the lowest thoracic drainage volume, the earliest first fecal passage, and the lowest length of hospital stay and hospitalization expenses. The incidence of pneumonia was the highest in Group 3. All postoperative outcomes of nutritional conditions were worse by a significant margin in Group 3. The authors concluded that it is safe and valid to start early enteral nutrition within 48 h in postoperative esophageal cancer patients. A combination of preoperative feeding and postoperative early enteral nutrition should be recommended to achieve continuous nutritional support with minimum interruption of enteral feedings.

Early enteral nutrition is often started using a nasogastric feeding tube or jejunostomy catheter. Although ERAS program recommends starting oral feeding early, there are concerns about anastomotic leakage in addition to nausea, vomiting, and aspiration after esophagectomy. In recent years, with the spread of minimally invasive esophagectomy, the early resumption of oral feeding has become a consideration. An RCT comparing early and late oral feeding was performed for patients undergoing minimally invasive McKeown esophagectomy with cervical esophagogastric anastomosis [66]. The early and late oral feeding groups started a liquid diet on the first and seventh postoperative days, respectively, while taking care to prevent aspiration. One hundred and forty patients were assigned to each group, and postoperative cardiac, respiratory, and gastrointestinal complications and quality of life were evaluated. The early oral feeding group was non-inferior to the late oral feeding group in terms of cardiac, respiratory, and gastrointestinal complications (30.0% in the early group vs. 32.9% in the late group). Compared with the late group, the early group had a significantly shorter time to first flatus ($p = 0.001$) and first bowel movement ($p < 0.001$). Compared with the late group, the early group had a significantly shorter length of postoperative stay. Two weeks after esophagectomy, global quality of life, physical function, emotional function, and social function were significantly higher in patients in the early group than in patients in the late group. The rates of anastomotic leak in the early group and late group were 3.6% (5/140) and 4.3% (6/140), respectively. A recent systematic review showed that the incidence of anastomotic leakage was not significantly different between early oral feeding (postoperative days 1–4) and traditional late oral feeding (postoperative days 6–8). Furthermore, the incidence of pneumonia and overall postoperative complications were lower in the early oral feeding group than in the traditional late oral feeding group [67]. Thus, current evidence indicates that early oral feeding following esophagectomy may be safe and effective. It may be the preferred mode of nutrition following esophagectomy. However, more high-quality studies are still needed to further validate.

14.7 Perioperative Multidisciplinary Team Approach

The essence of the ERAS program is to implement evidence-based comprehensive perioperative management and maximize patient recovery, thereby reducing postoperative complications, shortening hospital stays, and facilitating social reintegration. The ERAS program is a patient-centered, surgeon-led system that combines anesthesia, nursing, nutrition, psychology, and other aspects. Therefore, in order to implement an ERAS program, it is essential that medical team members from various professions, including not only surgeons but also anesthesiologists, nurses, nutritionists, pharmacists, physiotherapists, dentists, psychologists, and others, participate in medical care that makes use of the characteristics and strengths of each profession. By having a multidisciplinary medical team involved from the time of esophageal cancer diagnosis, patient information can be shared between each profession, making it possible to provide a more appropriate perioperative environment. The perioperative multidisciplinary team approach begins with a comprehensive check-up for surgery from the patient's first visit. Nutritional status, drinking and smoking status, social background, psychological issues, dental screening, oral cleaning, and others are evaluated, and a comprehensive geriatric assessment may be useful, especially for elderly patients. Most patients with advanced esophageal cancer receive neoadjuvant therapy; therefore, it is recommended that a perioperative multidisciplinary team be involved during the neoadjuvant therapy period. It is important for each professional to continuously intervene throughout the perioperative period, tailored to the patient's condition, in order to achieve better outcomes.

There have been some promising reports from high-volume centers in Japan regarding the multidisciplinary team approach for esophageal cancer patients. The total adverse event rate during neoadjuvant chemotherapy decreased significantly in the multidisciplinary team approach group compared with the conventional approach group [68]. Among the adverse events, the grade of the oral toxicity scale was also significantly improved and weight loss was suppressed in the group of multidisciplinary team approach that started before neoadjuvant chemotherapy. The introduction of a multidisciplinary team approach reduced the incidence of postoperative complications, particularly the incidence of postoperative pneumonia [69]. Another report showed that the incidence of postoperative pneumonia and atrial fibrillation was significantly lower in the perioperative multidisciplinary team group than in the non-perioperative multidisciplinary team group (pneumonia 6% vs. 19%, $p = 0.027$, atrial fibrillation 14% vs. 29%, $p = 0.037$) [70]. In particular, the incidence of pneumonia after the start of dietary intake was significantly lower with the intervention of a perioperative multidisciplinary team program that included swallowing evaluation, dental screening, and professional dental cleaning (3% vs. 16%, $p = 0.012$).

Although the facilities and personnel available to esophageal cancer patients vary by institution, implementing an ideal ERAS program requires maximum preparation and effort from a multidisciplinary medical team.

14.8 Practicable Example of ERAS Program for Esophagectomy

An ERAS program for esophagectomy aligned with clinical practice is shown in Fig. 14.5. Preoperative nutritional intervention requires particular caution in patients with significant dysphagia. Rapidly administering high-energy nutrition to patients who have been in a prolonged state of starvation carries the risk of serious complications such as refeeding syndrome, lactic acidosis, and nonocclusive mesenteric ischemia. Monitoring dehydration, serum electrolytes (phosphorus, potassium, magnesium, etc.), and blood glucose, start with a low-calorie intake of 10 kcal/kg/day and gradually increase the energy intake over 4–5 days to reach the target energy level. Initiate a multidisciplinary team approach early, including exercise therapy intervention, swallowing rehabilitation, oral care, and counseling, to prepare for future esophageal surgery. In recent years, preoperative therapy has become the gold standard for resectable advanced esophageal cancer. Therefore, continued nutritional and exercise interventions during neoadjuvant therapy are likely to contribute to reducing perioperative complications. Immediately after minimally invasive esophageal surgery, the endotracheal tube is removed, and physical therapy and respiratory rehabilitation are initiated the day after surgery. Removing chest drains by postoperative day 3 and encouraging early ambulation contribute to preventing postoperative pulmonary complications. For nutritional management, initiate

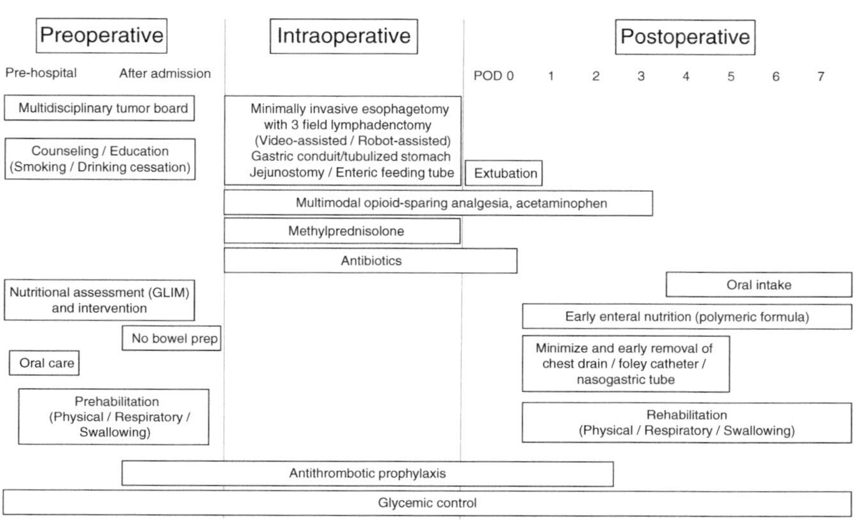

Fig. 14.5 Practicable example of ERAS program

polymeric formula via an enteric tube at a composition of 1 kcal/mL and a rate of 20 mL/h starting on postoperative day 1. As intestinal peristalsis normalizes, the enteral feeding rate is gradually increased by 10–20 mL/h daily, aiming for complete enteral nutrition management by the 5th postoperative day. If there are no complications such as recurrent laryngeal nerve palsy, pneumonia, or delirium, oral nutrition is initiated around the 4th postoperative day. Adherence to the ERAS program enables the implementation of a high-quality, standardized clinical pathway.

References

1. Takeuchi H, Ando M, Tsubosa Y, et al. A randomized controlled phase iii trial comparing thoracoscopic esophagectomy and open esophagectomy for thoracic esophageal cancer: Jcog1409 (Monet trial). J Clin Oncol. 2024;42(3_suppl):249.
2. Zhang Y, Dong D, Cao Y, et al. Robotic versus conventional minimally invasive esophagectomy for esophageal cancer: a meta-analysis. Ann Surg. 2023;278(1):39–50.
3. Takeuchi H, Miyata H, Gotoh M, et al. A risk model for esophagectomy using data of 5354 patients included in a Japanese nationwide web-based database. Ann Surg. 2014;260(2):259–66.
4. Kajiwara Y, Takahashi A, Ueno H, et al. Annual report on national clinical database 2020 for gastroenterological surgery in Japan. Ann Gastroenterol Surg. 2023;7(3):367–406.
5. Bardram L, Funch-Jensen P, Jensen P, Crawford ME, Kehlet H. Recovery after laparoscopic colonic surgery with epidural analgesia, and early oral nutrition and mobilisation. Lancet. 1995;345(8952):763–4.
6. Kehlet H. Multimodal approach to control postoperative pathophysiology and rehabilitation. Br J Anaesth. 1997;78(5):606–17.
7. Kehlet H, Mogensen T. Hospital stay of 2 days after open sigmoidectomy with a multimodal rehabilitation programme. Br J Surg. 1999;86(2):227–30.
8. Lau CS, Chamberlain RS. Enhanced recovery after surgery programs improve patient outcomes and recovery: a meta-analysis. World J Surg. 2017;41(4):899–913.
9. Low DE, Allum W, De Manzoni G, et al. Guidelines for perioperative care in esophagectomy: enhanced recovery after surgery (eras((r))) society recommendations. World J Surg. 2019;43(2):299–330.
10. Zhao G, Cao S, Cui J. Fast-track surgery improves postoperative clinical recovery and reduces postoperative insulin resistance after esophagectomy for esophageal cancer. Support Care Cancer. 2014;22(2):351–8.
11. Chen L, Sun L, Lang Y, et al. Fast-track surgery improves postoperative clinical recovery and cellular and humoral immunity after esophagectomy for esophageal cancer. BMC Cancer. 2016;16:449.
12. Li W, Zheng B, Zhang S, Chen H, Zheng W, Chen C. Feasibility and outcomes of modified enhanced recovery after surgery for nursing management of aged patients undergoing esophagectomy. J Thorac Dis. 2017;9(12):5212–9.
13. Yao R, Zhang T, Zhang J, et al. Effects of postoperative enteral nutrition combined with adjuvant radiotherapy on inflammatory response, nutrition, healing and prognosis in patients receiving radical surgery for esophageal carcinoma. J BUON. 2019;24(4):1673–8.
14. Shen Y, Chen X, Hou J, et al. The effect of enhanced recovery after minimally invasive esophagectomy: a randomized controlled trial. Surg Endosc. 2022;36(12):9113–22.
15. Kennelly P, Davey MG, Griniouk D, Calpin G, Donlon NE. Evaluating the impact of enhanced recovery after surgery protocols following oesophagectomy: a systematic review and meta-analysis of randomised clinical trials. Dis Esophagus. 2025;38(1):doae118.
16. Bouillanne O, Morineau G, Dupont C, et al. Geriatric nutritional risk index: a new index for evaluating at-risk elderly medical patients. Am J Clin Nutr. 2005;82(4):777–83.

17. Garth AK, Newsome CM, Simmance N, Crowe TC. Nutritional status, nutrition practices and post-operative complications in patients with gastrointestinal cancer. J Hum Nutr Diet. 2010;23(4):393–401.
18. Mariette C, De Botton ML, Piessen G. Surgery in esophageal and gastric cancer patients: what is the role for nutrition support in your daily practice? Ann Surg Oncol. 2012;19(7):2128–34.
19. Senesse P, Assenat E, Schneider S, et al. Nutritional support during oncologic treatment of patients with gastrointestinal cancer: who could benefit? Cancer Treat Rev. 2008;34(6):568–75.
20. Yamana I, Takeno S, Shimaoka H, et al. Geriatric nutritional risk index as a prognostic factor in patients with esophageal squamous cell carcinoma -retrospective cohort study. Int J Surg. 2018;56:44–8.
21. Feng JF, Chen QX. Significance of the prognostic nutritional index in patients with esophageal squamous cell carcinoma. Ther Clin Risk Manag. 2014;10:1–7.
22. Kubo N, Sakurai K, Tamura T, et al. The impact of geriatric nutritional risk index on surgical outcomes after esophagectomy in patients with esophageal cancer. Esophagus. 2019;16(2):147–54.
23. Matsumoto H, Okamoto Y, Kawai A, et al. Prognosis prediction for postoperative esophageal cancer patients using Onodera's prognostic nutritional index. Nutr Cancer. 2017;69(6):849–54.
24. Migita K, Matsumoto S, Wakatsuki K, et al. The prognostic significance of the geriatric nutritional risk index in patients with esophageal squamous cell carcinoma. Nutr Cancer. 2018;70(8):1237–45.
25. Nakatani M, Migita K, Matsumoto S, et al. Prognostic significance of the prognostic nutritional index in esophageal cancer patients undergoing neoadjuvant chemotherapy. Dis Esophagus. 2017;30(8):1–7.
26. Yoshida N, Harada K, Baba Y, et al. Preoperative controlling nutritional status (conut) is useful to estimate the prognosis after esophagectomy for esophageal cancer. Langenbeck's Arch Surg. 2017;402(2):333–41.
27. Ignacio de Ulíbarri J, González-Madroño A, de Villar NG, et al. Conut: a tool for controlling nutritional status. First validation in a hospital population. Nutr Hosp. 2005;20(1):38–45.
28. Haverkort EB, Binnekade JM, Busch OR, van Berge Henegouwen MI, de Haan RJ, Gouma DJ. Presence and persistence of nutrition-related symptoms during the first year following esophagectomy with gastric tube reconstruction in clinically disease-free patients. World J Surg. 2010;34(12):2844–52.
29. Cederholm T, Jensen GL, Correia M, et al. Glim criteria for the diagnosis of malnutrition - a consensus report from the global clinical nutrition community. Clin Nutr. 2019;38(1):1–9.
30. Kondrup J, Rasmussen HH, Hamberg O, Stanga Z. Nutritional risk screening (nrs 2002): a new method based on an analysis of controlled clinical trials. Clin Nutr. 2003;22(3):321–36.
31. Brown D, Loeliger J, Stewart J, et al. Relationship between global leadership initiative on malnutrition (glim) defined malnutrition and survival, length of stay and post-operative complications in people with cancer: a systematic review. Clin Nutr. 2023;42(3):255–68.
32. Wang P, Chen X, Liu Q, Liu X, Li Y. Good performance of the global leadership initiative on malnutrition criteria for diagnosing and classifying malnutrition in people with esophageal cancer undergoing esophagectomy. Nutrition. 2021;91–92:111420.
33. Yoshida N, Baba Y, Shigaki H, et al. Preoperative nutritional assessment by controlling nutritional status (conut) is useful to estimate postoperative morbidity after esophagectomy for esophageal cancer. World J Surg. 2016;40(8):1910–7.
34. Takagi K, Buettner S, Ijzermans JNM, Wijnhoven BPL. Systematic review on the controlling nutritional status (conut) score in patients undergoing esophagectomy for esophageal cancer. Anticancer Res. 2020;40(10):5343–9.
35. Fang P, Yang Q, Zhou J, et al. The impact of geriatric nutritional risk index on esophageal squamous cell carcinoma patients with neoadjuvant therapy followed by esophagectomy. Front Nutr. 2022;9:983038.
36. Zhou J, Fang P, Li X, et al. Prognostic value of geriatric nutritional risk index in esophageal carcinoma: a systematic review and meta-analysis. Front Nutr. 2022;9:831283.

37. Kanda M, Fujii T, Kodera Y, Nagai S, Takeda S, Nakao A. Nutritional predictors of postoperative outcome in pancreatic cancer. Br J Surg. 2011;98(2):268–74.
38. Migita K, Takayama T, Saeki K, et al. The prognostic nutritional index predicts long-term outcomes of gastric cancer patients independent of tumor stage. Ann Surg Oncol. 2013;20(8):2647–54.
39. Mohri Y, Inoue Y, Tanaka K, Hiro J, Uchida K, Kusunoki M. Prognostic nutritional index predicts postoperative outcome in colorectal cancer. World J Surg. 2013;37(11):2688–92.
40. Pinato DJ, North BV, Sharma R. A novel, externally validated inflammation-based prognostic algorithm in hepatocellular carcinoma: the prognostic nutritional index (pni). Br J Cancer. 2012;106(8):1439–45.
41. Sakurai K, Ohira M, Tamura T, et al. Predictive potential of preoperative nutritional status in long-term outcome projections for patients with gastric cancer. Ann Surg Oncol. 2016;23(2):525–33.
42. Sakai M, Sohda M, Miyazaki T, et al. Association of preoperative nutritional status with prognosis in patients with esophageal cancer undergoing salvage esophagectomy. Anticancer Res. 2018;38(2):933–8.
43. Weimann A, Braga M, Carli F, et al. Espen practical guideline: clinical nutrition in surgery. Clin Nutr. 2021;40(7):4745–61.
44. Odelli C, Burgess D, Bateman L, et al. Nutrition support improves patient outcomes, treatment tolerance and admission characteristics in oesophageal cancer. Clin Oncol (R Coll Radiol). 2005;17(8):639–45.
45. Rüfenacht U, Rühlin M, Wegmann M, Imoberdorf R, Ballmer PE. Nutritional counseling improves quality of life and nutrient intake in hospitalized undernourished patients. Nutrition. 2010;26(1):53–60.
46. Ligthart-Melis GC, Weijs PJ, te Boveldt ND, et al. Dietician-delivered intensive nutritional support is associated with a decrease in severe postoperative complications after surgery in patients with esophageal cancer. Dis Esophagus. 2013;26(6):587–93.
47. Shen Y, Zhou Y, He T, Zhuang X. Effect of preoperative nutritional risk screening and enteral nutrition support in accelerated recovery after resection for esophageal cancer. Nutr Cancer. 2020;73:1–6.
48. Matsui R, Sagawa M, Sano A, et al. Impact of perioperative immunonutrition on postoperative outcomes for patients undergoing head and neck or gastrointestinal cancer surgeries: a systematic review and meta-analysis of randomized controlled trials. Ann Surg. 2024;279(3):419–28.
49. Mudge LA, Watson DI, Smithers BM, Isenring EA, Smith L, Jamieson GG. Multicentre factorial randomized clinical trial of perioperative immunonutrition versus standard nutrition for patients undergoing surgical resection of oesophageal cancer. Br J Surg. 2018;105(10):1262–72.
50. Markar S, Mariette C, Bonnetain F, et al. Immunonutrition to improve the quality of life of upper gastrointestinal cancer patients undergoing neoadjuvant treatment prior to surgery (neoimmune): double-blind randomized controlled multicenter clinical trial. Dis Esophagus. 2025;38(1):doae113.
51. Mingliang W, Zhangyan K, Fangfang F, Huizhen W, Yongxiang L. Perioperative immunonutrition in esophageal cancer patients undergoing esophagectomy: the first meta-analysis of randomized clinical trials. Dis Esophagus. 2020;33(4):doz111.
52. Fearon K, Arends J, Baracos V. Understanding the mechanisms and treatment options in cancer cachexia. Nat Rev Clin Oncol. 2013;10(2):90–9.
53. Chen LK, Woo J, al Assantachai P e. Asian working group for sarcopenia: 2019 consensus update on sarcopenia diagnosis and treatment. J Am Med Dir Assoc. 2020;21(3):300–307.e302.
54. Park A, Orlandini MF, Szor DJ, Junior UR, Tustumi F. The impact of sarcopenia on esophagectomy for cancer: a systematic review and meta-analysis. BMC Surg. 2023;23(1):240.
55. Jogiat UM, Sasewich H, Turner SR, et al. Sarcopenia determined by skeletal muscle index predicts overall survival, disease-free survival, and postoperative complications in resectable esophageal cancer: a systematic review and meta-analysis. Ann Surg. 2022;276(5):e311–8.
56. Fang P, Zhou J, Xiao X, et al. The prognostic value of sarcopenia in oesophageal cancer: a systematic review and meta-analysis. J Cachexia Sarcopenia Muscle. 2023;14(1):3–16.

57. Oguma J, Ozawa S, Ishiyama K, Daiko H. Clinical significance of sarcopenic dysphagia for patients with esophageal cancer undergoing esophagectomy: a review. Ann Gastroenterol Surg. 2022;6(6):738–45.
58. Minnella EM, Awasthi R, Loiselle SE, Agnihotram RV, Ferri LE, Carli F. Effect of exercise and nutrition prehabilitation on functional capacity in esophagogastric cancer surgery: a randomized clinical trial. JAMA Surg. 2018;153(12):1081–9.
59. Guinan EM, Forde C, O'Neill L, et al. Effect of preoperative inspiratory muscle training on physical functioning following esophagectomy. Dis Esophagus. 2019;32(2):doy091.
60. Valkenet K, Trappenburg JCA, Ruurda JP, et al. Multicentre randomized clinical trial of inspiratory muscle training versus usual care before surgery for oesophageal cancer. Br J Surg. 2018;105(5):502–11.
61. Molenaar CJL, Minnella EM, Coca-Martinez M, et al. Effect of multimodal prehabilitation on reducing postoperative complications and enhancing functional capacity following colorectal cancer surgery: the prehab randomized clinical trial. JAMA Surg. 2023;158(6):572–81.
62. Reintam Blaser A, Starkopf J, al Alhazzani W e. Early enteral nutrition in critically ill patients: Esicm clinical practice guidelines. Intensive Care Med. 2017;43(3):380–98.
63. Peng J, Cai J, Niu ZX, Chen LQ. Early enteral nutrition compared with parenteral nutrition for esophageal cancer patients after esophagectomy: a meta-analysis. Dis Esophagus. 2016;29(4):333–41.
64. Manba N, Koyama Y, al Kosugi S e. Is early enteral nutrition initiated within 24 hours better for the postoperative course in esophageal cancer surgery? J Clin Med Res. 2014;6(1):53–8.
65. Wang G, Chen H, Liu J, Ma Y, Jia H. A comparison of postoperative early enteral nutrition with delayed enteral nutrition in patients with esophageal cancer. Nutrients. 2015;7(6):4308–17.
66. Sun HB, Li Y, Liu XB, et al. Early oral feeding following McKeown minimally invasive esophagectomy: an open-label, randomized, controlled, noninferiority trial. Ann Surg. 2018;267(3):435–42.
67. Mei LX, Liang GB, Dai L, Wang YY, Chen MW, Mo JX. Early versus the traditional start of oral intake following esophagectomy for esophageal cancer: a systematic review and meta-analysis. Support Care Cancer. 2022;30(4):3473–83.
68. Shirakawa Y, Noma K, Maeda N, et al. Early intervention of the perioperative multidisciplinary team approach decreases the adverse events during neoadjuvant chemotherapy for esophageal cancer patients. Esophagus. 2021;18(4):797–805.
69. Watanabe M, Mine S, Nishida K, et al. Improvement in short-term outcomes after esophagectomy with a multidisciplinary perioperative care team. Esophagus. 2016;13(4):337–42.
70. Kawata S, Hiramatsu Y, Shirai Y, et al. Multidisciplinary team management for prevention of pneumonia and long-term weight loss after esophagectomy: a single-center retrospective study. Esophagus. 2020;17(3):270–8.

Neoadjuvant and Adjuvant Therapy

15

Satoru Matsuda

15.1 Introduction

Surgery has improved the survival rates of patients with advanced squamous cell carcinoma (SCC) of the thoracic esophagus [1]. Radical surgery for esophageal cancer accompanied by extensive lymphadenectomy was established in leading institutions in Japan in the mid-1980s [2]. Further improvement of the 5-year survival rates through surgery alone seemed challenging, even in high-volume centers in Asia, as esophagectomy with extensive lymph node dissection was highly invasive and lacked control of systemic diseases. Therefore, optimization of multimodal treatments for localized and resectable clinical stage II/III esophageal cancer has been one of the most debated topics in this field [3], with many reports on this subject emerging over the past decades.

The results of clinical trials in Western countries were deemed directly applicable to clinical practice in Asian cases of esophageal cancer due to significant East–West differences in treatment approaches [4]. These differences include the varying distribution of main histological types, such as SCC or adenocarcinoma (ADC), the surgeons' philosophies regarding cancer surgery—focused on loco-regional or local tumor control—and the survival outcomes of the surgery-alone groups. Therefore, many Asian physicians treating patients with esophageal SCC (ESCC) hesitate to directly apply the currently available Western evidence—largely derived from studies on ADC—to clinical practice in Asia.

The Japan Esophageal Oncology Group (JEOG), a subgroup of the Japan Clinical Oncology Group (JCOG) [5], has conducted consecutive randomized controlled trials (RCTs) aimed at developing new surgical adjuvant therapies. These studies have led to clinical fruition in the development of new state-of-the-art treatments for ESCC in Japan [6] and have been incorporated as new evidence in the Esophageal

S. Matsuda (✉)
Department of Surgery, Keio University School of Medicine, Tokyo, Japan
e-mail: s.matsuda.a8@keio.jp

Y. Kitagawa et al. (eds.), *Esophageal Squamous Cell Carcinoma*,
https://doi.org/10.1007/978-981-92-2611-5_15

Cancer Practice Guidelines edited by the Japan Esophageal Society [7, 8]. This chapter begins with the findings of these JCOG studies, particularly regarding ESCC, and reviews and discusses the results of studies on esophageal cancer conducted outside of Japan.

15.2 Adjuvant and Neoadjuvant Therapy for ESCC in Japan

15.2.1 Historical Changes in Surgical Adjuvant Therapy of ESCC in Japan

15.2.1.1 Preoperative and Postoperative Radiotherapy

Preoperative radiotherapy was the prevailing treatment modality for esophageal cancer when the JEOG was first established in the 1970s. It was widely believed that this approach would lead to improvements in resectability (esophagectomy) and prevent local tumor recurrence [9]. The first JEOG phase III RCT (1978–1981) compared 30 Gy of preoperative radiotherapy combined with a tegafur suppository to 30 Gy of preoperative radiotherapy combined with a bleomycin injection. The survival rate in the preoperative radiotherapy plus tegafur group was better than that in the preoperative radiotherapy plus bleomycin group; furthermore, the postoperative morbidity and mortality in the bleomycin group were notably worse [10].

In the 1970s, during the era of preoperative radiotherapy, one group highlighted the advantages of postoperative radiotherapy, citing reduced operative morbidity and improved survival based on a retrospective comparison with controls [11]. Therefore, the second JEOG RCT (JCOG8201, 1981–1983) was conducted to determine which mode of radiotherapy—preoperative or postoperative—provided better survival outcomes [12]. This study compared preoperative radiotherapy (30 Gy) plus postoperative radiotherapy (24 Gy) with postoperative radiotherapy alone (50 Gy). The survival rate in the surgery plus postoperative radiotherapy alone group was significantly better than that in the surgery plus pre- and post-operative radiotherapy group (Fig. 15.1). As a result, there was a general shift away from preoperative radiotherapy, leading to a change in the timing of the multimodal approach to esophageal cancer from before to after surgery.

15.2.1.2 Postoperative Chemotherapy (Adjuvant Chemotherapy [aCT])

Postoperative Radiotherapy vs. Postoperative Chemotherapy

Cisplatin has been available as a key drug for treating esophageal cancer in Japan since the early 1980s. The third JEOG RCT (JCOG8503, 1984–1987) was conducted to determine which postoperative therapy—radiotherapy or chemotherapy—provided better survival [13]. The study compared postoperative radiotherapy (50 Gy) with postoperative chemotherapy (70 mg/m^2 of cisplatin plus 3 mg/m^2 of vindesine; two courses). The cisplatin plus vindesine regimen was adopted because it was the standard treatment for non-small cell lung cancer at the time, prior to the

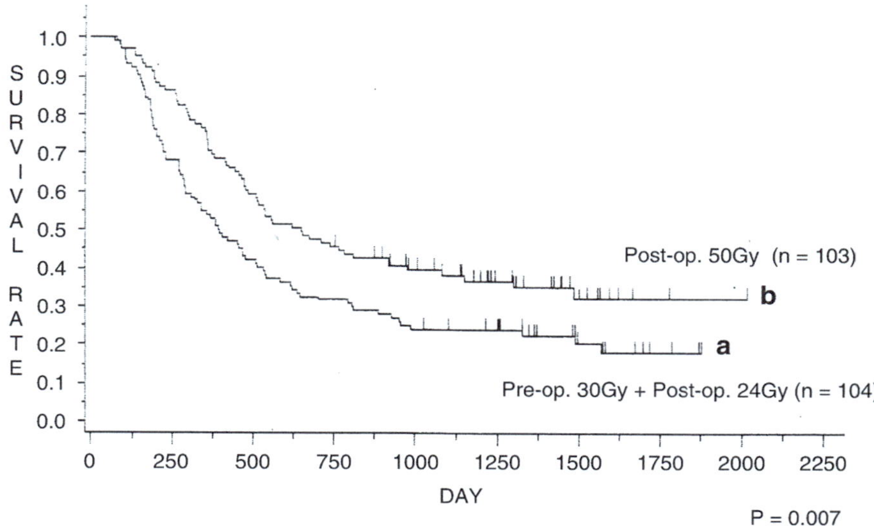

Fig. 15.1 Preoperative vs. postoperative radiotherapy. The survival rate in the pre- plus post-operative radiotherapy group (**a**) was significantly lower than that in the postoperative radiotherapy alone group (**b**)

popularity of cisplatin plus 5-fluorouracil (FU), a regimen later known as CF. Although no significant difference in the 5-year overall survival (OS) rate was observed between the two groups (Fig. 15.2), the results suggested that postoperative chemotherapy, including cisplatin, was not inferior to postoperative radiotherapy, the standard treatment modality at that time. As a result, aCT gained common acceptance as an adjuvant therapy for ESCC in Japan.

Additive Effect on Survival of Postoperative aCT over Surgery Alone

Esophageal cancer surgery demonstrated improved quality of lymphadenectomy, including specific dissection of the cervico-upper mediastinal nodes, which became standard practice in Japan in the late 1980s. Therefore, in the fourth JEOG RCT (JCOG8806, 1988–1991), it was deemed necessary to assess whether aCT conferred a survival benefit for patients undergoing radical surgery for esophageal cancer [14]. The study compared surgery alone with surgery plus aCT (70 mg/m^2 of cisplatin plus 3 mg/m^2 of vindesine; two courses) and showed no significant difference in the 5-year OS rate between the two groups (Fig. 15.3). Based on this result, surgery alone became the standard of care for ESCC at that time.

The combination of CF in patients with advanced esophageal cancer demonstrated greater efficacy than cisplatin and vindesine, based on our experience from two phase II studies. Consequently, the fifth JEOG RCT (JCOG9204, 1992–1997) was initiated to determine whether aCT using CF had an additive effect on survival in patients undergoing radical surgery alone for pathologic stage II or III SCC, excluding T4 [15]. The study compared surgery alone with surgery plus aCT

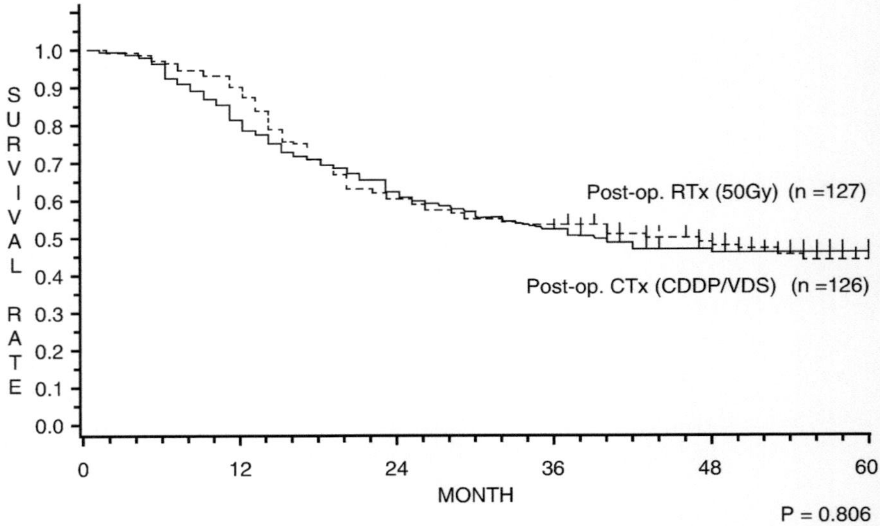

Fig. 15.2 Postoperative radiotherapy vs. postoperative chemotherapy. The 5-year survival rate was 44% in the postoperative radiotherapy group and 42% in the postoperative chemotherapy group, showing no significant difference between the two groups

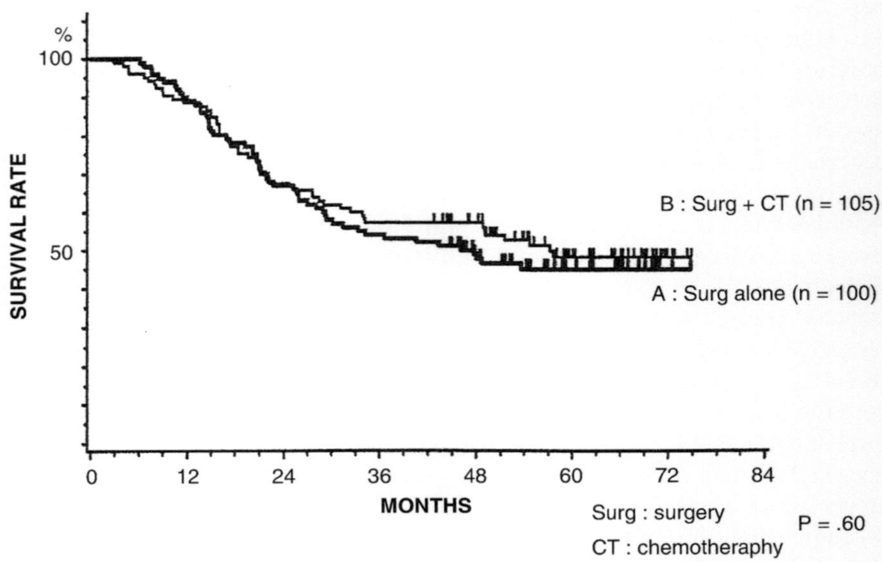

Fig. 15.3 Surgery alone vs. postoperative chemotherapy (cisplatin + vindesine). The 5-year survival rate was 45% in the surgery-alone group and 48% in the postoperative chemotherapy group, showing no significant difference between the two groups

(80 mg/m^2 of cisplatin on day 1 plus 800 mg/m^2 of 5-FU on days 1–5; two courses). The 5-year disease-free survival rates (primary endpoint) were 45% in the surgery-alone group (122 patients) and 55% in the postoperative chemotherapy group (120 patients; $p = 0.04$), while the 5-year OS rates were 52% and 61%, respectively ($p = 0.13$). Postoperative chemotherapy significantly reduced risk in the subgroup with lymph node metastasis (Fig. 15.4a, b). Based on these data, aCT using CF was considered the standard of care for patients with ESCC in the early 2000s.

15.2.1.3 Preoperative Chemotherapy (Neoadjuvant Chemotherapy [nCT])

Although aCT was considered the standard of care for esophageal cancer patients in Japan, preoperative treatment remained more common in Western countries due to the invasiveness of esophageal cancer surgery and the associated high morbidity [16]. Therefore, the positive impact of preoperative chemotherapy on survival in patients with esophageal cancer, when compared to surgery alone or postoperative chemotherapy, remains controversial. Details regarding this controversy are described in the following subchapter. The sixth JEOG RCT (JCOG9907, 2000–2006) was initiated to determine the optimal perioperative timing for chemotherapy (i.e., before or after surgery) in patients with locally advanced ESCC [17]. In the study, eligible patients with clinical stage II or III SCC, excluding T4, were randomly assigned to undergo surgery either preceded (Pre group) or followed (Post group) by chemotherapy (80 mg/m^2 of cisplatin on day 1 plus 800 mg/m^2 of 5-FU, continuous infusion [c.i.] over days 1–5; two courses with a 3-week interval). The primary endpoint, progression-free survival, did not reach the discontinuation boundary; however, OS in the Pre group (164 patients) was superior to that in the Post group (166 patients; $p = 0.01$). Updated analyses showed that the 5-year OS was 43% in the Post group and 55% in the Pre group (hazard ratio [HR], 0.73; 95% confidence interval [CI], 0.54–0.99; $p = 0.04$; Fig. 15.5a, b). Though renal dysfunction after surgery in the Pre group was slightly higher than that in the Post group, nCT did not increase the risk of complications or hospital mortality after surgery [18]. There are three possible reasons for the superior preoperative chemotherapy outcomes. First, some patients achieved downstaging through nCT. While the proportion of patients with clinical stage II disease was similar in the two groups, the proportion with pathological stage II or lower was greater in the Pre group. Second, complete resection (R0) was slightly more frequent in the Pre group than in the Post group. Third, the rate of protocol treatment completion was significantly higher in the Pre group than in the Post group, with 85.4% of Pre group patients undergoing treatment according to the protocol, which included two courses of chemotherapy and R0 resection, compared to only 75.0% of patients in the Post group.

Based on these results, nCT with CF was regarded as the standard of care for patients with stage II/III SCC [19]. Thus, the optimal perioperative timing for surgical adjuvant therapy was once again established to occur before surgery.

The results of the subgroup analyses in JCOG9907 showed that nCT was more effective in clinical stage II or T1–2 cases compared to stage III or T3, specifically in relatively early-stage patients. Furthermore, the lower rates of single

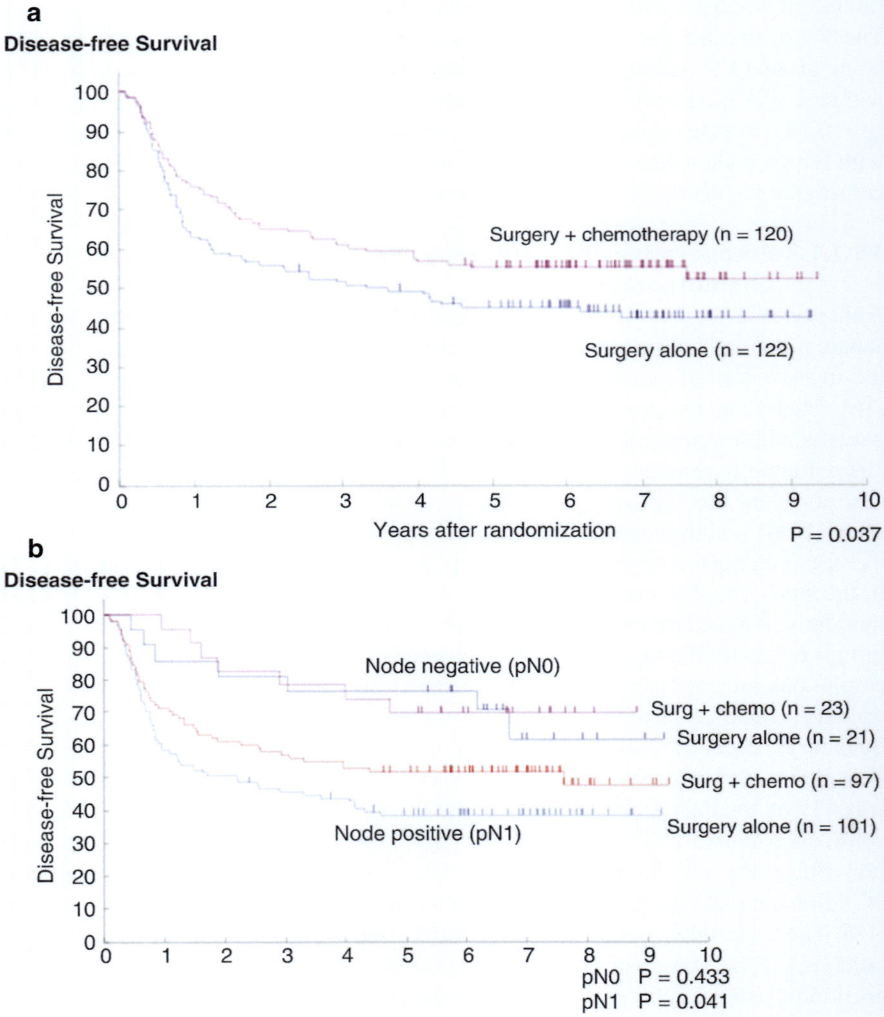

Fig. 15.4 (**a**) Surgery alone vs. postoperative chemotherapy (cisplatin +5-FU). Disease-free survival curves of all registered patients. The 5-year disease-free survival rates were 45% in patients who underwent surgery alone and 55% in those with surgery plus chemotherapy ($p = 0.037$). (**b**) Surgery alone vs. postoperative chemotherapy (pN0/pN1). In the pN0 subgroup, the 5-year disease-free survival was 76% in the surgery-alone group and 70% in the surgery plus chemotherapy group ($p = 0.433$); in the pN1 subgroup, it was 38% in the surgery-alone group and 52% in the surgery plus chemotherapy group ($p = 0.041$)

loco-regional recurrence at 31% and 25% among tumor recurrence cases in each group may be attributed to our meticulous surgical procedure. The results of our study suggest that nCT using CF is a viable strategy when sufficient local tumor control is achieved through aggressive surgical procedures. However, if local tumor

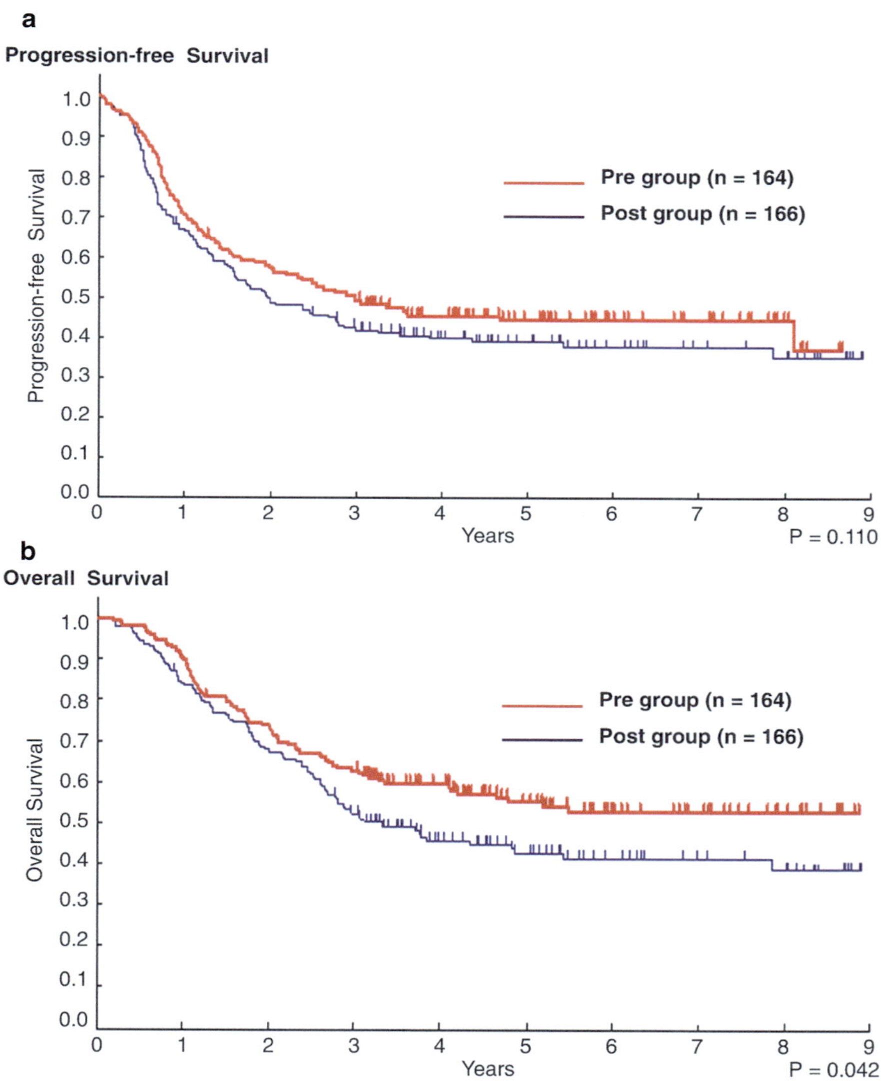

Fig. 15.5 (**a**) Progression-free survival. Preoperative vs. postoperative chemotherapy. Pre group = preoperative chemotherapy (nCT), Post group = postoperative chemotherapy (aCT). No significant difference in progression-free survival was observed between the two groups. (**b**) Overall survival. Preoperative vs. postoperative chemotherapy. Pre group = preoperative chemotherapy (nCT), Post group = postoperative chemotherapy (aCT). The 5-year OS rate was 43% in the Post group and 55% in the Pre group ($p = 0.04$)

control is insufficient, more aggressive adjuvant therapies, such as preoperative neoadjuvant chemoradiotherapy (nCRT) aimed at local tumor control or intensive nCT focused on systemic disease control, may be more preferable. Docetaxel is one of the most promising drugs for esophageal cancer. The exploratory trial of preoperative chemotherapy using docetaxel plus CF (DCF) for locally advanced ESCC demonstrated a good response rate (61.5%) with no treatment-related deaths. DCF is believed to have potential as a standard nCT regimen, as demonstrated by a randomized phase II study [20]. Nonetheless, the clinical question of whether nCT or nCRT is superior remains to be clarified.

Based on these background features, the JEOG launched a three-arm RCT, JCOG1109, in 2012 to confirm the superiority of DCF and chemoradiotherapy with CF (CF-RT) over CF as preoperative therapy for locally advanced ESCC in terms of OS [21]. Patients in arm A received two courses of preoperative CF (80 mg/m^2 of cisplatin on day 1 plus 800 mg/m^2 of 5-FU, c.i. on days 1–5) repeated every 3 weeks. Patients in arm B received three courses of preoperative DCF (70 mg/m^2 docetaxel on day 1 plus 70 mg/m^2 of cisplatin on day 1 plus 750 mg/m^2 of 5-FU, c.i. on days 1–5) repeated every 3 weeks. Patients in arm C received preoperative chemoradiotherapy (41.4 Gy/23 fractions) with two courses of CF (75 mg/m^2 of cisplatin on day 1 plus 1000 mg/m^2 of 5-FU, c.i. on days 1–4) repeated every 4 weeks (Fig. 15.6). Either transthoracic open esophagectomy or minimally invasive esophagectomy was acceptable in three arms.

JCOG1109 enrolled 601 patients with resectable ESCC; the patients' backgrounds were well balanced among the three study groups, including the performance status and clinical stage. The neoadjuvant DCF group showed superior

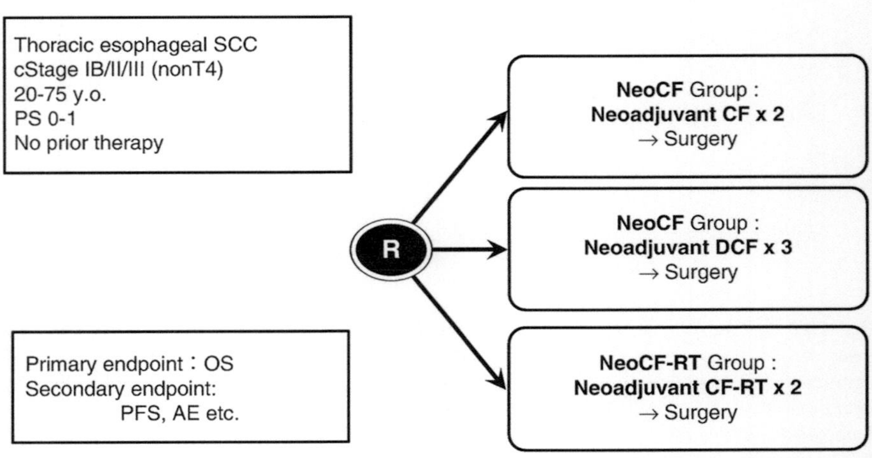

Fig. 15.6 Three-arm phase III trial comparing cisplatin plus 5-FU (CF) vs. docetaxel, cisplatin plus 5-FU (DCF) vs. radiation therapy with CF (CF-RT) as preoperative therapy for locally advanced esophageal cancer (JCOG1109, NExT Study)

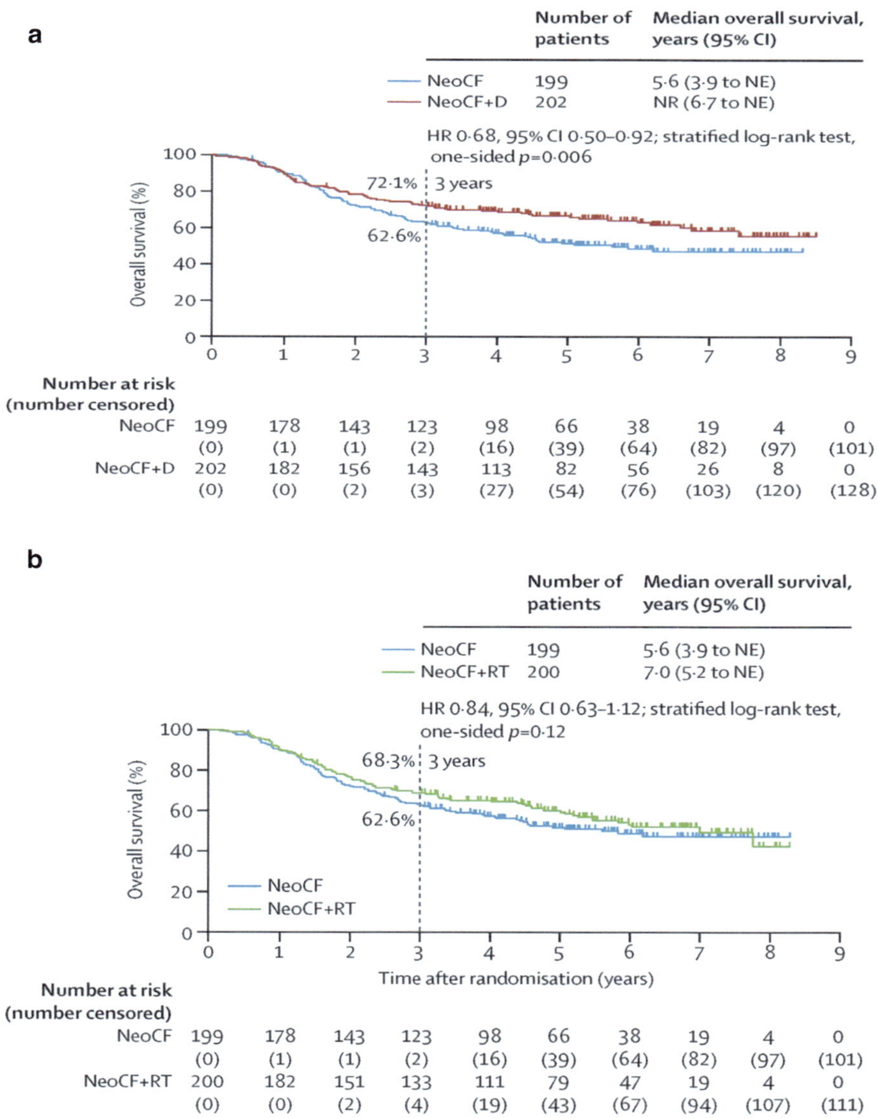

Fig. 15.7 (**a**) Overall survival rates for the NeoCF+D and NeoCF groups. (**b**) Overall survival rates for the NeoCF+RT and NeoCF groups

3-year OS compared to the neoadjuvant CF group (HR, 0.68; 95% CI, 0.50–0.92; $P = 0.006$; Fig. 15.7). In contrast, the HR (95% CI) in the neoadjuvant CF plus radiation (CF-RT) therapy group was 0.84 (0.63–1.12; $P = 0.12$), indicating no superiority over neoadjuvant CF therapy. The progression-free survival showed a trend similar to that of the OS, with an HR of 0.67 (95% CI, 0.51–0.88) for the neoadjuvant DCF vs. neoadjuvant CF groups and 0.77 (95% CI, 0.59–1.01) for the neoadjuvant CF-RT vs. neoadjuvant CF groups [22].

In terms of adverse events during neoadjuvant treatment, the DCF group had a higher proportion of patients who developed leukopenia (grade 3 or higher neutropenia in 85.2% of patients and febrile neutropenia (FN) in 16.3% of patients) compared to the CF and CF-RT groups. However, the administration of prophylactic antibiotics reduced the severity of FN, resulting in a completion rate of 84.7% in the DCF group.

In terms of the histological response, the pathologic complete response rate (pCR) rates were 2.2% for CF, 18.6% for DCF, and 36.7% for CF-RT, which were similar to the results of previous phase II studies. The DCF group showed better long-term results, indicating that the pCR rate and survival were not proportional. The rate of mortality due to other causes was higher in the CF-RT group within 5–8 years after surgery. Considering that approximately 30% of the patients in the CF-RT group died due to other causes, further detailed studies are required to elucidate the correlation between CF-RT and late adverse events.

Following this study, neoadjuvant DCF therapy plus surgery has become the new standard treatment strategy, as outlined in the 2022 edition of the Esophageal Cancer Treatment Guidelines developed by the Japan Esophageal Society [7, 8]. Furthermore, a real-world validation of the efficacy of neoadjuvant DCF therapy compared to that of neoadjuvant CF therapy using data collected from 85 centers certified by the Japanese Esophageal Association for Esophageal Surgery, including the external validation of the JCOG1109 trial, showed that OS (HR, 0.868; 95% CI: 0.770–0.978; $P = 0.\ 002$) and recurrence-free survival (RFS; HR, 0.845; 95% CI, 0.761–0.949; $P = 0.004$) were significantly longer in the DCF group compared to that in the CF group [23]. Subgroup analysis by age revealed that the superiority of DCF therapy over CF therapy in terms of survival was maintained in patients aged ≤75 years; however, no significant difference in OS or RFS was observed between CF and DCF therapies in patients aged >75 years. Postoperative pneumonia occurred in 21 out of 68 patients (30.9%) in the DCF group, and its incidence tended to be higher in the DCF group compared to that in the CF group (18 out of 88 patients [20.9%]; $P = 0.221$). The real-world data do not indicate the superiority of DCF therapy over CF therapy in patients aged over 75 years, and CF therapy should be considered a treatment option for nCT. Results from additional validation studies showed that postoperative infective complications (IC) are a negative prognostic factor of OS and RFS, with a more pronounced negative impact in patients aged >75 years [24]. When the patients were further stratified by chemotherapeutic regimen, using the CF/IC (−) group as a reference, patients aged >75 years in the DCF/IC (+) group showed significantly shorter OS with an HR of 2.551.

15.2.2 Future Perspectives on Neoadjuvant and Adjuvant Therapy for ESCC in Japan

With the advent of immunotherapy, its safety and efficacy were investigated in the adjuvant setting. In the CheckMate-577 trial, which evaluated the efficacy and safety of nivolumab as adjuvant therapy following nCRT and surgery, the median DFS times for stage II/III esophageal and esophagogastric junction cancer patients who underwent R0 resection after cCRT were 22.4 months in the nivolumab group (95% CI, 16.6–34.0) and 11.0 months in the placebo group (95% CI, 8.3–14.3); it was significantly better in the nivolumab group (HR, 0.69; 96.4% CI, 0.56–0.86; $P < 0.001$) [25]. Grades 3–4 treatment-related adverse events occurred in 71 out of 532 patients (13%) in the nivolumab group and 15 out of 260 patients (6%) in the placebo group. The rates of treatment discontinuation due to investigational drug-related adverse events were 9% in the nivolumab group and 3% in the placebo group. Additionally, grades 3–4 immune-related adverse events occurred in >1% of patients in the nivolumab group.

As a result, nCRT plus adjuvant nivolumab has become the standard treatment strategy in Western countries. However, when the survival outcomes of patients without adjuvant treatment in the CheckMate-577 study were compared to those in the DCF group in JCOG1109, a significant difference in long-term results was observed. The 3-year OS in the JCOG1109 study was 72.1%, whereas that in the CheckMate-577 was approximately 30%, as indicated by its survival curve. While we must exercise caution due to the differing timing of patient enrollment between these two studies, the long-term difference between JCOG1109 and CheckMate 577 was evident. Therefore, the effectiveness of adjuvant nivolumab therapy for patients who received nCT plus surgery remains debatable.

As an alternative treatment option for adjuvant therapy, results of the PIECE study—a phase II trial evaluating the efficacy and safety of additional S-1 administration as an adjuvant therapy after R0 resection in patients who had undergone surgery after nCT—were reported [26]. After 6 months of S-1 treatment as adjuvant therapy for cStage IB- ESCC patients III (excluding those with T4 disease) who received neoadjuvant CF therapy, the 3-year RFS was 72.3% (90% CI, 59.9–81.5), while the 3-year OS was 85.0% (90% CI, 73.9–91.6). The grade 3 or higher adverse events with an incidence of 10% or greater were neutropenia (13.2%), anorexia (13.2%), and diarrhea (10.5%); no treatment-related deaths were reported. While the results of this single-arm phase II study should be interpreted with caution, adjuvant S-1 therapy may be a promising option for adjuvant therapy following nCT and surgery.

Based on the results of the CheckMate-577 and PIECE trials, nivolumab or S-1 may be useful as adjuvant chemotherapy after nCT + surgery. JEOG is running a three-arm phase III clinical trial to evaluate the comparative clinical benefits of postoperative nivolumab or S-1 vs. no treatment and follow-up in patients with ESCC who have undergone radical surgery after cCT and failed to achieve a pCR [27].

The clinical significance of adding immune-checkpoint inhibitors (ICIs) to preoperative chemotherapy has been evaluated to improve the prognosis. The JCOG1804E (FRONTiER) study, a phase I trial examining the efficacy and safety of neoadjuvant CF or DCF plus nivolumab, is underway. In cohorts A and B, in which the efficacy of neoadjuvant CF plus nivolumab was examined, R0 resection was achieved in 92.3% of patients without treatment interruption, with a pCR rate of 33.3% in cohort A [28]. In cohorts C and D, where the efficacy of neoadjuvant DCF plus nivolumab therapy was examined, R0 resection was achieved in 91.7% of patients without treatment interruption, with pCR observed in one patient (16.7%) in cohort C and three patients (50.0%) in cohort D [28]. The results suggest that ICI combination therapy is well tolerated and promising.

In addition, a phase II study evaluating camrelizumab, an ICI developed in China, reported promising results with a 39.2% pCR rate (pT0N0), including lymph node metastases [29]. Hence, intensified preoperative treatment, including ICI, should be developed for esophageal cancer patients.

15.3 Adjuvant and Neoadjuvant Therapy for ESCC Outside Japan

Table 15.1 presents a comprehensive overview of the literature-based evidence on adjuvant and neoadjuvant therapies for ESCC within and outside Japan.

15.3.1 Adjuvant Therapy for ESCC

Studies on literature-based reviews of aCT for ESCC are limited. The French Association for Surgical Research conducted an RCT comparing surgery alone to aCT using CF for patients with ESSC [30]. Before randomization, 120 patients were separated into two groups: those undergoing curative complete resection and those undergoing palliative resection, which involved leaving residual macroscopic or microscopic tumor tissue. Chemotherapy included a maximum of eight courses (minimum of six courses) of cisplatin (80 mg/m^2 on day 1 or 30 mg/m^2 × 5 days) and 5-FU (1000 mg/m^2 × 5 days) administered within 1.5 months after surgery. The OS was similar in the two groups, with almost identical medians of 13 months in the aCT group (52 patients) and 14 months in the surgery-alone group (68 patients). The survival curves were similar in the curative resection and palliative resection strata, regardless of chemotherapy. Based on these data, it was concluded that CF following surgery is not beneficial for patients with ESCC.

Korean group conducted a prospective study of aCT (60 mg/m^2 of cisplatin on day 1 plus 1000 mg/m^2 of 5-FU, c.i. over days 1–4; three courses) in N1 resectable ESCC patients and compared the results with a historical control group that underwent curative resection alone during the same period [31]. The 3-year DFS rate was 47.6% in the adjuvant group and 35.6% in the surgery-alone group ($p = 0.049$). The researchers concluded that aCT could prolong DFS in node-positive patients and recommended that postoperative treatment strategies for esophageal cancer patients be guided by lymph node status, consistent with the findings of the JCOG9204 trial. A meta-analysis consisting of 11 studies (three RCTs, including JCOG 8806 and 9204, and eight non-RCTs) in patients with resectable ESCC compared surgery plus adjuvant chemotherapy vs. surgery alone [32]. The findings indicated that patients with stage III–IV disease could benefit from adjuvant chemotherapy in terms of the

Table 15.1 Overview of the literature-based evidence on adjuvant and neoadjuvant therapies for ESCC

First author	Accrual period	Stages enrolled	Chemotherapy	Radiotherapy	Surgery	No. of patients + CT, CRT surg. alone		Survival + CT, CRT surg. alone		p value
Adjuvant CT vs. surgery alone										
Pouliquen X 29 (FASR)	1987–1992	Excluding T4, N0	Cisplatin (100 mg/m^2) 5-FU (1000 mg/m^2) × 6–8 cycles		TTE	68	52	MST: 12 mo	MST: 12 mo	NS
Ando 15 (JCOG)	1992–1997	IIA, IIB, III, IVa	Cisplatin (80 mg/m^2) 5-FU (800 mg/m^2) × 2 cycles		TTE	120	122	5y-DFS: 55%	5y-DFS: 45%	0.037
Lee 30	1998–2003	IIb, III, Iva	Cisplatin (60 mg/m^2) 5-FU (1000 mg/m^2) × 3 cycles		TTE	40	52 (historical control)	3y-DFS: 47.6%	3y-DFS: 35.6%	0.049
Neoadjuvant CT vs. surgery alone										
Law 32	1989–1995	Excluding T4 and stage IV	Cisplatin (100 mg/m^2) 5-FU (500 mg/m^2) × 2 cycles		TTE	74	73	MST: 16.8 mo	MST: 13 mo	0.17
Ancona 33	1992–1997	IIA, IIB, and III	Cisplatin (100 mg/m) 5-FU (1000 mg/m^2) × 2 cycles		TTE	48	48	5y-OS: 34%	5y-OS: 22%	0.55
Kelsen 34, 35 (RTOG)	1990–1995	I, II, and III	Cisplatin (100 mg/m^2) 5-FU (1000 mg/m^2) × 3 cycles		TTE and THE	213 (54%; ADC)	227 (53%; ADC)	MST: 14.9 mo	MST: 16.1 mo	0.53 SCC/ADC NC/NC
MRC 36, 37	1992–1998	Resectable tumor	Cisplatin (80 mg/m^2) 5-FU (1000 mg/m^2) × 2 cycles		TTE and THE	400 (66%; ADC)	402 (67%; ADC)	MST: 16.8 mo	MST: 13.3 mo	0.004 HR: SCC/ADC 0.78/0.78
Neoadjuvant CT vs. adjuvant CT										
Ando 17 (JCOG)	2000–2006	IIA, IIB, and III	Cisplatin (80 mg/m^2) 5-FU (800 mg/m^2) × 2 cycles		TTE	Pre-op 164	Post-op 166	Pre-op 5y-OS: 55%	Post-op 5y-OS: 43%	0.04

(continued)

Table 15.1 (continued)

First author	Accrual period	Stages enrolled	Chemotherapy	Radiotherapy	Surgery	No. of patients + CT, CRT surg. alone	Survival + CT, CRT surg. alone		*p* value	
Neoadjuvant CRT vs. surgery alone										
Nygaad 46	1983–1988	I, II, III	Cisplatin (20 mg/m^2) × 5 Bleomycin (10 mg/m^2) × 5 × 2 cycles	35 Gy	TTE	26	15	MST: Not stated	MST: Not stated	0.3
Le Prise 45	1988–1991	I, II	Cisplatin (100 mg/m^2) 5-FU (600 mg/m^2) × 2 cycles	20 Gy	Not stated	41	45	1y-OS: 46.6%	1y-OS: 46.7%	0.56
Apinop 43	1986–1992	IIB, III	Cisplatin (100 mg/m^2) 5-FU (1000 mg/m^2) × 2 cycles	40 Gy	TTE	35	34	MST: 9.7 mo	MST: 7.4 mo	0.4
Bosset 44	1986–1992	I, II	Cisplatin (80 mg/m^2) × 2 cycles	37 Gy	TTE	143	139	MST: 18.6 mo	MST: 18.6 mo	0.78
Lee 47	1999–2002	IIA, IIB, III	Cisplatin (60 mg/m^2) 5-FU (1000 mg/m^2) × 2 cycles	45.6 Gy	TTE	51	50	MST: 28.2 mo	MST: 27.3 mo	0.69 study stopped
Yang 48	2007–2014	IIB and III	Cisplatin (75 mg/m^2) Vinorelbine (25 mg/m^2 × 2) × 2 cycles	40 Gy	TTE	224	227	MST: 100.1 mo	MST: 66.5 mo	0.025
Shapiro 49(CROSS Gr)	2004–2008	IIA, IIB, and III	Carboplatin (AUC 2) Paclitaxel (50 mg/m^2) × 23 days	41.4 Gy	TTE and THE	178 (75%; ADC)	188 (75%; ADC)	MST: 48.6 mo	MST: 24.0 mo	0.003

Neoadjuvant triplet CT vs doublet CT										
Kato 22	2012–2018	IB, II, III	DTX (70 mg/m^2) Cisplatin (70 mg/m^2) 5-FU (750 mg/m^2) × 3 cycles	CF Cisplatin (80 mg/m^2) 5- (800 mg/m^2) × 2 cycles	TTE	DCF 199	CF 202	DCF 3y-OS: 72%	CF 3y-OS: 63%	0.006
Neoadjuvant chemoradiotherapy plus surgery followed by adjuvant nivolumab vs placebo										
Kelly 25	2016–2019	Non-pCR	Nivo 240 mg every 2 weeks for 16 weeks, followed by 480 mg every 4 weeks	Placebo	TTE	Nivo 532	Placebo 626	Median DFS: 22.4 mo	Median DFS: 11.0 mo	<0.001

CT chemotherapy, *CRT* chemoradiotherapy, *SCC* squamous cell carcinoma, *ADC* adenocarcinoma, *TTE* transthoracic esophagectomy, *THE* transhiatal esophagectomy, *5-FU* 5- fluorouracil

3-year OS, while those with positive lymph nodes may experience improved 5-year DFS.

With the advent of immunotherapy, its safety and efficacy were investigated in the adjuvant setting. In the CheckMate-577 trial, which evaluated the efficacy and safety of nivolumab as adjuvant therapy after nCRT plus surgery, the median DFS was significantly better in the nivolumab group than in the placebo group [25]. Consequently, cCRT plus adjuvant nivolumab became the standard treatment strategy in Western countries.

15.3.2 Neoadjuvant Therapy for ESCC

Numerous reports have focused on neoadjuvant therapies for esophageal cancer patients with both SCC and ADC histologies.

15.3.2.1 nCT for ESCC

In a study in Hong Kong, Law et al. compared the effects of surgery alone to nCT (100 mg/m^2 of cisplatin on day 1 plus 500 mg/m^2 of 5-FU, c.i. over days 1–5; two courses) plus surgery for resectable ESCC [33]. Most patients had a tumor in the middle third of the esophagus, and the preferred surgical procedure was transthoracic esophagectomy with mediastinal lymphadenectomy. The cancer-free survival rate (primary endpoint) was 13 months in the surgery-alone group (73 patients) and 16.8 months in the nCT group (74 patients; $p = 0.17$). The researchers concluded that survival with nCT was not superior to that in the surgery-alone group. However, they suggested a potential survival advantage for patients who underwent nCT and emphasized the need for reliable predictors, noting that chemo-responders fare better than nonresponders.

In Italy, Ancona et al. compared surgery alone with nCT (100 mg/m^2 of cisplatin on day 1 plus 1000 mg/m^2 of 5-FU, c.i. over days 1–5; two courses) plus surgery for stage II/III ESCC [34]. The transthoracic esophagectomy plus two-field lymphadenectomy procedure was adopted in the study. The 5-year OS (primary endpoint) was 22% in the surgery-alone group (48 patients) and 34% in the nCT group (48 patients; $p = 0.55$). The researchers concluded that patients with clinically resectable ESCC who underwent neoadjuvant chemotherapy (nCT) and achieved a pathological complete response (pCR) experienced improved long-term survival. They also emphasized the importance of significant efforts to identify patients likely to respond to nCT.

Two pivotal RCTs in terms of nCT are known worldwide, the RTOG trial (a US intergroup study) and the MRC trial (UK and the Netherlands); both SCC and ADC histological types were included in these trials. Kelsen and four study group investigators compared surgery alone to nCT (100 mg/m^2 of cisplatin on day 1 plus 1000 mg/m^2 of 5-FU, c.i. over days 1–5; three courses) plus surgery followed by two cycles of postoperative chemotherapy in operable esophageal cancer cases [35]. More than 50% of patients (53% in the surgery-alone group and 54% in the preoperative chemotherapy group) were diagnosed with ADC, and both transthoracic and transhiatal esophagectomy were performed as the surgical procedures without limiting the extent of lymphadenectomy. The median survival was 16.1 months in the surgery-alone group (227 patients) and 14.9 months in the nCT group (213 patients; $p = 0.53$). No differences in survival were observed between patients with SCC and those with ADC. The researchers concluded that nCT plus CF did not improve OS among patients with SCC or ADC. Furthermore, in a long-term update, they reported that the median survival times were 1.3 years for patients receiving nCT vs. 1.3 years for those undergoing surgery alone [36]. The outcomes described were similar to those of other researchers, with an objective response to nCT being associated with improved survival.

Investigators in the Medical Research Council Oesophageal Cancer Working Party compared surgery alone to nCT (80 mg/m^2 of cisplatin on day 1 plus 1000 mg/m^2 of 5-FU, c.i. over days 1–4; two courses) plus surgery for resectable esophageal cancer [37]. Two-thirds of patients (67% in the surgery-alone group and 66% in the nCT group) were diagnosed with ADC, and the surgical procedure was chosen by the operating surgeon. The median survival rate was 13.3 months in the surgery-alone group (402 patients) and 16.8 months in the nCT group (400 patients; $p = 0.004$), with 2-year survival rates of 34% and 43%, respectively. The HRs for treatment effect in patients with SCC and ADC were similar, indicating that the effects of treatment were similar for both histological types. The researchers concluded that nCT improved survival in patients with resectable esophageal cancer. In the long-term update results of the trial, the 5-year survival was 17.1% in the surgery-alone group and 23.0% in the nCT group, with consistent treatment effects observed in both histological types [38]. They emphasized that nCT is an essential standard of care for patients with resectable esophageal cancer.

One of the most common failures in these two pivotal studies was local recurrence. The result of combined therapies cannot be discussed without considering the surgical procedure and its quality [39]. The two pivotal studies demonstrated completely different conclusions; therefore, the benefit of nCT, even when limited to patients with ESCC, was controversial prior to our latest JCOG9907 study. Therefore, there appears to be no current worldwide consensus on the optimal neoadjuvant approach. Preoperative chemoradiotherapy followed by surgery is an accepted standard of care in the United States, where ADC constitutes the majority of patients with esophageal cancer [40, 41]. Conversely, the United Kingdom follows preoperative chemotherapy as the standard of care based on the results of the MRC study [42]. However, preoperative chemoradiotherapy is considered the standard of care in the French treatment guidelines [43]. Even in Europe, there is no consensus on the optimal neoadjuvant approach.

15.3.2.2 nCRT for ESCC

Numerous RCTs comparing nCRT followed by surgery to surgery alone have been reported over the past three decades. Among them, four trials focused on ESCC in the 1990s showed no survival benefit attributed to nCRT [44–47]. In the 2000s, a Korean group compared surgery alone with nCRT (CF plus 45.6 Gy of radiotherapy in 38 fractions) followed by surgery for stage II/III ESCC. A transthoracic esophagectomy with en bloc lymphadenectomy was performed. The median survival was

27.3 months in the surgery-alone group (50 patients) and 28.2 months in the nCRT group (51 patients; $p = 0.69$), with 2-year survival rates of 51% and 49%, respectively. This trial was discontinued due to the unexpectedly high drop-out rate for esophagectomy and resultant excessive loco-regional failure rate in the nCRT group. Therefore, the researchers concluded that nCRT provided no survival benefit for resectable ESCC [48]. In another study, a Chinese collaborative group compared surgery alone to nCRT (cisplatin and vinorelbine plus 40.0 Gy of radiotherapy in 20 fractions) followed by surgery for potentially resectable thoracic ESCC [49]. A transthoracic esophagectomy with two-field lymphadenectomy was performed. The median OS was 100.1 months in the nCRT group (224 patients) and 66.5 months in the surgery-alone group (227 patients; $p < 0.001$), with 3-year OS rates of 69.1% and 58.9%, respectively. The researchers concluded that nCRT improved survival among patients with locally advanced ESCC, with acceptable and manageable adverse events.

A Dutch group (CROSS Group) compared surgery alone to nCRT (carboplatin and paclitaxel plus 41.4 Gy of radiotherapy in 23 fractions) followed by surgery for potentially curable SCC (23%) or ADC (75%) of the esophagus or the esophagogastric junction [50]. A transthoracic esophagectomy with two-field lymphadenectomy was performed. A transhiatal resection was preferred for tumors involving the esophagogastric junction. The median survival rate was 48.6 months for the nCRT group (178 patients) and 24.0 months for the surgery-alone group (188 patients; $p = 0.003$); the corresponding values were 81.6 months and 21.1 months, respectively, for patients with SCC, with 5-year OS rates of 47% and 33%, respectively. The researchers concluded that nCRT improved survival in patients with potentially curable esophageal or esophagogastric junction cancer, regardless of the histological subtype. The results of this study supported nCRT as the standard of care for locally advanced esophageal cancer in Western countries, where ADC is the predominant histological type. However, in Asian countries, criticism has arisen due to the relatively small subset of SCC patients included and the low R0 resection rate in the surgery-alone group.

Several meta-analyses have been conducted due to the inconsistent results from RCTs comparing neoadjuvant therapy to surgery alone for locally advanced esophageal cancer. Two out of six meta-analyses on nCRT did not show a significant survival benefit in patients with resectable esophageal cancer [51]. This discordance can be critiqued due to the heterogeneity of trials included in the meta-analyses. The most recent meta-analysis by Sjoquist et al. [52] included 12 RCTs comparing nCRT vs. surgery alone, with a total of 1854 patients; a significant survival benefit was evident for nCRT, with an HR of 0.78 (95% CI, 0.70–0.88; $p < 0.0001$). In the subgroup analysis, the HR was 0.80 (95% CI, 0.68–0.93, $p = 0.004$) for SCC and 0.75 (95% CI, 0.59–0.95, $p = 0.02$) for ADC. This updated meta-analysis provided stronger evidence for a survival benefit than the former meta-analysis conducted by the same group [53]. The analysis also compared nCT vs. nCRT and demonstrated a non-statistically significant survival benefit for nCRT (HR, 0.88; 95% CI, 0.76–1.01; $p = 0.07$). Therefore, controversy remains over which approach is more beneficial, nCT or nCRT [28]. An RCT comparing nCT (3 cycles of CF, 91 patients including 25 SCC patients) with nCRT (concurrent 40 Gy radiotherapy, 90 patients including 25 SCC patients) was conducted in Sweden and Norway [54]. The study revealed that the addition of radiotherapy to nCT resulted in higher pCR and R0 resection rates, without significantly affecting survival.

A network meta-analysis enables the evaluation of treatments that have not been directly or indirectly compared and the ranking of multiple treatments based on their efficacy. The result of a network meta-analysis including 27 eligible RCTs demonstrated that nCRT was the best treatment, followed by nCT and surgery alone [55]. A subgroup analysis based on histology in this network meta-analysis showed that both nCRT and nCT were effective and superior to adjuvant therapies for improving survival in patients with SCC.

15.4 Future Perspectives of Perioperative Treatment and Potential of the Organ Preservation Approach

The important role of individualized treatment for esophageal cancer has long been emphasized [56]. In the field of surgery, individualizing lymph node dissection by applying sentinel node navigation has been proposed as a rational approach to minimize the extent of lymphadenectomy [57]. In the field of multimodal treatments, identifying chemo- and radio-responders is crucial, given that histological complete response can predict longer DFS and OS outcomes, as described in the previous sections. If it were possible to predict responders, unnecessary toxicity and time wasted on unnecessary preoperative chemotherapy or chemoradiotherapy could be avoided, allowing for the implementation of rational radical surgery.

The response rate for the preoperative therapy of EC has dramatically improved. More cases are achieving pCR with preoperative treatment alone due to advancements in chemotherapy [22]. Hence, identifying pCR preoperatively and preserving the esophagus will remarkably benefit the patient. The two primary esophageal preservation strategies include definitive CRT (dCRT) for advanced cancer and active surveillance after nCRT. The JCOG0909 trial is a single-arm, non-randomized study of the efficacy and safety of dCRT (75 mg/m^2 of cisplatin and 1000 mg/m^2 of 5-FU + 50.4 Gy) in 94 patients with cStage II/III ESCC [58]. Patients were assessed for response after dCRT, and those with a CR or partial response received up to two additional CF therapy courses. They proceeded with salvage surgery if the response indicated stable or progressive disease. The study revealed a 3-year survival rate of 74.2% (90% CI, 65.9–80.8) and an esophagectomy-free survival rate of 63.6% (95% CI, 52.9–72.4). A RCT (NEEDS trial) is currently ongoing in Europe, comparing surgery after dCRT (platin-taxane or platin-fluoropyrimidine + 50 or 50.4 Gy) to the CROSS regimen [59].

The SANO trial is a study of active surveillance after nCRT. In this trial, patients who achieved clinical CR (cCR) with the CROSS regimen were randomly assigned to active surveillance or surgery [60]. The 2-year OS for active surveillance was 74% (95% CI, 69–78), which was non-inferior to that for standard surgery at 71% (95% CI, 62–78) based on a one-sided 95% boundary of 7% lower [61]. If active surveillance with selective surgery after nCRT for esophageal cancer results in OS that is non-inferior compared to standard oesophagectomy, it may be implemented as a standard of care.

All of the aforementioned esophageal preservation studies employed conventional methods to evaluate the efficacy of perioperative therapy. They contribute to some degree of stratification, but remain unsatisfactory. In particular, esophagectomy was performed on patients who did not react to chemotherapy after dCRT, including two with pCR, in the JCOG 0909 trial. Furthermore, only 35% of patients on active surveillance in the SANO trial maintained a cCR, raising questions about the value of these assessments. With continued advancements in neoadjuvant treatment and testing modalities to identify suitable candidates for organ preservation, the individualized approach that includes organ preservation will become the new standard for treating ESCC.

References

1. Ando N, Ozawa S, Kitagawa Y, Shinozawa Y, Kitajima M. Improvement in the results of surgical treatment of advanced squamous esophageal carcinoma during 15 consecutive years. Ann Surg. 2000;232(2):225–32.
2. Akiyama H, Tsurumaru M, Udagawa H, Kajiyama Y. Radical lymph node dissection for cancer of the thoracic esophagus. Ann Surg. 1994;220(3):364–72. discussion 372–3.
3. Mariette C, Piessen G, Triboulet J-P. Therapeutic strategies in oesophageal carcinoma: role of surgery and other modalities. Lancet Oncol. 2007;8(6):545–53.
4. Law S, Wong J. Changing disease burden and management issues for esophageal cancer in the Asia-Pacific region. J Gastroenterol Hepatol. 2002;17(4):374–81.
5. Fukuda H. Development of cancer cooperative groups in Japan. Jpn J Clin Oncol. 2010;40(9):881–90.
6. Ando N. Progress in multidisciplinary treatment for esophageal cancer in Japan as reflected in JCOG studies. Esophagus. 2011;8(3):151–7.
7. Kitagawa Y, Ishihara R, Ishikawa H, Ito Y, Oyama T, Oyama T, et al. Esophageal cancer practice guidelines 2022 edited by the Japan esophageal society: part 1. Esophagus. 2023;20(3):343–72.
8. Kitagawa Y, Ishihara R, Ishikawa H, Ito Y, Oyama T, Oyama T, et al. Esophageal cancer practice guidelines 2022 edited by the Japan Esophageal Society: part 2. Esophagus. 2023;20(3):373–89.
9. Akakura I, Nakamura Y, Kakegawa T, Nakayama R, Watanabe H, Yamashita H. Surgery of carcinoma of the esophagus with preoperative radiation. Chest. 1970;57(1):47–57.
10. Cooperative Clinical Study Group for Esophageal Carcinoma. Multidisciplinary treatment for esophageal carcinoma. Jpn J Clin Oncol. 1983;13:417–24.
11. Kasai M. Surgical treatment for carcinoma of the esophagus. J Jpn Surg Soc. 1980;81:845–53.
12. Iizuka T, Ide H, Kakegawa T, Sasaki K, Takagi I, Ando N, et al. Preoperative radioactive therapy for esophageal carcinoma. Randomized evaluation trial in eight institutions. Chest. 1988;93(5):1054–8.
13. Japanese Esophageal Oncology Group. A comparison of chemotherapy and radiotherapy as adjuvant treatment to surgery for esophageal carcinoma. Chest. 1993;104(1):203–7.
14. Ando N, Iizuka T, Kakegawa T, Isono K, Watanabe H, Ide H, et al. A randomized trial of surgery with and without chemotherapy for localized squamous carcinoma of the thoracic esophagus: the Japan Clinical Oncology Group Study. J Thorac Cardiovasc Surg. 1997;114(2):205–9.

15. Ando N, Iizuka T, Ide H. Surgery plus chemotherapy compared with surgery alone for localized squamous cell carcinoma of the thoracic esophagus: a Japan clinical oncology group study-JCOG 9204. J Clin Oncol. 2003;24:4592–6.
16. Kleinberg L, Forastiere AA. Chemoradiation in the management of esophageal cancer. J Clin Oncol. 2007;25(26):4110–7.
17. Ando N, Kato H, Shinoda M. A randomized trial of postoperative adjuvant chemotherapy with cisplatin and 5-fluorouracil versus neoadjuvant chemotherapy for localized squamous cell carcinoma of the thoracic esophagus (JCOG 9907). Ann Surg Oncol. 2012;19:68–74.
18. Hirao M, Ando N, Tsujinaka T. Japan esophageal oncology group/Japan clinical oncology group: influence of preoperative chemotherapy for advanced thoracic esophageal squamous cell carcinoma on perioperative complications. Br J Surg. 2011;98:1735–41.
19. Tsukada Y, Higashi T, Shimada H, Kikuchi Y, Terahara A. The use of neoadjuvant therapy for resectable locally advanced thoracic esophageal squamous cell carcinoma in an analysis of 5016 patients from 305 designated cancer care hospitals in Japan. Int J Clin Oncol. 2018;23(1):81–91.
20. Hara H, Tahara M, Daiko H, Kato K, Igaki H, Kadowaki S, et al. Phase II feasibility study of preoperative chemotherapy with docetaxel, cisplatin, and fluorouracil for esophageal squamous cell carcinoma. Cancer Sci. 2013;104(11):1455–60.
21. Nakamura K, Kato K, Igaki H. Three-arm phase III trial comparing cisplatin plus 5-FU (CF) versus docetaxel, cisplatin plus 5-FU (DCF) versus radiation therapy with CF (CF-RT) as preoperative therapy for locally advanced esophageal cancer (JCOG1109, NExT study). Jpn J Clin Oncol. 2013;43:752–5.
22. Kato K, Machida R, Ito Y, Daiko H, Ozawa S, Ogata T, et al. Doublet chemotherapy, triplet chemotherapy, or doublet chemotherapy combined with radiotherapy as neoadjuvant treatment for locally advanced oesophageal cancer (JCOG1109 NExT): a randomised, controlled, open-label, phase 3 trial. Lancet. 2024;404(10447):55–66.
23. Matsuda S, Kitagawa Y, Takemura R, Okui J, Okamura A, Kawakubo H, et al. Real-world evaluation of the efficacy of neoadjuvant DCF over CF in esophageal squamous cell carcinoma: propensity score-matched analysis from 85 authorized institutes for esophageal cancer in Japan: propensity score-matched analysis from 85 authorized institutes for esophageal cancer in Japan. Ann Surg. 2023;278(1):e35–42.
24. Matsuda S, Kitagawa Y, Okui J, Okamura A, Kawakubo H, Takemura R, et al. Old age and intense chemotherapy exacerbate negative prognostic impact of postoperative complication on survival in patients with esophageal cancer who received neoadjuvant therapy: a nationwide study from 85 Japanese esophageal centers. Esophagus. 2023;20(3):445–54.
25. Kelly RJ, Ajani JA, Kuzdzal J, Zander T, Van Cutsem E, Piessen G, et al. Adjuvant nivolumab in resected esophageal or gastroesophageal junction cancer. N Engl J Med. 2021;384(13):1191–203.
26. Nomura M, Yamaguchi T, Chin K, Hato S, Kato K, Baba E, et al. Phase II trial of adjuvant S-1 following neoadjuvant chemotherapy and surgery in patients with locally advanced esophageal squamous cell carcinoma: the PIECE trial. Ann Surg Oncol. 2025;32(1):302–11.
27. Kita R, Matsuda S, Nomura M, Machida R, Sasaki K, Kato K, et al. Protocol digest of a randomized controlled phase III study comparing surgery alone versus adjuvant nivolumab versus adjuvant S-1 for locally advanced oesophageal squamous cell carcinoma with no pathological complete response after neoadjuvant chemotherapy followed by curative esophagectomy: Japan Clinical Oncology Group study JCOG2206 (SUNRISE trial). Jpn J Clin Oncol. 2024;54(2):212–6.
28. Hamilton E, Vohra RS, Griffiths EA. What is the best neoadjuvant regimen prior to oesophagectomy: chemotherapy or chemoradiotherapy? Int J Surg. 2014;12(3):196–9.
29. Liu J, Yang Y, Liu Z, Fu X, Cai X, Li H, et al. Multicenter, single-arm, phase II trial of camrelizumab and chemotherapy as neoadjuvant treatment for locally advanced esophageal squamous cell carcinoma. J Immunother Cancer. 2022;10(3):e004291.
30. Pouliquen X, Levard H, Hay JM, McGee K, Fingerhut A, Langlois-Zantin O. 5-Fluorouracil and cisplatin therapy after palliative surgical resection of squamous cell carcinoma of the

esophagus. A multicenter randomized trial. French Associations for Surgical Research. Ann Surg. 1996;223(2):127–33.

31. Lee J, Lee KE, Im YH. Adjuvant chemotherapy with 5-fuorouracil and cisplatin in lymph node-positive thoracic esophageal squamous cell carcinoma. Ann Thorac Surg. 2005;80:1170–5.
32. Zhang S-S, Yang H, Xie X, Luo K-J, Wen J, Bella AE, et al. Adjuvant chemotherapy versus surgery alone for esophageal squamous cell carcinoma: a meta-analysis of randomized controlled trials and nonrandomized studies. Dis Esophagus. 2014;27(6):574–84.
33. Law S, Fok M, Chow S, Chu KM, Wong J. Preoperative chemotherapy versus surgical therapy alone for squamous cell carcinoma of the esophagus: a prospective randomized trial. J Thorac Cardiovasc Surg. 1997;114(2):210–7.
34. Ancona E, Ruol A, Santi S. Only pathologic complete response to neoadjuvant chemotherapy improves significantly the long term survival of patients with resectable esophageal squamous cell carcinoma. Final report of randomized, controlled trial of preoperative chemotherapy versus surgery alone. Cancer. 2001;91:2165–74.
35. Kelsen DP, Ginsberg R, Pajak TF, Sheahan DG, Gunderson L, Mortimer J, et al. Chemotherapy followed by surgery compared with surgery alone for localized esophageal cancer. N Engl J Med. 1998;339(27):1979–84.
36. Kelsen DP, Winter KA, Gunderson LL, Mortimer J, Estes NC, Haller DG, et al. Long-term results of RTOG trial 8911 (USA intergroup 113): a random assignment trial comparison of chemotherapy followed by surgery compared with surgery alone for esophageal cancer. J Clin Oncol. 2007;25(24):3719–25.
37. Medical Research Council Oesophageal Cancer Working Party. Surgical resection with or without preoperative chemotherapy in oesophageal cancer: a randomised controlled trial. Lancet. 2002;359:1727–33.
38. Allum WH, Stenning SP, Bancewicz J, Clark PI, Langley RE. Long-term results of a randomized trial of surgery with or without preoperative chemotherapy in esophageal cancer. J Clin Oncol. 2009;27(30):5062–7.
39. Zheng Y, Li Y, Liu X. Reevaluation of neoadjuvant chemotherapy for esophageal squamous cell carcinoma a meta - analysis of randomized controlled trials over the past 20 years. Medicine. 2015;94:e1102.
40. Almhanna K, Strosberg JR. Multimodality approach for locally advanced esophageal cancer. World J Gastroenterol. 2012;18(40):5679–87.
41. Merkow RP, Bilimoria KY, McCarter MD, Chow WB, Ko CY, Bentrem DJ. Use of multimodality neoadjuvant therapy for esophageal cancer in the United States: assessment of 987 hospitals. Ann Surg Oncol. 2012;19(2):357–64.
42. Pennathur A, Gibson MK, Jobe BA, Luketich JD. Oesophageal carcinoma. Lancet. 2013;381(9864):400–12.
43. Bedenne L, Vincent J, Jouve J-L. Is surgery always necessary in esophageal cancer? Esophagus. 2011;8(1):3–7.
44. Apinop C, Puttisak P, Preecha N. A prospective study of combined therapy in esophageal cancer. Hepato-Gastroenterology. 1994;41(4):391–3.
45. Bosset JF, Gignoux M, Triboulet JP, Tiret E, Mantion G, Elias D, et al. Chemoradiotherapy followed by surgery compared with surgery alone in squamous-cell cancer of the esophagus. N Engl J Med. 1997;337(3):161–7.
46. Le Prise E, Etienne PL, Meunier B, Maddern G, Ben Hassel M, Gedouin D, et al. A randomized study of chemotherapy, radiation therapy, and surgery versus surgery for localized squamous cell carcinoma of the esophagus. Cancer. 1994;73(7):1779–84.
47. Nygaard K, Hagen S, Hansen HS. Preoperative radiotherapy prolongs survival in operable esophageal carcinoma: a randomized, multicenter study of preoperative radiotherapy and chemotherapy. The second Scandinavian trial in esophageal cancer. World J Surg. 1992;16:1104–9.
48. Lee J-L, Park SI, Kim S-B, Jung H-Y, Lee GH, Kim J-H, et al. A single institutional phase III trial of preoperative chemotherapy with hyperfractionation radiotherapy plus surgery versus surgery alone for resectable esophageal squamous cell carcinoma. Ann Oncol. 2004;15(6):947–54.

49. Yang H, Liu H, Chen Y, Zhu C, Fang W, Yu Z, et al. Neoadjuvant chemoradiotherapy followed by surgery versus surgery alone for locally advanced squamous cell carcinoma of the esophagus (NEOCRTEC5010): a phase III multicenter, randomized, open-label clinical trial. J Clin Oncol. 2018;36(27):2796–803.
50. Shapiro J, Van Lanschot J, Hulshof M. Neoadjuvant chemoradiotherapy plus surgery versus surgery alone for esophageal or junctional cancer (CROSS): long-term results of a randomized controlled trial. Lancet Oncol. 2015;16:1090–8.
51. Wijnhoven B, Van Lanschot J, Tilanus HW. Neoajuvant chemoradiotherapy for esophageal cancer: a review of meta-analyses. World J Surg. 2009;33:2606–14.
52. Sjoquist KM, Burmeister BH, Smithers BM, Zalcberg JR, Simes RJ, Barbour A, et al. Survival after neoadjuvant chemotherapy or chemoradiotherapy for resectable oesophageal carcinoma: an updated meta-analysis. Lancet Oncol. 2011;12(7):681–92.
53. Gebski V, Burmeister B, Smithers BM, Foo K, Zalcberg J, Simes J, et al. Survival benefits from neoadjuvant chemoradiotherapy or chemotherapy in oesophageal carcinoma: a meta-analysis. Lancet Oncol. 2007;8(3):226–34.
54. Klevebro F, Alexandersson von Döbeln G, Wang N, Johnsen G, Jacobsen A-B, Friesland S, et al. a randomized clinical trial of neoadjuvant chemotherapy versus neoadjuvant chemoradiotherapy for cancer of the oesophagus or gastro-oesophageal junction. Ann Oncol. 2016;27(4):660–7.
55. Pasquali S, Yim G, Vohra RS, Mocellin S, Nyanhongo D, Marriott P, et al. Survival after neoadjuvant and adjuvant treatments compared to surgery alone for resectable esophageal carcinoma: a network meta-analysis. Ann Surg. 2017;265(3):481–91.
56. Kitajima M, Kitagawa Y. Surgical treatment of esophageal cancer - the advent of the era of individualization. N Engl J Med. 2002;347:1705–8.
57. Takeuchi H, Kitagawa Y. Sentinel node navigation surgery in esophageal cancer. Ann Gastroenterol Surg. 2019;3(1):7–13.
58. Takeuchi H, Ito Y, Machida R, Kato K, Onozawa M, Minashi K, et al. A single-arm confirmatory study of definitive chemoradiation therapy including salvage treatment for clinical stage II/III esophageal squamous cell carcinoma (JCOG0909 study). Int J Radiat Oncol Biol Phys. 2022;114(3):454–62.
59. Nilsson M, Olafsdottir H, Alexandersson von Döbeln G, Villegas F, Gagliardi G, Hellström M, et al. Neoadjuvant chemoradiotherapy and surgery for esophageal squamous cell carcinoma versus definitive chemoradiotherapy with salvage surgery as needed: the study protocol for the randomized controlled NEEDS trial. Front Oncol. 2022;12:917961.
60. Eyck BM, van der Wilk BJ, Noordman BJ, Wijnhoven BPL, Lagarde SM, Hartgrink HH, et al. Updated protocol of the SANO trial: a stepped-wedge cluster randomised trial comparing surgery with active surveillance after neoadjuvant chemoradiotherapy for oesophageal cancer. Trials. 2021;22(1):345.
61. van der Wilk BJ, Eyck BM, Wijnhoven BPL, Lagarde SM, Rosman C, Noordman BJ, et al. Neoadjuvant chemoradiotherapy followed by active surveillance versus standard surgery for oesophageal cancer (SANO trial): a multicentre, stepped-wedge, cluster-randomised, non-inferiority, phase 3 trial. Lancet Oncol. 2025;26(4):425–36.

Chemotherapy, Immunotherapy, and Chemoradiotherapy

16

Shun Yamamoto, Hiroshi Imazeki, and Ken Kato

16.1 Purpose and Evaluation of Chemotherapy

Chemotherapy has many roles in the treatment of esophageal squamous cell carcinoma (ESCC). It has been used for patients with advanced or recurrent cancer to prolong survival and/or alleviate the symptoms caused by cancer, and it has also been used for perioperative therapy combined with surgery to increase the complete resection rate and improve survival. At the same time, chemotherapy has been used with radiation therapy as definitive chemoradiotherapy (CRT) for localized ESCC. Responses to chemotherapy may be evaluated via endoscopy, computed tomography, magnetic resonance imaging, and other modalities, which are the same modalities used at diagnosis, as described in Chaps. 3, 4, and 7. There is no current consensus on the optimal follow-up duration, although evaluation frequencies of every 2 or 3 months for advanced cancer and evaluations at every course for neoadjuvant chemotherapy or CRT are the usual manner.

16.2 Cytotoxic Agents Used for Esophageal Squamous Cell Carcinoma

Various agents have been reported as effective for ESCC, but most of these studies were phase I and II studies and included only a small population. While these results were investigational, they provided support for consideration of combination therapy with new drugs. 5-Fluorouracil (5-FU), bleomycin, mitomycin, cisplatin (CDDP), and taxanes have been used most frequently because of their activity and synergistic effect with radiation and other drugs (Table 16.1).

S. Yamamoto · H. Imazeki · K. Kato (✉)
Department of Head and Neck, Esophageal Medical Oncology, National Cancer Center Hospital, Chuo-ku, Tokyo, Japan
e-mail: shuyamam@ncc.go.jp; himazeki@ncc.go.jp; kenkato@ncc.go.jp

Y. Kitagawa et al. (eds.), *Esophageal Squamous Cell Carcinoma*,
https://doi.org/10.1007/978-981-92-2611-5_16

Table 16.1 Single-agent cytotoxic chemotherapy for advanced esophageal cancer

Agent/trial name	Histology and number of pts	Treatment line	Regimen	Response (%)	PFS (m)	MST (m)	References
5-FU	SCC 26	1st	5-FU 500 mg/m^2 × 5 days/q5wks	15	3.4	NA	[1]
S-1	SCC 20	2nd or 3rd	S-1 40–60 mg × twice daily day 1–28/q6wks	25	3.3	10.8	[2]
S-1	SCC11	2nd or 3rd	S-1 40–60 mg × twice daily day 1–28/q6wks	22.2	3.0	11.7	[3]
Cisplatin	SCC 44	1st	Cisplatin 100 mg/m^2/q3wks	19	4.1	6.4	[5]
Carboplatin	SCC 11	1st	NA	9	NA	NA	[6]
Carboplatin	SCC 18	1st	Carboplatin 130 mg/m^2/day days 1, 3, 5	0	NA	NA	[7]
Nedaplatin	SCC 29	1st or 2nd	Nedaplatin 100 mg/m^2/q4wks	51.7	NA	NA	[8]
Paclitaxel	SCC18 AC32	1st	Paclitaxel 250 mg/m^2/q3wks	SCC28 AC34	3.9	13.2	[10]
Paclitaxel	SCC20 AC66	1st、2nd	Paclitaxel 80 mg/m^2 Day 1, 8, 15, 22/q4wks	12	3.1	9.0	[11]
Paclitaxel	SCC 52	2nd	Paclitaxel 100 mg/m^2 Day 1, 8, 15, 22, 29, 35/q7wks	44.2	3.9	10.4	[12]
Docetaxel	AC 41	1st	Docetaxel 100 mg/m^2/q3wks	17	NA	NA	[13]
Docetaxel	AC 22	1st or 2nd	Docetaxel 75 mg/m^2/q3wks	1st 18 2nd 0	NA	3.4	[14]
Docetaxel	SCC35 AC 3	1st or 2nd	Docetaxel 70 mg/m^2/q3wks	1st 36 2nd 16	4.7	8.1	[15]
OGSG1201	SCC 80	2nd	Paclitaxel 100 mg/m^2 Day 1, 8, 15, 22, 29, 35/q7wks Docetaxel 70 mg/m^2/q3wks	25.6 7.7	4.4 2.1	8.8 7.3	[16]
Bleomycin	SCC 29	1st	NA	14	NA	NA	[17]
Bleomycin	SCC + AC 20	1st	NA	20	NA	NA	[18]
Bleomycin	SCC 14	1st	NA	0	NA	NA	[19]
Ifosfamide	SCC 32	1st or 2nd	Ifosfamide 1.5 g/m^2 × 5 days	7	NA	NA	[21]
Gemicitabine	SCC6 AC14	1st	Gemcitabine 1250 mg/m^2 Day 1, 8, 15/q4wks	0	2	5	[22]

Vindesine	SCC26	1st	Vindesine 3.0 mg/m^2 weekly	17.3	NA	NA	[23]
Vindesine	SCC 9	1st or 2nd	vindesine 4.0 mg/m^2/q2wks	22.2	NA	NA	[24]
Vindesine	SCC 52	1st	Vindesine 3 mg/m^2 weekly	27	NA	NA	[25]
Vinorelbine	SCC 46	1st or 2nd	Vinorelbine 25 mg/m^2 weekly	1st 20 2nd 6	NA	6.0	[26]
Etoposide	SCC 26	1st	Etoposide 200 mg/m^2 day 1, 2, 3/q3wks	19	4.0	NA	[27]
Irinotecan	SCC10 AC3	1st or 2nd	Irinotecan 125 mg/m^2 Day 1, 8, 15, 22/q6wks	15	3.8	6.1	[30]
Methotorexate	SCC 26	1st	Methotrexate 40 mg/m^2 weekly	12	NA	3.2	[1]
Doxorubicin	SCC 20	1st	Doxorubicin 60 mg/m^2/q3wks	5	NA	1.8	[1]

Pts patients, *PFS* progression-free survival, *MST* median survival time, *SCC* squamous cell carcinoma, *AC* adenocarcinoma, *NA* not available, *wks* weeks, *5-FU* 5-fluorouracil

16.2.1 Fluoropyrimidine

Fluoropyrimidines, including 5-FU and S-1, were used as a key drug for decades. Efficacy of 5-FU as a single agent is modest. A response rate of 15% was observed in treated ESCC [1]. S-1, an oral fluoropyrimidine preparation combining tegafur, gimeracil, and oteracil potassium in a molar ratio of 1:0.4:1, showed response rate for treated ESCC that was reported to be 22%–25% [2, 3].

16.2.2 Platinum Agents

Platinum agents, such as cisplatin (CDDP), carboplatin, nedaplatin, and oxaliplatin, were used as a key drug for ESCC. As monotherapy, CDDP is administered at doses of 50–120 mg/m^2 every 3–4 weeks; the cumulative response rate for ESCC was 21% [4, 5]. In a randomized phase II trial, addition of CDDP to 5-FU (CF) was compared to CDDP monotherapy administered at 100 mg/m^2 every 3 weeks in 92 patients with ESCC. Although the response rate was higher in the combination group (35% vs. 19%), survival was similar in both groups (monotherapy vs. combination: 33 weeks vs 28 weeks) [5]. Carboplatin, a second-generation platinum analogue, showed response rate of 0%–14% [6, 7]. Oxaliplatin, a third-generation platinum derivative, has been evaluated mainly in combination regimens for esophageal cancer. Nedaplatin, a second-generation platinum derivative, showed that monotherapy at 100 mg/m^2 via intravenous infusion every 4 weeks, 5 partial responses (55.6%) were observed in 9 patients [8].

16.2.3 Taxanes

Paclitaxel promotes the stabilization of microtubules, and it is a cell cycle-specific agent affecting cells in the G2/M phase, showing activity for ESCC by monotherapy [9–11]. A phase II study of a weekly paclitaxel schedule at a dose of 100 mg/m^2 administered via 1-h intravenous infusion on days 1, 8, 15, 29, and 36 every 7 weeks for treated ESCC showed an overall response rate of 43.1% [12]. Docetaxel at doses of 75–100 mg/m^2 administered every 3 weeks showed a response rate of approximately 20% in untreated adenocarcinoma [13, 14]. For ESCC, a phase II trial of docetaxel at a dose of 70 mg/m^2 administered every 3 weeks showed that response rate was reported to be 16% for pretreated patients and 36% for untreated patients [15]. A randomized phase II trial showed superiority of overall survival (OS) in paclitaxel compared to docetaxel as salvage-line treatment (median survival time [MST]: 8.8 months vs 7.3 months) [16].

16.2.4 Other Cytotoxic Agents

Other drugs have been evaluated for ESCC as single agents, and they have demonstrated antitumor activity, with response rates of 0%–42%; these include bleomycin [17–20] methotrexate [1], ifosfamide [21], gemcitabine [22], doxorubicin [1], vindesine [23–25], vinorelbine [26], etoposide [27–29], and irinotecan [30].

16.3 Combination Cytotoxic Chemotherapy

Because of the limited activity of single-agent chemotherapy, most of the drugs described above have also been tested in combination regimens. Another randomized trial in 24 patients with esophageal cancer, including 19 patients with ESCC, also failed to show a meaningful survival benefit with cyclophosphamide and doxorubicin combination therapy. Although these randomized trials did not show a survival benefit with combination therapy, combination regimens with 5-FU, CDDP, and newer agents have been used for the treatment of ESCC (Table 16.2).

16.3.1 Combination with Platinum Agents

CDDP-based combinations appear to be the most studied regimen and demonstrate the most favorable response activity. CF is the most frequently used regimen, but the schedules vary. Although a randomized trial did not show benefit of CF over outcomes with CDDP monotherapy [5], CDDP (80–100 mg/m^2 on day 1) and 5-FU (800–1000 mg/m^2/day continuous infusion for 4–5 days) repeated every 3–4 weeks has been the standard regimen for ESCC. Other trials with smaller population and different treatment schedules showed response rates of 30%–35% and MST of 5.5–12.0 months [5, 31–35]. Phase II with 60 mg/m^2 CDDP intravenously on day 1 and 1250 mg/m^2 capecitabine orally twice daily on days 1–14, repeated every 3 weeks, showed the overall response rate of 57.8%, and MST of 11.2 months [36].

Oxaliplatin has been used in combination with 5-FU and leucovorin primarily for colorectal cancer, as the FOLFOX regimen. A response rate of 23.2% and MST of 7.7 months was reported in a phase II trial [37, 38]. Capecitabine combined with oxaliplatin (XELOX) was evaluated in a phase II trial with a schedule of 120 mg/m^2 oxaliplatin administered intravenously on day 1 and 1000 mg/m^2 capecitabine administered orally twice daily on days 1–14. Among 64 patients with ESCC, the overall response rate was 43.8%, and the MST was 10 months [39].

Nedaplatin was also evaluated in combination with 5-FU. JCOG9905-DI, a phase II trial with 42 patients with ESCC, showed a response rate of 39.5% response rate and MST of 8.8 months [40].

The combination of CDDP with vinorelbine [41] or with gemcitabine [42] showed response rate of 33.8%–40%.

Table 16.2 Combination cytotoxic chemotherapy for advanced esophageal cancer

Agent/trial name	Histology and number of Pts	Treatment line	Regimen	Response (%)	PFS (m)	MST (m)	References
5-FU+cisplatin	SCC 44	1st	Cisplatin 100 mg/m^2 day 1 5-FU 1000 mg/m^2/day day 1–5/q3wks	35	6.2	7.6	[5]
5-FU+ cisplatin	SCC 72	1st	Cisplatin 20 mg/m^2 day 1–5 5-FU 1000 mg/m^2/day day 1–5/q4wks	NA	NA	12	[31]
5-FU+ cisplatin	SCC 39	1st	Cisplatin 70 mg/m^2 day 1 5-FU 700 mg/m^2/day day 1–5/q3wks	35.9	Responders 3.5	Responders 9.5	[32]
5-FU+ cisplatin	SCC 36	1st	Cisplatin 20 mg/m^2 day 1–5 5-FU 800 mg/m^2/day day 1–5/q4wks	33.3	NA	7.5	[33]
5-FU+ cisplatin +leucovorin	SCC 5 AC 5	1st	Cisplatin 50 mg/m^2 day 1 5-FU 2000–2600 mg/m^2/day day 1, 8 Leucovorin 500 mg/m^2/day day 1, 8/q2wks	40	NA	10.6	[34]
5-FU+ cisplatin	SCC 30	1st	Cisplatin 100 mg/m^2 day 1 5-FU 1000 mg/m^2/day day 1–5/q4wks	13	3.6	5.5	[35]
Capecitabine + cisplatin	SCC 45	1st	Capecitabine 1250 mg/m^2 twice a day 1–14 Cisplatin 60 mg/m^2/day day 1/q3wks	57.8	4.7	11.2	[36]
FOLFOX	SCC 56	1st	Oxaliplatin 100 mg/m^2 day 1 Leucovorin 400 mg/m^2 day 1 5-FU 400 mg/m^2 day 1 iv 5-FU 2400 mg/m^2 day 1–2 46 h div	23.2	4.4	7.7	[37]
XELOX	SCC 64	1st or 2nd	Capecitabine 1000 mg/m^2 twice daily day 1–14 oxaliplatin 120 mg/m^2 day 1/q3wks	43.8	4.0	10.0	[39]
5-FU+nedaplatin	SCC 42	1st	5-FU 800 mg/m^2/day day 1–5 nedaplatin 90 mg/m^2 day 1/q4wks	39.5	2.5	8.8	[40]
Vinorelbine+ cisplatin	SCC 71	1at	Vinorelbine 25 mg/m^2/day day 1, 8 Cisplatin 80 mg/m^2/day day 1/q3wks	33.8	3.6	6.8	[41]

Gemcitabine + cisplatin	SCC 12 AC 24	1st	Gemcitabine 800 mg/m^2/day day 2, 9, 16 Cisplatin 50 mg/m^2/day day 1, 8/q4wks	SCC42 AC 41	NA	9.8	[42]
Paclitaxel +carboplatin	SCC 13 AC 22	1st	Paclitaxel 200 mg/m^2/day day 1 Carboplatin AUC5mg/h/ml/q3wks	SCC 31 AC 50	3.4	8.8	[43]
Paclitaxel +cisplatin	SCC 30 AC33	1at	Paclitaxel 100–200 mg/m^2/day day 1 Cisplatin 60 mg/m^2 day 1/q2wks	SCC 48 AC 59	NA	NA	[44]
Paclitaxel +cisplatin	SCC 14 AC 6		Paclitaxel 90 mg/m^2/day day 1 Cisplatin 50 mg/m^2 day 1/q2wks	SCC 50 AC 17	NA	7	[45]
Paclitaxel +cisplatin	SCC 39	1st	Paclitaxel 175 mg/m^2/day day 1 Cisplatin 75 mg/m^2 day 1/q3wks	48.5	7	13	[46]
Nab-paclitaxel +cisplatin	SCC 33	1st	Nab-paclitaxel 250 mg/m^2/day day 1 Cisplatin 75 mg/m^2 day 1/q3wks	60.6	6.2	15.5	[47]
Paclitaxel +nedaplatin	SCC 36 AC 3	1st	Paclitaxel 175 mg/m^2/day day 1 Nedaplatin 80 mg/m^2 day 1/q3wks	SCC 44.5 AC 33.3	6.1	10.3	[48]
Paclitaxel +nedaplatin	SCC 46 AC 2	1st	Paclitaxel 175 mg/m^2/day day 1 Nedaplatin 80 mg/m^2 day 1/q3wks	41.7	6.1	11.5	[49]
Paclitaxel +nedaplatin	SCC 39	1st	Paclitaxel 175 mg/m^2/day day 1 Nedaplatin 80 mg/m^2 day 1/q3wks	46.1	7.1	12.4	[50]
Capecitabine +paclitaxel	SCC 32	1st or 2nd	Capecitabine 900 mg/m^2 twice daily day 1–14 Paclitaxel 80 mg/m^2/day day 1, 8/q3wks	56.3	5.2	11.7	[51]
Docetaxel +cisplatin	SCC 38	2nd	Docetaxel 70 mg/m^2/day day 1 Cisplatin 75 mg/m^2 day 1/q3wks	34.2	4.5	7.4	[52]
Docetaxel + nedaplatin	SCC 12	2nd	Docetaxel 30–40 mg/m^2/day day 1, 15 Nedaplatin 70–90 mg/m^2 day 1/q4wks	25	NA	NA	[53]
Docetaxel + nedaplatin	SCC 48	2nd	Docetaxel 30 mg/m^2/day day 1 Nedaplatin 50 mg/m^2 day 1/q2wks	27.1	3.1	5.9	[54]
Docetaxel + nedaplatin	SCC 12	2nd	Docetaxel 50 mg/m^2/day day 1, 8 Nedaplatin 50 mg/m^2 day8/q3wks	0	2.0	7.8	[55]

(continued)

Table 16.2 (continued)

Agent/trial name	Histology and number of Pts	Treatment line	Regimen	Response (%)	PFS (m)	MST (m)	References
Docetaxel + nedaplatin	SCC 9	2nd	Docetaxel 50–60 mg/m^2/day day 1 Nedaplatin 70 mg/m^2 day 1/q4wks	22	2.1	9.5	[56]
Paclitaxel +5-FU+cisplatin	SCC 31 AC 30	1st	Paclitaxel 175 mg/m^2/day day 1 5-FU 750–1000 mg/m^2 daily Cisplatin 20 mg/m^2 weekly/q5wks	SCC 50 AC 46	5.7	10.8	[58]
Docetaxel +5-FU+cisplatin	SCC 39	1st	Docetaxel 50 mg/m^2/day day 1 5-FU 700 mg/m^2/day day 1–5 Cisplatin 70 mg/m^2 day 1/q3wks	66.6	7.0	13.0	[59]
Docetaxel +5-FU+cisplatin	SCC 18	1st	Docetaxel 30–40 mg/m^2/day day 1 5-FU 400 mg/m^2/day day 1–5 Cisplatin 40 mg/m^2 day 1/q2wks	88.9	NA	NA	[60]
Docetaxel +5-FU+cisplatin	SCC 30	1st	Docetaxel 60 mg/m^2/day day 1 5-FU 800 mg/m^2/day day 1–5 Cisplatin 60 mg/m^2 day 1/q3–4wks	72	NA	8.9	[61]
Docetaxel +5-FU+cisplatin	SCC 40	1st	Docetaxel 70 mg/m^2/day day 1 5-FU 700 mg/m^2/day day 1–5 Cisplatin 70 mg/m^2 day 1/q3wks	72.5	14	1-year 74.6	[62]
Docetaxel +5-FU+cisplatin	SCC 29	1st	Docetaxel 50 mg/m^2/day day 1 5-FU 700 mg/m^2/day day 1–5 Cisplatin 70 mg/m^2 day 1/q3wks	34.5	2.8	10.4	[63]

JCOG0807	SCC 55	1st	Docetaxel 30 mg/m²/day day 1, 15 5-FU 800 mg/m²/day day 1–5 Cisplatin 80 mg/m² day 1/q4wk	62	5.8	11.1	[64]
JCOG1314	SCC 230, AC 10	1st	Docetaxel 30 mg/m²/day day 1, 15 5-FU 800 mg/m²/day day 1–5 Cisplatin 80 mg/m² day 1/q4wk	52.8	6.0	16.2	[65]
			5-FU 800 mg/m²/day day 1–5 Cisplatin 80 mg/m² day 1/q4wk	45.6	5.2	14.8	
Docetaxel+5-FU +nedaplatin	SCC 43	1st	Docetaxel 75 mg/m²/day day 1 5-FU 375 mg/m²/day day 1 5-FU 2600 mg/m²/day 1–2 46 h div Nedaplatin 100 mg/m² day 1/q3wks	62.8	6.6	10.2	[66]
Doxorubicin +5-FU+cisplatin	SCC 41	1st	Doxorubicin 30 mg/m²/day day 1 5-FU 700 mg/m²/day day 1–5 Cisplatin 14 mg/m²/day day 1–5/q4wks	43.9	5.0	7.6	[67]

Pts patients, *PFS* progression-free survival, *MST* median survival time, *SCC* squamous cell carcinoma, *AC* adenocarcinoma, *NA* not available, *wks* weeks, *5-FU* 5-fluorouracil

16.3.2 Combination with Taxanes

Paclitaxel and carboplatin, which have been used for many cancers, have been reported to be effective for ESCC. Among 35 patients, an objective response was observed in 43%, and the MST was 8 months [43]. Prospective trials which evaluate paclitaxel and CDDP combination therapy with ESCC reported response rate of 40.0%–57.8% and MST of 7.0–13.0 months [44–46]. Nab-paclitaxel is a novel, solvent-free paclitaxel that uses albumin to deliver paclitaxel, thus avoiding the need for solvents such as polyoxymethylene, castor oil, and ethanol. In 33 patients with ESCC, a higher response rate (60.6%) and longer survival time (15.5 months) were reported with the combination of nab-paclitaxel and CDDP [47]. Another platinum combination of nedaplatin and paclitaxel was reported to have response rates of 40%–46.1% and MST of 10.3–12.4 months [48–50].

The combination of paclitaxel and capecitabine, an oral fluoropyrimidine, showed that response rate was 75% and MST was 14.5 months in the first-line treatment, and 45% and 8.5 months as the second-line treatment [51].

A phase II trial that included 35 patients with ESCC treated with docetaxel (70 mg/m^2) and CDDP (75 mg/m^2) on day 1, repeated every 3 weeks. The overall response rate was 34.2%, with a 2.6% complete response rate. Median progression-free survival (PFS) and MST were 4.5 months and 7.4 months [52]. Many small studies have evaluated nedaplatin and docetaxel combination regimens as the second-line treatment. The response rates were 0%–27.1%, and median PFS and MST were reported to be approximately 2 months and 7 months [53–57].

16.3.3 Triplet Combinations

Triplet combination regimens showed higher response rates compared to doublet regimens. The triplet of paclitaxel combined with CF as the first-line treatment showed the response rate of 54% in patients with ESCC, with a 20% complete response rate [58].

The combination of CF and docetaxel has shown response rates of 44.3%–88.9% and MST of 8.9–14 months [59–64]. From the result of JCOG0807, biweekly docetaxel in combination with 5-FU and cisplatin showed response rate of 62% and MST of 11.1 months. From the result of randomized phase III trial (JCOG1314), which compared biweekly DCF to CF as a first line chemotherapy, no significant survival benefit was observed with biweekly DCF compared to CF (MST: 16.2 months vs 14.8 months, HR 0.90 [95% CI, 0.68 to 1.19]; $P = 0.23$), although an improvement of PFS was noted (median PFS: 6.0 months vs 5.2 months, HR, 0.68 [95% CI, 0.52 to 0.88]) [65]. Nedaplatin may sometimes be used as a substitute for CDDP in patients with renal or cardiac dysfunction. Among 43 patients, including 13 patients with adenocarcinoma, the combination of 5-FU, nedaplatin, and docetaxel resulted in a 62.78% response rate and MST of 10.2 months [66].

Another triplet combination of 5-FU, CDDP, and doxorubicin, which has been used in gastric adenocarcinoma, was as ECF regimen, also evaluated in patients with ESCC. Doxorubicin was administered on day 1 at 30 mg/m^2; CDDP, on days 1–5 at 14 mg/m^2; and 5-FU, on days 1–5 at 700 mg/m^2. Among 41 patients with ESCC, the response rate was 43.9%, and MST was 10.1 months [67].

16.4 Chemoradiotherapy

The role of CRT varies. CRT has proven effective against resectable/unresectable ESCC. The Radiation Therapy Oncology Group (RTOG) trial 85–01 demonstrated the superiority of CRT with CF, and concurrent irradiation (50.4 Gy) over radiotherapy alone (64 Gy) in patients with T1–3N0-1 M0 esophageal cancer. The final outcome showed a 5-year survival rate of 26% in the CRT arm compared with 0% in the radiation-alone arm [68]. Therefore, CRT is recognized as the standard noninvasive treatment for patients with localized ESCC who opt for nonsurgical treatment (Table 16.3).

16.4.1 Definitive Chemoradiotherapy for Resectable Esophageal Cancer

CRT has been clinically indicated for patients with resectable ESCC who refuse surgical resection. In a retrospective analysis, 55 patients with T1–3NanyM0 ESCC, who received CRT with CF and concurrent 60-Gy irradiation, showed a complete response rate of 70% and a 5-year survival rate of 46%, suggesting comparable outcomes with surgery [69]. A phase II trial (JCOG9708) was conducted in Japan for stage I esophageal cancer. Among 73 patients, 63 (87.5%) achieved a complete response, and the 5-year survival rate was 75.5% [70]. Residual (12.5%) or recurrent (41%) disease was observed, but curative resection was achieved in most of these cases via endoscopy or surgery. Based on the results of JCOG0502, the parallel-group controlled trial of esophagectomy versus CRT in patients with stage I ESCC, the 5-year survival rate was 86.5% for esophagectomy arm and 85.5% for CRT arm. Though this comparison was not randomized, adjusted hazard ratio was 1.052 (95%CI: 0.674–1.640) [71]. CRT would be considered as one of the standard care for stage I ESCC.

JCOG9906, a phase II study of CRT for stage II/III ESCC, showed promising activity with a complete response rate of 62.2% and a 5-year survival rate of 36.8% [72]. In JCOG9906, radiotherapy was delivered using megavoltage (≥6 MV) X-rays; a total dose of 60 Gy was administered in 30 fractions with 40 Gy of elective lymph node irradiation. Acute toxicities were mild, but there were 4 treatment-related deaths (5.3%) related to late toxicities. Most of these events occurred several years after CRT. Moreover, a high mortality rate of 8%–11% was seen in patients who underwent “salvage” surgery for residual or recurrent disease after completion of CRT [73–75]. The late toxicities and higher mortality rate might be caused by the extended field of irradiation, which corresponds to the dissected area in an extended radical surgery. RTOG 94–05 demonstrated that a higher irradiation dose (64.8 Gy)

Table 16.3 Chemoradiotherapy for esophageal cancer

Trial name	Stage histology	Regimen	Radiation dose (Gy)	CRR (%)	Survival (%)	References
RTOG85–01	Stage I/II/III SCC, AC	Radiation alone	64	NA	5-year 0	[68]
		5-FU 1000 mg/m² day 1–4, 29–32 Cisplatin 75 mg/m² day 1, 29	50.4	NA	5-year 26	
RTOG95–04	Stage I/II/III SCC, AC	5-FU1000mg/m² day 1–4, 29–32 Cisplatin 75 mg/m² day 1, 29	50.4	NA	2-year 31	[76]
		5-FU1000mg/m² day 1–4, 29–32 Cisplatin 75 mg/m² day 1, 29	64.8	NA	2-year 40	
JCOG9708	Stage Ib SCC	5-FU 700 mg/m²day 1–4, 29–32 Cisplatin 70 mg/m² day 1, 29	60	87.5	5-year 75.5	[70]
JCOG0502	Stage Ib SCC	Esophagectomy + two-three field lymph node dissection	–	–	5-year 86.5	[71]
		5-FU 700 mg/m² day 1–4, 29–32 Cisplatin 70 mg/m² day 1, 29	60		5-year 85.5	
JCOG9906	Stage II/III SCC	5-FU 400 mg/m² day 1–5, 8–12, 36–40, 43–47 Cisplatin 40 mg/m² day 1, 8, 36, 43	60	62.2	3-year 44.7	[72]
mRTOG	Stage II/III SCC	5-FU 1000 mg/m² day 1–4, 29–32 Cisplatin 75 mg/m² day 1, 29	50.4	70.6	3-year 63.8	[77]
JCOG0909	Stage II/III SCC	5-FU 1000 mg/m² day 1–4, 29–32 Cisplatin 75 mg/m² day 1, 29	50.4	58.5	3-year 74.2	[78]
PRODIGE5	Stage I-IVA SCC, AC	5-FU 1000 mg/m² day 1–4, 29–32 Cisplatin 75 mg/m² day 1, 29	50	41.3	3-year 26.9	[82]
		Oxaliplatin 85 mg/m² day 1, 15, 29 Leucovorin 200 mg/m² day 1, 15, 29 Bolus 5-FU 400 mg/m² day 1, 15, 29 Infusional 5-FU 1600 mg/m² day 1–3, 15–17, 29–31	50	41.0	3-year 19.9	

JCOG9516	Unresectable local SCC	5-FU 700 mg/m² day 1–4, 29–32 Cisplatin 70 mg/m² day 1, 29	60	15	2-year 31.5	[84]
KDOG0501	Unresectable local SCC	5-FU 400 mg/m² day 1–5, 15–19, 29–33 Cisplatin 40 mg/m² day 1,15, 29 docetaxel 20–40 mg/m² day 1, 15, 29	61.2	42.1	1-year 63.2	[86]
NOBEL	Stage I-IVB SCC	5-FU 1000 mg/m² day 1–4, 29–32 Cisplatin 75 mg/m² day 1, 29 Nivolumab 240 mg/body, q2wks	50.4	Resectable 84	1-year Resectable 100	[110]
				Unresectable 56	1-year Unresectable 81.3	
TENERGY	Unresectable local SCC	5-FU 700 mg/m² day 1–4, 29–32 Cisplatin 70 mg/m² day 1, 29 Atezolizumab 1200 mg/q4wks (after CRT)	60	42.1	1-year 65.8	[121]
SKYSCRAPER-07	Unresectable local SCC Without PD after platinum-based CRT	Tiragolumab 600 mg/q3wks Atezolizumab 1200 mg/q3wks	Definitivedose	–	1-year 76.8	[123]
		Placebo Atezolizumab 1200 mg/q3wks		–	1-year 83.3	
		Placebo Placebo		–	1-year 75.1	

SCC squamous cell carcinoma, *AC* adenocarcinoma, *PD* progressive disease, *NA* not available, *wks* weeks, *5-FU* 5-fluorouracil, *CRR* complete response rate in CRT did not result in improved survival and local control as compared to a standard dose (50.4 Gy) due to lower tolerability and higher toxicity in 64.8Gy arm [76]. A phase II study of CRT for patients with stage II/III ESCC included 2 courses of 5-FU infusion (1000 mg/m^2) on days 1–4 and a 2-h infusion of CDDP (75 mg/m^2) on day 1, with concurrent radiotherapy at a dose of 50.4 Gy, was conducted for Japanese patients [77]. Although the radiation dose was reduced, the efficacy was comparable to previous report, and late toxicities greater than grade 3 were lower than those of previous reports. In the JCOG0909, among the ninety-four patients with stage II/III ESCC, salvage endoscopic resection and surgery were performed in 5 (5%) and 25 patients (27%). R0 resection of salvage surgery was achieved in 19 (76%) without any operative mortality [78].

Other combination regimens with concurrent irradiation have been evaluated. Stomatitis or esophagitis caused by 5-FU may sometimes occur during CRT with CF. The combination of paclitaxel and carboplatin has also been used as neoadjuvant CRT or definitive CRT [79, 80]. Although there is no robust evidence, this regimen has shown non-inferior antitumor activity and reduced non-hematologic toxicity [81].

FOLFOX was evaluated in PRODIGE5, a phase III study that included 85% patients with ESCC. FOLFOX with radiation therapy did not show superiority compared to CRT with CF, but a lower frequency of renal toxicity and treatment-related death was observed in the FOLFOX radiation arm [82]. Despite the increased incidence of peripheral neuropathy, the FOLFOX radiation regimen is considered as a standard regimen for ESCC because of its convenience.

16.4.2 Chemoradiotherapy for Unresectable Locally Advanced Esophageal Cancer

CRT is the only treatment modality with a potentially curative intent for unresectable locally advanced ESCC. From the results of prospective trial, 15%–33% of complete response rate and approximately 20% of 3-year survival rate were reported in the patients with clinical T4 and/or M1 only in cervical lymph nodes who received CF with concurrent 60-Gy irradiation [83–85].

The triplet combination of CF and docetaxel, which consisted of 400 mg/m^2 5-FU on days 1–5, 40 mg/m^2 CDDP on day 1, and 20–40 mg/m^2 docetaxel on day 1 repeated every 2 weeks, with concurrent irradiation of 61.2 Gy for T4 ESCC, was conducted as a phase I study [86]. The overall response rate was 89.5%, including a complete response rate of 42.1%. Docetaxel, CDDP, and 5-FU with radiation showed promising efficacy, but relatively larger number of severe adverse events, for example, esophagitis and febrile neutropenia, are critical for practical use.

Fistula formation between the esophagus and the neighboring structures, such as the aorta or the airway, is highly associated with death and termination of treatment. Esophageal fistula was observed in 22% of patients who enrolled in the JCOG0303 trial, which was related to poor survival [87]. Induction chemotherapy with DCF before CRT may reduce the risk of fistula formation even in T4 disease. A phase II study of induction DCF followed by CRT revealed no fistula formation among 48 ESCC patients with T4 and/or unresectable supraclavicular lymph node metastasis. Conversion surgery was performed 41.7% of patients, and R0 resection was achieved in 39.6% of patients [88]. Phase III trial, which compared CRT with induction DCF followed by surgery or CRT, has completed enrollment and is awaiting results [89].

16.5 Chemotherapy or Chemoradiotherapy with Targeted Agents

Since the 2000s, many targeted agents have been approved for the treatment of lung, colorectal, breast, and other cancers. Results from preclinical or translational studies may help identify optimal targets related to cancer invasion, proliferation, and oncogenesis. Recently, many molecular targets have been evaluated for clinical use on the basis of the genetic findings of ESCC (Table 16.4).

16.5.1 Antihuman Epidermal Growth Factor Receptor Inhibitors

Epidermal growth factor receptor (EGFR) is one of the therapeutic targets of ESCC. High levels of EGFR protein expression have been detected in 50%–70% of ESCC cases via immunohistochemical analysis, and gene amplification of *EGFR* has been observed in 7%–31% of ESCC cases [90–92]. Overexpression of EGFR may correlate with invasion and poor prognosis [93]. Rare mutations in *EGFR* and *KRAS* have also been reported [94, 95].

Two types of EGFR inhibitory therapy, an antibody and tyrosine kinase inhibitors (TKI), were evaluated in patients with ESCC. Gefitinib, an orally active EGFR TKI, showed 2.8% partial response and 27.8% of stable disease among ESCC patients. Median PFS and MST were 2 and 5.5 months [96]. Erlotinib, another oral EGFR TKI, showed 15% of partial response and 13.3% of stable disease in ESCC patients. The median time to progression was 3.3 months [97]. No correlation of the EGFR status and the degree of expression with erlotinib efficacy could be established, possibly because of the small number of patients. A large phase III trial that compared the effect of gefitinib alone to placebo in patients with esophageal cancer by considering disease progression following standard chemotherapy was conducted in England. Totally, there were no significant differences between two groups [98]. Totally, the efficacy of EGFR TKIs is modest and limited to ESCC. The patients with copy number gain of EGFR were reported to have benefited from EGF TKI by the TRANS-COS study [99].

Cetuximab, an anti-EGFR monoclonal chimeric antibody, was evaluated for the treatment of ESCC in combination with CF as the first-line treatment. From the result of randomized phase II trial comparing daily CF with or without 250 mg/m^2 cetuximab administered weekly for untreated ESCC, there was no significant adding effect of cetuximab, though a trend toward longer PFS (5.9 months vs.

Table 16.4 Targeted agents for esophageal cancer

Agent/trial name	Histology and number of pts	Treatment line	Regimen	Response (%)	PFS (m)	MST (m)	References
Gefitinib	SCC 27 AC 9	2nd	Gefitinib 500 mg/day	2.8	2	5.5	[96]
Erlotinib	SCC 13 AC 17	2nd	Erlotinib 150 mg/day	SCC 15 AC 0	SCC 3.3 AC 1.6	SCC 8.2 AC 11.2	[97]
Gefitinib	SCC 107 AC 340	2nd	Placebo	0.4	1.17	3.60	[98]
			Gefitinib 500 mg/day	3.1	1.60	3.73	
Cetuximab	SCC 30	1st	5-FU 1000 mg/m^2 day 1–5 Cisplatin 100 mg/m^2 day 1/q4wks	30%	3.9	5.5	[35]
	SCC 32		5-FU 1000 mg/m^2 day 1–5 Cisplatin 100 mg/m^2 day 1/q4wks Cetuximab 250 mg/m^2 weekly (after a loading dose of 400 mg/m^2)	34%	5.9	9.5	
SCOPE1	SCC 96 AC 32	cT1–4 N0-1M0 1st	Capecitabine 625 mg/m^2 twice daily day 1–84 Cisplatin 60 mg/m^2 day 1, 22, 43, 64 Radiation 50Gy	NA	21.6	25.4	[100]
	SCC 92 AC 33		Capecitabine 625 mg/m^2 twice daily day 1–84 Cisplatin 60 mg/m^2 day 1, 22, 43, 64 Radiation 50Gy Cetuximab 250 mg/m^2 weekly (after a loading dose of 400 mg/m^2)	NA	15.9	22.1	

RTOG0436	SCC 59 AC 79	cT1N1M0 cT2-4NanyM0 cTanyNanyM1a 1st	Paclitaxel 25 mg/m^2 day 1, 8, 15, 22, 29, 36 Cisplatin 50 mg/m^2 day 1, 8, 15, 22, 29, 36 Radiation 50.4Gy	CRR SCC 64 AC 54	NA	2-year survival SCC 43% AC 41%	[101]
	SCC 54 AC 74		Paclitaxel 25 mg/m^2 day 1, 8, 15, 22, 29, 36 Cisplatin 50 mg/m^2 day 1, 8, 15, 22, 29, 36 Raiation 50.4Gy Cetuximab 250 mg/m^2 weekly (after a loading dose of 400 mg/m^2)	CRR SCC 59 AC 53	NA	2-year survival SCC 46% AC 43%	
POWER	SCC 73	1st	Panitumumab 9 mg/kg day 1 5-FU 1000 mg/m^2 day 1–4 Cisplatin 100 mg/m^2 day 1/q3wks	35.6	5.3	9.4	[102]
	SCC 73		5-FU 1000 mg/m^2 day 1–4 Cisplatin 100 mg/m^2 day 1/q3wks	37.0	5.8	10.2	

Pts patients, *PFS* progression-free survival, *MST* median survival time, *SCC* squamous cell carcinoma, *AC* adenocarcinoma, *NA* not available, *wks* weeks, *5-FU* 5-fluorouracil, *CRR* complete response rate

3.9 months) and OS (9.5 months vs. 5.5 months) was observed in the cetuximab arm [35]. The phase II/III trial (SCOPE1), which compared capecitabine and CDDP with radiotherapy, with or without cetuximab, showed that OS was significantly worse in the CRT plus cetuximab group than in the CRT group (hazard ratio = 1.53; $p = 0.035$) [100] due to toxicities in cetuximab group. In a phase III trial (RTOG0436), weekly concurrent paclitaxel and CDDP plus radiotherapy at a dose of 50.4 Gy with cetuximab was compared to that without cetuximab. The superiority of cetuximab group was not shown with the 1-year and 2-year survival rates of 64% and 44% in the cetuximab group and 65% and 42% in the non-cetuximab group, respectively. These tendencies were the same among patients in both histological groups [101].

Panitumumab is a fully human immunoglobulin (IgG) 2 monoclonal antibody targeting EGFR. A phase III trial (POWER) comparing CF versus CF plus panitumumab as the first-line chemotherapy in patients with ESCC showed that treatment-related deaths occurred more frequently in the CF plus panitumumab group (23.6% versus 4.3%, $p = 0.0012$) and no improvement of OS was observed in the CF plus panitumumab group (median OS: 9.4 months in the CF plus panitumumab group versus 10.2 months in the CF group, HR = 1.17; $p = 0.43$) [102].

Sym004 is a 1:1 mixture of two antibodies targeting nonoverlapping epitopes of the epidermal growth factor receptor that antagonize ligand binding and induce receptor downregulation and have greater growth inhibition than cetuximab in preclinical models. From the result of expansion cohort of Sym004 phase I trial, 16.7% of 30 patients achieved objective response, and disease control rate was 56.7% for refractory ESCC patients [103].

Nimotuzumab, a humanized antibody directed against epidermal growth factor receptor, was evaluated adding effect with concurrent CRT for locally advanced ESCC patients. Nimotuzumab is less likely to induce skin toxicities because nimotuzumab has relatively low affinity, and bivalent binding are required for stable attachment of nimotuzumab to cellular surface. Randomized phase II named NICE trial showed tendency for survival benefit of nimotuzumab with CRT arm with MST of 15.9 months compared to CRT arm with MST of 11.5 months [104]. Safety of CF and nimotuzumab with radiation was confirmed in Japanese patients [105].

Amivantamab, a bispecific monoclonal antibody targeting EGFR and MET, is evaluated for treating advanced sloid tumor including ESCC, objective response rate and disease control rate were 10.7% and 67.9% [106].

In addition, necitumumab, a fully humanized monoclonal antibody targeting EGFR, is being developed for treating advanced ESCC and gastric cancer with EGFR amplification (jRCT2031240655).

16.5.2 Immune-Checkpoint Inhibitors

Immune-checkpoint inhibitors became the key drug for most cancer types. Inhibitory immune checkpoint molecules (e.g., programmed cell death ligand 1 [PD-L1], cytotoxic T lymphocyte–associated antigen 4 [CTLA-4], lymphocyte activation gene-3 [LAG-3]), and stimulatory immune checkpoint molecules (e.g., CD40L, OX40, inducible T-cell costimulatory [ICOS]) play a role in maintaining immunological homeostasis. In ESCC tumors, PD-L1 expression is observed in 18.4%–82.8%, associated with poor survival [107] (Table 16.5).

Nivolumab, a human IgG4 monoclonal antibody against PD-1, was evaluated in a single-arm, multicenter phase II trial (ATTRACTION-1) for ESCC that failed to fluoropyrimidine, platinum, and taxane-based treatments [108]. Nivolumab showed response rate of 17% and MST of 10.8 months. A global phase III trial (ATTRACTION-3), which compared nivolumab versus docetaxel or paclitaxel for treated ESCC refractory to fluoropyrimidine and platinum, showed superiority of OS (MST: 10.9 months vs 8.4 months; HR 0.77, 95% CI 0.62–0.96; $p = 0.019$) [109]. In addition, a global randomized phase III trial (CheckMate 648) showed superiority of OS in CF plus nivolumab compared to CF (MST: 13.2 months vs 10.7 months; HR 0.74; 99.1% CI, 0.58 to 0.96; $P = 0.002$) for untreated advanced ESCC [110].

As for combination with definitive CRT, a phase II trial has evaluated the efficacy and safety of definitive CRT with nivolumab (UMIN000035889). The complete response rate was reached 84% for resectable cases, and 56.3% for unresectable cases, and incidence of pneumonitis remained within an acceptable range [111].

Pembrolizumab, a humanized IgG4 monoclonal antibody against PD-1, was evaluated in a multicohort phase Ib trial (KEYNOTE-028) for patients with PD-L1-positive advanced solid tumors. In the esophageal cancer cohort, response rate was 30% [112]. Additionally, a phase II trial (KEYNOTE-180), which evaluates the efficacy of pembrolizumab for heavily treated esophageal cancer, showed objective response rate of 14.3% in ESCC and 5.2% in adenocarcinoma [113]. A global phase III trial (KEYNOTE-181) was conducted to compare pembrolizumab versus the investigator's choice chemotherapy (paclitaxel, docetaxel, or irinotecan) as the second-line treatment in patients with esophageal cancer, but there was no superiority of OS in pembrolizumab compared to cytotoxic agents among patients with PD-L1 positive and patients with ESCC, in intent to treat cohort as primary endpoints. Only among patients with PD-L1-positive ESCC, pembrolizumab showed better tendency of OS compared to cytotoxic agents (MST: 10.3 months vs 6.7 months) [114]. A global randomized phase III trial (KEYNOTE-590) showed superiority of OS in CF plus pembrolizumab compared to CF (MST: 12.4 months vs 9.8 months; HR 0.73 [0.62–0.86]; $p < 0.0001$) for untreated advanced esophageal cancer [115].

For advanced ESCC, PD-1/PD-L1 blockade is important role to control tumor progression, other PD-1/PD-L1 blockade drugs, such as tislelizumab [116, 117], camrelizumab [118, 119], toripalimab [120], sintilimab [121], and serplulimab [122], showed clinically meaningful benefits for advanced ESCC.

Atezolizumab, the anti-PD-1 antibody, has demonstrated high efficacy as sequential use after definitive CRT in the phase II trial [123], based on the rationale of the PACIFIC trial for non-small cell lung carcinoma.

Dual immune checkpoint inhibition has been investigated to enhance the efficacy of immune checkpoint inhibitor monotherapy. A randomized phase 3 trial (CheckMate 648) showed superiority of OS in nivolumab plus

Table 16.5 Immune-checkpoint inhibitor for esophageal cancer

Agent/trial name	Histology and number of pts	Treatment line	Regimen	Response (%)	PFS (m)	MST (m)	References
ATTRACTION-1	SCC 65	3rd	Nivolumab 3 mg/kg/q2wks	17.2	1.5	10.78	[108]
ATTRACTION-3	SCC419	2nd	Nivolumab 3 mg/kg/q2wks	19	1.7	10.9	[109]
			Paclitaxel or docetaxel	22	3.4	8.4	
CheckMate 648	SCC 970	1st	Nivolumab 3 mg/kg, q2wks Ipilimumab 1 mg/kg, q6wks	28	2.9	12.7	[110]
			Nivolumab 240 mg/body, q2wks 5-FU 800 mg/m^2 day 1–5 Cisplatin 80 mg/m^2 day 1/q4wks	47	5.8	13.2	
			5-FU 1000 mg/m^2 day 1–5 Cisplatin 80 mg/m^2 day 1/q4wks	27	5.6	10.7	
KEYNOTE-180	SCC 63 AC 58	3rd	Pembrolizumab 200 mg/q3wks	SCC 14 AC 5	SCC 2.1 AC 1.9	SCC 6.8 AC 3.9	[113]
KEYNOTE-181	CPS ≥10,107 CPS <10,201	2nd	Pembrolizumab 200 mg/q3wks	CPS ≥10 23	CPS ≥10 2.6	CPS ≥10 9.3	[114]
	CPS ≥10,115 CPS <10,196		Paclitaxel 80–100 mg/m^2 day 1, 8, 15/q4wks Docetaxel 75 mg/m^2/q3wks Irinotecan 180 mg/m^2/q2wks	CPS ≥10 7	CPS ≥10 3.0	CPS ≥10 6.7	
KEYNOTE-590	SCC 548, AC 201	1st	Pembrolizumab 200 mg/body 5-FU 800 mg/m^2 day 1–5 Cisplatin 80 mg/m^2 day 1/q3wks	45.0	6.3	12.4	[115]
			5-FU 800 mg/m^2 day 1–5 Cisplatin 80 mg/m^2 day 1/q3wks	29.3	5.8	9.8	
RARTIONALE-302	SCC 512	2nd	Tislelizumab 200 mg/q3wks	20.3	1.6	8.6	[116]
			Paclitaxel 135–175 mg/m^2 day 1/q3wks Docetaxel 75 mg/m^2/q3wks Irinotecan 125 mg/m^2 day 1, 8/q3wks	9.5	2.1	6.3	

RATIONALE-306	SCC 649	1st	Tislelizumab 200 mg/q3wks 5-FU 750–800 mg/m² day 1–5 or Cape 1000 mg/m² day 1–14, Paclitaxel 175 mg/m² day 1/q3wks Cisplatin 60–80 mg/m² day 1 or Oxaliplatin 130 mg/m² day 1/q3wks	63	7.3	17.2	[117]
			5-FU 750–800 mg/m² day 1–5 or Cape 1000 mg/m² day 1–14, Paclitaxel 175 mg/m² day 1/q3wks Cisplatin 60–80 mg/m² day 1 or Oxaliplatin 130 mg/m² day 1/q3wks	42	5.6	10.6	
ESCORT	SCC 457	2nd	Camrelizumab 200 mg/q3wks	20.2	1.9	8.3	[118]
			Docetaxel 75 mg/m²/q3wks Irinotecan 180 mg/m²/q2wks	6.4	1,9	6.2	
ESCORT-1st	SCC 596	1st	Camrelizumab 200 mg/body Paclitaxel 175 mg/m² day 1 Cisplatin 75 mg/m² day 1/q3wks	72.1	6.9	15.3	[119]
			Paclitaxel 175 mg/m² day 1 Cisplatin 75 mg/m² day 1/q3wks	62.1	5.6	12.0	
JUPITER-6	SCC 514	1st	Toripalimab 240 mg/body Paclitaxel 175 mg/m² day 1 Cisplatin 75 mg/m² day 1/q3wks	69.3	5.7	17	[120]
			Paclitaxel 175 mg/m² day 1 Cisplatin 75 mg/m² day 1/q3wks	52.1	5.5	11	
ORIENT-15	SCC 659	1st	Sintilimab 3 mg/kg or 200 mg/body Paclitaxel 175 mg/m² day 1 Cisplatin 75 mg/m² day 1/q3wks	66	7.2	16.7	[121]
			Paclitaxel 175 mg/m² day 1 Cisplatin 75 mg/m² day 1/q3wks	45	5.7	12.5	

(continued)

Table 16.5 (continued)

Agent/trial name	Histology and number of pts	Treatment line	Regimen	Response (%)	PFS (m)	MST (m)	References
HLX10–007-EC301	SCC 551	1st	Serplulimab 3 mg/kg 5-FU 1200 mg/m^2 day 1, 2 Cisplatin 50 mg/m^2 day 1/q2wks	57.6	5.8	15.3	[122]
			5-FU 1200 mg/m^{2}day 1, 2 Cisplatin 50 mg/m^2 day 1/q2wks	42.1	5.3	11.8	
SKYSCRAPER-08	SCC 461	1st	Atezolizumab 1200 mg/body Tiragolumab 600 mg/body Paclitaxel 175 mg/m^2 day 1 Cisplatin 60–80 mg/m^2 day 1/q3wks	59.7	6.2	15.7	[124]
			Paclitaxel 175 mg/m^2 day 1 Cisplatin 60–80 mg/m^2 day 1/q3wks	45.5	5.4	11.1	
LEAP-014	SCC 850	1st	Lenvatinib 8 mg (consolidation 20 mg)/body Pembrolizumab 400 mg/body day 1 CF or TP/q3wks or FOLFOX/q2wks	62.2	7.2	17.6	[130]
			Pembrolizumab 400 mg/body day 1 CF or TP/q3wks or FOLFOX/q2wks	54.8	6.9	15.5	

CPS Combined Positive Score of PD-L1

ipilimumab (anti-CTLA-4 antibody) compared to in CF (MST: 12.7 months vs 10.7 months; HR 0.78; 98.2% CI, 0.62 to 0.98; $P = 0.01$) for untreated advanced ESCC [110].

TIGIT is an immune checkpoint molecule, and anti-TIGIT antibody, such as tiragolumab, was developed. The global randomized phase III trial (SKYSCRAPER-08) showed superiority of OS in tiragolumab plus atezolizumab, taxane, platinum compared to taxane plus platinum (MST: 15.7 months vs 11.1 months; HR: 0.70; 95% CI: 0.55, 0.88; $P = 0.0024$) for untreated advanced ESCC [124]. Nevertheless, tiragolumab plus atezolizumab as maintenance therapy after definitive CRT could not show superiority of investigator accessed PFS (median PFS: 20.8 months vs 16.6 months; HR 0.82; 95%CI, 0.65 to 1.03, $P = 0.0947$) and OS (MST: 38.6 months vs 36.4 months; HR 0.91; 95% CI, 0.70 to 1.18; $P = 0.4772$) compared to placebo plus placebo in phase III trial (SKYSCRAPER-07) in locally advanced unresetable setting. Although atezolizumab plus placebo demonstrated statistical superiority over the tiragolumab plus atezolizumab arm (HR, 1.36; 95% CI, 1.03–1.80; $P = 0.0314$), formal statistical testing between the atezolizumab plus placebo and placebo plus placebo arms was not performed according to the hierarchical testing plan, since the primary PFS endpoint was not met for tiragolumab plus atezolizumab versus placebo plus placebo [125].

16.5.3 Other Potential Molecular Targets

Antiangiogenesis is also a potential therapeutic target. Vascular endothelial growth factor-A expression is seen in 24%–93% of ESCC cases [126]. The overexpression of vascular endothelial growth factor isoforms has been shown to correlate significantly with poor prognosis in ESCC [126–128]. Apatinib is oral multi-kinase inhibitor, including antiangiogenetic pathway, which showed survival benefit for later lines of gastric cancer. Phase II trial of apatinib for ESCC showed efficacy with a response rate of 24.2% and a disease control rate of 74.2% [128]. Regorafenib, a multi-kinase TKI, combined with nivolumab showed higher response rate (43%) for the ICI naïve ESCC patients [129]. Lenvatinib, an oral multiple kinase inhibitor targeting vascular endothelial growth factor receptor, was promising drug. However, a randomized phase III trial (LEAP-014) showed no superiority of OS in lenvatinib plus pembrolizumab, fluoropyrimidine, platinum compared to pembrolizumab plus fluoropyrimidine, platinum (MST: 17.6 months vs 15.5 months) for untreated advanced ESCC [130].

BKM120, an oral pan-class I PI3K inhibitor, showed modest activity for ESCC patients with DCR of 51.2% and PFS of 2.3 months. PI3K pathway activation was observed in patients with good clinical response [131].

TAS120, an oral FGFR inhibitor, showed promising efficacy, such as response rate of 76.9% in combination with immune checkpoint inhibitor and CF for untreated advanced esophageal cancer [132].

16.6 Future Directions

There are two main streams of new treatment development for advanced ESCC. First, one is molecular targeted agent plus immune checkpoint inhibitor combination therapy. LEAP-014 did not show clinical improvement of adding lenvatinib to pembrolizumab plus doublet chemotherapy; TAS120 plus immune checkpoint inhibitor combination therapy showed promising results at the first-line and salvage-line treatments in the phase I/II trials. The other is antibody-drug conjugate (ADC). In advanced ESCC, some molecules such as B7-H3, TROP2, HER2, and nectin-4 show high expression. Several ADCs have been developed targeting B7-H3 and TROP2. Ifanatamab deruxtecan is an ADC consisting of anti B7-H3 antibody and topoisomerase I inhibitor. A randomized phase III trial comparing ifanatamab deruxtecan with cytotoxic agents as second-line treatment for advanced ESCC (IDeate-Esophageal01) and a phase I trial which is evaluating ifanatamab deruxtecan plus pembrolizumab with or without cytotoxic agents as first-line treatment for advanced ESCC (KEYMAKER-06E) are ongoing. Sacituzumab tirumotecan is an ADC consisting of anti TROP-2 antibody and topoisomerase I inhibitor. A randomized phase I/II trial comparing sacituzumab tirumotecan with cytotoxic agent as second-line treatment for advanced ESCC (KEYMAKER-06B) is ongoing. Trastuzumab deruxtecan is an ADC consisting of anti-B7-H3 antibody and topoisomerase I inhibitor. A multicohort phase II trial (HERALD) showed objective response rate was 50.0% in HER2 amplification advanced EC [133]. Enfortumab vedotin is an ADC consisting of anti-Nection-4 antibody and monomethyl auristatin E. A phase II trial showed objective response rate was 18.2% in treated advanced ESCC [134]. These clinical trials might improve the prognosis of advanced ESCC.

References

1. Ezdinli EZ, Gelber R, Desai DV, et al. Chemotherapy of advanced esophageal carcinoma: Eastern Cooperative Oncology Group experience. Cancer. 1980;46:2149–53.
2. Akutsu Y, Kono T, Uesato M, et al. S-1 monotherapy as second- or third-line chemotherapy for unresectable and recurrent esophageal squamous cell carcinoma. Oncology. 2013;84:305–10.
3. Ito T, Honma Y, Hirano H, et al. S-1 monotherapy after failure of platinum plus 5-fluorouracil chemotherapy in recurrent or metastatic esophageal carcinoma. Anticancer Res. 2019;39:3931–6.
4. Panettiere FJ, Leichman LP, Tilchen EJ, et al. Chemotherapy for advanced epidermoid carcinoma of the esophagus with single-agent cisplatin: final report on a Southwest Oncology Group study. Cancer Treat Rep. 1984;68:1023–4.
5. Bleiberg H, Conroy T, Paillot B, et al. Randomised phase II study of cisplatin and 5-fluorouracil (5-FU) versus cisplatin alone in advanced squamous cell oesophageal cancer. Eur J Cancer. 1997;33:1216–20.
6. Mannell A, Winters Z. Carboplatin in the treatment of oesophageal cancer. S Afr Med J. 1989;76:213–4.
7. Queisser W, Preusser P, Mross KB, et al. Phase II evaluation of carboplatin in advanced esophageal carcinoma. A trial of the phase I/II study Group of the Association for Medical Oncology of the German Cancer Society. Onkologie. 1990;13:190–3.

8. Taguchi T, Wakui A, Nabeya K, et al. A phase II clinical study of cis-diammine glycolato platinum, 254-S, for gastrointestinal cancers. 254-S Gastrointestinal Cancer Study Group. Gan To Kagaku Ryoho. 1992;19:483–8.
9. Rowinsky EK, Cazenave LA, Donehower RC. Taxol: a novel investigational antimicrotubule agent. J Natl Cancer Inst. 1990;82:1247–59.
10. Ajani JA, Ilson DH, Daugherty K, et al. Activity of taxol in patients with squamous cell carcinoma and adenocarcinoma of the esophagus. J Natl Cancer Inst. 1994;86:1086–91.
11. Ilson DH, Wadleigh RG, Leichman LP, et al. Paclitaxel given by a weekly 1-h infusion in advanced esophageal cancer. Ann Oncol. 2007;18:898–902.
12. Kato K, Tahara M, Hironaka S, et al. A phase II study of paclitaxel by weekly 1-h infusion for advanced or recurrent esophageal cancer in patients who had previously received platinum-based chemotherapy. Cancer Chemother Pharmacol. 2011;67:1265–72.
13. Einzig AI, Neuberg D, Remick SC, et al. Phase II trial of docetaxel (Taxotere) in patients with adenocarcinoma of the upper gastrointestinal tract previously untreated with cytotoxic chemotherapy: the Eastern Cooperative Oncology Group (ECOG) results of protocol E1293. Med Oncol. 1996;13:87–93.
14. Heath EI, Urba S, Marshall J, et al. Phase II trial of docetaxel chemotherapy in patients with incurable adenocarcinoma of the esophagus. Investig New Drugs. 2002;20:95–9.
15. Muro K, Hamaguchi T, Ohtsu A, et al. A phase II study of single-agent docetaxel in patients with metastatic esophageal cancer. Ann Oncol. 2004;15:955–9.
16. Yamamoto S, Kawakami H, Kii T, et al. Randomized phase II study of docetaxel versus paclitaxel in patients with esophageal squamous cell carcinoma refractory to fluoropyrimidine- and platinum-based chemotherapy: OGSG1201. Eur J Cancer. 2021;154:307–15.
17. Tancini G, Bajetta E, Bonadonna G. Bleomycin alone and in combination with methotrexate in the treatment of carcinoma of the esophagus. Tumori. 1974;60:65–71.
18. Bonadonna G, De Lena M, Monfardini S, et al. Clinical trials with bleomycin in lymphomas and in solid tumors. Eur J Cancer. 1972;8:205–15.
19. Ravry M, Moertel CG, Schutt AJ, et al. Treatment of advanced squamous cell carcinoma of the gastrointestinal tract with bleomycin (NSC-125066). Cancer Chemother Rep. 1973;57:493–5.
20. Mannell A, Becker PJ, Melissas J, et al. Intubation v. dilatation plus bleomycin in the treatment of advanced oesophageal cancer. The results of a prospective randomized trial. S Aft J Surg. 1986;24:15–9.
21. Nanus DM, Kelsen DP, Lipperman R, et al. Phase II trial of ifosfamide in epidermoid carcinoma of the esophagus: unexpectant severe toxicity. Investig New Drugs. 1988;6:239–41.
22. Sandler AB, Kindler HL, Einhorn LH, et al. Phase II trial of gemcitabine in patients with previously untreated metastatic cancer of the esophagus or gastroesophageal junction. Ann Oncol. 2000;11:1161–4.
23. Kelsen DP, Bains M, Cvitkovic E, et al. Vindesine in the treatment of esophageal carcinoma: a phase II study. Cancer Treat Rep. 1979;63:2019–21.
24. Bedikian AY, Valdivieso M, Bodey GP, et al. Phase II evaluation of vindesine in the treatment of colorectal and esophageal tumors. Cancer Chemother Pharmacol. 1979;2:263–6.
25. Bezwoda WR, Derman DP, Weaving A, et al. Treatment of esophageal cancer with vindesine: an open trial. Cancer Treat Rep. 1984;68:783–5.
26. Conroy T, Etienne PL, Adenis A, et al. Phase II trial of vinorelbine in metastatic squamous cell esophageal carcinoma. European Organization for Research and Treatment of Cancer Gastrointestinal Treatment Cancer Cooperative Group. J Clin Oncol. 1996;14:164–70.
27. Harstrick A, Bokemeyer C, Preusser P, et al. Phase II study of single-agent etoposide in patients with metastatic squamous-cell carcinoma of the esophagus. Cancer Chemother Pharmacol. 1992;29:321–2.
28. Coonley CJ, Bains M, Heelan R, et al. Phase II study of etoposide in the treatment of esophageal carcinoma. Cancer Treat Rep. 1983;67:397–8.

29. Radice PA, Bunn PA Jr, Ihde DC. Therapeutic trials with VP-16-213 and VM-26: active agents in small cell lung cancer, non-Hodgkin's lymphomas, and other malignancies. Cancer Treat Rep. 1979;63:1231–9.
30. Mühr-Wilkenshoff F, Hinkelbein W, Ohnesorge I, et al. A pilot study of irinotecan (CPT-11) as single-agent therapy in patients with locally advanced or metastatic esophageal carcinoma. Int J Color Dis. 2003;18:330–4.
31. Levard H, Pouliquen X, Hay JM, et al. 5-Fluorouracil and cisplatin as palliative treatment of advanced oesophageal squamous cell carcinoma. A multicentre randomised controlled trial. The French Associations for Surgical Research. Eur J Surg. 1998;164:849–57.
32. Iizuka T, Kakegawa T, Ide H, et al. Phase II evaluation of cisplatin and 5-fluorouracil in advanced squamous cell carcinoma of the esophagus: a Japanese Esophageal Oncology Group Trial. Jpn J Clin Oncol. 1992;22:172–6.
33. Hayashi K, Ando N, Watanabe H, et al. Phase II evaluation of protracted infusion of cisplatin and 5-fluorouracil in advanced squamous cell carcinoma of the esophagus: a Japan Esophageal Oncology Group (JEOG) Trial (JCOG9407). Jpn J Clin Oncol. 2001;31:419–23.
34. Caroli-Bosc FX, Van Laethem JL, Michel P, et al. A weekly 24-h infusion of high-dose 5-fluorouracil (5-FU) +leucovorin and bi-weekly cisplatin (CDDP) was active and well tolerated in patients with non-colon digestive carcinomas. Eur J Cancer. 2001;37:1828–32.
35. Lorenzen S, Schuster T, Porschen R, et al. Cetuximab plus cisplatin-5-fluorouracil versus cisplatin-5-fluorouracil alone in first-line metastatic squamous cell carcinoma of the esophagus: a randomized phase II study of the Arbeitsgemeinschaft Internistische Onkologie. Ann Oncol. 2009;20:1667–73.
36. Lee J, Im YH, Cho EY, et al. A phase II study of capecitabine and cisplatin (XP) as first-line chemotherapy in patients with advanced esophageal squamous cell carcinoma. Cancer Chemother Pharmacol. 2008;62:77–84.
37. Wang J, Chang J, Yu H, et al. A phase II study of oxaliplatin in combination with leucovorin and fluorouracil as first-line chemotherapy in patients with metastatic squamous cell carcinoma of esophagus. Cancer Chemother Pharmacol. 2013;71:905–11.
38. Mauer AM, Kraut EH, Krauss SA, et al. Phase II trial of oxaliplatin, leucovorin, and fluorouracil in patients with advanced carcinoma of the esophagus. Ann Oncol. 2005;16:1320–5.
39. Qin TJ, An GL, Zhao XH, et al. Combined treatment of oxaliplatin and capecitabine in patients with metastatic esophageal squamous cell cancer. World J Gastroenterol. 2009;15:871–6.
40. Kato K, Muro K, Ando N, et al. A phase II study of nedaplatin and 5-fluorouracil in metastatic squamous cell carcinoma of the esophagus: the Japan Clinical Oncology Group (JCOG) Trial (JCOG 9905-DI). Esophagus. 2014;11:183–8.
41. Conroy T, Etienne PL, Adenis A, et al. Vinorelbine and cisplatin in metastatic squamous cell carcinoma of the oesophagus: response, toxicity, quality of life and survival. Ann Oncol. 2002;13:721–9.
42. Kroep JR, Pinedo HM, Giaccone G, et al. Phase II study of cisplatin preceding gemcitabine in patients with advanced oesophageal cancer. Ann Oncol. 2004;15:230–5.
43. El-Rayes BF, Shields A, Zalupski M, et al. A phase II study of carboplatin and paclitaxel in esophageal cancer. Ann Oncol. 2004;15:960–5.
44. van der Gaast A, Kok TC, Kerkhofs L, et al. Phase I study of a biweekly schedule of a fixed dose of cisplatin with increasing doses of paclitaxel in patients with advanced oesophageal cancer. Br J Cancer. 1999;80:1052–7.
45. Petrasch S, Welt A, Reinacher A, et al. Chemotherapy with cisplatin and paclitaxel in patients with locally advanced, recurrent or metastatic oesophageal cancer. Br J Cancer. 1998;78:511–4.
46. Zhang X, Shen L, Li J, et al. A phase II trial of paclitaxel and cisplatin in patients with advanced squamous-cell carcinoma of the esophagus. Am J Clin Oncol. 2008;31:29–33.
47. Shi Y, Qin R, Wang ZK, et al. Nanoparticle albumin-bound paclitaxel combined with cisplatin as the first-line treatment for metastatic esophageal squamous cell carcinoma. Onco Targets Ther. 2013;6:585–91.

48. Gong Y, Ren L, Zhou L, et al. Phase II evaluation of nedaplatin and paclitaxel in patients with metastatic esophageal carcinoma. Cancer Chemother Pharmacol. 2009;64:327–33.
49. Cao W, Xu C, Lou G, et al. A phase II study of paclitaxel and nedaplatin as first-line chemotherapy in patients with advanced esophageal cancer. Jpn J Clin Oncol. 2009;39:582–7.
50. He YF, Ji CS, Hu B, et al. A phase II study of paclitaxel and nedaplatin as front-line chemotherapy in Chinese patients with metastatic esophageal squamous cell carcinoma. World J Gastroenterol. 2013;19:5910–6.
51. Yun T, Han JY, Lee JS, et al. Phase II study of weekly paclitaxel and capecitabine in patients with metastatic or recurrent esophageal squamous cell carcinoma. BMC Cancer. 2011;11:385.
52. Shim HJ, Cho SH, Hwang JE, et al. Phase II study of docetaxel and cisplatin chemotherapy in 5-fluorouracil/cisplatin pretreated esophageal cancer. Am J Clin Oncol. 2010;33:624–8.
53. Yoshioka T, Sakayori M, Kato S, et al. Dose escalation study of docetaxel and nedaplatin in patients with relapsed or refractory squamous cell carcinoma of the esophagus pretreated using cisplatin, 5-fluorouracil, and radiation. Int J Clin Oncol. 2006;11:454–60.
54. Kanai M, Matsumoto S, Nishimura T, et al. Retrospective analysis of 27 consecutive patients treated with docetaxel/nedaplatin combination therapy as a second-line regimen for advanced esophageal cancer. Int J Clin Oncol. 2007;12:224–7.
55. Jin J, Xu X, Wang F, et al. Second-line combination chemotherapy with docetaxel and nedaplatin for Cisplatin-pretreated refractory metastatic/recurrent esophageal squamous cell carcinoma. J Thorac Oncol. 2009;4:1017–21.
56. Akutsu Y, Shuto K, Kono T, et al. A phase I/II study of second-line chemotherapy with fractionated docetaxel and nedaplatin for 5-FU/cisplatin-resistant esophageal squamous cell carcinoma. Hepato-Gastroenterology. 2012;59:2095–8.
57. Kajiura S, Hosokawa A, Yoshita H, et al. Phase I study of docetaxel plus nedaplatin in patients with metastatic or recurrent esophageal squamous cell carcinoma after cisplatin plus 5-fluorouracil treatment. Am J Clin Oncol. 2013;39:13–7.
58. Ilson DH, Ajani J, Bhalla K, et al. Phase II trial of paclitaxel, fluorouracil, and cisplatin in patients with advanced carcinoma of the esophagus. J Clin Oncol. 1998;16:1826–34.
59. Takahashi H, Arimura Y, Yamashita K, et al. Phase I/II study of docetaxel/cisplatin/fluorouracil combination chemotherapy against metastatic esophageal squamous cell carcinoma. J Thorac Oncol. 2010;5:122–8.
60. Tanaka Y, Yoshida K, Sanada Y, et al. Biweekly docetaxel, cisplatin, and 5-fluorouracil (DCF) chemotherapy for advanced esophageal squamous cell carcinoma: a phase I dose-escalation study. Cancer Chemother Pharmacol. 2010;66:1159–65.
61. Osaka Y, Shinohara M, Hoshino S, et al. Phase II study of combined chemotherapy with docetaxel, CDDP, and 5-FU for highly advanced esophageal cancer. Anticancer Res. 2011;31:633–8.
62. Yamasaki M, Miyata H, Tanaka K, et al. Multicenter phase I/II study of docetaxel, cisplatin, and fluorouracil combination chemotherapy in patients with advanced or recurrent squamous cell carcinoma of the esophagus. Oncology. 2011;80:307–13.
63. Tamura S, Imano M, Takiuchi H, et al. Phase II study of docetaxel, cisplatin, and 5-fluorouracil (DCF) for metastatic esophageal cancer (OGSG 0403). Anticancer Res. 2012;32:1403–8.
64. Hironaka S, Tsubosa Y, Mizusawa J, et al. Phase I/II trial of 2-weekly docetaxel combined with cisplatin plus fluorouracil in metastatic esophageal cancer (JCOG0807). Cancer Sci. 2014;105:1189–95.
65. Tsushima T, Hironaka S, Tsubosa Y, et al. First-line docetaxel once every 2 weeks with cisplatin plus fluorouracil for metastatic esophageal cancer: a multicenter, randomized controlled phase III study (JCOG1314, MIRACLE). JCO Oncol Adv. 2025;2:e2500064.
66. Guo JF, Zhang B, Wu F, et al. A phase II trial of docetaxel plus nedaplatin and 5-fluorouracil in treating advanced esophageal carcinoma. Chin J Cancer. 2010;29:321–4.
67. Honda M, Miura A, Izumi Y, et al. Doxorubicin, cisplatin, and fluorouracil combination therapy for metastatic esophageal squamous cell carcinoma. Dis Esophagus. 2010;23:641–5.

68. Cooper JS, Guo MD, Herskovic A, et al. Chemoradiotherapy of locally advanced esophageal cancer: long-term follow-up of a prospective randomized trial (RTOG 85-01). Radiation Therapy Oncology Group. JAMA. 1999;281:1623–7.
69. Hironaka S, Ohtsu A, Boku N, et al. Nonrandomized comparison between definitive chemoradiotherapy and radical surgery in patients with T(2-3)N(any) M(0) squamous cell carcinoma of the esophagus. Int J Radiat Oncol Biol Phys. 2003;57:425–33.
70. Kato H, Sato A, Fukuda H, et al. A phase II trial of chemoradiotherapy for stage I esophageal squamous cell carcinoma: Japan Clinical Oncology Group Study (JCOG9708). Jpn J Clin Oncol. 2009;39:638–43.
71. Kato K, Ito Y, Nozaki I, et al. Parallel-group controlled trial of surgery versus chemoradiotherapy in patients with stage I esophageal squamous cell carcinoma. Gastroenterology. 2021;161:1878–86.
72. Kato K, Muro K, Minashi K, et al. Phase II study of chemoradiotherapy with 5-fluorouracil and cisplatin for stage II-III esophageal squamous cell carcinoma: JCOG trial (JCOG 9906). Int J Radiat Oncol Biol Phys. 2011;81:684–90.
73. Tachimori Y, Kanamori N, Uemura N, et al. Salvage esophagectomy after high-dose chemoradiotherapy for esophageal squamous cell carcinoma. J Thorac Cardiovasc Surg. 2009;137:49–54.
74. Swisher SG, Wynn P, Putnam JB, et al. Salvage esophagectomy for recurrent tumors after definitive chemotherapy and radiotherapy. J Thorac Cardiovasc Surg. 2002;123:175–83.
75. Meunier B, Raoul J, Le Prisé E, et al. Salvage esophagectomy after unsuccessful curative chemoradiotherapy for squamous cell cancer of the esophagus. Dig Surg. 1998;15:224–6.
76. Minsky BD, Pajak TF, Ginsberg RJ, et al. INT 0123 (radiation therapy oncology group 94-05) phase III trial of combined-modality therapy for esophageal cancer: high-dose versus standard-dose radiation therapy. J Clin Oncol. 2002;20:1167–74.
77. Kato K, Nakajima TE, Ito Y, et al. Phase II study of concurrent chemoradiotherapy at the dose of 50.4 Gy with elective nodal irradiation for stage II-III esophageal carcinoma. Jpn J Clin Oncol. 2013;43(6):608–15.
78. Takeuchi H, Ito Y, Machida R, et al. A single-arm confirmatory study of definitive chemoradiation therapy including salvage treatment for clinical stage II/III esophageal squamous cell carcinoma (JCOG0909 study). Int J Radiat Oncol Biol Phys. 2022;114:454–62.
79. van Hagen P, Hulshof MC, van Lanschot JJ, et al. Preoperative chemoradiotherapy for esophageal or junctional cancer. N Engl J Med. 2012;366:2074–84.
80. Safran H, Suntharalingam M, Dipetrillo T, et al. Cetuximab with concurrent chemoradiation for esophagogastric cancer: assessment of toxicity. Int J Radiat Oncol Biol Phys. 2008;70:391–5.
81. Münch S, Pigorsch SU, Devečka M, et al. Comparison of definite chemoradiation therapy with carboplatin/paclitaxel or cisplatin/5-fluoruracil in patients with squamous cell carcinoma of the esophagus. Radiat Oncol. 2018;13:139.
82. Conroy T, Galais MP, Raoul JL, et al. Definitive chemoradiotherapy with FOLFOX versus fluorouracil and cisplatin in patients with oesophageal cancer (PRODIGE5/ACCORD17): final results of a randomised, phase 2/3 trial. Lancet Oncol. 2014;15:305–14.
83. Ohtsu A, Boku N, Muro K, et al. Definitive chemoradiotherapy for T4 and/or M1 lymph node squamous cell carcinoma of the esophagus. J Clin Oncol. 1999;17:2915–21.
84. Ishida K, Ando N, Yamamoto S, et al. Phase II study of cisplatin and 5-fluorouracil with concurrent radiotherapy in advanced squamous cell carcinoma of the esophagus: a Japan Esophageal Oncology Group (JEOG)/Japan Clinical Oncology Group Trial (JCOG9516). Jpn J Clin Oncol. 2004;34:615–9.
85. Shinoda M, Ando N, Kato K, et al. Randomized study of low-dose versus standard-dose chemoradiotherapy for unresectable esophageal squamous cell carcinoma (JCOG0303). Cancer Sci. 2015;106:407–12.
86. Higuchi K, Koizumi W, Tanabe S, et al. A phase I trial of definitive chemoradiotherapy with docetaxel, cisplatin, and 5-fluorouracil (DCF-R) for advanced esophageal carcinoma: Kitasato digestive disease & oncology group trial (KDOG 0501). Radiother Oncol. 2008;87:398–404.

87. Tsushima T, Mizusawa J, Sudo K, et al. Risk factors for esophageal fistula associated with chemoradiotherapy for locally advanced unresectable esophageal cancer: a supplementary analysis of JCOG0303. Medicine (Baltimore). 2016;95(20):e3699.
88. Yokota T, Kato K, Hamamoto Y, et al. Phase II study of chemoselection with docetaxel plus cisplatin and 5-fluorouracil induction chemotherapy and subsequent conversion surgery for locally advanced unresectable oesophageal cancer. Br J Cancer. 2016;115(11):1328–34.
89. Terada M, Hara H, Daiko H, et al. Phase III study of tri-modality combination therapy with induction docetaxel plus cisplatin and 5-fluorouracil vs definitive chemoradiotherapy for locally advanced unresectable squamous cell carcinoma of the thoracic esophagus. Jpn J Clin Oncol. 2019;49:1055–60.
90. Kato H, Arao T, Matsumoto K, et al. Gene amplification of EGFR, HER2, FGFR2 and MET in esophageal squamous cell carcinoma. Int J Oncol. 2013;42:1151–8.
91. Sunpaweravong P, Sunpawervong S, Puttawibul P, et al. Epidermal growth factor receptor and cyclin D1 are independently amplified and overexpressed in esophageal squamous cell carcinoma. J Cancer Res Clin Oncol. 2005;131:111–9.
92. Yang YL, Xu KL, Zhou Y, et al. Correlation of epidermal growth factor receptor overexpression with increased epidermal growth factor receptor gene copy number in esophageal squamous cell carcinomas. Chin Med J. 2012;125:450–4.
93. Hanawa M, Suzuki S, Dobashi Y, et al. EGFR protein overexpression and gene amplification in squamous cell carcinomas of the esophagus. Int J Cancer. 2006;118:1173–80.
94. Ku GY, Ilson DH. Esophagogastric cancer: targeted agents. Cancer Treat Rev. 2010;36:235–48.
95. Boone J, van Hillegersberg R, Offerhaus GJ, et al. Targets for molecular therapy in esophageal squamous cell carcinoma: an immunohistochemical analysis. Dis Esophagus. 2009;22:496–504.
96. Janmaat ML, Gallegos-Ruiz M, Rodriguez JA, et al. Predictive factors for outcome in a phase II study of gefitinib in second-line treatment of advanced esophageal cancer patients. J Clin Oncol. 2006;24:1612–9.
97. Ilson DH, Kelsen D, Shah M, et al. A phase 2 trial of erlotinib in patients with previously treated squamous cell and adenocarcinoma of the esophagus. Cancer. 2011;117:1409–14.
98. Ferry DR, Dutton SJ, Mansoor W, et al. Phase III multicentre, randomised, double-blind, placebo-controlled trial of gefitinib versus placebo in esophageal cancer progressing after chemotherapy, COG (Cancer Oesophagus Gefitinib). Ann Oncol. 2012;23:ixe1–30.
99. Petty RD, Dahle-Smith A, Stevenson DAJ, et al. Gefitinib and EGFR gene copy number aberrations in esophageal cancer. J Clin Oncol. 2017;35(20):2279–87.
100. Crosby T, Hurt CN, Falk S, et al. Chemoradiotherapy with or without cetuximab in patients with oesophageal cancer (SCOPE1): a multicentre, phase 2/3 randomised trial. Lancet Oncol. 2013;14:627–37.
101. Suntharalingam M, Winter K, Ilson D, et al. Effect of the addition of cetuximab to paclitaxel, cisplatin, and radiation therapy for patients with esophageal cancer: the NRG oncology RTOG 0436 phase 3 randomized clinical trial. JAMA Oncol. 2017;3:1520–8.
102. Moehler M, Maderer A, Thuss-Patience PC, et al. Cisplatin and 5-fluorouracil with or without epidermal growth factor receptor inhibition panitumumab for patients with non-resectable, advanced or metastatic oesophageal squamous cell cancer: a prospective, open-label, randomised phase III AIO/EORTC trial (POWER). Ann Oncol. 2020;31:228–35.
103. Kojima T, Yamazaki K, Kato K, et al. Phase I dose-escalation trial of Sym004, an anti-EGFR antibody mixture, in Japanese patients with advanced solid tumors. Cancer Sci. 2018;109(10):3253–62.
104. de Castro Junior G, Segalla JG, de Azevedo SJ, et al. A randomised phase II study of chemoradiotherapy with or without nimotuzumab in locally advanced oesophageal cancer: NICE trial. Eur J Cancer. 2018;88:21–30.
105. Kato K, Ura T, Koizumi W, et al. Nimotuzumab combined with concurrent chemoradiotherapy in Japanese patients with esophageal cancer: a phase I study. Cancer Sci. 2018;109:785–93.
106. Kotani D, Yamaguchi K, Kato K, et al. A phase 2, open-label study of amivantamab in patients with previously treated advanced or metastatic gastric or esophageal cancer. J Clin Oncol. 2024;42(Supple 3):363.

107. Guo W, Wang P, Li N, et al. Prognostic value of PD-L1 in esophageal squamous cell carcinoma: a meta-analysis. Oncotarget. 2018;9:13920–33.
108. Kudo T, Hamamoto Y, Kato K, et al. Nivolumab treatment for oesophageal squamous-cell carcinoma: an open-label, multicentre, phase 2 trial. Lancet Oncol. 2017;18:631–9.
109. Kato K, Cho BC, Takahashi M, et al. Nivolumab versus chemotherapy in patients with advanced oesophageal squamous cell carcinoma refractory or intolerant to one prior chemotherapy (ATTRACTION-3): a randomised, open-label, phase 3 trial. Lancet Oncol. 2019;20:1506–17.
110. Doki Y, Ajani JA, Kato K, et al. Nivolumab combination therapy in advanced esophageal squamous-cell carcinoma. N Engl J Med. 2022;386:449–62.
111. Muto M, Nomura M, Sakanaka K, et al. Effect of nivolumab combined with definitive chemoradiotherapy on response rate for esophageal cancer: an immune active intrinsic subtype could be its biomarker—the NOBEL trial. J Clin Oncol. 2024;42:4068.
112. Doi T, Piha-Paul SA, Jalal SI, et al. Safety and antitumor activity of the anti-programmed death-1 antibody pembrolizumab in patients with advanced esophageal carcinoma. J Clin Oncol. 2018;36:61–7.
113. Shah MA, Kojima T, Hochhauser D, et al. Efficacy and safety of pembrolizumab for heavily pretreated patients with advanced, metastatic adenocarcinoma or squamous cell carcinoma of the esophagus: the phase 2 KEYNOTE-180 study. JAMA Oncol. 2018;5:546–50.
114. Kojima T, Shah MA, Muro K, et al. Randomized phase III KEYNOTE-181 study of pembrolizumab versus chemotherapy in advanced esophageal cancer. J Clin Oncol. 2020;38:4138–48.
115. Sun JM, Shen L, Shah MA, et al. Pembrolizumab plus chemotherapy versus chemotherapy alone for first-line treatment of advanced oesophageal cancer (KEYNOTE-590): a randomised, placebo-controlled, phase 3 study. Lancet. 2021;398:759–71.
116. Shen L, Kato K, Kim SB, et al. Tislelizumab versus chemotherapy as second-line treatment for advanced or metastatic esophageal squamous cell carcinoma (RATIONALE-302): a randomized phase iii study. J Clin Oncol. 2022;40:3065–76.
117. Xu J, Kato K, Raymond E, et al. Tislelizumab plus chemotherapy versus placebo plus chemotherapy as first-line treatment for advanced or metastatic oesophageal squamous cell carcinoma (RATIONALE-306): a global, randomised, placebo-controlled, phase 3 study. Lancet Oncol. 2023;24:483–95.
118. Huang J, Xu J, Chen Y, et al. Camrelizumab versus investigator's choice of chemotherapy as second-line therapy for advanced or metastatic oesophageal squamous cell carcinoma (ESCORT): a multicentre, randomised, open-label, phase 3 study. Lancet Oncol. 2020;21:832–42.
119. Luo H, Lu J, Bai Y, et al. Effect of camrelizumab vs placebo added to chemotherapy on survival and progression-free survival in patients with advanced or metastatic esophageal squamous cell carcinoma: the ESCORT-1st randomized clinical trial. JAMA. 2021;326:916–25.
120. Wang ZX, Cui C, Yao J, et al. Toripalimab plus chemotherapy in treatment-naïve, advanced esophageal squamous cell carcinoma (JUPITER-06): a multicenter phase 3 trial. Cancer Cell. 2022;40:277–88.
121. Lu Z, Wang J, Shu Y, et al. Sintilimab versus placebo in combination with chemotherapy as first line treatment for locally advanced or metastatic oesophageal squamous cell carcinoma (ORIENT-15): multicentre, randomised, double blind, phase 3 trial. BMJ. 2022;377:e068714.
122. Song Y, Zhang B, Xin D, et al. First-line serplulimab or placebo plus chemotherapy in PD-L1-positive esophageal squamous cell carcinoma: a randomized, double-blind phase 3 trial. Nat Med. 2023;29:473–82.
123. Bando H, Kumagai S, Kotani D, et al. Atezolizumab following definitive chemoradiotherapy in patients with unresectable locally advanced esophageal squamous cell carcinoma-a multicenter phase 2 trial (EPOC1802). Nat Cancer. 2025;6:445–59.
124. Hsu CH, Lu Z, Gao S, et al. SKYSCRAPER-08: a phase III, randomized, double-blind, placebo-controlled study of first-line (1L) tiragolumab (tira) + atezolizumab (atezo) and chemotherapy (CT) in patients (pts) with esophageal squamous cell carcinoma (ESCC). J Clin Oncol. 2024;24(supple 3):245.

125. Chau I, Cho BC, Chen M-H, et al. SKYSCRAPER-07: a phase III, randomised study of atezolizumab (atezo) with or without tiragolumab (tira) in patients (pts) with unresectable esophageal squamous cell carcinoma (ESCC) that has not progressed following definitive concurrent chemoradiotherapy (dCRT). Ann Oncol. 2025;35:1043.
126. Möbius C, Freire J, Becker I, et al. VEGF-C expression in squamous cell carcinoma and adenocarcinoma of the esophagus. World J Surg. 2007;31:1768–72.
127. Uchida S, Shimada Y, Watanabe G, et al. In oesophageal squamous cell carcinoma vascular endothelial growth factor is associated with p53 mutation, advanced stage and poor prognosis. Br J Cancer. 1998;77:1704–9s.
128. Li J, Wang L. Efficacy and safety of apatinib treatment for advanced esophageal squamous cell carcinoma. Onco Targets Ther. 2017;10:3965–9.
129. Bai LY, Chiu CF, Kadowaki S, et al. A phase II study of regorafenib in combination with nivolumab in patients with recurrent or metastatic solid tumors: results of the ESCC cohort. Ann Oncol. 2022;33. supple 7:S1101–2.
130. Sun JM, Kim SB, Ogata T, et al. Lenvatinib plus pembrolizumab and chemotherapy vs pembrolizumab and chemotherapy in untreated advanced metastatic esophageal squamous cell carcinoma: the randomized phase 3 LEAP-014 study. Ann Oncol. 2025;20:2709–21.
131. Kojima T, Kato K, Hara H, et al. Phase II study of BKM120 in patients with advanced esophageal squamous cell carcinoma (EPOC1303). Esophagus. 2022;19:702–10.
132. Yamamoto S, Muro K, Nishio K, et al. Phase 1b study of Futibatinib plus Pembrolizumab in patients with esophageal carcinoma: updated results of antitumor activity and tolerability results in combination with chemotherapy. Ann Oncol. 2023;34(supple 2):S861–2.
133. Yagisawa M, Taniguchi H, Satoh T, et al. Trastuzumab deruxtecan in advanced solid tumors with human epidermal growth factor receptor 2 amplification identified by plasma cell-free DNA testing: a multicenter, single-arm, phase Ii basket trial. J Clin Oncol. 2024;42:3817–25.
134. Muro K, Chin K, Maron SB, et al. Enfortumab vedotin (EV) in previously treated gastric/esophageal cancers cohorts of EV-202. J Clin Oncol. 2024;42(supple 16):4046.

17 Radiation Therapy

Yoshinori Ito

17.1 Indications of Radiotherapy

Although surgery is the principal curative therapy for resectable esophageal cancer, definitive chemoradiotherapy (CRT) is a treatment option in an attempt to preserve the esophagus since favorable treatment results were reported from clinical trials [1–5]. And resection of a cervical esophageal cancer would require a laryngoesophagectomy, so definitive CRT is also a treatment option in an attempt to preserve the larynx in addition to the esophagus. For locally advanced unresectable esophageal cancer (T4 cases), definitive CRT is a standard therapy from favorable results [6–8]. Prophylactic CRT for patients with pT1b or pT1a involving lymphovascular invasion after endoscopic resection could be a treatment option from favorable result of clinical trial [9, 10]. And radiotherapy alone is a treatment option since many patients with esophageal cancer are elderly, of poor PS or have metastases at presentation. Radiotherapy is also useful to palliate dysphagia or pain.

17.2 Radiation Therapy Techniques

17.2.1 Simulation

During simulation, the patient lies supine with arms by their sides or with arms above their head in the case of considering to use the lateral or oblique beam arrangements. For cervical esophageal tumor, an immobilization mask should be used to minimize variation in daily setup. Computed tomography (CT)-based planning is recommended. The patient is placed on the CT simulator in the treatment

Y. Ito (✉)
Department of Radiation Oncology, Showa Medical University School of Medicine, Tokyo, Japan
e-mail: yito@med.showa-u.ac.jp

Y. Kitagawa et al. (eds.), *Esophageal Squamous Cell Carcinoma*,
https://doi.org/10.1007/978-981-92-2611-5_17

position, and a scan of the entire area of interest with margin is obtained. At minimum, 3–5 mm slices should be used, allowing accurate tumor characterization, as well as improved quality of digitally reconstructed radiographs. The tumor and normal tissue structures are then outlined on each slice on the treatment planning system, enabling a three-dimensional treatment plan to be generated. Four-dimensional (4D) CT scan may be appropriate to assess tumoral motion and facilitate appropriate margin placement on the target volumes, particularly in the setting of high-precision radiotherapy.

17.2.2 Treatment Planning

17.2.2.1 Target Volume Delineation

Gross Tumor Volumes (GTV)

The primary tumor in the esophagus is defined as GTVp based on the examinations, including barium swallow, upper esophagogastroduodenoscopy (EGD), endoscopic ultrasonography (EUS), and CT scan. The endoscopic diagnosis with iodine staining is essential for detecting the superficial cancer and intraepithelial spread of the advanced cancer. In the treatment of the superficial cancer, endoscopic metal clips are inserted in the esophageal wall near the proximal and distal ends of the primary tumor as fiducial markers before radiotherapy treatment planning (Fig. 17.1a).

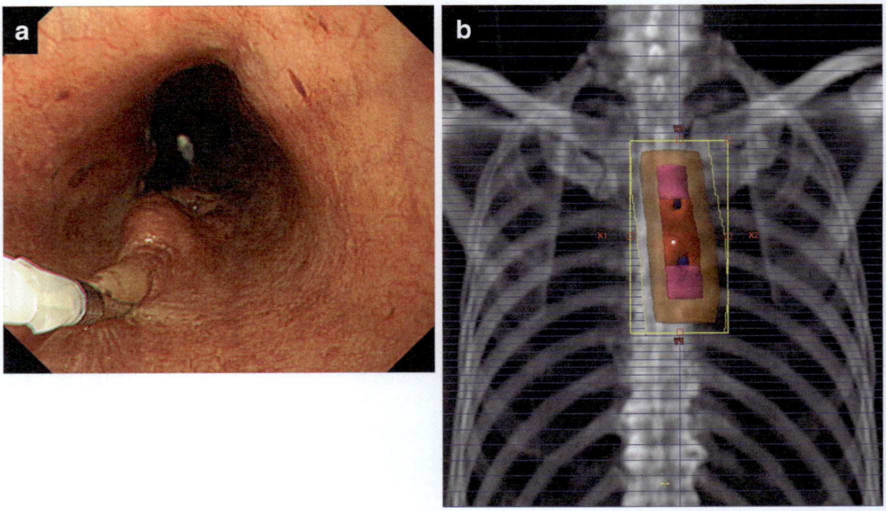

Fig. 17.1 (**a, b**) Example 3D-treatment planning for a cT1bN0 middle thoracic esophagus tumor (**a**) Endoscopic insertion of metal clips in the esophageal wall near the proximal and distal end of the primary tumor. (**b**) Target volume of local radiotherapy planning. Metal clips (blue), GTV of primary tumor (red), CTV of primary tumor (pink); GTV plus 2 cm margin proximally and distally along the length of the esophagus, PTV (orange)

Diagnostic PET/CT has more recently been integrated into radiation treatment planning of esophageal cancer and definition of GTV [11]. The metastatic lymph nodes are defined as GTVn mainly based on the CT scan and palpitation. Similarly, EUS may detect enlarged nodes that need to be included. It is difficult to evaluate the metastatic lymph nodes accurately by the tumor size. In a study from Kyoto University, the optimal size criterion for both CT and MR in the detection of cervical and mediastinal lymph node metastases is 5 mm for short-axis diameter [12].

Clinical Target Volume (CTV)

CTVp is defined as the GTVp with 2–4 cm expansion proximally and distally along the length of the esophagus. The intent is to extend the margin along the length of the esophagus to provide a margin for coverage of the submucosal extension of the tumor. One pathological analysis of 34 surgical specimens of ESCC showed the mean microscopic spread beyond the gross tumor was 10.5 ± 13.5 mm proximally, and 10.6 ± 8.1 mm distally, and placement of a 3-cm margin proximally and distally on the primary tumor would cover microscopic disease extension in 94% of cases [13].

CTVn is defined as the GTVn with a 0–0.5 cm margin in all directions.

The regional lymph nodes are defined as CTVsubclinical (CTVs) for each primary site in the treatment of elective nodal irradiation. Several pathological analyses of surgical specimens of ESCC reported that the rate of positive lymph nodes per number of cases were 47–70% and patterns of involved nodal spread were different from each primary site [14–16] (Fig. 17.2). Even if clinical T1bN0 cases, the rate of positive lymph node was 27.0% based on the pathological analysis of surgical specimens of ESCC [17]. Retrospective analysis from Japan showed that elective nodal irradiation (ENI) was effective for regional lymph node failure [18].

	Primary site		
	Upper thoracic tumor	Middle thoracic tumor	Lower thoracic tumor
Cervical	46.3%	29.2%	27.2%
Uppermediastinal	46.3%	35.7%	29.6%
Middle mediastinal	22.0%	32.7%	39.5%
Lowermediastinal	7.3%	16.1%	35.8%
Abdominal	12.2%	39.9%	74.1%

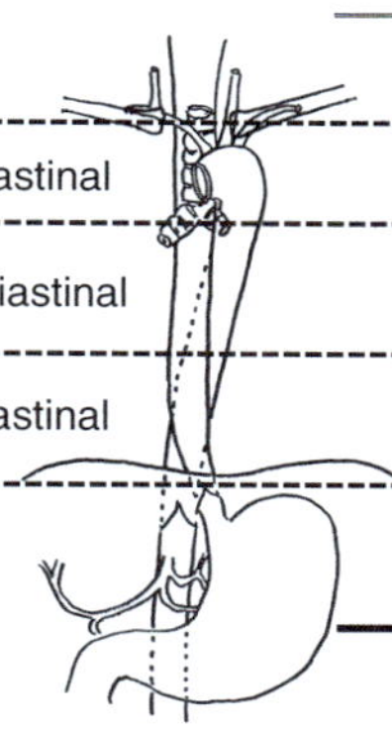

Fig. 17.2 Location and frequency of nodal involvement (%) by ESCC according to the site of primary site. (From Akiyama H, et al. [14])

Guidelines 2024 for the treatment of esophageal cancer in Japan show the inclusion of regional lymph nodes in CTVs for each primary site (Table 17.1) (Fig. 17.3a–d) [19]. Typically, the regional lymph nodes include bilateral supraclavicular fossae, superior mediastinal, and subcarinal lymph nodes for carcinoma of the cervical esophagus and upper thoracic esophagus (Fig. 17.4a). Mid jugular lymph nodes are also included for carcinoma of the cervical esophagus. And the regional lymph nodes include superior mediastinal, subcarinal, middle mediastinal, lower mediastinal, and perigastric lymph nodes for carcinoma of the middle or lower thoracic esophagus (Fig. 17.4b). Celiac axis lymph nodes are also included for carcinoma of the lower thoracic esophagus. There is no consensus about inclusion of regional lymph nodes in CTVs for each primary site. Although ENI yields to prevent or

Table 17.1 Regional lymph nodes defined as CTVs for each primary site

Primary site	Regional lymph nodes
Cervical esophagus	Mid jugular lymph nodes, supraclavicular lymph nodes, superior mediastinal lymph nodes, subcarinal lymph nodes
Upper thoracic esophagus	Supraclavicular lymph nodes, superior mediastinal lymph nodes, subcarinal lymph nodes
Middle thoracic esophagus	Superior mediastinal lymph nodes, subcarinal lymph nodes, middle mediastinal lymph nodes, lower mediastinal lymph nodes, perigastric lymph nodes
Lower thoracic esophagus	Superior mediastinal lymph nodes, middle mediastinal lymph nodes, lower mediastinal lymph nodes, perigastric lymph nodes, Celiac lymph nodes

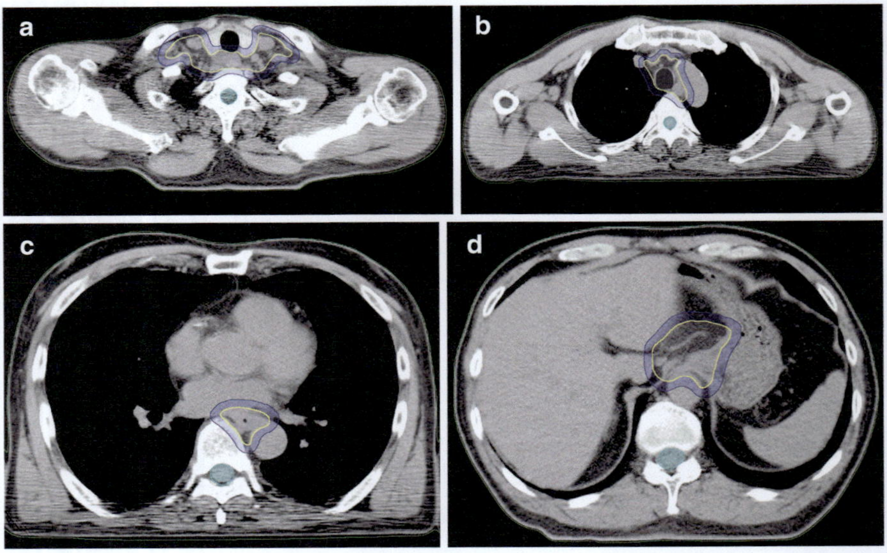

Fig. 17.3 Example of target volume delineation of CTV of elective nodal region. CTVs (yellow), PTVs (blue)

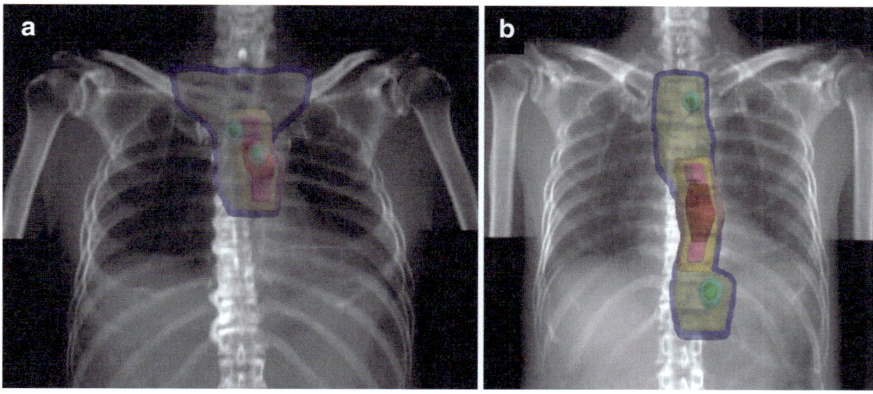

Fig. 17.4 (**a, b**) Examples of target volume with elective nodal region in the 3D-treatment planning for cT3N1 thoracic esophagus tumor (**a**) For cancer of the upper thoracic esophagus. (**b**) For cancer of the middle or lower thoracic esophagus. GTV of primary tumor (red), GTV of metastatic lymph nodes (green), CTV of primary tumor (pink), CTV of elective nodal region (yellow), Initial PTV (blue), boost PTV (orange and cyan)

delay regional node failure, recent randomized controlled trials have demonstrated no survival difference compared with involved-field irradiation (IFI) [20, 21]. For cT1bN0M0 ESCC treated with CRT, randomized controlled trial (JCOG1904) is currently ongoing to determine whether ENI is superior to IFI in preventing locoregional recurrence [22].

Planning Target Volume (PTV)

Planning target volume (PTV) is defined as clinical target volume (CTV) with a 1–2 cm margin in craniocaudal direction and a 0.5–1 cm margin in the lateral direction to account for respiratory organ motion and daily setup error. Report of evaluating the respiratory motion of distal esophageal tumor using 4D-CT showed that a radical margin of 0.8 cm and an axial margin of ±1.8 cm would provide tumor motion coverage for 95% of the cases [23].

17.2.2.2 Field Design

In the treatment of target to the primary tumor and involved lymph nodes only, beam arrangement in 3D-CRT uses a multi-field technique such as a three- to six-field arrangement (Fig. 17.1b). By contrast in the treatment including the elective nodal irradiation, anteroposterior (AP)/posteroanterior (PA) fields are used up to 40–45 Gy followed by off-cord boost fields. For cervical esophageal tumor, right anterior oblique (RAO) and left anterior oblique (LAO) with wedged pairs are usually used as off-cord boost fields. For upper, middle, and lower esophageal tumors, RAO and left posterior oblique (LPO) are usually used as off-cord boost fields. At the beginning of initial treatment for a middle or lower thoracic esophagus tumor, a multi-field technique such as a four-field arrangement (AP/PA/RAO/LPO) is recommended, considering the cardiac toxicity (Fig. 17.5a). However, it is necessary to

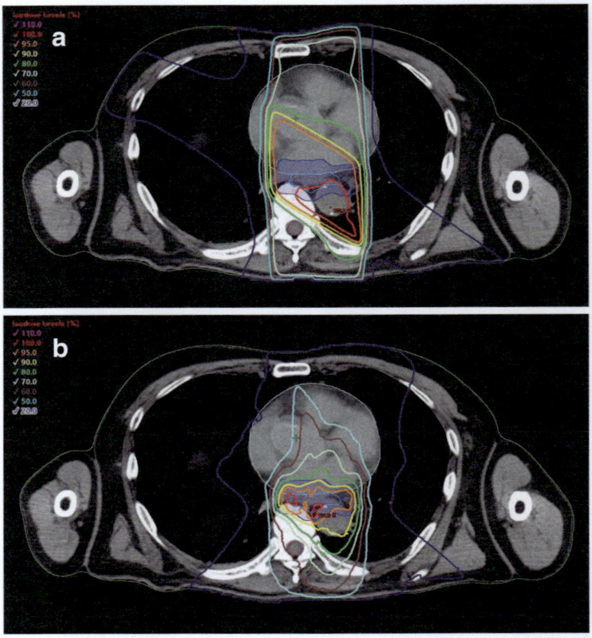

Fig. 17.5 (**a, b**) Example of dose distribution of treatment planning for a middle thoracic esophageal tumor (**a**) 3D-CRT plan with a four-field technique (beam weights arrangement of 180 cGy per fraction; anterior 60 cGy, posterior 70 cGy, obliques 25 cGy). (**b**) IMRT (VMAT) plan

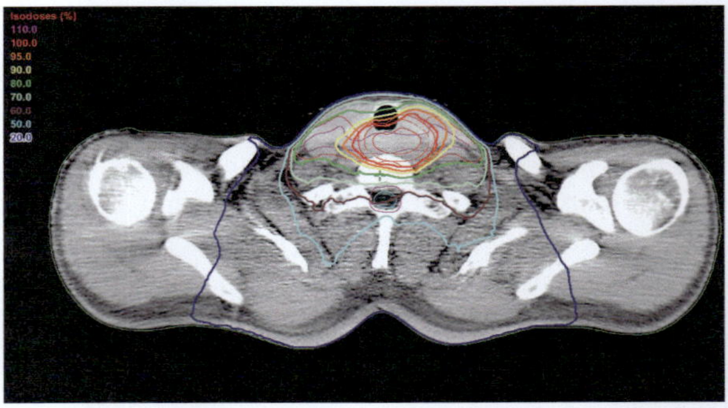

Fig. 17.6 Dose distribution of IMRT plan for a cervical esophagus tumor

minimize the volume of the irradiated lung (beam weight; AP/PA > > obliques) to minimize lung toxicity. In the case of the existence of hot spot, such as >110% of the prescribed radiation dose, the field-in-field technique is considered to improve the conformity of the dose distribution. Currently, intensity-modulated radiotherapy (IMRT) has been considered. IMRT can further improve the conformity of the dose distribution by sparing the adjacent normal structures such as spinal cord, lung, and heart to help meet dose constraints (Figs. 17.5b and 17.6). A retrospective analysis showed that, compared with 3D-CRT, IMRT was associated with improved survival and a lower risk of radiation pneumonitis after definitive CRT for esophageal cancer [24].

17.2.2.3 Dose and Fractionation

Conventional daily dosing at 1.8–2.0 Gy fraction is standard. In the treatment of radiotherapy alone, 60–70 Gy at 1.8–2 Gy per fraction is standard radiation dose. In the treatment of CRT, based on the result of a randomized trial intergroup (INT) 0123 demonstrated that no significant difference in overall survival (OS) and local/regional control between the 50.4 Gy arm and the 64.8 Gy arm among patients (85% SCC) treated with concurrent 5-FU and cisplatin chemotherapy for nonsurgical therapy [25], standard dose of radiotherapy for esophageal cancer is usually 50–50.4 Gy at 1.8–2 Gy per fraction in the definitive setting. In recent randomized controlled trials, dose escalation of radiotherapy has failed to improve OS or local control compared with standard fractionation and has been associated with increased toxicity [26–28]. In the neoadjuvant setting, 40–50.4 Gy at 1.8–2 Gy per fraction is standard radiation dose. And in the prophylactic setting, 41.4 Gy at 1.8 Gy per fraction is used in clinical trial [9, 10].

17.2.2.4 Dose Constraints

In radiotherapy treatment planning of esophageal cancer, normal-tissue tolerance should always be considered. Accurate delineation of adjacent organs, including lungs, spinal cord, heart, kidneys, and liver, is important. And it is necessary to evaluate the dose-volume histogram (DVH) analyses for each organ (Fig. 17.7). Several studies have demonstrated that dosimetric parameters derived from DVH are associated with organ toxicity after treatment of esophageal cancer. According

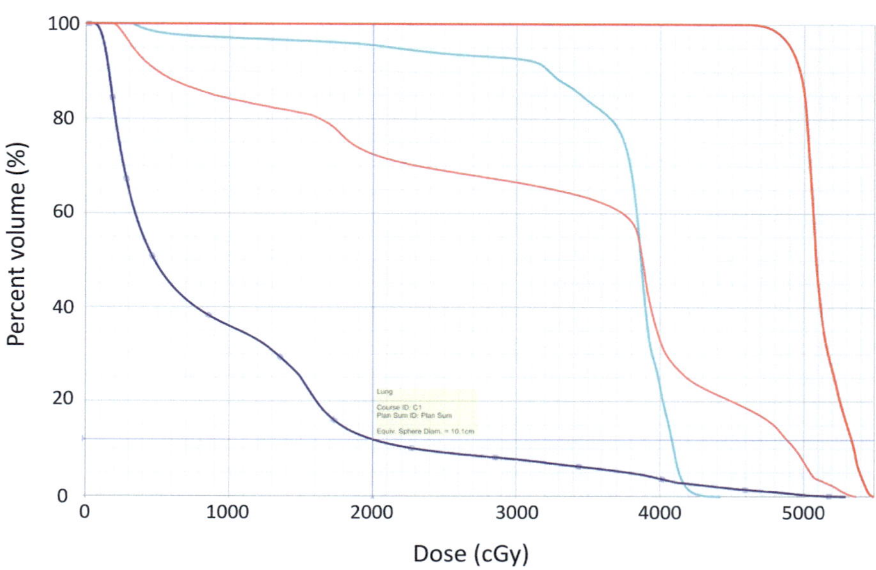

Fig. 17.7 DVH analysis of a four-field technique for a middle thoracic esophagus tumor (50.4 Gy in 28 fractions with elective nodal irradiation of 41.4 Gy). Boost PTV (red), Total lung (blue), Heart (pink), Spinal cord (cyan)

to the National Comprehensive Cancer Network Practice Guidelines, organ-specific dose constraints are defined as follows [29]. For the lungs, the recommended constraints are lung V40 (the percentage of lung volume receiving ≥40 Gy) ≤ 10%, V30 ≤ 15%, V20 ≤ 20%, V10 ≤ 40%, and V5 ≤ 50%, with the mean lung dose maintained below 20 Gy. The maximum dose to the spinal cord is generally limited to 45 Gy. For the heart, it is recommended that heart V30 be ≤10% and that the mean heart dose be kept below 30 Gy. For the kidneys, the recommended constraints are kidney V20 ≤ 33% and a mean kidney dose below 18 Gy. For the liver, a liver V30 ≤ 33% and a mean liver dose below 25 Gy are recommended. For the stomach, the mean dose should be kept below 45 Gy, and the maximum dose should not exceed 54 Gy. For the bowel, the maximum dose is similarly limited to less than 54 Gy, with an additional constraint of bowel V45 < 195 cc.

17.2.3 Brachytherapy

Brachytherapy involves intraluminal placement of a radioactive source into the esophagus with an intraorally or intranasally inserted applicator and permits treatment of a localized area of the esophagus to high radiation doses with relative sparing of surrounding structures. This technique may be used alone or in combination with external beam radiotherapy with or without chemotherapy. The indication of brachytherapy is the treatment of superficial esophageal cancer for curative intent in Japan (local control rate: 79–85%) [30–36]; on the other hand, it is used to relief symptom such as dysphagia for palliative intent in the treatment of advanced esophageal cancer in Western countries [37, 38]. Brachytherapy can be administered by two general methods: low-dose rate (LDR) brachytherapy and high-dose rate (HDR) brachytherapy. Modern HDR brachytherapy equipment delivers radiation much faster than 12 Gy/h, permitting the delivery of a planned dose within minutes compared with LDR sources, which require many hours or days. As a general rule of HDR brachytherapy, the diameter of the balloon applicator should be 15–20 mm. The whole length of the tumor and 2 cm above and below the lesion are included in the target volume. The reference dose point is set at a depth of 5 mm of the esophageal submucosa (5 mm beyond the wall of the balloon surface). There is no definite consensus about the optimal dose of intraluminal brachytherapy for esophageal cancer. In Japan, 50–60 Gy external beam radiotherapy followed by 8–12 Gy in two-four fractions (3–4 Gy per fraction), HDR brachytherapy is generally used. It was reported that a higher dose per fraction is associated with the risk of esophageal ulcer and perforation [30]. Dose of 4 Gy or less per fraction by HDR brachytherapy and dose of 6 Gy or less per fraction by LDR brachytherapy once or twice a week is recommended in Japan [32]. The American Brachytherapy Society (ABS) recommends an HDR dose of 10 Gy in two fractions, prescribed at 1 cm from the source, to boost 50 Gy EBRT [39]. Figure 17.8 illustrates the dose distribution and 3D-view in the treatment planning of HDR-brachytherapy.

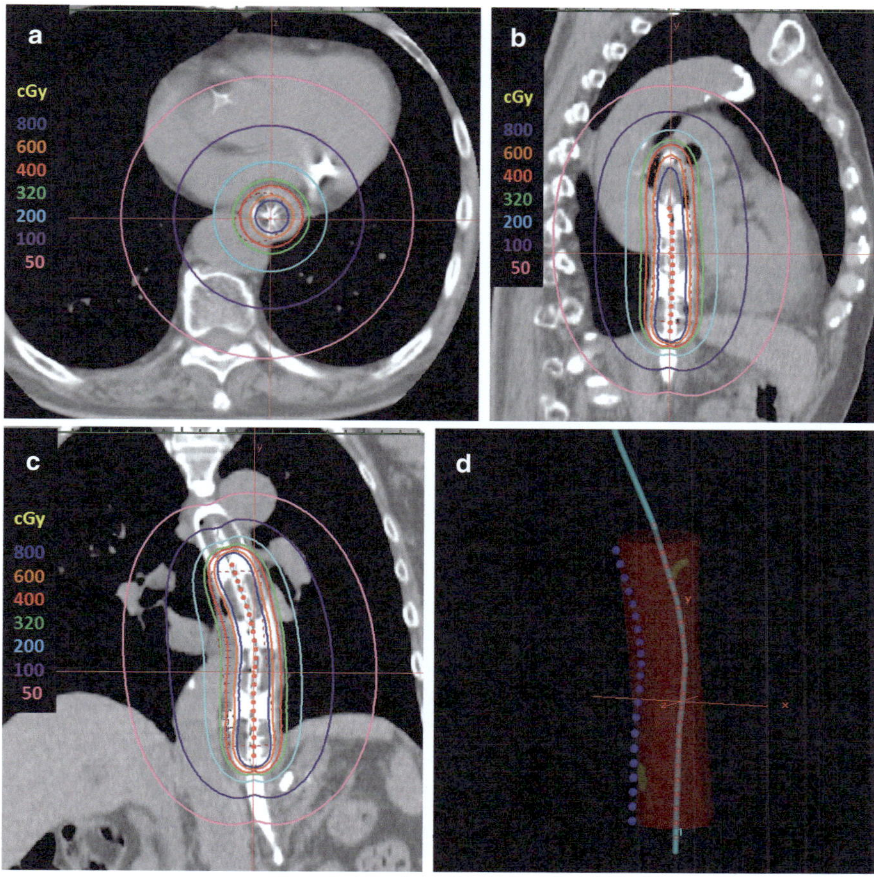

Fig. 17.8 (**a–d**) Dose distribution of intraluminal brachytherapy for a cT1bN0 middle thoracic esophagus tumor. Prescription dose: 400 cGy at a depth of 5 mm of the esophageal submucosa as the reference dose point. (**a**) Axial view. (**b**) sagittal view. (**c**) coronal view, (**d**) 3D-view. Metal clips (green), High risk CTV (red): GTV plus 2 cm margin proximally and distally along the length of the esophagus, reference dose point (blue), catheter (cyan), dwell points (red)

17.3 Treatment Results

17.3.1 Radiotherapy Alone

Radiation therapy alone has usually been delivered when lesions are deemed inoperable because of tumor extent or medical contraindications. In general, patients receiving radiation as a sole treatment modality have a median survival of 6–12 months and 5-year OS of <10%. In a review of 49 early series involving more than 8400 patients (100% SCC) treated with radiation therapy alone, OS rates at 1,

2, and 5 years were 18%, 8%, and 6%, respectively [40]. According to the Comprehensive Registry of Esophageal Cancer in Japan by the Japan Esophageal Society for the 2015–2017 surveys (patients treated between 2009 and 2011, 97% SCC), the 5-year OS rate was 23.2% and the rates in patients with cStage 0–1, II, III, and IV disease were 41.8%, 18.5%, 9.3%, and 13.9%, respectively [41]. As a result of clinical trial, Radiation Therapy Oncology Group (RTOG) trial (RTOG8501) comparing combined chemotherapy with 5-FU and cisplatin with radiotherapy (50 Gy) versus radiotherapy alone (64 Gy) showed that 3-year OS with radiotherapy alone was 0% [1–3]. In a prospective trial of radiotherapy alone (66 Gy) for patients older than 80 years old with T1-3N0M0 squamous cell carcinoma of the thoracic esophagus, median survival time and 3-year OS rate were 30 months and 39%, respectively [42]. These favorable results were due to patient selection, including earlier stage (non-T4N0; 35% T1N0) compared to RTOG8501.

17.3.2 Chemoradiotherapy

The landmark trial establishing the superiority of concurrent CRT to radiation therapy alone was RTOG8501. Herskovic and colleagues reported the results of this randomized trial comparing combined chemotherapy with 5-FU and cisplatin with radiotherapy (50 Gy) versus radiotherapy alone (64 Gy) for esophageal cancer (88% SCC) [1]. The median survival in patients treated by radiation alone was 8.9 months compared with 12.5 months for those treated with combined therapy, with 2-year OS rate 10% versus 38%; the incidence of local recurrence decreased from 24% to 16%, and the 2-year distant metastasis rate decreased from 26% to 12%. Updated results showed that at 5 years, OS rates were 26% and 0%, respectively, for CRT and radiation therapy alone [2, 3].

17.3.2.1 Chemoradiotherapy for Unresectable Locally Advanced Esophageal Cancer

For locally advanced unresectable esophageal cancer, CRT is standard treatment with potentially curative intent. Results of clinical trials of definitive CRT for T4 tumors are shown in Table 17.2 [6–8, 25, 43–54]. INT0123, a randomized clinical trial compared standard-dose 50.4 Gy to high-dose 64.8 Gy with both concurrent 5-FU and cisplatin chemotherapy for patients with clinical T1-4N0–1 M0 esophageal cancer [21]. This study was closed after an interim analysis showed no probability of superiority in the high-dose arm. No significant difference in median survival (18.1 vs. 13 months), 2-year OS (40% vs. 31%), or local-regional failure/persistence of disease (52% vs. 56%) was seen between the standard-dose and high-dose arms. In a single institute phase II trial of CRT with 5-FU and cisplatin and 60 Gy irradiation for patients with clinical T4 and/or M1 lymph node ESCC, complete response (CR) rate was 33%, and median survival time and 3-year OS rate were 9 months and 23%, respectively [6]. Another clinical trials of 5-FU and cisplatin and 60 Gy irradiation for patients including clinical T4 showed that CR rate was 15–33% and 2-year, 3-year OS rates were 27%–46% and 23%–30%, respectively

Table 17.2 Results of clinical trials of definitive CRT for ESCC including T4

Author	cStage	Pathology: rate of SCC (%)	No. of pt.	Regimen	CR rate	Survival
INT0123 [25] (USA)	T1-4N0-1 (T4: 8%)	86	109 109	FP + 50.4 Gy FP + 64.8 Gy	NR NR	2y: 31% 2y: 40%
Ohtsu [6] (Japan)	T4/M1Lym (T4: 67%)	100	54	FP + 60 Gy	33%	1y: 41% 3y: 23%
Nishimura [7] (Japan)	T4/M1Lym (T4: 100%)	100	28	FP + 60 Gy	32%	StageIII;2y: 27% StageIV;1y: 23%
JCOG9516 [8] (Japan)	T4/M1lym (T4: 100%)	100	60	FP + 60 Gy	15%	2y: 31.5%
JCOG0303 [43] (Japan)	T4/M1lym (T4: 75%)	100	71 71	FP + 60 Gy Low dose FP + 60 Gy	0%[a] 1.4%[a]	3y: 30% 3y: 26%
KROSG0101/ JROSG021 [44, 45] (Japan)	Stage II-IVA (T4: 44%)	100	46 45	FP + 60 Gy Low dose FP + 60 Gy	NR NR	2y: 46%, 5y: 35% 2y: 44%, 5y: 22%
Shahl [46] (Germany)	T3-4N0-1 (T4: 17%)	100	86 86	FLEP→EP + 60 Gy FLEP→EP + 40 Gy + S	NR NR	3y: 55% 3y: 58%
PRODIGE5/ ACCORD17 [47] (France)	StageI-IVA (T4: NR)	86	133 134	FP + 50 Gy FOLFOX+50 Gy	43% 43%	3y: 26.9% 3y: 19.9%
SCOPE1 [48] (UK)	StageI-III (T4: NR)	73	129 129	CP + 50 Gy CP + Cetuximab+50 Gy		2y: 56.0% 2y: 41.3%
RTOG0436 [49] (USA)	T1N1/ T2-4N0-1/ M1a (T4: 18%)	37	169 159	CDDP+PTX + 50.4 Gy CDDP+PTX + Cetuximab+50.4 Gy	57.9% 56.3%	2y: 44.0%, 3y: 27.9% 2y: 44.9%, 3y: 33.8%
KDOG0501 [50] (Japan)	T4/M1lym (T4: 69%)	100	42	DCF + 50.4 Gy, 61.2 Gy	52.4%	1y: 66.1%, 3y: 43.9%

(continued)

Table 17.2 (continued)

Author	cStage	Pathology: rate of SCC (%)	No. of pt.	Regimen	CR rate	Survival
NICE trial [51] (Brazil)	T3-4N0-1/ M1a (T4: 33%)	93	107	FP + 50.4 Gy FP + Nimotuzumab+50.4 Gy	33.3%[b] 47.2%[b]	MST: 11.5 months MST: 15.9 months
Sateke [52] (Japan)	T4/M1lym (T4: 61%)	100	33	DCF → FP + 60 Gy	39.4%	1y: 78.8%, 3y: 40.4%
Yokota [53, 54] (Japan)	T4/M1lym (T4: 90%)	98	48	DCF →CS if resectable →FP + 60 Gy → CS if resectable	23.5% (no CS group)	1y: 67.9%, 3y: 46.6%
NOBEL trial [57] (Japan)	StageI-IVB (T4: 17%)	100	42	FP + Nivolimab+50.4 y → Nivolumab	73%	1y: 92.7%

CRT chemoradiotherapy, *SCC* squamous cell carcinoma, *CR* complete response, *INT* intergroup, *JCOG* Japan Clinical Oncology Group, *KROSG* Kyoto Radiation Oncology Study Group, *JROSG* Japanese Radiation Oncology Study Group, *PRODIGE* Partenariat de Recherche en Oncologie Digestive, *ACCORD* Actions Concertées dans les Cancers Colo-Rectaux et Digestifs, *SCOPE* Study of Chemoradiotherapy in OesoPhageal cancer with Erbitux), *KDOG* Kitasato digestive disease & oncology group, *S* surgery, *FP* 5-FU+cisplatin, *FLEP* 5-FU+leucovorin+etoposide+cisplatin, *FOLFOX* 5-FU+oxaliplatin+leucovorin, *EP* etoposide+cisplatin, *CP* capecitabine+cisplatin, *CDDP* cisplatin, *DCF* docetaxel+cisplatin+5-FU, *NR* not reported, *MST* median survival time, *CS* conversion surgery

[a]Endoscopic complete response

[b]Only one point assessment of tumor response

[7, 8, 43–45]. Other combination regimens using new drugs (paclitaxel, docetaxel, oxaliplatin, S-1, capecitabine, cetuximab, and nimotuzumab) with concurrent radiotherapy have been evaluated [47–56]. Furthermore, clinical trials aimed at improving treatment efficacy are being conducted to evaluate the combination of CRT with immune checkpoint inhibitors (nivolumab, pembrolizumab, tislelizumab, durvalumab, and atezolizumab) [57–61]. Recently, another treatment strategy including intensive induction chemotherapy (docetaxel, cisplatin, and 5-FU; DCF) have been evaluated [52–54]. Multidisciplinary treatment in which surgery or CRT was performed after intensive induction chemotherapy has been shown to yield favorable outcomes, with OS rate of 67.9% at 1-year and 46.6% at 3-year [53, 54]. JCOG1510, randomized controlled trial comparing this multidisciplinary treatment to definitive CRT, is now ongoing [62].

17.3.2.2 Chemoradiotherapy for Resectable Esophageal Cancer

Definitive CRT is a treatment option in an attempt to preserve the esophagus for resectable esophageal cancer. Results of clinical trials of definitive CRT for resectable esophageal cancer are shown in Table 17.3 [1–5, 55, 56, 63, 68–73]. For stage I esophageal cancer, Japan Clinical Oncology Group (JCOG) 9708, a phase II trial of CRT with 5-FU and cisplatin and 60 Gy irradiation against primary tumor only was conducted (Fig. 17.1b). CR rate was 87.5%, and the 5-year OS rate was 75.5% [4]. Recently, results of the parallel group-controlled trial of esophagectomy versus CRT for stage I (T1b) esophageal cancer (JCOG0502) were reported [63]. CRT consisted of 5-FU and cisplatin and 60 Gy irradiation against primary tumor, the same as JCOG9708 regimen. The 3-year and 5-year OS rates were 94.7% and 86.5% in esophagectomy arm (209 patients), and 93.1% and 85.5% in CRT arm (159 patients), which results were comparable with esophagectomy. CR rate was 87.3%, and 3-year and 5-year esophagectomy-free survival rates were 88.7% and

Table 17.3 Results of clinical trials of definitive CRT for resectable ESCC

Author	cStage	Pathology: rate of SCC	No. of pt.	Regimen	CR rate	Survival
RTOG8501 [1–3] (USA)	T1-3N0-1	88%	62 134	64 Gy FP + 50 Gy	NR NR	2y: 10%, 5y: 0% 2y: 38%, 5y: 26%
Bedenne [56] (France)	T3N0-1	89%	130 129	FP + 30 Gy or 46 Gy →FP + 15Gy or 20 Gy FP + 30 Gy or 46 Gy →S	NR NR	3y: 34% 3y: 29%
JCOG9708 [4] (Japan)	Stage I	100%	72	FP + 60 Gy	87.5%	4y: 80.5%
JCOG0502 [63] (Japan)	Stage I (T1b)	100%	159	FP + 60 Gy	87.3%	3y: 93.1% 5y: 85.5%

(continued)

Table 17.3 (continued)

Author	cStage	Pathology: rate of SCC	No. of pt.	Regimen	CR rate	Survival
JCOG9906 [5] (Japan)	Stage II/ III	100%	76	FP + 60 Gy	62.2%	3y: 44.7% 5y: 36.8%
Kato [68] (Japan)	Stage II/ III	98%	51	FP + 50.4 Gy	70.6%	1y: 88.2% 3y: 63.8%
JCOG0604 [55] (Japan)	Stage II/ III	100%	44	S-1+cisplatin+50.4 Gy	59.5%	3y: 61.9%
RTOG0246 [69, 70] (USA)	Stage II/ III	27%	41	TPF → FP + 50.4 Gy +selective S	36.6%	1y: 71% 5y: 36.6%
JCOG0909 [71, 72] (Japan)	Stage II/ III	100%	94	FP + 50.4 Gy ±salvage treatment	58.5%	3y: 74.2% 5y: 64.5%
CROC trial [73] (Japan)	Stage I-III	100%	90	DCF →FP + 50.4 Gy if RR →S if LPR or PR	89.8% (CRT group)	1y: 96.6% 3y: 74.1%

CRT chemoradiotherapy, *SCC* squamous cell carcinoma, *CR* complete response, *RTOG* Radiation Therapy Oncology Group, *JCOG* Japan Clinical Oncology Group, *FP* 5-FU+cisplatin, *S* surgery, *TPF* Paclitaxel+cisplatin+5-FU, *DCF* docetaxel+cisplatin+5-FU, *RR* remarkable response, *LPR* limited partial response, *PR* poor response, *NR* not reported

80.4% in CRT arm. Most of residual or recurrent diseases after CRT were curatively resected by endoscopy or surgery. Several reports showed the efficacy of these salvage treatments after definitive CRT [64–67]. For stage II/III esophageal cancer, JCOG9906, a phase II trial of CRT with 5-FU and cisplatin and 60 Gy irradiation with elective lymph nodal irradiation showed promising activity with 62.2% of CR rate and 36.8% of 5-year OS rate [5]. Acute toxicities were mild, but there were four treatment-related deaths (5.3%) caused by late toxicities. Moreover, 8–15% of high mortality rate was seen in patients who underwent salvage surgery for residual or recurrent disease after CRT [65, 66]. Late toxicity and higher mortality rate might be caused by the extensive radiation field and daily treatment of AP/PA opposite fields. Therefore, a phase II trial of CRT with 5-FU and cisplatin and concurrent radiotherapy 50.4 Gy using of multiple field technique with reducing both the radiation dose and the volume of heart within the radiation field for stage II/III esophageal cancer was conducted [68]. At a median follow-up of 29.4 months, late toxicities, which were greater than grade 3, were observed in 5.9% of pneumonitis only. The CR rate was 70.6%, and 3-year OS rate was 63.8%. As a development of the esophagus-preserving approach, a phase II study of induction chemotherapy followed by definitive CRT with selective salvage surgery for stage II/III esophageal cancer (27% SCC) was conducted (RTOG0246) [69, 70]. CR rate was 36.6%. Salvage surgery was performed in 44%. Treatment-related death after surgery occurred in 4.8%. The 1-year and 5-year OS rates were 71% and 36.6%. Recently, a single-arm confirmatory study of definitive CRT including salvage treatment for stage II/III esophageal carcinoma (JCOG0909) was reported [71, 72]. CRT consisted of 5-FU and cisplatin and 50.4 Gy irradiation with elective nodal irradiation of 41.4 Gy. For residual or recurrent disease after CRT, salvage endoscopic resection or surgery was performed based on the prespecified criteria. CR rate was 58.8%. Salvage endoscopic resection and surgery were performed in 5% and 27%. R0 resection of salvage surgery was achieved in 76%. Treatment-related death after surgery occurred in 4.0%. The OS rates were 74.2% at 3 years and 64.5% at 5 years, while the esophagectomy-free survival rates were 63.6% at 3 years and 54.9% at 5 years. Grade 3 late toxicities were observed in only 9.6%. Organ-preservation strategies based on chemotherapy-based selection using intensive induction chemotherapy are also being developed. In the phase II trial (CROC trial) of patients with stage I-III ESCC, those with a remarkable response after induction DCF subsequently received CRT with 5-FU and cisplatin and 50.4 Gy irradiation, resulting in a 3-year OS of 74.1% and a 3-year esophagectomy-free survival rate of 45.3% [73].

17.3.2.3 Prophylactic Chemoradiotherapy

A single-arm confirmatory study of endoscopic resection followed by selective CRT for stage I esophageal carcinoma (JCOG0508) was reported [9, 10]. Patients with cT1bN0 (SM1-2) esophageal cancer, which was estimated to be treatable endoscopically, were treated with endoscopic resection, and prophylactic CRT was performed for patients with pathologically confirmed complete resection who had pT1a with positive vascular invasion or pT1b. CRT consisted of 5-FU and cisplatin and 41.4 Gy irradiation for regional lymph nodes. The OS rates were 90.7% at 3 years and 89.7% at 5 years. Grade 3 late toxicities were observed in 3.1% only.

17.3.2.4 Neoadjuvant Chemoradiotherapy

Several randomized trials comparing surgery alone to neoadjuvant CRT were conducted, and the results were conflicting (Table 17.4) [74–82]. Bosset and colleagues reported a European Organisation for Research and Treatment of Cancer (EORTC)

Table 17.4 Results of clinical trials of neoadjuvant chemoradiotherapy for ESCC

Author	Pathology: rate of SCC	Regimen	No. of pt.	Suvival	p-value
Bosset [74] (France)	100%	S	139	MST: 18.6 M	0.78
		FP + 37 Gy + S	143	MST: 18.6 M	
Urba [75] (USA)	25%	S	50	MST: 17.6 M	0.15
		FP + VBL + 40 Gy + S	50	MST: 16.9 M	
Lee [76] (Korea)	100%	S	51	MST: 27.3 M	0.69
		FP + 45.6 Gy (HF) + S	50	MST: 28.2 M	

(continued)

Table 17.4 (continued)

Author	Pathology: rate of SCC	Regimen	No. of pt.	Suvival	p-value
Burmeister [77] (trans-Tasman)	38%	S	128	MST: 19.3 M	> 0.05
		FP + 35 Gy + S	128	MST: 22.2 M	
CALGB9781 [78] (USA)	25%	S	30	5y: 16%	0.002
		FP + 50.4 Gy + S	26	5y: 39%	
CROSS study [79, 80] (Netherland)	23%	S	188	3y: 44%, 5y: 33%	0.003
		PTX + CBDCA+41.4 Gy + S	178	3y: 58%, 5y: 47%	
NEOCRETEC5010 [81, 82] (China)	100%	S	227	3y: 57.8%, 49.1%	0.03
		CDDP+VNR + 40 Gy + S	224	3y: 65.8%, 5y: 59.9%	
JCOG1109 [86] (Japan)	98%	FP + S	199	3y: 62.6%	
		DCF + S	202	3y: 72.1%	0.006 (FP vs. DCF)
		FP + 41.4 Gy + S	200	3y: 68.3%	0.12 (FP vs. CRT)
Tang [87] (China)	100%	PTX + CDDP+S	132	3y: 64.1%	0.28
		PTX + CDDP+40 Gy + S	132	3y: 54.9%	
CheckMate577 [88, 89] (international collaboration)	29%	nCRT+S	262	3y: 50%, 5y: 41%	0.106
		nCRT+S → Nivolumab	532	3y: 57%, 5y: 46%	
SANO trial [91] (Netherland)	23%	PTX + CBDCA+41.4 Gy			
		→active surveillance	198	2y: 74%	0.55
		→S	111	2y: 71%	

SCC squamous cell carcinoma, *MST* median survival time, *S* surgery, *FP* 5-FU+cisplatin, *VBL* vinblastine, *HF* hyperfraction, *PTX* paclitaxel, *CBDCA* carboplatin, *CDDP* cisplatin, *VNR* vinorelbine, *nCRT* neoadjuvant chemoradiotherapy, *MST* median survival time, *M* months, *OS* overall survival

trial randomizing 282 patients with squamous cell carcinoma of the esophagus to either surgery alone or preoperative therapy using concurrent cisplatin chemotherapy with radiation therapy [74]. Outcomes showed patients receiving neoadjuvant therapy experienced a significant improvement in disease-free survival, cancer-related mortality, margin-negative resection, and local control; however, no improvement in OS was seen versus patients undergoing surgery alone. Results of the largest randomized trial assessing neoadjuvant CRT in the treatment of esophageal cancer (23% SCC) showed a significant survival benefit in patients receiving preoperative CRT [79, 80]. A pathological CR rate was 29% in patients receiving preoperative therapy. Median survival was 49.4 months in patients receiving CRT versus 24.0 months in surgery alone, with a significant improvement in 3-year OS (58% vs. 44%). Updated results showed that at 5 years, OS rates were 47% and 33%, respectively, for neoadjuvant CRT and surgery alone [80]. Several meta-analyses have been performed concerning neoadjuvant therapy for esophageal cancer. Sjoquist and colleagues conducted an updated meta-analysis comparing neoadjuvant CRT and neoadjuvant chemotherapy, demonstrating that neoadjuvant CRT was associated with an absolute 2-year OS benefit of 8.7% in terms of all-cause mortality [83]. with survival benefits similar between squamous cell carcinoma and adenocarcinoma patients. Another meta-analysis demonstrated that neoadjuvant CRT significantly increased rates of pathologic CR/R0 resection in both adenocarcinoma and squamous cell carcinoma patients compared to neoadjuvant chemotherapy alone. A significant increase in 3-year OS was seen only in squamous cell carcinoma patients (56.8% vs. 42.8%), whereas in adenocarcinoma patients, no significant difference was seen (46.3% vs. 41%) [84]. Currently, neoadjuvant CRT is accepted as the standard treatment for locally advanced esophageal cancer in Western countries. However, there is no randomized trial performed comparing neoadjuvant CRT to surgery alone or neoadjuvant chemotherapy in Japan. Therefore, neoadjuvant CRT for resectable esophageal cancer is investigational in Japan. Hashimoto and colleagues conducted a first multi-institutional phase II trial of neoadjuvant CRT for stage II/III esophageal cancer in Japan and reported promising activity with 41% of pathological CR rate and 70.8% of 3-year OS [85]. Recently, results of JCOG1109, a three-arm randomized controlled trial compared neoadjuvant 5-FU and cisplatin to neoadjuvant 5-FU and cisplatin and radiotherapy or neoadjuvant DCF, followed by esophagectomy with regional lymph node dissection for stage I–III esophageal cancer (98% SCC) in Japan, were conducted [86]. At a median follow-up of 50.7 months, compared with the neoadjuvant 5-FU and cisplatin group, the 3-year OS rate was significantly higher in the neoadjuvant DCF group (72.1% vs. 62.6%), but not in the neoadjuvant CRT group (68.3%). Another randomized control trial compared neoadjuvant paclitaxel and cisplatin to neoadjuvant paclitaxel and cisplatin and radiotherapy, followed by minimally invasive esophagectomy for T3-4aN0-1 M0 ESCC in China [87]. Compared with neoadjuvant chemotherapy, neoadjuvant CRT improved pathological CR rates (28% vs. 3%), but failed to improve OS (3-year, 64% vs. 55%). As the development of adjuvant treatment following surgery after neoadjuvant chemoradiotherapy, a randomized controlled trial, CheckMate 577, was conducted comparing adjuvant nivolumab with placebo in patients with resected (R0) stage II/III esophageal or gastroesophageal junction cancer (29% SCC) who had residual pathological disease after neoadjuvant CRT [88, 89]. At a median follow-up of 24 months, adjuvant nivolumab significantly improved disease-free survival compared with placebo (median, 22 vs. 11 months), with consistent benefits observed across all patient subgroups, including histology, tumor location, initial and posttreatment disease stage, and PD-L1 expression status [88].

With a median follow-up of 78.3 months, adjuvant nivolumab also demonstrated a non-statistically significant trend toward improved OS compared with placebo (5-year OS, 46% vs. 41%) [89]. As a preoperative treatment strategy aimed at conversion surgery in patients with T4b esophageal cancer, a randomized phase II trial comparing neoadjuvant DCF with neoadjuvant 5-FU and cisplatin and 50.4 Gy irradiation was conducted [90]. At a median follow-up of 24 months, 2-year OS rate was higher in the CRT group (55.1%) compared to the chemotherapy group (34.7%). Local and regional lymph node recurrence in patients undergoing R0 resection was significantly higher in the chemotherapy group compared to the CRT group (local: 30% vs. 8%, regional: 37% vs. 8%). An important clinical question is whether surgery is necessary, with the aim of esophageal preservation, in patients with locally advanced esophageal cancer who achieve a clinical CR after initial CRT. In a stepped-wedge, cluster-randomized, noninferiority phase III trial (SANO trial), compared neoadjuvant carboplatin and paclitaxel and 41.4 Gy irradiation followed by active surveillance to standard surgery for locally advanced potentially resectable esophageal cancer was conducted in the Netherlands [91]. OS after active surveillance for esophageal cancer (22% SCC) was non-inferior compared with standard surgery after 2 years (2-year OS, 75% vs. 70%). Patients who underwent active surveillance followed by postponed surgery demonstrated a similar frequency of postoperative complications (82% vs. 84%) and postoperative mortality (4% vs. 5%) compared with those who underwent immediate standard surgery.

17.3.3 Palliative Therapy

Palliative radiotherapy is also useful for relief of symptoms such as dysphagia and pain, and impairment of the patient's quality of life. Palliative treatment regimens range from 30 Gy over 2 weeks to 50 Gy over 5 weeks or up to 60 Gy over 6 weeks, with up to 80% relief of pain and dysphagia [92]. Many studies report a 60% to >80% rate of relief from dysphagia with radiation. Coia and colleagues reported that nearly half of patients with baseline dysphagia experienced an improvement in swallowing within 2 weeks of treatment initiation [93]. By the completion of the sixth week, 80% or more of patients experienced improvement. A median time to maximal improvement was approximately 1 month. Palliative CRT is likely preferable to radiation alone for patients with advanced-stage esophageal carcinoma who have a good performance status. Retrospective analysis showed that 75% of stage IVB patients treated with 5-FU and cisplatin and 40 Gy irradiation improved dysphagia score [94]. Penniment and colleagues reported a Trans-Tasman Radiation Oncology Group (TROG) trial (TROG 03.01) randomizing 220 patients with advanced/metastatic esophageal cancer (26% SCC) to receive 35 Gy in 15 fractions (or 30 Gy in 10 fractions) with or without the addition of concurrent 5-FU and cisplatin [95]. No significant differences in dysphagia relief (45% vs. 35%) and median OS (6.9 vs. 6.7 months) were seen between the CRT group and the radiotherapy group. As to toxicity, there were significant differences in grade 3–4 acute toxicity (36% vs. 16%) between the CRT group and the radiotherapy group. Intraluminal brachytherapy has also been used for palliation of dysphagia [39]. The previously described randomized trial from the Netherlands comparing intraluminal brachytherapy to stent placement showed that although patients undergoing stenting experienced a more rapid improvement in dysphagia, long-term palliation was significantly improved in patients treated with brachytherapy [38]. A meta-analysis of prospective studies of brachytherapy encompassing 623 patients concluded that brachytherapy was a highly effective and relatively safe treatment option that was currently underused. However, the severe adverse event rate was 23% (stenosis 12%, fistula development 8%) [96].

17.4 Toxicity of Radiotherapy

Acute adverse events are esophagitis, dermatitis, weight loss, fatigue, and anorexia. Nausea and vomiting are relatively common, particularly in patients with lower esophageal tumor. Most patients experience esophagitis and dysphagia. Many symptoms resolve within 1–2 weeks of treatment completion. Radiation pneumonitis is subacute, generally occurs 2–6 months after radiation therapy completion. Usually, most patients have no symptoms. Common symptoms include nonproductive cough, fever, dyspnea, and, more uncommonly, respiratory distress. Late adverse events are pericardial effusion, pleural effusion, esophageal strictures, fistula formation, and hemorrhage [97]. And hypothyroidism may occur in case of including the thyroid within radiation field [45]. In a Japanese study, long-term analysis of 78 patients with complete remission treated with definitive CRT (cisplatin and 5-FU with 60 Gy) for squamous cell carcinoma revealed grade 2, 3, and 4 late pericarditis occurring in 6%, 5%, and 1% of patients, respectively; grade 4 heart failure in 2 patients; grade 2, 3, and 4 pleural effusion development in 5%, 6%, and 0% of patients, respectively; and grade 2, 3, and 4 radiation pneumonitis development in 1%, 2%, and 0% of patients, respectively [98]. Another analysis from Japan using fields inclusive of supraclavicular, mediastinal, and celiac regions up to a dose of 60 Gy with concurrent cisplatin and 5-FU showed a 2-year cumulative incidence of late, high-grade cardiopulmonary toxicities for patients ≥75 years of 29% versus 3% in younger patients. They concluded that older patients may not tolerate extensive radiation fields [99]. In JCOG9906, late toxicities included grade 3/4 esophagitis (13%), pericardial (16%), and pleural (9%) effusions, and radiation pneumonitis (4%), which caused 4 deaths [5]. These high incidences of late toxicities might be caused by extensive radiation field and daily treatment of AP/PA opposite fields. Recently, to reduce the late cardiac toxicity, use of multiple field technique with reducing both the radiation dose and the volume of heart within the radiation field is recommended while keeping the volume of the irradiated lung at a lower percentage [9, 10, 68, 71, 72]. About half of the esophageal strictures are due to local persistent or local recurrence. For benign strictures, dilation results in palliation in the majority of patients. Tumor involvement of the trachea, aorta, or lung can lead to fistula formation during or after radiotherapy. Regarding brachytherapy, combination CRT with HDR-brachytherapy was associated with a high risk of life-threatening toxicities including esophageal ulcer, fistula, and perforation [35, 100–102]. And intubation with metallic stents before or during radiotherapy was associated with a high risk of life-threatening complications (Grade 3–5: 51%, Grade 5: 21%) such as hematemesis, esophageal fistula, and pneumonitis [103]. Samual and colleagues reported the outcome of patients with and without esophageal stenting before radiotherapy treated with concurrent CRT at a median dose of 50.4 Gy [104]. Of the 103 patients, there were significant differences in grade 3 or higher acute toxicities including esophagitis, dehydration, and anorexia, between the stent group and no-stent group (71% vs. 27%). And after propensity score matching, the stent patients had a worse median OS compared with the no-stent patients (11.5 vs. 22.0 months).

17.5 New Radiation Treatment Modalities

New radiotherapy techniques such as IMRT, proton beam therapy (PBT), and carbon-ion radiotherapy (CIRT) permit concentration of the radiation dose on the tumor with avoidance of critical organs such as the heart, lung, and spinal cord. These techniques may allow dose escalation in the treatment of esophageal cancer. In recent years, volumetric modulated arc therapy (VMAT) has been increasingly used as a type of IMRT, delivering radiation continuously during gantry rotation with simultaneous modulation of dose rate, gantry speed, and multileaf collimator position to achieve highly conformal dose distributions. PBT and CIRT take advantage of Bragg peak property to allow dose localization at the tumor while avoiding critical organs. In addition, CIRT that utilizes heavy-ion beams has a high relative biological effectiveness (RBE) with high linear transfer. In a treatment planning comparison study of photon radiotherapy and PBT for esophageal cancer, PBT was reported to significantly reduce the mean doses to the heart and lungs [105, 106]. Lin and colleagues analyzed data from 580 patients who underwent neoadjuvant CRT using 3D-CRT, IMRT, or PBT, and reported that the mean heart dose was significantly lower with PBT (22.4 ± 6.7 Gy) compared with 3D-CRT (28.4 ± 7.4 Gy) and IMRT (28.4 ± 7.4 Gy), as was the mean lung dose, which was 6.1 ± 2.6 Gy with PBT versus 10.5 ± 3.9 Gy with 3D-CRT and 9.5 ± 3.2 Gy with IMRT [106]. Regarding clinical outcomes, Mizumoto and colleagues reported the results of locally advanced ESCC using protons with or without photons to a total dose of 70–98 GyE [107]. Of 51 patients, 40 (78%) showed a CR (T1, T2: 100%; T3: 77%; T4: 38%). And the 5-year local control rate was 38.0%, and 5-year OS rate was 21.1%. As a late toxicity, one patient died due to hemorrhage from an esophageal ulcer at the site of irradiation without recurrence. However, there were no other non-hematologic toxicities of grade ≥ 3 including lung and heart toxicity. Ishikawa and colleagues also reported the toxicities and outcomes of 40 patients treated with proton-beam therapy concurrently combined with chemotherapy consisting of 5-FU and cisplatin for ESCC [108]. A total dose of 60 GyE was delivered, and an additional boost of 4–10 GyE was given when residual tumors were suspected. Of 40 patients, 31 (78%) showed a CR (stage I: 88%; stage II: 89%; stage III: 56%). The

2-year local control rate was 66.4%, and 2-year OS rate was 75.1%. As a late toxicity, no cardiopulmonary toxicities of grade 3 or higher were observed. In a randomized phase IIB trial comparing CRT using IMRT or PBT in patients with cStage I-III esophageal cancer (11% SCC), Lin and colleagues demonstrated a lower incidence of grade ≥ 3 late adverse events with PBT compared with IMRT (4.4% vs. 8.2%), while the 3-year OS rates were similar between the two groups (51.2% vs. 50.8%, respectively) [109]. Furthermore, Wang and colleagues reported that the 5-year incidence of cardiac function decline after treatment was 21% in the IMRT group and 13% in the PBT group, showing a trend toward a lower incidence with PBT ($p = 0.053$); notably, when the analysis was restricted to patients with pre-existing cardiac disease, the incidence was significantly lower in the PBT group than in the IMRT group (14% vs. 32%, $p = 0.018$) [110]. Currently, two randomized controlled trials comparing PBT with photon radiotherapy for esophageal cancer are ongoing: one in the United States (NRG-GI006), which evaluates definitive CRT, and the other in Europe (PROTECT), which investigates neoadjuvant CRT.

In a treatment planning comparison study of 3D-CRT, VMAT, and CIRT for patients with stage I esophageal cancer, CIRT was reported to reduce radiation doses to the heart and lungs [111]. Akutsu and colleagues conducted a phase I/II clinical trial of preoperative CIRT for ESCC [112]. Thirty-one patients were enrolled, and the radiation dose was escalated from 28.8 GyE up to 36.8 GyE. 12 (38.7%) patients achieved a pathological CR. The 3- and 5-year OS rates in the stage I cases were 81% and 61%, and were 85% and 77% for the stage II cases, and 43% and 29% for the stage III cases, respectively. One case (3.2%) in 35.2 GyE presented Grade 3 of postoperative acute respiratory distress syndrome, and there were no late toxicities. Subsequently, a phase I/II dose-escalation trial of CIRT was conducted in patients with stage I (cT1bN0M0) ESCC, in which the radiation dose was escalated stepwise from 48.0 GyE in 12 fractions over 3 weeks to 50.4 GyE in 12 fractions over 3 weeks [113]. A total of 30 patients were enrolled, and among the 25 patients who received ≥45.6 Gy, favorable outcomes were achieved, with a complete response rate of 92% and a 5-year overall survival rate of 80.0%. In terms of safety, grade ≥ 3 acute adverse events included esophagitis in 6.7%, pneumonitis in 3.3%, and neutropenia in 6.7% of patients, while no grade ≥ 3 late adverse events were observed. However, these new approaches remain investigational, and the results of ongoing and future clinical trials of advanced high-precision radiotherapy are awaited to further clarify the efficacy and safety of these novel techniques and technologies in prospective settings.

References

1. Herskovic A, Martz K, Al-Sarraf M, et al. Combined chemotherapy and radiotherapy compared with radiotherapy alone in patients with cancer of the esophagus. N Engl J Med. 1992;326:1593–8.
2. Al-Sarraf M, Martz K, Herskovic A, et al. Progress report of combined chemoradiotherapy versus radiotherapy alone in patients with esophageal cancer: an intergroup study. J Clin Oncol. 1997;15:277–84.

3. Cooper JS, Guo MD, Herskovic A, et al. Chemoradiotherapy of locally advanced esophageal cancer: long-term follow-up of a prospective randomized trial (RTOG 85-01). Radiation therapy oncology group. JAMA. 1999;281:1623–7.
4. Kato H, Sato A, Fukuda H, et al. A phase II trial of chemoradiotherapy for stage I esophageal squamous cell carcinoma: Japan clinical oncology group study (JCOG9708). Jpn J Clin Oncol. 2009;39:638–43.
5. Kato K, Muro K, Minashi K, Gastrointestinal oncology study group of the Japan clinical oncology group (JCOG), et al. Phase II study of chemoradiotherapy with 5-fluorouracil and cisplatin for stage II-III esophageal squamous cell carcinoma: JCOG trial (JCOG 9906). Int J Radiat Oncol Biol Phys. 2011;81:684–90.
6. Ohtsu A, Boku N, Muro K, et al. Definitive chemoradiotherapy for T4 and/or M1 lymph node squamous cell carcinoma of the esophagus. J Clin Oncol. 1999;17:2915–21.
7. Nishimura Y, Suzuki M, Nakamatsu K, et al. Prospective trial of concurrent chemoradiotherapy with protracted infusion of 5-fluorouracil and cisplatin for T4 esophageal cancer with or without fistula. Int J Radiat Oncol Biol Phys. 2002;53:134–9.
8. Ishida K, Ando N, Yamamoto S, et al. Phase II study of cisplatin and 5-fluorouracil with concurrent radiotherapy in advanced squamous cell carcinoma of the esophagus: a Japan esophageal oncology group (JEOG)/Japan clinical oncology group trial (JCOG9516). Jpn J Clin Oncol. 2004;34:615–9.
9. Minashi K, Nihei K, Mizusawa J, et al. Efficacy of endoscopic resection and selective chemoradiotherapy for stage I esophageal squamous cell carcinoma. Gastroenterology. 2019;157:382–90.
10. Nihei K, Minashi K, Yano T, et al. Final analysis of diagnostic endoscopic resection followed by selective Chemoradiotherapy for stage I esophageal cancer: JCOG0508. Gastroenterology. 2023;164:296–9.
11. Leong T, Everitt C, Yuen K, et al. A prospective study to evaluate the impact of FDG-PET on CT-based radiotherapy treatment planning for oesophageal cancer. Radiother Oncol. 2006;78:254–61.
12. Mizowaki T, Nishimura Y, Shimada Y, et al. Optimal size criteria of malignant lymph nodes in the treatment planning of radiotherapy for esophageal cancer: evaluation by computed tomography and magnetic resonance imaging. Int J Radiat Oncol Biol Phys. 2007;36:1091–8.
13. Gao XS, Qiao X, Wu F, et al. Pathological analysis of clinical target volume margin for radiotherapy in patients with esophageal and gastroesophageal junction carcinoma. Int J Radiat Oncol Biol Phys. 2007;67:389–96.
14. Akiyama H, Tsurumaru M, Udagawa H, et al. Radical lymph node dissection for cancer of the thoracic esophagus. Ann Surg. 1994;220:364–73.
15. Huang W, Li B, Gong H, et al. Pattern of lymph node metastases and its implication in radiotherapeutic clinical target volume in patients with thoracic esophageal squamous cell carcinoma: a report of 1077 cases. Radiother Oncol. 2010;95:229–33.
16. Tachimori Y, Nagai Y, Kanamori N, et al. Pattern of lymph node metastases of esophageal squamous cell carcinoma based on the anatomical lymphatic drainage system. Dis Esophagus. 2011;24:33–8.
17. Akutsu Y, Kato K, Igaki H, et al. The prevalence of overall and initial lymph node metastases in clinical T1N0 thoracic esophageal cancer: from the results of JCOG0502, a prospective multicenter study. Ann Surg. 2016;264:1009–15.
18. Onozawa M, Nihei K, Ishikura S, et al. Elective nodal irradiation (ENI) in definitive chemoradiotherapy (CRT) for squamous cell carcinoma of the thoracic esophagus. Radiother Oncol. 2009;92:266–9.
19. Jingu K, Nihei K, Ito Y, et al. Radiotherapy treatment planning for esophageal cancer: JASTRO guidelines 2024 for radiotherapy treatment planning. J Radiat Res. 2025;66:354–64.
20. Lyu J, Yisikandaer A, Li T, et al. Comparison between the effects of elective nodal irradiation and involved-field irradiation on long-term survival in thoracic esophageal squamous cell carcinoma patients: a prospective, multicenter, randomized, controlled study in China. Cancer Med. 2020;9:7460–8.

21. Zhang J, Li M, Zhang K, et al. Concurrent chemoradiotherapyof different radiation doses and different irradiation fields for locally advanced thoracic esophageal squamous cell carcinoma: a randomized, multicenter, phase III clinical trial. Cancer Commun (Lond). 2024;44:1173–88.
22. Sasaki K, Nomura M, Kato K, et al. A phase III randomized controlled trial comparing local field with additional prophylactic irradiation in chemoradiotherapy for clinical-T1bN0M0 esophageal cancer: ARMADILLO trial (JCOG1904). Jpn J Clin Oncol. 2024;54:103–7.
23. Yaremko BP, Guerrero TM, McAleer MF, et al. Determination of respiratory motion for distal esophagus cancer using four-dimensional computed tomography. Int J Radiat Oncol Biol Phys. 2008;70:145–53.
24. Lan K, Zhu J, Zhang J, et al. Propensity score-based comparison of survival and radiation pneumonitis after definitive chemoradiation for esophageal cancer: intensity-modulated radiotherapy versus three-dimensional conformal radiotherapy. Radiother Oncol. 2020;149:228–35.
25. Minsky BD, Pajak TF, Ginsberg RJ, et al. INT 0123 (radiation therapy oncology group 94-05) phase III trial of combined-modality therapy for esophageal cancer: high-dose versus standard-dose radiation therapy. J Clin Oncol. 2002;20:1167–74.
26. Hulshof MCCM, Geijsen ED, Rozema T, et al. Randomized study on dose escalation in definitive chemoradiation for patients with locally advanced esophageal cancer (ARTDECO study). J Clin Oncol. 2021;39:2816–24.
27. Xu Y, Dong B, Zhu W, et al. A phase III multicenter randomized clinical trial of 60 Gy versus 50 Gy radiation dose in concurrent chemoradiotherapy for inoperable esophageal squamous cell carcinoma. Clin Cancer Res. 2022;28:1792–9.
28. You J, Zhu S, Li J, et al. High-dose versus standard-dose intensity-modulated radiotherapy with concurrent paclitaxel plus carboplatin for patients with thoracic esophageal squamous cell carcinoma: a randomized, multicenter, open-label, phase 3 superiority trial. Int J Radiat Oncol Biol Phys. 2023;115:1129–37.
29. National Comprehensive Cancer Network (NCCN). Practice guidelines in oncology for esophageal and Esophagogastric junction cancers. Version 1. 2025.
30. Akagi Y, Hirokawa Y, Kagemoto M, et al. Optimum fractionation for high-dose-rate endoesophageal brachytherapy following external irradiation of early stage esophageal cancer. Int J Radiat Oncol Biol Phys. 1999;43:525–30.
31. Ishikawa H, Nonaka T, Sakurai H, et al. Usefulness of intraluminal brachytherapy combined with external beam radiation therapy for submucosal esophageal cancer: long-term follow-up results. Int J Radiat Oncol Biol Phys. 2010;76:452–9.
32. Nemoto K, Yamada S, Nishio M, JASTRO Study Group, et al. Results of radiation therapy for superficial esophageal cancer using the standard radiotherapy method recommended by the Japanese society of therapeutic radiology and oncology (JASTRO) study group. Anticancer Res. 2006;26(2B):1507–12.
33. Nishimura Y, Okuno Y, Ono K, et al. External beam radiation therapy with or without high-dose-rate intraluminal brachytherapy for patients with superficial esophageal carcinoma. Cancer. 1999;86:220–8.
34. Okawa T, Dokiya T, Nishio M, et al. Multi-institutional randomized trial of external radiotherapy with and without intraluminal brachytherapy for esophageal cancer in Japan. Japanese society of therapeutic radiology and oncology (JASTRO) study group. Int J Radiat Oncol Biol Phys. 1999;45:623–8.
35. Yamada K, Murakami M, Okamoto Y, et al. Treatment results of chemoradiotherapy for clinical stage I (T1N0M0) esophageal carcinoma. Int J Radiat Oncol Biol Phys. 2006;64:1106–11.
36. Yorozu A, Dokiya T, Oki Y, et al. Curative radiotherapy with high-dose-rate brachytherapy boost for localized esophageal carcinoma: dose-effect relationship of brachytherapy with the balloon type applicator system. Radiother Oncol. 1999;51:133–9.
37. Bergquist H, Wenger U, Johnsson E, et al. Stent insertion or endoluminal brachytherapy as palliation of patients with advanced cancer of the esophagus and gastroesophageal junction. Results of a randomized, controlled clinical trial. Dis Esophagus. 2005;18:131–9.

38. Homs MY, Steyerberg EW, Eijkenboom WM, et al. Single-dose brachytherapy versus metal stent placement for the palliation of dysphagia from oesophageal cancer: multicentre randomized trial. Lancet. 2004;364:1497–504.
39. Gaspar LE, Nag S, Herskovic A, et al. American brachytherapy society (ABS) consensus guidelines for brachytherapy of esophageal cancer. Clinical research committee, American brachytherapy society, Philadelphia, PA. Int J Radiat Oncol Biol Phys. 1997;38:127–32.
40. Earlam R, Cunha-Melo JR. Oesophageal squamous cell carcinoma: II. A critical review of radiotherapy. Br J Surg. 1980;67:457–61.
41. Toh Y, Numasaki H, Tachimori Y, et al. Current status of radiotherapy for patients with thoracic esophageal cancer in Japan, based on the comprehensive registry of esophageal cancer in Japan from 2009 to 2011 by the Japan esophageal society. Esophagus. 2020;17:25–32.
42. Kawashima M, Kagami Y, Toita T, et al. Prospective trial of radiotherapy for patients 80 years of age or older with squamous cell carcinoma of the thoracic esophagus. Int J Radiat Oncol Biol Phys. 2006;64:1112–21.
43. Shinoda M, Ando N, Kato K, Japan Clinical Oncology Group, et al. Randomized study of low-dose versus standard-dose chemoradiotherapy for unresectable esophageal squamous cell carcinoma (JCOG0303). Cancer Sci. 2015;106:407–12.
44. Nishimura Y, Mitsumori M, Hiraoka M, et al. A randomized phase II study of cisplatin/5-FU concurrent chemoradiotherapy for esophageal cancer: short-term infusion versus protracted infusion chemotherapy (KROSG0101/JROSG021). Radiother Oncol. 2009;92:260–5.
45. Nishimura Y, Hiraoka M, Koike R, et al. Long-term follow-up of a randomized phase II study of cisplatin/5-FU concurrent chemoradiotherapy for esophageal cancer (KROSG0101/JROSG021). Jpn J Clin Oncol. 2012;42:807–12.
46. Stahl M, Stuschke M, Lehmann N, et al. Chemoradiation with and without surgery in patients with locally advanced squamous cell carcinoma of the esophagus. J Clin Oncol. 2005;23:2310–7.
47. Conroy T, Galais MP, Raoul JL, Fédération Francophone de Cancérologie Digestive and UNICANCER-GI Group, et al. Definitive chemoradiotherapy with FOLFOX versus fluorouracil and cisplatin in patients with oesophageal cancer (PRODIGE5/ACCORD17): final results of a randomised, phase 2/3 trial. Lancet Oncol. 2014;15:305–14.
48. Crosby T, Hurt CN, Falk S, et al. Chemoradiotherapy with or without cetuximab in patients with oesophageal cancer (SCOPE1): a multicentre, phase 2/3 randomised trial. Lancet Oncol. 2013;14:627–37.
49. Suntharalingam M, Winter K, Ilson D, et al. Effect of the addition of cetuximab to paclitaxel, cisplatin, and radiation therapy for patients with esophageal cancer: the NRG oncology RTOG 0436 phase 3 randomized clinical trial. JAMA Oncol. 2017;3:1520–8.
50. Higuchi K, Komori S, Tanabe S, Kitasato Digestive Disease and Oncology Group, et al. Definitive chemoradiation therapy with docetaxel, cisplatin, and 5-fluorouracil (DCF-R) in advanced esophageal cancer: a phase 2 trial (KDOG 0501-P2). Int J Radiat Oncol Biol Phys. 2014;89:872–9.
51. de Castro JG, Segalla JG, de Azevedo SJ, et al. A randomised phase II study of chemoradiotherapy with or without nimotuzumab in locally advanced oesophageal cancer: NICE trial. Eur J Cancer. 2018;88:21–30.
52. Satake H, Tahara M, Mochizuki S, et al. A prospective, multicenter phase I/II study of induction chemotherapy with docetaxel, cisplatin and fluorouracil (DCF) followed by chemoradiotherapy in patients with unresectable locally advanced esophageal carcinoma. Cancer Chemother Pharmacol. 2016;78:91–9.
53. Yokota T, Kato K, Hamamoto Y, et al. Phase II study of chemoselection with docetaxel plus cisplatin and 5-fluorouracil induction chemotherapy and subsequent conversion surgery for locally advanced unresectable oesophageal cancer. Br J Cancer. 2016;115:1328–34.
54. Yokota T, Kato K, Hamamoto Y, et al. A 3-year overall survival update from a phase 2 study of chemoselection with DCF and subsequent conversion surgery for locally advanced unresectable esophageal cancer. Ann Surg Oncol. 2020;27:460–7.

55. Tahara M, Fuse N, Mizusawa J, et al. Phase I/II trial of chemoradiotherapy with concurrent S-1 and cisplatin for clinical stage II/III esophageal carcinoma (JCOG 0604). Cancer Sci. 2015;106:1414–20.
56. Bedenne L, Michel P, Bouché O, et al. Chemoradiation followed by surgery compared with chemoradiation alone in squamous cancer of the esophagus: FFCD 9102. J Clin Oncol. 2007;25:1160–8.
57. Nomura M, Sakanaka K, Shimizu J, et al. Nivolumab with definitive chemoradiotherapy for oesophageal squamous cell carcinoma: a phase II trial (NOBEL trial). eClinicalMedicine. 2026;91:103689.
58. Shah MA, Bennouna J, Doi T, et al. KEYNOTE-975 study design: a phase III study of definitive chemoradiotherapy plus pembrolizumab in patients with esophageal carcinoma. Future Oncol. 2021;17:1143–53.
59. Yu R, Wang W, Li T, et al. RATIONALE 311: tislelizumab plus concurrent chemoradiotherapy for localized esophageal squamous cell carcinoma. Future Oncol. 2021;17:4081–9.
60. Wang L, Chen M, Kato K, et al. A phase 3 randomized, double-blind, placebo-controlled, multicenter, global study of durvalumab with and after chemoradiotherapy in patients with locally advanced, unresectable esophageal squamous cell carcinoma: KUNLUN. J Clin Oncol. 2022;40:TPS373.
61. Chau I, Cho BC, Chen MH, et al. SKYSCRAPER-07: a phase III, randomised study of atezolizumab with or without tiragolumab in patients with unresectable esophageal squamous cell carcinoma that has not progressed following definitive concurrent chemoradiotherapy. Ann Oncol. 2025;36:S1181–2.
62. Terada M, Hara H, Daiko, et al. Phase III study of tri-modality combination therapy with induction docetaxel plus cisplatin and 5-fluorouracil versus definitive chemoradiotherapy for locally advanced unresectable squamous-cell carcinoma of the thoracic esophagus (JCOG1510: TRIANgLE). Jpn J Clin Oncol. 2019;49:1055–60.
63. Kato K, Ito Y, Nozaki I, et al. Parallel-group controlled trial of surgery versus chemoradiotherapy in patients with stage I esophageal squamous cell carcinoma. Gastroenterology. 2021;161:1878–86.
64. Makazu M, Kato K, Takisawa H, et al. Feasibility of endoscopic mucosal resection as salvage treatment for patients with local failure after definitive chemoradiotherapy for stage IB, II, and III esophageal squamous cell cancer. Dis Esophagus. 2014;27:42–9.
65. Swisher SG, Wynn P, Putnam JB, et al. Salvage esophagectomy for recurrent tumors after definitive chemotherapy and radiotherapy. J Thorac Cardiovasc Surg. 2002;123:175–83.
66. Tachimori Y, Kanamori N, Uemura N, et al. Salvage esophagectomy after high-dose chemoradiotherapy for esophageal squamous cell carcinoma. J Thorac Cardiovasc Surg. 2009;137:49–54.
67. Yano T, Muto M, Hattori S, et al. Long-term results of salvage endoscopic mucosal resection in patients with local failure after definitive chemoradiotherapy for esophageal squamous cell carcinoma. Endoscopy. 2008;40:717–21.
68. Kato K, Nakajima TE, Ito Y, et al. Phase II study of concurrent chemoradiotherapy at the dose of 50.4 Gy with elective nodal irradiation for stage II-III esophageal carcinoma. Jpn J Clin Oncol. 2013;43:608–15.
69. Swisher SG, Winter KA, Komaki RU, et al. A phase II study of a paclitaxel-based chemoradiation regimen with selective surgical salvage for resectable locoregionally advanced esophageal cancer: initial reporting of RTOG 0246. Int J Radiat Oncol Biol Phys. 2012;82:1967–72.
70. Swisher SG, Moughan J, Komaki RU, et al. Final results of NRG oncology RTOG 0246: an organ-preserving selective resection strategy in esophageal cancer patients treated with definitive chemoradiation. J Thorac Oncol. 2017;12:368–74.
71. Takeuchi H, Ito Y, Machida R, et al. A single-arm confirmatory study of definitive chemoradiation therapy including salvage treatment for clinical stage II/III esophageal squamous cell carcinoma (JCOG0909 study). Int J Radiat Oncol Biol Phys. 2022;114:454–62.

72. Ito Y, Takeuchi H, Ogawa G, et al. Final analysis of single-arm confirmatory study of definitive chemoradiotherapy including salvage treatment in patients with clinical stage II/III esophageal carcinoma (JCOG0909). J Clin Oncol. 2020;38:4545.
73. Katada C, Yokoyama T, Watanabe A, et al. Optimizing organ-preservation strategies through chemotherapy-based selection in esophageal squamous cell carcinoma: results from the CROC multi-institutional phase 2 clinical trial. Int J Radiat Oncol Biol Phys. 2024;120:1353–62.
74. Bosset JF, Gignoux M, Triboulet JP, et al. Chemoradiotherapy followed by surgery compared with surgery alone in squamous-cell cancer of the esophagus. N Engl J Med. 1997;337:161–7.
75. Urba SG, Orringer MB, Turrisi A, et al. Randomized trial of preoperative chemoradiation versus surgery alone in patients with locoregional esophageal carcinoma. J Clin Oncol. 2001;19:305–13.
76. Lee JL, Park SI, Kim SB, et al. A single institutional phase III trial of preoperative chemotherapy with hyperfractionation radiotherapy plus surgery versus surgery alone for resectable esophageal squamous cell carcinoma. Ann Oncol. 2004;15:947–54.
77. Burmeister BH, Smithers BM, Gebski V, Trans-Tasman Radiation Oncology Group, Australasian Gastro-Intestinal Trials Group, et al. surgery alone versus chemoradiotherapy followed by surgery for resectable cancer of the oesophagus: a randomised controlled phase III trial. Lancet Oncol. 2005;6:659–68.
78. Tepper J, Krasna MJ, Niedzwiecki D, et al. Phase III trial of trimodality therapy with cisplatin, fluorouracil, radiotherapy, and surgery compared with surgery alone for esophageal cancer: CALGB 9781. J Clin Oncol. 2008;26:1086–92.
79. van Hagen P, Hulshof MC, van Lanschot JJ, CROSS Group, et al. Preoperative chemoradiotherapy for esophageal or junctional cancer. N Engl J Med. 2012;366:2074–84.
80. Shapiro J, van Lanschot JJB, Hulshof MCCM, CROSS Study Group, et al. Neoadjuvant chemoradiotherapy plus surgery versus surgery alone for oesophageal or junctional cancer (CROSS): long-term results of a randomised controlled trial. Lancet Oncol. 2015;16:1090–8.
81. Yang H, Liu H, Chen Y, et al. Neoadjuvant chemoradiotherapy followed by surgery versus surgery alone for locally advanced squamous cell carcinoma of the esophagus (NEOCRTEC5010): a phase III multicenter, randomized, open-label clinical trial. J Clin Oncol. 2018;36:2796–803.
82. Yang H, Liu H, Chen Y, et al. Long-term efficacy of neoadjuvant chemoradiotherapy plus surgery for the treatment of locally advanced esophageal squamous cell carcinoma: the NEOCRTEC5010 randomized clinical trial. JAMA Surg. 2021;156:721–9.
83. Sjoquist KM, Burmeister BH, Smithers BM, Australasian Gastro-Intestinal Trials Group, et al. Survival after neoadjuvant chemotherapy or chemoradiotherapy for resectable oesophageal carcinoma: an updated meta-analysis. Lancet Oncol. 2011;12:681–92.
84. Deng HY, Wang WP, Wang YC, et al. Neoadjuvant chemoradiotherapy or chemotherapy? A comprehensive systematic review and meta-analysis of the options for neoadjuvant therapy for treating oesophageal cancer. Eur J Cardiothorac Surg. 2017;51:421–31.
85. Hashimoto J, Kato K, Ito Y, et al. Phase II feasibility study of preoperative concurrent chemoradiotherapy with cisplatin plus 5-fluorouracil and elective lymph node irradiation for clinical stage II/III esophageal squamous cell carcinoma. Int J Clin Oncol. 2019;24:60–7.
86. Kato K, Machida R, Ito Y, et al. Doublet chemotherapy, triplet chemotherapy, or doublet chemotherapy combined with radiotherapy as neoadjuvant treatment for locally advanced oesophageal cancer (JCOG1109 NExT): a randomised, controlled, open-label, phase 3 trial. Lancet. 2024;404:55–66.
87. Tang H, Wang H, Fang Y, et al. Neoadjuvant chemoradiotherapy versus neoadjuvant chemotherapy followed by minimally invasive esophagectomy for locally advanced esophageal squamous cell carcinoma: a prospective multicenter randomized clinical trial. Ann Oncol. 2023;34:163–72.
88. Kelly RJ, Ajani JA, Kuzdzal J, et al. Adjuvant Nivolumab in resected esophageal or gastroesophageal junction cancer. N Engl J Med. 2021;384:1191–203.

89. Kelly RJ, Ajana JA, Kuzdzal J, et al. Adjuvant nivolumab in resected esophageal or gastroesophageal junction cancer following neoadjuvant chemoradiotherapy: first results of overall survival from CheckMate 577. J Clin Oncol. 2025;43:4S.
90. Yamasaki M, Miyata H, Yamashita K, et al. Chemoradiotherapy versus triplet chemotherapy as initial therapy for T4b esophageal cancer: survival results from a multicenter randomized phase 2 trial. Br J Cancer. 2023;129:54–60.
91. van der Wilk BJ, Eyck BM, Wijnhoven BPL, et al. Neoadjuvant chemoradiotherapy followed by active surveillance versus standard surgery for oesophageal cancer (SANO trial): a multicentre, stepped-wedge, cluster-randomised, non-inferiority, phase 3 trial. Lancet Oncol. 2025;26:425–36.
92. Rosenberg JC, Franklin R, Steiger Z. Squamous cell carcinoma of the thoracic esophagus: an interdisciplinary approach. Curr Probl Cancer. 1981;5:1–52.
93. Coia LR, Soffen EM, Schultheiss TE, et al. Swallowing function in patients with esophageal cancer treated with concurrent radiation and chemotherapy. Cancer. 1993;71:281–6.
94. Ikeda E, Kojima T, Kaneko K, et al. Efficacy of concurrent chemoradiotherapy as a palliative treatment in stage IVB esophageal cancer patients with dysphagia. Jpn J Clin Oncol. 2011;41:964–2.
95. Penniment MG, De Ieso PB, Harvey JA, TROG 03.01/CCTG ES.2 group, et al. Palliative chemoradiotherapy versus radiotherapy alone for dysphagia in advanced oesophageal cancer: a multicentre randomised controlled trial (TROG 03.01). Lancet Gastroenterol Hepatol. 2018;3:114–24.
96. Fuccio L, Mandolesi D, Farioli A, et al. Brachytherapy for the palliation of dysphagia owing to esophageal cancer: a systematic review and meta-analysis of prospective studies. Radiother Oncol. 2017;122:332–9.
97. Nemoto K, Takai Y, Ogawa Y, et al. Fatal hemorrhage in irradiated esophageal cancer patients. Acta Oncol. 1998;37:259–62.
98. Ishikura S, Nihei K, Ohtsu A, et al. Long-term toxicity after definitive chemoradiotherapy for squamous cell carcinoma of the thoracic esophagus. J Clin Oncol. 2003;21:2697–702.
99. Morota M, Gomi K, Kozuka T, et al. Late toxicity after definitive concurrent chemoradiotherapy for thoracic esophageal carcinoma. Int J Radiat Oncol Biol Phys. 2009;75:122–8.
100. Brunner TB, Rupp A, Melzner W, et al. Esophageal cancer. A prospective phase II study of concomitant-boost external-beam chemoradiation with a top-up endoluminal boost. Strahlenther Onkol. 2008;184:15–22.
101. Gaspar LE, Winter K, Kocha WI, et al. A phase I/II study of external beam radiation, brachytherapy, and concurrent chemotherapy for patients with localized carcinoma of the esophagus (radiation therapy oncology group study 9207): final report. Cancer. 2000;88:988–95.
102. Kumar S, Dimri K, Khurana R, et al. A randomised trial of radiotherapy compared with cisplatin chemo-radiotherapy in patients with unresectable squamous cell cancer of the esophagus. Radiother Oncol. 2007;83:139–47.
103. Nishimura Y, Nagata K, Katano S, Japanese Society for Esophageal Diseases, et al. Severe complications in advanced esophageal cancer treated with radiotherapy after intubation of esophageal stents: a questionnaire survey of the Japanese society for esophageal diseases. Int J Radiat Oncol Biol Phys. 2003;56:1327–32.
104. Francis SR, Orton A, Thorpe C, et al. Toxicity and outcomes in patients with and without esophageal stents in locally advanced esophageal cancer. Int J Radiat Oncol Biol Phys. 2017;99:884–94.
105. Nonaka T, Kawashiro S, Ishikawa H, et al. Concurrent chemoradiotherapy using proton beams can reduce cardiopulmonary morbidity in esophageal cancer patients: a systematic review. Esophagus. 2023;20:605–16.
106. Lin SH, Merrell KW, Shen J, et al. Multi-institutional analysis of radiation modality use and postoperative outcomes of neoadjuvant chemoradiation for esophageal cancer. Radiother Oncol. 2017;123:376–81.
107. Mizumoto M, Sugahara S, Nakayama H, et al. Clinical results of proton-beam therapy for locoregionally advanced esophageal cancer. Strahlenther Onkol. 2010;186:482.

108. Ishikawa H, Hashimoto T, Moriwaki T, et al. Proton beam therapy combined with concurrent chemotherapy for esophageal cancer. Anticancer Res. 2015;35:1757–62.
109. Lin SH, Hobbs BP, Verma V, et al. Randomized phase IIB trial of proton beam therapy versus intensity-modulated radiation therapy for locally advanced esophageal cancer. J Clin Oncol. 2020;38:1569–79.
110. Wang X, Palaskas NL, Yusur SW, et al. Incidence and onset of severe cardiac events after radiotherapy for esophageal cancer. J Thorac Oncol. 2020;15:1682–90.
111. Takakusagi Y, Yoshida D, Kusano Y, et al. Dosimetric comparison between carbon-ion radiotherapy and photon radiotherapy for stage I esophageal cancer. In Vivo. 2021;35:447–52.
112. Akutsu Y, Yasuda S, Nagata M, et al. A phase I/II clinical trial of poperative short-course carbon-ion radiotherapy for patients with squamous cell carcinoma of the esophagus. J Surg Oncol. 2012;105:750–5.
113. Isozaki T, Ishikawa H, Yasuda S, et al. A phase I/II trial of definitive carbon ion radiotherapy for clinical T1bN0M0 esophageal squamous cell carcinoma. Int J Radiat Oncol Biol Phys. 2023;117:416–21.

Hong Kong Experiences

18

Claudia Wong and Simon Law

18.1 Introduction

Esophageal cancer is the eleventh most common cancer and the seventh leading cause of cancer deaths in the world [1]. There has been a divergence of histological cell type between the East and West. In Western countries, adenocarcinoma has increased dramatically in incidence in the past 30 years, closely related to rising prevalence of obesity, gastro-esophageal reflux disease, and Barrett's esophagus. In Asia, esophageal squamous cell carcinoma (ESCC) remains the predominant cell type; more than 80% of esophageal cancer is squamous cell in origin. There has not been a convincing rise in incidence of true adenocarcinoma of the esophagus (Siewert type I) in Asia. In Hong Kong, ESCC accounts for more than 90% of all esophageal cancers.

There has been advancement of technology in diagnosis, staging, and treatment of this highly lethal disease in the last few decades. In Hong Kong, more than 70% of esophageal cancer patients are diagnosed at stage III/IV. Diagnosis at an earlier stage can improve the outcome and prognosis. Accurate staging allows optimal stage-directed therapeutic strategy. Multimodality treatment methods, such as neo-adjuvant chemotherapy or chemoradiation with surgery, have gained popularity, and outcomes have improved compared with surgical resection alone. The authors will summarize the treatment strategies and experience at The University of Hong Kong.

C. Wong · S. Law (✉)
Division of Esophageal and Upper Gastrointestinal Surgery, Department of Surgery, The University of Hong Kong, Pokfulam, Hong Kong
e-mail: slaw@hku.hk

Y. Kitagawa et al. (eds.), *Esophageal Squamous Cell Carcinoma*,
https://doi.org/10.1007/978-981-92-2611-5_18

18.2 Diagnosis

When diagnosed at an early stage, the prognosis of ESCC is significantly better. The rate of detection of early tumors is higher in countries where uptake of endoscopy for early cancer diagnosis and screening is high, such as in Japan. In Hong Kong, there is no screening program, but at the authors' institution, high-risk patients are offered screening endoscopy, in particular those with a history of head and neck cancers [2, 3]. Chromoendoscopy with Lugol's iodine solution and optical chromo-endoscopy, such as narrow band imaging with magnifying endoscopy, are routinely utilized for screening. Since 2011, the authors' institution has performed surveillance endoscopy for patients who had a history of head and neck cancers. Among these patients, 6.3% had screening-detected neoplastic lesions, and 3.9% had ESCC or dysplastic lesions amendable to endoscopic treatment (unpublished data).

18.3 Investigations

Once the diagnosis is confirmed, investigations are directed to (1) accurate staging of disease, and (2) assessment of co-morbidities and operative risk. Based on the information obtained, an appropriate therapeutic strategy can be formulated for each individual. The algorithm in patient evaluation is shown in Fig. 18.1.

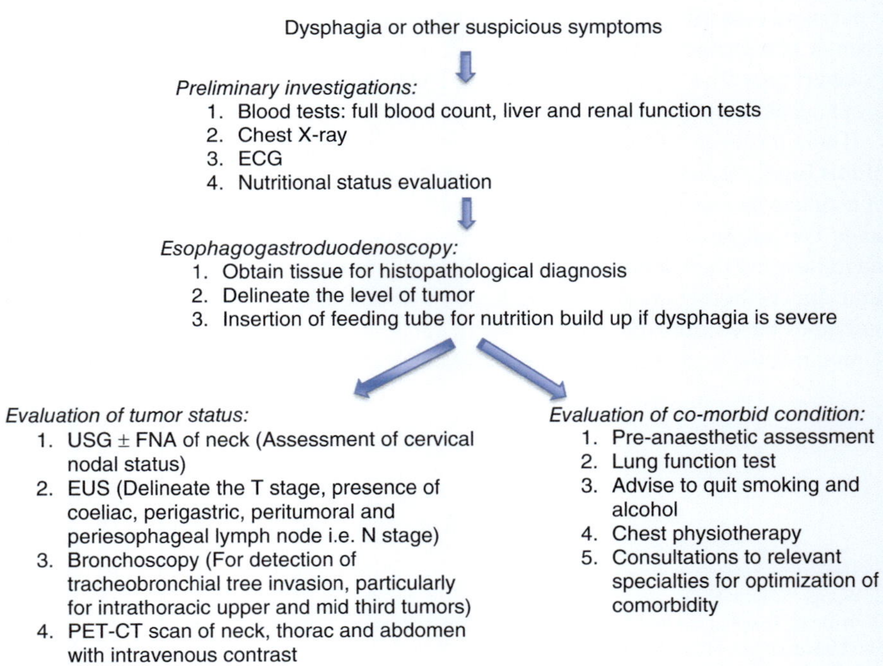

Fig. 18.1 Evaluation of patients suffering from cancer of the esophagus

18.3.1 Staging

Clinical staging follows the American Joint Committee on Cancer Staging (AJCC) TNM classification system. In addition to endoscopy, bronchoscopy [4], percutaneous ultrasound of the neck with or without fine-needle aspiration (FNA) cytology, endoscopic ultrasonography (EUS) with or without fine-needle aspiration [5], 2-(^{18}F) fluoro-2-deoxy-D-glucose (FDG) positron emission tomography (PET) / computed tomography (CT) scan are routinely employed.

Since the 1960s, bronchoscopic examination has been routine practice for patients with esophageal cancer at the authors' institution, initially by rigid, and later with flexible bronchoscope [6, 7]. This is especially important for tumors that are located in the middle and upper portions of the esophagus. In one study, the reported complication rate was 0.95% (4 out of 525 patients). Airway involvement by tumor contraindicates surgical resection. In a handful of anecdotal cases, response to chemoradiation therapy resulted in disappearance of tumor involvement, leading to subsequent successful resection, but this is an exception rather than the rule.

Percutaneous ultrasonography with or without fine needle aspiration is crucial to delineate the nodal status of the cervical region, and this is routinely performed. Diagnosis of cervical nodal metastases is important from a therapy point of view. Prior to the seventh edition of the AJCC staging classification, cervical nodal metastases were regarded as stage IV disease, although our policies have been in line with the Japanese guidelines to treat them as regional nodal metastases [8]. Chemotherapy or chemoradiation is usually given and followed by surgery if restaging demonstrates potentially curatively resectable disease.

We have been using endoscopic ultrasound (EUS) for staging since the 1990s [5]. The sensitivity and specificity of EUS in detecting the depth of esophageal involvement are 89% and 96%, respectively, whereas the respective figures for nodal status are 85% and 86% [5]; results that are comparable with other reports [9–11]. In recent years, we have been using the miniaturized ultrasound catheter probes (12.5 MHz mini probe), mainly because a substantial proportion of our patients have un-traversable tumor stenosis for conventional dedicated radial endo-ultrasonic endoscope.

In Hong Kong, FDG-PET is a routine investigation for ESCC; it is used in most of our patients although one limitation is that the scan is still not publicly funded and is self-financed. In those who could not afford a PET scan, only contrast CT scans are available. In an early study, we found that the maximum standard uptake value (SUVmax) correlated with nodal status (N+ vs. N- disease) on PET scan, the T stage measured by EUS, the pathological T stage after surgical resection, the pathological overall stage, as well as the chance of a R0 resection [12].

In a series of 244 patients from 2007–2012, we found that the SUVmax correlated with the T stage of disease; the mean SUVmax values for T1, 2, 3, and 4 tumors were 2.74, 4.55, 12.9, and 13.6, respectively. In addition, an SUVmax of 7.3 or more predicted a T3/4 tumor with a sensitivity of 90.1% and specificity of 95%. For nodal metastases, our experience with PET scan has an accuracy of diagnosing positive nodal spread of 70.3%. The tendency, however, is to underestimate false-negative nodes, while the predictive value of a metabolically active node is generally high. For patients who undergo neoadjuvant therapy, our policy is to repeat a PET/CT at 4 weeks post-therapy before a decision is made for surgical resection.

18.3.2 Patient Pretreatment Evaluation

Accurate tumor staging guides stage-directed therapy. In addition to tumor stage, careful pretreatment risk evaluation is important in selecting the appropriate patients for surgery.

The physiological reserve is an important factor to evaluate for potential surgical candidate. The assessment is generally based on surgeons' experience and intuition rather than an exact science. Objective score systems are available to help assess operative risk and patient selection [13, 14]. In our multivariate analysis of predictive factors for morbidity and mortality after esophagectomy, advanced age was predictive of both pulmonary complications and postoperative death. Patients with a tumor location in the superior mediastinal segment were also at risk of pulmonary complications [15]. In addition to routine blood tests for work-up, specific tests would include a pulmonary spirometric function test, and in selected patients, an echocardiogram and coronary angiography or stress thallium test. In our experience, there is not much in general that can be done to improve the existing physiological fitness of patients, with perhaps the exception of cardio-revascularization by angioplasty or stenting in those with critical coronary artery stenosis. In such patients, double antiplatelet agents such as aspirin and Clopidogrel may be required after coronary intervention. Neoadjuvant therapy is often given in these patients, aiming to downstage the tumor. It would allow the patient to recover from the cardiac procedure. Modern coronary intervention frequently allows the stopping of Clopidogrel at 1-month post-procedure. Aspirin can be continued in the perioperative period.

18.3.3 Patient Pre-habilitation and Preparation for Surgery

Postoperative management starts with preoperative evaluation and optimization. Enhanced Recovery After Surgery (ERAS) programs have been employed successfully in many institutions and are shown to improve outcomes. Major guidelines are published for its adoption [16–18]. The protocol used at the authors' institution is shown in Table 18.1.

The following preoperative measures should be instituted:

- Cessation of smoking and alcohol intake.
- Incentive spirometry and chest physiotherapy +/− prehabilitation program.
- Optimization of bronchodilator therapy in patients with asthma or significant chronic obstructive airway disease.

Table 18.1 Perioperative management.

Preoperative	
Preoperative counseling	
Nutritional assessment	Nasogastric tube feeding for those with significant stenosis of the esophagus, and oral supplement in those at risk of malnutrition
Preoperative exercise	General and incentive spirometry + pre-habilitation program
Stop smoking and alcohol intake	
Chest physiotherapy	
Carbohydrate loading on day of surgery	No solid food 6 h before and fluid 2 h before surgery. Carbohydrate loading night before and finishes 2 h before surgery
No need for bowel preparation unless colonic interposition is planned	
Intraoperative	
Prophylactic antibiotics	
DVT prophylaxis	Mechanical ± pharmacological
Judicious use of intraoperative fluids	
Avoid hypothermia	
Minimally invasive surgery if possible	
Epidural analgesia	
Postoperative	
Nutrition	POD1 carbohydrate drink, gradual advancement to soft diet by POD5 (if no vocal cord palsy and assessment by speech therapist shows no risk of aspiration) PPN/TPN in those at nutritional risk and oral intake insufficient
Nasogastric tube	Removal on POD 1 (if no vocal cord palsy and assessment by speech therapist shows no risk of aspiration)
Analgesia	Epidural analgesia/patient-controlled analgesia/multimodal analgesia
Chest drain	Single closed small caliber drain (19Fr Blake drain, which does not require underwater seal), removal POD 3–4 when output <200–300 ml per day
Early mobilization	From POD1, supervised by physiotherapist
Urinary catheter	Early removal as soon as close monitoring of urine output is not essential
Intravenous fluid	Balanced intravenous fluid to avoid over- and under-hydration
DVT prophylaxis	

DVT deep vein thrombosis, *POD* post-operation day, *PPN/TPN* peripheral parenteral nutrition/total parenteral nutrition

- In patients with high-grade esophageal tumor stenosis, a fine-bore nasogastric tube can be placed for nutritional support while workup is performed, and it is preferable over parenteral nutrition, gastrostomy, or jejunostomy feeding. Oral nutritional supplementation is given [19].
- Diabetic control should be optimized.

- Immediate preoperative preparations include prophylactic antibiotics to be given at anesthesia indication and deep vein thrombosis prophylaxis. Bowel preparation is not necessary unless a colonic interposition is intended.
- Preoperative patient education and counselling.

18.4 Treatment

Surgical resection and radical radiotherapy used to be the only two treatment options for esophageal cancer. Advances in endoscopic technology have made endoscopic treatment for early cancer possible. Improvements in chemotherapy and radiotherapy also increase the choice of therapeutic options. The management algorithm for ESCC at The University of Hong Kong is shown in Fig. 18.2.

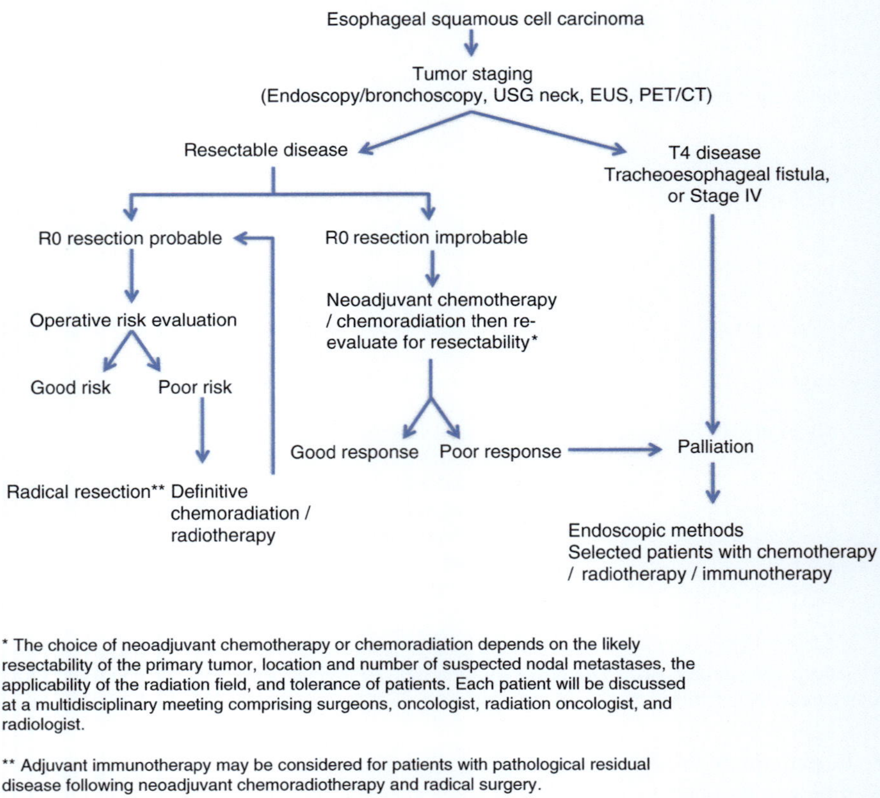

Fig. 18.2 Management protocol of patients with cancer of the esophagus at The University

18.4.1 Endoscopic Treatment for Early Cancer

Early ESCC is defined as tumor that is limited to the mucosa or submucosa. In Hong Kong, most ESCC patients are diagnosed at an advanced stage. The number of patients suitable for endoscopic treatment is therefore small. The indications for endoscopic treatment generally follow the guidelines from Japan [20]. Distinguishing m1/2 disease (where the chance of nodal metastases is negligible) from deeper lesions is often difficult. Deep invasions are not uncommonly missed with superficial biopsies and careful endoscopic examination. We practice endoscopic mucosal resection (EMR) or endoscopic submucosal dissection (ESD) to assess the lesions in detail pathologically before deciding on further treatments. Radiofrequency Ablation (RFA) is also an option over EMR/ESD, especially in treating long-segment and circumferential early cancers/neoplastic lesions. Studies have boasted lower stricture rates and complete response rates of up to 80–97% [21–24]. The safety of radiofrequency ablation (RFA) remains debatable in the context of treating ESCC. Compared to other endoscopic methods, RFA does not allow detailed histological assessment of depth of neoplastic lesions, hence harbors risk of undertreatment.

18.4.2 Neoadjuvant or Adjuvant Treatment

Neoadjuvant and adjuvant therapy for esophageal cancer has been controversial. Policies on their use vary widely in different countries. Preoperative chemotherapy is the standard-of-care in Japan and is commonly used in the United Kingdom [25–27], while in the United States, chemoradiation is more widely practiced [28–30]. With the published ChemoRadiotherapy for Esophageal cancer followed by Surgery Study (CROSS) from Europe, neoadjuvant chemoradiotherapy is liberally adopted at the authors' unit [31]. Currently, both chemotherapy and chemoradiotherapy are implemented as preoperative treatment strategies.

Historically, in Hong Kong, we have investigated different treatment strategies in treating esophageal cancer in addition to surgical resection alone. An early randomized trial looked at the impact of postoperative radiotherapy after esophagectomy. It was found that while postoperative radiotherapy did not lead to an overall improvement in survival, in those with palliative resections, the addition of radiotherapy reduced the chance of death from local-regional recurrence, especially from tracheobronchial recurrence [32]. The technique of radiotherapy was suboptimal by modern standards, the fractionation was high (3 Gy per fraction), and a few deaths resulted from the deleterious effects on the gastric conduit, even including perforation. This might have affected the overall survival results. Postoperative radiotherapy is not widely practiced worldwide, perhaps with the exception of some centers in China, where improved survival can be shown in selected patient populations [33, 34].

In the early 1990's, our focus shifted to preoperative chemotherapy. A randomized trial compared esophagectomy alone and two courses of preoperative cisplatin and 5-FU was carried out. Again, the overall survival benefit could not be demonstrated. A pathological complete response rate of 7% was achieved, and in those who responded well to chemotherapy, survival was superior to those who had surgery alone. Unfortunately, this was offset by those who responded poorly, whose survival was worse than the controls [35]. Attempts were made to identify predictors of response, but none was found to be reliable [36].

Chemoradiotherapy as neoadjuvant therapy has been investigated since the mid-1990s. A historical cohort comparison on patients treated with surgery alone and surgery with neoadjuvant chemoradiation demonstrated that the strategy of including chemoradiotherapy improved outcomes. The adoption of chemoradiation allowed better patient selection for curative surgery and resulted in more R0 resections by tumor downstaging [37]. The technique of radiotherapy has also improved over the years. Often Intensity-Modulated Radiation Therapy (IMRT) and 3-D conformal radiotherapy planning are used, replacing the traditional AP opposing radiation field.

In our earliest experience with chemoradiation, the most common chemotherapy regimen was cisplatin at 100 mg/m^2 on day 1 and then day 22 and continuous infusion of 5-fluorouracil at 500 mg/m^2 per day for 5 days from days 1–5 and days 22–26. Radiotherapy was given concurrently with a dose of 40Gy at 2 Gy per fraction. With this approach, tumor downstaging of 75% can be achieved. Pathological complete response rate in the primary tumor was up to 45%, and overall pathological complete response rate (including negative nodes) is 31% [38].

In response to the positive results of the CROSS trial [39], our choice of chemotherapeutic agents has widened to include taxanes since 2012. In a recent review of our own experience of treating ESCCs with the CROSS regime, pathological complete response rate was 33.3%. Median survival was 24.2 months. This is inferior to the original Dutch data in the CROSS trial, which reported a complete response rate of 49% in ESCC. The inclusion of patients with more advanced disease could have explained the discrepancy in results [40]. A study comparing the response of CROSS for ESCC in patients from Hong Kong, Taipei, Shanghai, and data from the Netherlands after propensity score matching showed that the response to nCRT in East Asia was poorer, regardless of patient, tumor, and treatment characteristics; the pCR rates were 27.8% and 43.6% in Asia and the Netherlands, respectively.

Patient selection seems essential to ensure good response and outcome. We conducted another study looking at a group of 40 patients with advanced nodal disease (stage M1a/M1b according to sixth edition of the AJCC—cervical and celiac lymph nodes, but considered loco-regional disease according to the seventh edition of AJCC) and still considered a potentially resectable disease. Chemoradiotherapy according to the CROSS regimen was given. Five (25%) patients developed distant metastases upon post-chemoradiation assessment; three patients were not operated on because of death before surgery, tracheoesophageal fistula, and patient refusal. Therefore, only 60% underwent esophagectomy, and R0 resection was achieved in 75% and pathological complete response in 15%. Median survival of the group was 11.1 months, and even for those who underwent esophagectomy was only 14 months [41]. It highlights the fact that promising trial results may not be reproducible in the real-world setting when it is more widely and less stringently applied. Certainly, better defining how chemoradiotherapy, such as CROSS, impacts treatment strategy is important [42, 43].

Research is still ongoing in Asia to find the optimal neoadjuvant therapy for ESCC. Reinforcement of conventional neoadjuvant chemotherapy with the addition of Docetaxel (triplet therapy) has been tested in Japan [44], prompted by the superiority of such over a combination of fluorouracil and cisplatin in locoregionally advanced head and neck cancer [45]. At the authors' institution, this combination is selectively applied in patients whose suspected nodal metastases' distribution is too extensive for effective radiation. This strategy has been adopted since early 2018. It is, however, the authors' impression that in those with bulky, clinically staged cT3+/4 lesions, radiotherapy is probably still more effective in bringing about enough downstaging to ensure an R0 resection. This depends more on the primary tumor than nodal metastases. The triplet regimen is also more toxic compared to the usual doublet regimens, and routinely G-CSF is given. Results of a randomized phase 3 three-arm trial in Japan comparing neoadjuvant cisplatin/5-FU, neoadjuvant triplet chemotherapy (Doxetaxel, Cisplatin, and 5-FU), and neoadjuvant radiation with doublet chemotherapy were published. Despite a substantially higher rate of pathological complete response, coupling nCRT did not demonstrate superior survival when compared with doublet chemotherapy alone in this study. Neoadjuvant DCF is associated with a superior 3-year overall survival when compared to doublet chemotherapy with a hazard ratio of 0.67. Treatment-related adverse events leading to termination of neoadjuvant therapy were more common in the triplet chemotherapy group [46]. Therefore, it is essential to carefully select patients who are in good condition, as they are more likely to tolerate the complete course of treatment and the subsequent surgery.

The timing of surgery after chemoradiation is an important consideration; when the interval between chemoradiation and surgery is short, the resultant pathological response rate may be affected because the tumor has not had a chance to degenerate, tissue inflammation may still be severe, and patients often need some time to recover physically from the treatment. On the other hand, if the interval is left too long, fibrosis may ensure, which may make dissection more difficult. More importantly, tumor may have more chance to regrow and metastasize. Our policy is to restage the patients at 4 weeks post-therapy, including endoscopy and PET / CT scan. Surgery is then performed around 6 to 10 weeks post-therapy.

At the authors' institution, the impact of time interval between neoadjuvant chemoradiation and surgery was studied in 107 ESCC patients. Patients were divided into two groups using 64 days from the completion of neoadjuvant therapy (median interval). When an R0 resection could be performed, the 3–year and 5-year survivals were better in the early surgery group than the delayed surgery group (3-year: 71.7% vs 56.5%, $p = 0.023$; 5-year: 71.7% vs 51%, $p = 0.032$).

On further analysis by reclassifying the patients into 3 interval groups, patients who underwent surgery within 40 days from completion of therapy had significantly lower R0 resection rate than those who had a longer wait till surgery (80 days: 74.2%, $p = 0.006$) [47]. Postoperative morbidity and mortality rates were not affected by the timing of surgery. Our previous data had also demonstrated the safety of neoadjuvant chemoradiation with regard to postoperative morbidity rates [15, 37].

The relationship between survival and interval to surgery after neoadjuvant therapy is an interesting observation, but the data require confirmation in a larger cohort. This factor needs consideration when surgery is planned.

The applicability of the AJCC staging system in the post-neoadjuvant chemoradiation setting has also been questioned. In one study, we showed that in patients without neoadjuvant therapy, there was an orderly relationship between the chance of finding nodal metastases with advancing pT stage. This was no longer true after chemoradiation. Applying the same TNM staging system may not be accurate enough to provide prognostic information [48]. Survival tends to be much poorer in postneoadjuvant therapy early stage ESCCs compared to the corresponding pathological stage groups without neoadjuvant therapy [49]. The latest eighth edition of the AJCC staging system addresses the dissimilarity in survival between treatment naïve and post-chemoradiation or chemotherapy ESCCs [50].

The percent of residual viable cells in the primary tumor, together with nodal status, were independent prognostic factors [38], while ypT stage was not. The cut-off point on the percent of residual viable cells and the interplay between other prognostic factors for better prognosis stratification warrant further investigation.

One major consideration of neoadjuvant therapy is how best to predict response. Much evidence has shown that those with pathological complete response had better survival [38, 51]. Chemotherapy and radiotherapy are not without morbidities, and subjecting patients to such treatments without significant effect will potentially cause harm, delay surgery, and increase the chance of tumor metastases while waiting for definitive treatment. However, no reliable clinical, biochemical, or molecular predictor exists. At the author's institution, using PET scans, SUVmax values were found to correlate with pathological complete response (pCR). In 52 patients who had undergone neoadjuvant chemoradiation and then resection, 21 (40.4%) achieved pCR. SUVmax value of the primary tumor at 1 month post-neoadjuvant therapy is independently predictive of pCR. However, the predictive value was only modest, sensitivity was 71%, specificity was 66.7%, positive predictive value was 75.9%, and negative predictive value was 60.9% [52]. PET scans were also only performed after completion of therapy and, therefore, limited their application. The use of PET scans to assess response during the early part of neoadjuvant therapy has some promise. Nonetheless, most of these reports to date studied chemotherapy-treated patients with substantial number being adenocarcinomas [53–55].

At the authors' institution, molecular pathways and blood-based assays are actively being studied to see if prediction of response is possible [56–60]. For example, specific microRNAs such as miR-193b are significantly elevated in good responders to chemoradiation with cisplastin/5-FU [61]. It is hoped that assays can be developed that have significant predictive value to guide treatment in the future, and even develop potential therapeutic targets to enhance sensitivity to chemotherapy [62].

In the event of a complete clinical response, is surgery still indicated? This is one of the latest areas of research. The concept of esophageal preservation, active surveillance, and salvage surgery only in the event of recurrence after a clinical complete response to neoadjuvant therapy is attractive [63, 64]. The Dutch Pre-SANO study has been published. It evaluated the accuracy of clinical response evaluation. Patients with potential complete response after chemoradiation underwent postponed surgery at 12–14 weeks with a presurgery second-stage clinical response evaluation, comprising fine needle aspiration of suspicious local-regional lymph nodes in addition to repeat endoscopic ultrasonography, bite-on-bite tumor biopsy, and PET-CT scan. The overall false negative rate of this approach to response evaluation was 10% for Chirieac modified tumor regression grades 3 and 4 tumors (more than 10% residual carcinoma) [64]. This has led to a randomized SANO trial. Under the study protocol, patients with clinical complete response were assigned to undergo either esophagectomy or active surveillance. It was demonstrated that the overall survival rate of the active surveillance was non-inferior to the surgery group, statistical differences in the disease-free survival and distant metastasis rates were also not demonstrated [65]. This study included squamous cell carcinoma and mostly adenocarcinoma. The biological behaviors of the two histological types are different. The question, hence, was whether results from the Pre-SANO and SANO trials could be applied to esophageal squamous cell carcinoma. To address the uncertainty, the authors' institution participated in a multicenter trial similar to the Pre-SANO trial but exclusively in squamous cell carcinoma (Pre-SINO trial). Using the same method of clinical response evaluation as described in the Pre-SANO trial, the false negative rate for detecting Chirieac modified tumor regression grades 3 and 4, and grades 1 and 2 tumors with ypN+ residual disease was 13.5% [66]. Liquid biopsy of circulating tumor cells (ctDNA) for surveillance of esophageal cancer is still under investigation, but has shown promise in detecting molecular residual disease. The addition of ctDNA as a diagnostic modality to the clinical response evaluation in a subset of patients resulted in a further reduction of false negative rate in detection of residual disease in the Pre-SINO trial. The role of ctDNA at this current point in time is still investigational, but results from this study provide a basis for its potential role in selecting patients for esophageal preservation strategies in the future.

Not until recent years, with the advent of oncological therapeutic agents, adjuvant therapy was not standard practice at the authors' institution, as mentioned earlier, due to the lack of supporting evidence. After the results of the Checkmate 577 trial became available, immunotherapy, namely nivolumab, has been adopted as adjuvant therapy for patients who underwent R0 resection following neoadjuvant chemoradiotherapy with pathological residual disease. The study demonstrated that the use of adjuvant nivolumab is associated with improved disease-free survival [67, 68]. However, immunotherapy is currently not publicly funded in the authors' locality and is not affordable for all. Its benefit has yet to be applied to all patients who fall into this category.

18.4.3 Surgery

Most patients seen at the authors' institution have advanced disease with co-morbidities. Early cancers are uncommon, and therefore most who come to surgery will have had neoadjuvant chemotherapy +/– radiotherapy. This has to be taken into account when operative strategies are planned.

18.4.3.1 Cervical Esophageal Cancer

Cervical ESCC justifies separate consideration. It accounts for 2–10% of all esophageal carcinomas, and by convention, this cancer is treated by pharyngo-laryngo-esophagectomy (PLE) with or without adjuvant radiotherapy. PLE with one-stage gastric pull-up was first described by GB Ong in 1960 from the authors' institution [69]. The original description of PLE involved a thoracotomy for esophageal mobilization. This was later modified so that a transhiatal approach was used without a thoracotomy. This was again changed when videoscopic-assisted thoracoscopy (VATS) became available [70, 71].

In recent years, laryngeal preservation has been the aim of treatment, and definitive chemoradiation therapy is generally preferred; surgery is reserved for those who respond suboptimally or when recurrence develops. While definitive chemoradiation is widely practiced, out data show that this type of strategy is not without drawbacks. Chemoradiation-related complications include mucositis, vocal cord palsies, esophageal stricture, carotid blowout, hypothyroidism, and hypoparathyroidism. Persistent dysphagia affects 29% of patients, and 38% eventually require surgery as salvage. Salvage surgery has suboptimal results, disease status, and prior heavy irradiation increases morbidities. In patients with locally advanced disease, especially in those with extra-esophageal extension, upfront surgery with postoperative radiotherapy as the preferred therapy should be carefully considered, in particular, the outcomes of PLE have also significantly improved over the last few decades [72–75]. Both the anastomotic leak and mortality rates were reduced to 9% [76]. Improvements in surgical technique including thoracoscopic esophageal mobilization, better perioperative care, and patient selection, all contributed to better results [70, 71, 77].

To reduce morbidity further, in patients with limited tumor extension into the intrathoracic esophagus, availability of the technique of free jejunal graft to replace the cervical esophagus has also reduced the need for PLE with total esophageal extirpation [77]. Less morbidity is expected as no thoracic phase and mediastinal dissection are needed. A significant number of patients with primary hypopharyngeal cancer or those with limited involvement of the cervical esophagus can undergo pharyngo-laryngo-cervical esophagectomy. Free jejunal graft is the preferred organ for reconstruction; it has a failure rate of 2% and anastomotic leak rate of 4.6% [76, 78, 79].

18.4.3.2 Intra-Thoracic Esophageal Cancer

The Approach to Resection

Our preferred surgical approach is a transthoracic one. In the past, a randomized trial comparing transthoracic and transhiatal approach for lower third tumors was conducted at the authors' institution [80]. No significant difference was found; the trial sample size was too small to be able to demonstrate any difference. The study was terminated because our focus then shifted to minimally invasive esophagectomy.

In Hong Kong, the application of minimally invasive surgical technology in esophagectomy commenced in the mid-1990s [81]. At the initial stage, thoracoscopic esophageal dissection was applied in lieu of open thoracotomy or transhiatal mobilization of the esophagus in PLE [70]. Then it was applied to intrathoracic esophageal cancers as well. Thoracoscopic esophageal mobilization with lymphadenectomy was carried out, combined with open laparotomy for gastric conduit preparation for cervical esophago-gastrostomy [82]. Our early hypothesis was that minimally invasive method had its maximum benefits in those with high risk of surgery, and such patients were preferentially selected. The early results, though acceptable, were not impressive [81]. This was because of the combination of high-risk patients, immature techniques, and suboptimal instrumentation. The uptake of minimally invasive esophagectomy (MIE) was thus slow. It was not until 2006 that we changed our policy and applied this surgical approach more broadly. In addition, laparoscopic gastric mobilization was introduced so that the whole procedure became totally minimally invasive. Our techniques have also improved, together with better instruments.

To date, we have performed such procedures in more than 500 patients. MIE is the approach in about 82% of our patients; in nearly 70% of these patients, prior neoadjuvant therapy has been applied (12.8% with chemotherapy and 49.4% with chemoradiotherapy). VATS esophagectomy with laparotomy was performed in 219 patients, totally MIE in 218. The median thoracoscopy time was 200 min, blood loss was 200 mls. Our conversion rate (VATS) was 12.6%, reflecting our policy of unselected choice of patients. In one patient, conversion was due to hemorrhage, while most were related to extensive lung adhesions or advanced post-chemoradiated tumors that were found to be unsafe to dissect. In a propensity score-matched analysis of VATS/MIE and conventional open esophagectomies, thoracoscopic approach improved lymph node yield. The median number of lymph nodes harvested was 35, compared to a significantly lower median of 21 nodes in open esophagectomies. It may be explained by better visualization, especially at the apex of the thoracic cavity, by thoracoscopy. There was also significant difference in pulmonary complication rate of 29% in the VATS/MIE group and 55.1% in open esophagectomy group. Long-term survival was not compromised [83]. Results from other trials across the world concur with our findings [81, 82]. Postoperative quality of life has also been demonstrated to be superior [84].

Extent of Resection and Lymphadenectomy

A curative (R0) resection implies histologically clear proximal, distal, and lateral margins. There is propensity of ESCC to have intramural and submucosal spread. Increasing the length of resection margin reduces the chance of a histologically positive resection margin. We advocate an in-situ proximal resection margin length of 10 cm to allow a less than 5% chance of anastomotic recurrence [85]. In our study, 28 (5.3%) out of 524 patients developed anastomotic recurrence; the length of the axial resection margin correlated with the chance of anastomotic recurrence [86]. A negative margin, however, may not totally preclude anastomotic recurrence. In our experience, anastomotic recurrence occurred in 10.2% of patients with positive resection margin compared to 4.9% in those with negative margin [85].

On lymphadenectomy, although extended mediastinal lymphadenectomy is practiced, cervical nodal dissection is not routinely performed at our institution. In patients with overt cervical nodal metastases, our policy is, in general, to treat with upfront chemotherapy +/− radiotherapy before surgical resection. In a study of 109 patients with cervical nodal metastases proven on ultrasound-guided FNA, survival was compared among those with stage IV disease by virtue of cervical nodal disease (AJCC sixth edition) and those with systemic metastases. The former group had significantly longer survival compared to the latter group; median survival was 9.8 months vs. 3 months. More importantly, in those with upfront chemoradiation and then esophagectomy, a median survival of 35 months was achieved [87]. In our experience, cervical lymphadenectomy after neoadjuvant chemoradiation often yields negative nodes on histological examination, but dissection around the recurrent laryngeal nerve may lead to a higher rate of vocal cord palsy. However, nodal dissection should still be performed because of the unreliable means of confirming the absence of metastases after chemoradiation.

In patients with no evidence of cervical nodal metastases on preoperative workup including PET/CT scan and ultrasound, routine cervical lymphadenectomy is not performed. Neck dissection can still be performed later should recurrence occur locally in the cervical region. In our study of recurrence patterns after esophagectomy without routine cervical lymphadenectomy, isolated recurrence in the neck was uncommon. We studied 108 patients who underwent curative resection for ESCC; 56 (52%) of them developed recurrence. There were 12 patients who had cervical nodal recurrence, only four of them had isolated recurrence in the neck. This implies that cervical nodal recurrence, if present, tends to be found together with other sites of recurrences, thus reducing the benefits of cervical lymphadenectomy [86].

Mediastinal dissection, however, is important, especially when future resection for nodal recurrence in the mediastinum is generally not possible after esophagectomy. Therefore, disease control at the time of esophagectomy must be maximized. In the era of neoadjuvant chemoradiation, dissection, especially around the recurrent laryngeal nerve, is difficult with increased risk of nerve injury. And again, prediction of residual positive disease is often unreliable. These factors have to be taken into account when lymph node dissection is considered. For each patient, the risks and benefits should be carefully balanced. As far as surgical technique is concerned, we do not limit MIE to patients without prior neoadjuvant chemoradiation. As stated above, approximately 50% of our patients would have had chemoradiation before esophagectomy. From a technical standpoint, judicious use of energy dissection devices is important to achieve the required lymphadenectomy without risking recurrent laryngeal nerve injury as well as airway injury.

Since 2014, intraoperative nerve conduction study is routinely carried out in esophagectomies at the authors' institution (Fig. 18.3). In our early experience, both intermittent nerve stimulation for mapping and continuous nerve monitoring were routinely used [88, 89]. Overall, the recurrent laryngeal nerve palsy rate was 22.2%, but only 5.2% persisted at 1 year [90]. Although there has not been an apparent reduction in nerve palsy rate since the implementation of this technique compared to our previous data, it might have been contributed by the more extensive lymphadenectomy along the recurrent laryngeal nerves since the use of intraoperative nerve monitoring. The use of this technology to safeguard recurrent laryngeal nerve injury is still investigational. Our current practice is intermittent nerve stimulation alone, as we have accumulated experience in extensive recurrent laryngeal nerve dissection over the years. Despite advancements in surgical precision enabled by minimally invasive surgery and intraoperative nerve conduction study as an adjunct, safeguarding the left recurrent laryngeal nerve still proves to be challenging even in high-volume institutions around the world, especially for patients post-chemoradiotherapy [91, 92]. In recent years, left recurrent nerve palsy rate at our institution is 14.4%. Overall recurrent nerve palsy rate is 19.6%, and 27% of which persisted for more than 6 months. So, overall persistent palsy rate is 5.3%.

Chylothorax after esophagectomy is not common but is associated with increased morbidity and prolonged hospitalization. Indocyanine green dye can be administered in various ways to enhance visualization of the thoracic duct, which is difficult to locate due to its inconspicuous structure and complex anatomical variations [93]. To the authors' experience, it is still uncertain whether the application of ICG in such context would reduce the incidence of chylothorax (Fig. 18.4).

18.4.3.3 Reconstruction

Restoration of the gastrointestinal tract continuity after esophagectomy has significant impact on immediate postoperative morbidity and long-term quality of life.

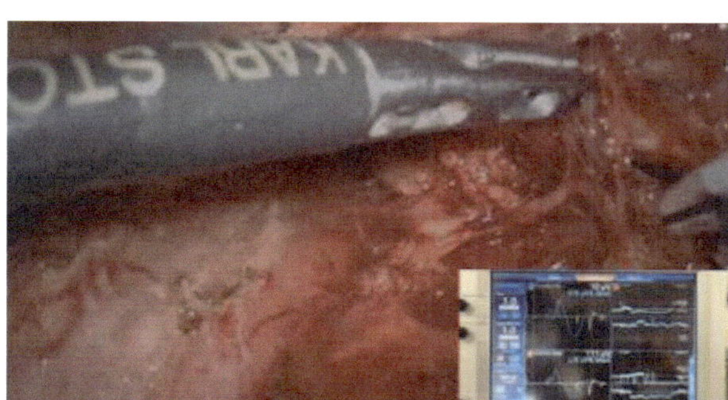

Fig. 18.3 Recurrent laryngeal nerve lymphadenectomy showing the effect on intraoperative continual nerve monitoring. Traction of the left recurrent laryngeal nerve results in an increase of the latency of nerve condition.

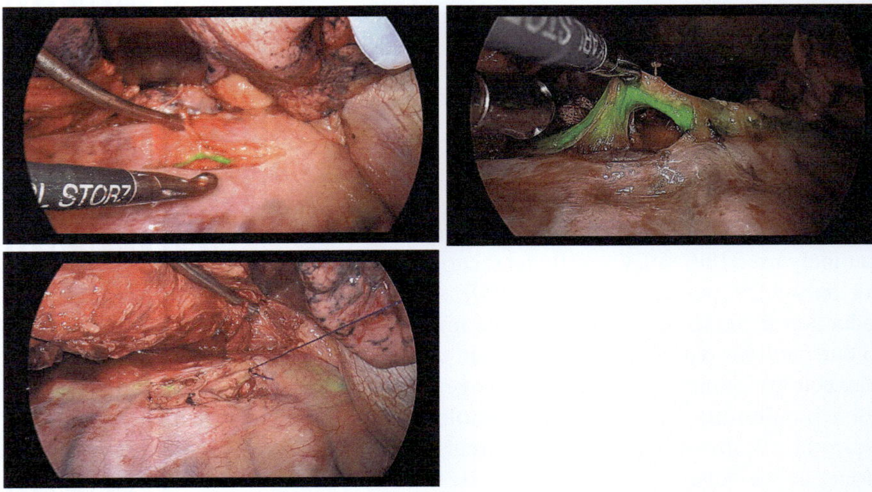

Fig. 18.4 Indocyanine green dye fluorescent enhancement of the thoracic duct during video-thoracoscopic-assisted esophagectomy. Top left: Exposed thoracic duct with ICG enhancement at the lower mediastinum; Top right: ICG-enhanced thoracic duct being isolated; Bottom: ICG-enhanced thoracic duct being ligated

The authors' institution has performed many studies on reconstructive techniques and their relationship to morbidity and mortality after esophagectomy.

A pyloric drainage procedure remains controversial. Pyloroplasty is a routine procedure during esophagectomy by the authors. In a randomized trial comparing outcomes after a Lewis-Tanner esophagectomy with or without a pyloroplasty, 13% of patients who did not have the drainage procedure had delayed gastric emptying [94]. A pyloromyotomy was shown to be as effective [95, 96]. Although meta-analyses have not proven the role of pyloroplasty and other factors are probably contributory to gastric emptying, based on our own experience, we perform pyloroplasty for all patients, except in those whose stomach length is short, and foregoing the pyloroplasty could preserve more length of the gastric conduit.

Our preferred conduit is the gastric tube because of its ease of preparation and reliability. Right ileo-colonic interposition is our second choice for esophageal replacement. Colonic interposition reconstruction is associated with higher morbidity rates, such as more blood loss, longer operating duration, and higher anastomotic leak rate [97]. In 57 patients who had colonic interpositions, the reasons for using the colon as the esophageal substitute were prior gastrectomy in 34 (59.6%), tumor involvement of the stomach in 18 (31.6%), presence of peptic ulcer in 3(5.3%), and for other reasons: 2(3.5%). Four patients (7%) developed ischemia and required re-exploration, nine (15.8%) had anastomotic leak, and two patients (3.5%) died within 30 days of surgery [98].

Our preferred route of reconstruction when cervical anastomosis is performed is the retrosternal route. We see several advantages over the posterior mediastinum as the route of reconstruction. Compared to the posterior mediastinal route, longer gastric conduit transit time in the retrosternal route was described, which did not translate into difference in dysphagic symptoms and quality of life of patients [99]. In our own experience, the use of retrosternal route is in fact associated with fewer emptying problems. It contrasts with the posterior mediastinal route, where the gastric conduit could flop into the right paravertebral space, resulting in distension or twisting (Fig. 18.5). In case of residual tumor left in the posterior mediastinum after resection, reconstruction via the retrosternal route prevents tumor ingrowth from recurrent disease. Postoperative radiotherapy can also be given to the tumor bed, avoiding injury to the gastric conduit. Another application of retrosternal route is when the reconstructive phase of the surgery precedes the resection phase. The conduit is brought up to the neck via the new surgical plane (retrosternal route) before the thoracotomy for tumor resection. This is a routine practice by the authors when a colonic interposition is planned.

It has been reported that retrosternal route is associated with increased cardiopulmonary morbidity[99], but in a meta-analysis, it was not associated with increased perioperative morbidity compared to reconstruction through the posterior mediastinum [100]. In our experience, no difference was found comparing the posterior mediastinal and retrosternal routes of reconstruction in intraoperative blood loss, operative duration, cardiopulmonary complications, leak, and mortality rates [101].

Much effort was made in studying the optimal esophageal anastomosis after esophagectomy. Anastomotic leak and stricture remain problematic areas in many centers around the world. The location and technique of anastomosis affect the outcomes of esophagectomy [102]. Anastomosis can be located in the neck or in the thoracic cavity. It is generally believed that cervical anastomosis is associated with a higher leak rate, but it is more easily managed and results in lower mortality rate

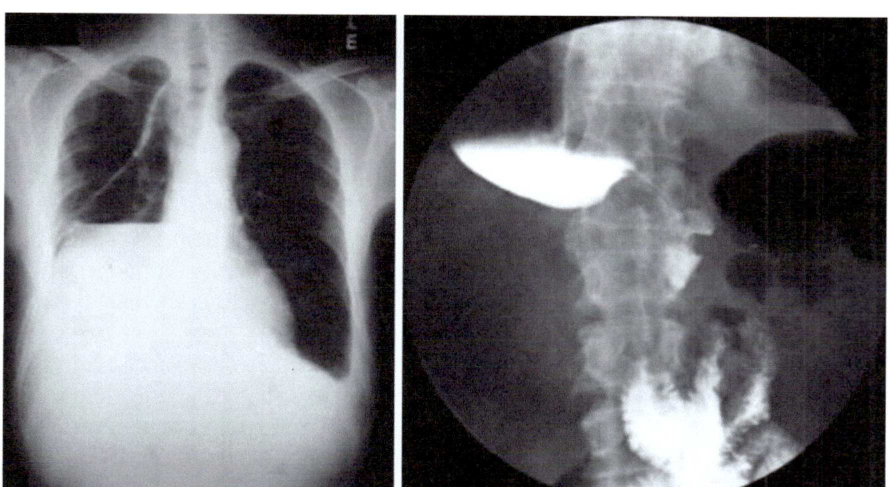

Fig. 18.5 Distended intrathoracic stomach as a result of a wide gastric tube rotated and flopping into the right paravertebral space. Right panel: Dilated stomach with the fluid level. Left panel: A contrast study showing the hold-up of contrast in the dilated stomach. This is not the site of the pyloroplasty

[103]. However, in our experience, a cervical anastomosis is no more likely to leak compared to its intra-thoracic counterpart, both occurring at around 4%. Mortality rates were also similar. If hand-sewn method is used, the stricture rate is also similar at around 10%.

The technique of anastomosis was studied in a randomized controlled trial comparing a circular stapling device and a hand-sewn method. Similar leak rates were found; 1.8% for hand-sewn and 5% for circular stapler [104]. The stricture rate, however, was fourfold with the stapling technique, 9.1% vs. 40% [104]. Our preferred way of anastomosis thus remains a one-layer hand-sewn method with a fine monofilament suture. The exception being a low mediastinal anastomosis performed via the abdomen for a gastric cardia lesion, where exposure for a hand-sewn method is generally inadequate. For these lesions, our experience has evolved from using circular stapler to linear stapling, which involves side-to-side anastomosis of the esophageal stump to the gastric conduit and stapled closure of the defect.

The authors' institution has previously reported the leak rate of below 5% and that most of the leaks were related to technical faults [14, 105] such as tension between the conduit and esophageal stump or conduit ischemia. The principles of management of leaks are early detection, maintenance of nutrition, and treatment of sepsis. Depending on the severity, general condition of the patient, and the location of the anastomosis, approaches to manage anastomotic leak vary. Most leaks from cervical anastomoses can be managed conservatively by drainage via cervical wound with or without nasogastric tube drainage and enteral nutrition via nasoduodenal tube. Our practice has been to deploy a negative pressure dressing system to the cervical surgical bed to facilitate drainage and promote healing by granulation. Surgical exploration for drainage is reserved for large-sized defects and leaks that do not respond to the strategy aforementioned. In patients with frank conduit ischemia, it is important to diagnose and explore early before actual leakage occurs and sepsis ensures. Immediate re-anastomosis is sometimes possible in stable patients with limited necrosis. Historically, a take-down of the ischemic stomach is necessary for most, and staged reconstruction is later carried out. In selected patients whose extent of conduit necrosis does not allow immediate re-anastomosis, intervening free jejunal flap reconstruction with manubrial resection to facilitate exposure may be performed. The use of indocyanine green fluorescent angiography is an increasingly useful adjunct in assessing conduit vascularity intraoperatively (Fig. 18.6). This should reduce the incidence of ischemic conduits and may be anastomotic leak rates as well [106].

Management of leaks has improved so that most patients are successfully salvaged. In the 1960s and 1970s, our leakage rate was 16%, and 61% of patients died, making a leak-related mortality of 9.8%; in the 1980s and 1990s, leakage rate was 3.5%, 35% of patients died, making a leak-related mortality rate of 1.2%. This subsequently improved to 3.2%, and there was no mortality [37, 105, 107].

18.4.3.4 Postoperative Management

The appropriate selection of surgical procedures, its meticulous execution, and perioperative care have a causal relationship with morbidity and mortality. For most

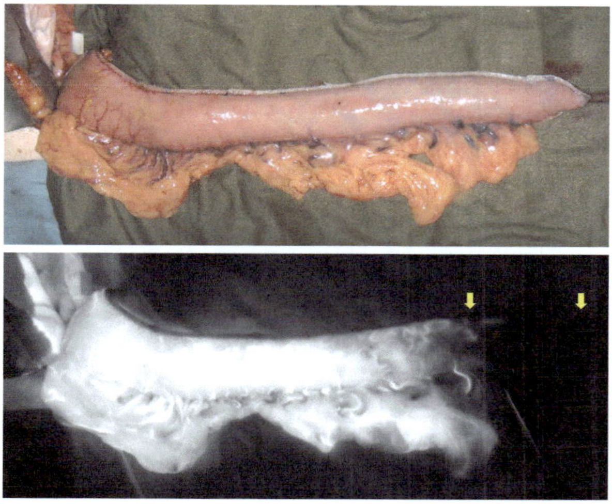

Fig. 18.6 Indocyanine green fluorescence showing poor perfusion at the tip of the gastric conduit (indicated by the arrows)

patients, a standardized clinical pathway is helpful, along the lines of ERAS protocol (Table 18.1):

- Most patients have endotracheal tube extubation in the recovery room, unless the surgery has been prolonged, complicated, or performed in high-risk patients.
- Epidural analgesia is most important in postoperative pain relief. It is continued for the first 4–5 days after surgery and can be replaced by patient-controlled analgesia or oral medications. Recently, a propensity score-matched analysis revealed that postoperative scheduled intravenous acetaminophen decreased the rate of opioid use and may contribute to ERAS program for esophagectomy [108].
- At the author's unit, the nasogastric tube is usually removed the day after surgery. Early removal of the tube results in more comfort and facilitates coughing. There is no need to replace the tube unless progressive dilatation of the gastroplasty is seen, but this is uncommon with a narrow gastric tube with a drainage procedure.
- All patients have a bronchoscopic examination on the first postoperative day to check for recurrent laryngeal nerve injury although this is unusual in the absence of superior mediastinal or cervical lymphadenectomy. Judicious use of intravenous fluid is also important to avoid over-hydration and pulmonary edema.
- Chest physiotherapy is instituted, and early ambulation is encouraged.
- Deep vein thrombosis prophylaxis is continued.
- Chest drain is removed on day 4–5 post operation, the daily output should be less than 200–300 ml per day.
- Liquid by mouth is started on day 1 post-operation; usually, a carbohydrate drink can be taken as sips of fluid. Generally, by days 3–4, patients can take a liquid diet freely. A soft diet is started on day 5 post-operation. The early oral intake does not increase the incidence of anastomotic leak and pneumonia*. An oral contrast study is not routine unless leakage is suspected or if there is evidence of

delayed gastric emptying. The author does not place feeding jejunostomy as a routine because early oral alimentation is successful in most patients, and most do not need supplementary nutritional support. Should oral intake be delayed, such as when anastomotic leak occurs, endoscopic placement of a nasoduodenal tube for feeding will suffice.

18.4.3.5 Other Morbidities and Mortality

In our experience, the commonest medical complications are atrial fibrillation and pulmonary morbidities (pneumonia, atelectasis, sputum retention, and respiratory failure). Atrial fibrillation affects about 20% of our patients. Although it is relatively benign and is easily controlled with appropriate anti-arrhythmic medications, it may be reflective of underlying more serious events, such as pneumonia, anastomotic leak, or conduit ischemia [109]. Among a cohort of 921 patients, 198 (22%) developed postoperative atrial fibrillation; pulmonary complications affected 42% of patients in the atrial fibrillation group compared to only 17% among the controls. Similarly, anastomotic leak was more common (6.9% vs. 1.4%, $p = 0.035$); surgical sepsis was also four times more frequent ($p = 0.001$). Occurrence of atrial fibrillation should prompt a search for an underlying cause. It is our policy to have a low threshold for performing endoscopy to look for complications with the anastomosis or conduit whenever such arrhythmia occurs, so that we can intervene early if required.

Pneumonia and respiratory failure occur in 15.9% of our patients and are responsible for 55% of the hospital mortality. A cohort study from our institution demonstrated that advanced age, tumor location above the tracheal bifurcation, and long operative duration were independent risk factors for pulmonary complications [15]. The chance of developing a major respiratory complication was twice in those older than 70 years, and the death rate was fourfold higher. Patients with a supra-carinal tumor had a 3.5 times higher risk of developing pulmonary complications when compared to tumors located more distally. The measures to reduce pulmonary complications include cessation of smoking preoperatively, early institution of chest physiotherapy, avoidance of recurrent laryngeal nerve injury, avoidance of fluid overload, use of smaller-sized chest tube, early ambulation, regular bronchoscopic toileting, and early tracheostomy should sputum retention be severe. Postoperative pain control with epidural analgesia is invaluable [110].

The hospital mortality rate in the 1980s in the authors' institution was 11%–15.5% [14, 111]. The respective figures reduced to 3.2% in the early 1990s and 1.1% in the late 1990s, respectively [15, 111]. Mortality rate since 2000 has remained below 3%. Surgical volume and experience have obvious positive impact on outcome.

18.4.3.6 Palliation

Various treatment modalities are available for palliation. Radiotherapy +/− chemotherapy is used in selected patients. Pain and dysphagia are the most frequent symptoms that need palliation in our patients. Pain anesthesiologists are often an integral part of our management. To palliate dysphagia, our preferred choice of endoscopic treatment is placement of self-expanding metallic stents (SEMS) [112]. Palliative resections and bypass procedures, such as the Kirschner bypass using gastric or colonic conduits, are seldom necessary nowadays [113, 114].

18.5 Summary

In Hong Kong, ESCC remains one of the most challenging cancers. Steady advances have been made in the last three decades in staging methods, surgery, and multimodality strategies. Like many centers in the world, a low mortality rate after esophagectomy has been achieved. Morbidity rates, however, remain substantial [115]. Although progress has been made in prolonging long-term survival, there is still much room for improvement. Owing to positive results from neoadjuvant therapy, watchful waiting after neoadjuvant therapy and salvage surgery on an as-needed basis in selected patients with good clinical response is being tested. Results from such research may allow finer individualization of treatment strategy in patients suffering from this highly lethal cancer, so that survival and quality of life can be optimized.

References

1. Bray F, Laversanne M, Sung H, et al. Global cancer statistics 2022: GLOBOCAN estimates of incidence and mortality worldwide for 36 cancers in 185 countries. CA Cancer J Clin. 2024;74(3):229–63.
2. Lo OS, Law S, Wei WI, et al. Esophageal cancers with synchronous or antecedent head and neck cancers: a more formidable challenge? Ann Surg Oncol. 2008;15(6):1750–6.
3. Poon RT, Law SY, Chu KM, Branicki FJ, Wong J. Multiple primary cancers in esophageal squamous cell carcinoma: incidence and implications. Ann Thorac Surg. 1998;65(6):1529–34.
4. Cheung HC, Siu KF, Wong J. A comparison of flexible and rigid endoscopy in evaluating esophageal cancer patients for surgery. World J Surg. 1988;12(1):117–22.
5. Fok M, Cheng SW, Wong J. Endosonography in patient selection for surgical treatment of esophageal carcinoma. World J Surg. 1992;16(6):1098–103. discussion 1103
6. Choi TK, Siu KF, Lam KH, Wong J. Bronchoscopy and carcinoma of the esophagus I. Findings of bronchoscopy in carcinoma of the esophagus. Am J Surg. 1984;147(6):757–9.
7. Choi TK, Siu KF, Lam KH, Wong J. Bronchoscopy and carcinoma of the esophagus II. Carcinoma of the esophagus with tracheobronchial involvement. Am J Surg. 1984;147(6):760–2.
8. Japan Esophageal S. Japanese classification of esophageal cancer, 11th edition: part I. Esophagus. 2017;14(1):1–36.
9. Puli SR, Reddy JB, Bechtold ML, Antillon D, Ibdah JA, Antillon MR. Staging accuracy of esophageal cancer by endoscopic ultrasound: a meta-analysis and systematic review. World J Gastroenterol. 2008;14(10):1479–90.
10. Lowe VJ, Booya F, Fletcher JG, et al. Comparison of positron emission tomography, computed tomography, and endoscopic ultrasound in the initial staging of patients with esophageal cancer. Mol Imaging Biol. 2005;7(6):422–30.
11. Dittler HJ, Bollschweiler E, Siewert JR. What is the value of endosonography in the preoperative staging of esophageal carcinoma? Dtsch Med Wochenschr. 1991;116(15):561–6.
12. Law S, Wong KH, Tong DK, Wong J. Standardized uptake value (SUV) in PET/CT for oesophageal cancer correlates with pathological stage and predicts R-category of resection. Gut. 2007;56((suppl)):A223.

13. Lagarde SM, Maris AK, de Castro SM, Busch OR, Obertop H, van Lanschot JJ. Evaluation of O-POSSUM in predicting in-hospital mortality after resection for oesophageal cancer. Br J Surg. 2007;94(12):1521–6.
14. Law SY, Fok M, Wong J. Risk analysis in resection of squamous cell carcinoma of the esophagus. World J Surg. 1994;18(3):339–46.
15. Law S, Wong KH, Kwok KF, Chu KM, Wong J. Predictive factors for postoperative pulmonary complications and mortality after esophagectomy for cancer. Ann Surg. 2004;240(5):791–800.
16. Findlay JM, Gillies RS, Millo J, Sgromo B, Marshall RE, Maynard ND. Enhanced recovery for esophagectomy: a systematic review and evidence-based guidelines. Ann Surg. 2014;259(3):413–31.
17. Low DE, Allum W, De Manzoni G, et al. Guidelines for perioperative care in esophagectomy: enhanced recovery after surgery (ERAS(®)) society recommendations. World J Surg. 2019;43(2):299–330.
18. Markar SR, Karthikesalingam A, Low DE. Enhanced recovery pathways lead to an improvement in postoperative outcomes following esophagectomy: systematic review and pooled analysis. Dis Esophagus. 2015;28(5):468–75.
19. Weimann A, Braga M, Carli F, et al. ESPEN practical guideline: clinical nutrition in surgery. Clin Nutr. 2021;40(7):4745–61.
20. Kitagawa Y, Uno T, Oyama T, et al. Esophageal cancer practice guidelines 2017 edited by the Japan esophageal society: part 2. Esophagus. 2019;16(1):25–43.
21. Chen WC, Wolfsen H. Role of radiofrequency ablation in esophageal squamous dysplasia and early neoplasia. Gastrointest Endosc. 2017;85(2):330–1.
22. Haidry RJ, Butt MA, Dunn J, et al. Radiofrequency ablation for early oesophageal squamous neoplasia: outcomes form United Kingdom registry. World J Gastroenterol. 2013;19(36):6011–9.
23. Bergman JJ, Zhang YM, He S, et al. Outcomes from a prospective trial of endoscopic radiofrequency ablation of early squamous cell neoplasia of the esophagus. Gastrointest Endosc. 2011;74(6):1181–90.
24. He S, Bergman J, Zhang Y, et al. Endoscopic radiofrequency ablation for early esophageal squamous cell neoplasia: report of safety and effectiveness from a large prospective trial. Endoscopy. 2015;47(5):398–408.
25. Allum WH, Stenning SP, Bancewicz J, Clark PI, Langley RE. Long-term results of a randomized trial of surgery with or without preoperative chemotherapy in esophageal cancer. J Clin Oncol. 2009;27(30):5062–7.
26. Medical Research Council Oesophageal Cancer Working G. Surgical resection with or without preoperative chemotherapy in oesophageal cancer: a randomised controlled trial. Lancet. 2002;359(9319):1727–33.
27. Ando N, Kato H, Igaki H, et al. A randomized trial comparing postoperative adjuvant chemotherapy with cisplatin and 5-fluorouracil versus preoperative chemotherapy for localized advanced squamous cell carcinoma of the thoracic esophagus (JCOG9907). Ann Surg Oncol. 2012;19(1):68–74.
28. Herskovic A, Martz K, al-Sarraf M, et al. Combined chemotherapy and radiotherapy compared with radiotherapy alone in patients with cancer of the esophagus. N Engl J Med. 1992;326(24):1593–8.
29. al-Sarraf M, Martz K, Herskovic A, et al. Progress report of combined chemoradiotherapy versus radiotherapy alone in patients with esophageal cancer: an intergroup study. J Clin Oncol. 1997;15(1):277–84.
30. Cooper JS, Guo MD, Herskovic A, et al. Chemoradiotherapy of locally advanced esophageal cancer: long-term follow-up of a prospective randomized trial (RTOG 85-01). Radiation Therapy Oncology Group. Jama. 1999;281(17):1623–7.
31. van Hagen P, Hulshof MC, van Lanschot JJ, et al. Preoperative chemoradiotherapy for esophageal or junctional cancer. N Engl J Med. 2012;366(22):2074–84.

32. Fok M, Sham JS, Choy D, Cheng SW, Wong J. Postoperative radiotherapy for carcinoma of the esophagus: a prospective, randomized controlled study. Surgery. 1993;113(2):138–47.
33. Chen J, Zhu J, Pan J, et al. Postoperative radiotherapy improved survival of poor prognostic squamous cell carcinoma esophagus. Ann Thorac Surg. 2010;90(2):435–42.
34. Xiao ZF, Yang ZY, Liang J, et al. Value of radiotherapy after radical surgery for esophageal carcinoma: a report of 495 patients. Ann Thorac Surg. 2003;75(2):331–6.
35. Law S, Fok M, Chow S, Chu KM, Wong J. Preoperative chemotherapy versus surgical therapy alone for squamous cell carcinoma of the esophagus: a prospective randomized trial. J Thorac Cardiovasc Surg. 1997;114(2):210–7.
36. Lam KY, Law S, Ma LT, Ong SK, Wong J. Pre-operative chemotherapy for squamous cell carcinoma of the oesophagus: do histological assessment and p53 overexpression predict chemo-responsiveness? Eur J Cancer. 1997;33(8):1221–5.
37. Law S, Kwong DL, Kwok KF, et al. Improvement in treatment results and long-term survival of patients with esophageal cancer: impact of chemoradiation and change in treatment strategy. Ann Surg. 2003;238(3):339–47. discussion 347–338
38. Tong DK, Law S, Kwong DL, Chan KW, Lam AK, Wong KH. Histological regression of squamous esophageal carcinoma assessed by percentage of residual viable cells after neoadjuvant chemoradiation is an important prognostic factor. Ann Surg Oncol. 2010;17(8):2184–92.
39. Shapiro J, van Lanschot JJB, Hulshof MCCM, et al. Neoadjuvant chemoradiotherapy plus surgery versus surgery alone for oesophageal or junctional cancer (CROSS): long-term results of a randomised controlled trial. Lancet Oncol. 2015;16(9):1090–8.
40. Eyck BM, Gao X, Yang Y, et al. Pathological response to neoadjuvant chemoradiotherapy for oesophageal squamous cell carcinoma: multicentre East Asian and Dutch database comparison. Br J Surg. 2022;109(12):1312–8.
41. Law TLK, Tong D, Chan WL, Chan DKK, Wong IYH, Chan SY, Kwong DLW, Law S. Neoadjuvant chemoradiotherapy in locoregionally advanced squamous cell cancer of the esophagus: beyond CROSS? Dis Esophagus. 2016;29:28A–9A.
42. Wong I, Law S. The CROSS road in neoadjuvant therapy for esophageal cancer: long-term results of CROSS trial. Transl Cancer Res. 2016;5(S3):S415–9.
43. Wong IY-H, Law S. Surgery in the era of neoadjuvant therapy for cancer of the esophagus. Esophagus. 2016;13(2):105–9.
44. Hara H, Tahara M, Daiko H, et al. Phase II feasibility study of preoperative chemotherapy with docetaxel, cisplatin, and fluorouracil for esophageal squamous cell carcinoma. Cancer Sci. 2013;104(11):1455–60.
45. Vermorken JB, Remenar E, van Herpen C, et al. Cisplatin, fluorouracil, and docetaxel in unresectable head and neck cancer. N Engl J Med. 2007;357(17):1695–704.
46. Kato K, Machida R, Ito Y, et al. Doublet chemotherapy, triplet chemotherapy, or doublet chemotherapy combined with radiotherapy as neoadjuvant treatment for locally advanced oesophageal cancer (JCOG1109 NExT): a randomised, controlled, open-label, phase 3 trial. Lancet. 2024;404(10447):55–66.
47. Tsang JS, Tong DKH, Lam KO, et al. Appropriate timing for surgery after neoadjuvant chemoradiation for esophageal cancer. Dis Esophagus. 2017;30(9):1–8.
48. Law S, Kwong DL, Wong KH, Kwok KF, Wong J. The effects of neoadjuvant chemoradiation on pTNM staging and its prognostic significance in esophageal cancer. J Gastrointest Surg. 2006;10(9):1301–11.
49. Rice TW, Gress DM, Patil DT, Hofstetter WL, Kelsen DP, Blackstone EH. Cancer of the esophagus and esophagogastric junction-major changes in the American joint committee on cancer eighth edition cancer staging manual. CA Cancer J Clin. 2017;67(4):304–17.
50. Rice TKBE, et al. Esophagus and esophagogastric junction. In: Amin ME, Greene FL, editors. AJCC cancer staging manual. 8th ed. New York: Springer; 2017b. p. 185–202.
51. Swisher SG, Hofstetter W, Wu TT, et al. Proposed revision of the esophageal cancer staging system to accommodate pathologic response (pP) following preoperative chemoradiation (CRT). Ann Surg. 2005;241(5):810–7. discussion 817–820

52. Yuan H, Tong DK, Vardhanabhuti V, Law SY, Chiu KW, Khong PL. PET/CT in the evaluation of treatment response to neoadjuvant chemoradiotherapy and prognostication in patients with locally advanced esophageal squamous cell carcinoma. Nucl Med Commun. 2016;37(9):947–55.
53. Weber WA, Ott K, Becker K, et al. Prediction of response to preoperative chemotherapy in adenocarcinomas of the esophagogastric junction by metabolic imaging. J Clin Oncol. 2001;19(12):3058–65.
54. Wong C, Law S. Predictive factors in the evaluation of treatment response to neoadjuvant chemoradiotherapy in patients with advanced esophageal squamous cell cancer. J Thorac Dis. 2017;9(Suppl 8):S773–80.
55. Lordick F, Ott K, Krause BJ, et al. PET to assess early metabolic response and to guide treatment of adenocarcinoma of the oesophagogastric junction: the MUNICON phase II trial. Lancet Oncol. 2007;8(9):797–805.
56. Lai KK, Chan KT, Choi MY, et al. 14-3-3σ confers cisplatin resistance in esophageal squamous cell carcinoma cells via regulating DNA repair molecules. Tumour Biol. 2016;37(2):2127–36.
57. Lau MC, Ng KY, Wong TL, et al. FSTL1 promotes metastasis and Chemoresistance in esophageal squamous cell carcinoma through NFκB-BMP signaling cross-talk. Cancer Res. 2017;77(21):5886–99.
58. Li B, Li J, Xu WW, et al. Suppression of esophageal tumor growth and chemoresistance by directly targeting the PI3K/AKT pathway. Oncotarget. 2014;5(22):11576–87.
59. Li B, Xu WW, Guan XY, et al. Competitive binding between Id1 and E2F1 to Cdc20 regulates E2F1 degradation and thymidylate synthase expression to promote esophageal cancer chemoresistance. Clin Cancer Res. 2016;22(5):1243–55.
60. Li B, Hong P, Zheng CC, et al. Identification of miR-29c and its target FBXO31 as a key regulatory mechanism in esophageal cancer chemoresistance: functional validation and clinical significance. Theranostics. 2019;9(6):1599–613.
61. Chan CM, Lai KKY, Ng EKO, et al. Serum microRNA-193b as a promising biomarker for prediction of chemoradiation sensitivity in esophageal squamous cell carcinoma patients. Oncol Lett. 2018;15(3):3273–80.
62. Chan D, Zhou Y, Chui CH, et al. Expression of insulin-like growth factor binding Protein-5 (IGFBP5) reverses cisplatin-resistance in esophageal carcinoma. Cells. 2018;7(10):143.
63. Bedenne L. Comparison of systemic surgery versus surveillance and rescue surgery in operable oesophageal cancer with a complete clinical response to radiochemotherapy (esostrate). https://wwwclinicaltrialsgov/ct2/show/NCT02551458. 2015.
64. Noordman BJ, Spaander MCW, Valkema R, et al. Detection of residual disease after neoadjuvant chemoradiotherapy for oesophageal cancer (preSANO): a prospective multicentre, diagnostic cohort study. Lancet Oncol. 2018;19(7):965–74.
65. van der Wilk BJ, Eyck BM, Wijnhoven BPL, et al. Neoadjuvant chemoradiotherapy followed by active surveillance versus standard surgery for oesophageal cancer (SANO trial): a multicentre, stepped-wedge, cluster-randomised, non-inferiority, phase 3 trial. Lancet Oncol. 2025;26(4):425–36.
66. Yang Y, Liu Z, Wong I, et al. Detecting residual disease after neoadjuvant chemoradiotherapy for oesophageal squamous cell carcinoma: the prospective multicentre preSINO trial. Br J Surg. 2025;112(2):znae342.
67. Kelly RJ, Ajani JA, Kuzdzal J, et al. Adjuvant Nivolumab in resected esophageal or gastroesophageal junction cancer. N Engl J Med. 2021;384(13):1191–203.
68. Kelly RJ, et al. Adjuvant nivolumab in resected esophageal or gastroesophageal junction cancer (EC/GEJC) following neoadjuvant chemoradiotherapy (CRT): first results of overall survival (OS) from CheckMate 577. J Clin Oncol. 2025;43:4000.
69. Ong GB, Lee TC. Pharyngogastric anastomosis after oesophago-pharyngectomy for carcinoma of the hypopharynx and cervical oesophagus. Br J Surg. 1960;48:193–200.
70. Law SY, Fok M, Wei WI, et al. Thoracoscopic esophageal mobilization for pharyngolaryngoesophagectomy. Ann Thorac Surg. 2000;70(2):418–22.

71. Cense HA, Law S, Wei W, et al. Pharyngolaryngoesophagectomy using the thoracoscopic approach. Surg Endosc. 2007;21(6):879–84.
72. Wei WI, Lam LK, Yuen PW, Wong J. Current status of pharyngolaryngo-esophagectomy and pharyngogastric anastomosis. Head Neck. 1998;20(3):240–4.
73. Lam KH, Wong J, Lim ST, Ong GB. Pharyngogastric anastomosis following pharyngolaryngoesophagectomy. Analysis of 157 cases. World J Surg. 1981;5(4):509–16.
74. Spiro RH, Bains MS, Shah JP, Strong EW. Gastric transposition for head and neck cancer: a critical update. Am J Surg. 1991;162(4):348–52.
75. Le Quesne LP, Ranger D. Pharyngolaryngectomy, with immediate pharyngogastric anastomosis. Br J Surg. 1966;53(2):105–9.
76. Wei WI, Lam LK, Yuen PW, Kwong D, Chan KW. Mucosal changes of the free jejunal graft in response to radiotherapy. Am J Surg. 1998;175(1):44–6.
77. Tong DK, Law S, Kwong DL, Wei WI, Ng RW, Wong KH. Current management of cervical esophageal cancer. World J Surg. 2011;35(3):600–7.
78. Chan JY, Liu LH, Wei WI. Early prediction of anastomotic leakage after free jejunal flap reconstruction of circumferential pharyngeal defects. J Plast Reconstr Aesthet Surg. 2013;66(3):376–81.
79. Chow VLY, Chan JYW, Law SYK. Esophagogastric preservation in the surgical management of proximal esophageal cancer. Ann Thorac Surg. 2019;108(4):1029–36.
80. Chu KM, Law SY, Fok M, Wong J. A prospective randomized comparison of transhiatal and transthoracic resection for lower-third esophageal carcinoma. Am J Surg. 1997;174(3):320–4.
81. Law S, Fok M, Chu KM, Wong J. Thoracoscopic esophagectomy for esophageal cancer. Surgery. 1997;122(1):8–14.
82. Law S, Wong J. Use of minimally invasive oesophagectomy for cancer of the oesophagus. Lancet Oncol. 2002;3(4):215–22.
83. Kwan Kit Chan D, Siu Yin Chan F, King Hung Tong D, et al. FA01.01: Minimally invasive approach results in better outcome compared to open esophagectomy-a propensity score matched analysis. Dis Esophagus. 2018;31(13):1.
84. Biere SS, van Berge Henegouwen MI, Maas KW, et al. Minimally invasive versus open oesophagectomy for patients with oesophageal cancer: a multicentre, open-label, randomised controlled trial. Lancet. 2012;379(9829):1887–92.
85. Law S, Arcilla C, Chu KM, Wong J. The significance of histologically infiltrated resection margin after esophagectomy for esophageal cancer. Am J Surg. 1998;176(3):286–90.
86. Law SY, Fok M, Wong J. Pattern of recurrence after oesophageal resection for cancer: clinical implications. Br J Surg. 1996;83(1):107–11.
87. Tong DK, Kwong DL, Law S, Wong KH, Wong J. Cervical nodal metastasis from intrathoracic esophageal squamous cell carcinoma is not necessarily an incurable disease. J Gastrointest Surg. 2008;12(10):1638–45. discussion 1645
88. Wong I, Tong DKH, Tsang RKY, et al. Continuous intraoperative vagus nerve stimulation for monitoring of recurrent laryngeal nerve during minimally invasive esophagectomy. J Vis Surg. 2017;3:9.
89. Tsang RK, Law S. Adaptation of continuous intraoperative Vagus nerve stimulation for monitoring of recurrent laryngeal nerve during minimally invasive Esophagectomy. World J Surg. 2016;40(1):137–41.
90. Wong I TR, Chan DKK, Wong CLY, Tong DKH, Chan FSY, Law SYK. Experience from 102 patients with continuous intraoperative vagus nerve stimulation during minimally invasive esophagectomy. International Society of Diseases of the Esophagus Scientific Congress Vienna. 2018: 689.
91. Chiu CH, Wen YW, Chao YK. Lymph node dissection along the recurrent laryngeal nerves in patients with oesophageal cancer who had undergone chemoradiotherapy: is it safe? Eur J Cardiothorac Surg. 2018;54(4):657–63.
92. Taniyama Y, Okamoto H, Sato C, et al. Prevention and management of recurrent laryngeal nerve palsy in minimally invasive esophagectomy: current status and future perspectives. J Clin Med. 2024;13(24):7611.

93. Peristeri DV, Baltatzis M. Real-time fluorescence imaging for thoracic duct identification during oesophagectomy: a systematic review of the literature. J Chest Surg. 2025;58(1):5–14.
94. Fok M, Cheng SW, Wong J. Pyloroplasty versus no drainage in gastric replacement of the esophagus. Am J Surg. 1991;162(5):447–52.
95. Lee YM, Law S, Chu KM, Wong J. Pyloroplasty in gastric replacement of the esophagus after esophagectomy: one-layer or two-layer technique? Dis Esophagus. 2000;13(3):203–6.
96. Law S, Cheung MC, Fok M, Chu KM, Wong J. Pyloroplasty and pyloromyotomy in gastric replacement of the esophagus after esophagectomy: a randomized controlled trial. J Am Coll Surg. 1997;184(6):630–6.
97. Davis PA, Law S, Wong J. Colonic interposition after esophagectomy for cancer. Arch Surg. 2003;138(3):303–8.
98. Tong DK, Law S, Chan SY. Operative outcomes of colonic interposition in the treatment of esophageal cancer: a three decades experience. Gastroenterology. 2012;142(5 Supplement 1):S-1075.
99. Gawad KA, Hosch SB, Bumann D, et al. How important is the route of reconstruction after esophagectomy: a prospective randomized study. Am J Gastroenterol. 1999;94(6):1490–6.
100. Urschel JD, Urschel DM, Miller JD, Bennett WF, Young JEM. A meta-analysis of randomized controlled trials of route of reconstruction after esophagectomy for cancer. Am J Surg. 2001;182:470–5.
101. Wong AC, Law S, Wong J. Influence of the route of reconstruction on morbidity, mortality and local recurrence after esophagectomy for cancer. Dig Surg. 2003;20(3):209–14.
102. Tong DK, Law S. Reconstruction after pharyngolaryngectomy and esophagectomy: challenges and outcomes. Japan Bronco-Esophagological Society. 2013;64(2):65–70.
103. Biere SS, Maas KW, Cuesta MA, van der Peet DL. Cervical or thoracic anastomosis after esophagectomy for cancer: a systematic review and meta-analysis. Dig Surg. 2011;28(1):29–35.
104. Law S, Fok M, Chu KM, Wong J. Comparison of hand-sewn and stapled esophagogastric anastomosis after esophageal resection for cancer: a prospective randomized controlled trial. Ann Surg. 1997;226(2):169–73.
105. Whooley BP, Law S, Alexandrou A, Murthy SC, Wong J. Critical appraisal of the significance of intrathoracic anastomotic leakage after esophagectomy for cancer. Am J Surg. 2001;181(3):198–203.
106. Wong ICS, Tong DKH, Chan DKK, Wong C, Law TT, Law S. Use of indocyanine green (ICG) fluorescence in minimally invasive esophagectomy to assess conduit vascularity. Gastroenterology. 2017b;152:S1243.
107. Lorentz T, Fok M, Wong J. Anastomotic leakage after resection and bypass for esophageal cancer: lessons learned from the past. World J Surg. 1989;13(4):472–7.
108. Ohkura Y, Shindoh J, Ueno M, Iizuka T, Haruta S, Udagawa H. A new postoperative pain management (intravenous acetaminophen: Acelio®) leads to enhanced recovery after esophagectomy: a propensity score-matched analysis. Surg Today. 2018;48(5):502–9.
109. Murthy SC, Law S, Whooley BP, Alexandrou A, Chu KM, Wong J. Atrial fibrillation after esophagectomy is a marker for postoperative morbidity and mortality. J Thorac Cardiovasc Surg. 2003;126(4):1162–7.
110. Tsui SL, Law S, Fok M, et al. Postoperative analgesia reduces mortality and morbidity after esophagectomy. Am J Surg. 1997;173(6):472–8.
111. Whooley BP, Law S, Murthy SC, Alexandrou A, Wong J. Analysis of reduced death and complication rates after esophageal resection. Ann Surg. 2001;233(3):338–44.
112. Tong DK, Law S, Wong KH. The use of self-expanding metallic stents (SEMS) is effective in symptom palliation from recurrent tumor after esophagogastrectomy for cancer. Dis Esophagus. 2010;23(8):660–5.
113. Whooley BP, Law S, Murthy SC, Alexandrou A, Chu KM, Wong J. The Kirschner operation in unresectable esophageal cancer: current application. Arch Surg. 2002;137(11):1228–32.
114. Wong J, Lam KH, Wei WI, Ong GB. Results of the Kirschner operation. World J Surg. 1981;5(4):547–52.
115. Low DE, Kuppusamy MK, Alderson D, et al. Benchmarking complications associated with Esophagectomy. Ann Surg. 2019;269(2):291–8.

Indian Experiences

19

C. S. Pramesh, Devayani Niyogi, Virendra Kumar Tiwari, Karthik Venkataramani, Apurva Ashok, Sabita Jiwnani, Madhavi Shetmahajan, and Priya Ranganathan

19.1 Introduction

Esophageal cancer is a morbid disease and globally is a major cause of cancer-related deaths [1]. Worldwide, squamous cell carcinoma is the commonest type of esophageal cancer, although there has been an exponential increase in the incidence of adenocarcinoma in the western world in the past three decades [2–5]. The overall disease spectrum has unique geographic distribution, with squamous cancers being common in Asia (countries like China, Iran, India, Japan, and Korea) and adenocarcinomas of the gastroesophageal junction and lower esophagus in North America and Europe [3–5].

C. S. Pramesh (✉) · D. Niyogi · V. K. Tiwari · K. Venkataramani · S. Jiwnani
Division of Thoracic Surgery, Department of Surgical Oncology, Tata Memorial Centre, Homi Bhabha National Institute, Mumbai, Maharashtra, India
e-mail: cspramesh@ncgindia.org

A. Ashok
Department of Surgical Oncology, Tata Medical Center, Kolkata, West Bengal, India

M. Shetmahajan · P. Ranganathan
Department of Anesthesiology, Critical Care and Pain, Tata Memorial Centre, Homi Bhabha National Institute, Mumbai, Maharashtra, India

Y. Kitagawa et al. (eds.), *Esophageal Squamous Cell Carcinoma*,
https://doi.org/10.1007/978-981-92-2611-5_19

19.2 Epidemiology, Etiology, Diagnosis and Staging of Squamous Esophageal Cancer in India

19.2.1 Epidemiology of Esophageal Cancer in India

In India, esophageal cancer is the fourth most common cancer in males and the fifth most common cancer in females, with an estimated incidence of over 70,000 new diagnoses in 2022 [2]. It is also the fifth most common cause of cancer-related deaths in India [2]. As in most parts of Asia, most esophageal cancers in India are squamous cell carcinoma [6, 7] although there has been a recent increase in the incidence of adenocarcinoma [8]. In a retrospective study [9] involving 1000 patients with esophageal cancer over 16 years, patients were divided into four cohorts of 4 years each. Lower esophageal cancers outnumbered the mid-esophageal cancers in the 4th cohort, though mid-esophageal cancers represented the most common site of malignancy overall. However, there have been no systematic prospective studies on the changing epidemiology and histopathological profile of esophageal cancer in India. Regional variations in the incidence of esophageal squamous cancer have been observed in India, with markedly higher rates seen in the Kashmir valley [10] and northeastern India [11]. Overall, approximately 80% of all esophageal cancers in India are squamous cancers, with 20% being adenocarcinomas.

19.2.2 Etiology

The common risk factors for esophageal squamous cell carcinoma (ESCC) in India include smoking, alcohol, combination of both, low socioeconomic status, deficiency of micronutrients, dietary factors, and intake of hot beverages. Various case control and other studies from certain areas of high incidence in India, such as the Kashmir valley, demonstrate that there are unique risk factors in these areas for the development of esophageal squamous carcinoma [12–17]. There have been several other studies from virtually all parts of the country evaluating various risk factors including tobacco, alcohol, tea drinking, and other nutritional factors [11, 18–26].

19.2.2.1 Tobacco Consumption

Tobacco consumption in India is peculiar in the sense that smokeless tobacco use is far more prevalent than smoked tobacco. Several smokeless tobacco products are popular and freely consumed across all age groups in India [27]. In a survey of over 300,000 adults, 30% used tobacco in some form, with over 20% using chewed tobacco or pan masala. Chewed tobacco is one of the important risk factors for squamous esophageal cancer [11, 18–21]. In a case-control study of 702 cases and over 1600 controls, Dar and colleagues found that cigarette smoking was not a major risk factor for esophageal cancer in the Kashmir valley [17]. However, the consumption of smokeless tobacco (nass) and hookah smoking were associated with a significantly increased risk [17]. Nass chewing had an increased risk of esophageal squamous cancer with an OR of 2.88. Ever-hookah smoking was associated with an increased risk of ESCC (OR 1.85; 95% CI = 1.41–2.44). They also found association between the intensity, duration, and cumulative amount of hookah smoking [17].

A study conducted in South India identified both smoked and chewed tobacco to be associated with an increased risk of squamous esophageal cancer, with risk ratios of 2.8 and 2.5, respectively [21]. Another study found a risk of 3.16 times associated with consumption of betel leaf with tobacco and 1.95 times with bidi smoking [18]. A case control study of 343 cases and 686 controls [19] found that chewing areca preparations was associated with an increased risk of developing cancer in the middle third of the esophagus; in contrast, chewing tobacco was associated with lesions in the lower third [19]. A study from the northeastern state of Assam (which has amongst the highest rates of esophageal cancer in India) found betel nut chewing to be associated with higher risks of developing esophageal cancer when compared to smoking and alcohol consumption [11]. The adjusted odds ratios for persons who chewed betel nut more than 20 times a day in comparison with non-chewers were 13.3 for males and 8.4 for females [11]. A meta-analysis of case-control studies reported areca nut use to be a significant and independent risk factor for esophageal squamous cancer with an odds ratio of 3.05. Areca nut chewing with smoked tobacco had an additive effect that increased the risk of esophageal cancer by a factor of 6.79 [28]. A case control study conducted at the authors' institute included 442 cases of esophageal cancer and 1628 hospital controls [20]. Data was collected on chewing, smoking, alcohol habits, and dietary habits. The results indicated a moderate 1.1 times excess risk for chewers of pan (betel-leaf) with tobacco, 1.8-fold excess risk for bidi smokers, and two-fold for cigarette smokers [20].

19.2.2.2 Alcohol

Alcohol consumption is not as common in India as it is in other parts of the world, both in frequency as well as quantity of consumption [29, 30]; however, it is one of the known etiological factors for esophageal cancer in India. In a case-control study conducted in South India with more than 500 patients with esophageal cancer and over 1700 controls, alcohol consumption was shown to increase the risk threefold [23]. A significant dose-response relationship was observed for the duration of drinking and average daily amount of alcohol consumption with ESCC. Among all types of alcohol analyzed, arrack, a locally brewed preparation, showed the highest risk—4.5 times that of the controls [23]. In another study conducted in South India, the risk was found to be 3.5 times higher with alcohol consumption [21]. In the study conducted in the authors' institute [20], alcohol was found to be associated with 1.8 times increased risk, while a case control study carried out in Kerala showed an increased risk of 2.33 for regular alcohol use [24].

19.2.2.3 Dietary Factors

It is widely recognized that a diet high in vegetables, fruits, and other plant-based foods and low in animal fats can reduce the risk of cancer [31]. In a case-control study, low consumption of green leafy vegetables, other vegetables, and consumption of alcohol were the three factors that were associated with increased risk for esophageal cancer [25]. Other researchers also found an increased risk with less consumption of green and leafy vegetables and fruits, and consuming more of spicy, fried, and hot food and beverages [18, 26]. A case control study done in Assam found a positive association between increased risk of esophageal cancer and consumption of spicy food, hot foods, and beverages, while green leafy vegetables and fruits were protective [11].

Consumption of salt tea has been associated with increased risk of esophageal cancer in Kashmir, where 90% of the cases had history of salt tea consumption [12]. The mechanism of carcinogenic activity of salt tea has been attributed to the presence of nitroso compounds, which get activated due to its peculiar method of brewing and presence of salt. Hyperthermic injury to the esophageal mucosa due to consumption at high temperatures may also be responsible [13]. Presence of higher levels of nitrosamines was found in the sun-dried vegetables and chillies, which are commonly consumed in Kashmir [32]. A study conducted in the authors' institute showed a fourfold higher risk with tea drinking [20]. They also found that consumption of fresh fish was associated with a 20% reduction in the risk.

A study conducted in Jammu with 200 case control pairs evaluated the role of dietary characteristics as risk factors for esophageal cancer [14]. Among the dietary and lifestyle risk factors, snuff was highest (OR = 3.86, 95% CI = 2.46–6.08) followed by salt tea (OR = 2.53, 95% CI = 1.49–4.29), smoking (OR = 1.97, 95% CI = 1.18–3.30), sundried food (OR = 1.77, 95% CI = 1.10–2.85) and red chilli (OR = 1.76, 95% CI = 1.07–2.89) [14]. Pickle consumption was associated with an odds ratio of 2.5 in a study conducted in South India [21].

19.2.2.4 Low Socioeconomic Status

Studies have associated esophageal squamous cell carcinoma risk with low socioeconomic status. A case-control study was conducted to assess the association of multiple indicators of socioeconomic status and esophageal squamous carcinoma risk in the Kashmir valley [15]. A total number of 703 histologically confirmed ESCC cases were matched with 1664 controls with respect to age, sex, and district of residence. Composite wealth scores were constructed based on the ownership of several appliances using multiple correspondence analyses. Higher education, living in a constructed house, use of liquefied petroleum gas and electricity for cooking, and higher wealth scores showed an inverse association with esophageal cancer risk. Compared to farmers, individuals who had government jobs or worked in the business sector were at lower risk of esophageal squamous cancer. They also found an inverse association between poor oral hygiene and increased risk of esophageal cancer, suggesting that oral hygiene could be used as a surrogate marker for socioeconomic status [15].

19.2.2.5 Genetic Factors

A study from Kashmir [33], which analyzed TP53 mutations in esophageal SCC in 55 patients, revealed the presence of mutations in 36.4% (20/55) tumors. Another study analyzed the interaction of various habit-related factors and polymorphism of

GSTM1/GSTT1 genes toward inducing promoter hypermethylation of multiple tumor suppressor genes [34]. In 112 cases with 130 matched controls, significantly higher methylation frequencies were observed in tobacco chewers than non-chewers for the genes under study ($p < 0.01$) [34].

Other studies have also found a high rate of protein overexpression and alterations in p53 gene expression in subjects with esophageal squamous cancer and correlated a higher expression with increased intake of chillies [35]. These results have been corroborated by other workers who showed that somatic chromosomal mutations, especially in exon 6 of Tp53 gene, among patients with esophageal cancer of an ethnically homogenous population of Kashmir valley are closely related to continued exposure to various common dietary risk factors, especially hot salty tea, meat, baked bread, and "Hakh," that are rich in nitrosoamines and familial cancer history [36].

19.2.2.6 Role of Human Papilloma Virus (HPV)

The role of Human papilloma virus as a causative factor for esophageal cancer is unclear. Various studies have demonstrated the presence of HPV in esophageal cancer specimens in the range of 15%–80% [37, 38]. Few studies in India have also demonstrated moderate to high HPV positivity rate, although the results are conflicting and the etiological role of this virus remains unclear. One small study evaluated the prevalence of HPV infection in ESCC tumors and adjoining mucosa in 23 patients with paired samples [39]. They found an HPV positivity rate of 87% in esophageal cancer patients, and higher rates were seen in smokers [39]. Another study identified HPV DNA in 46% of non-keratinizing squamous cell carcinomas of the esophagus and in none of the keratinizing squamous cell carcinomas or adenocarcinomas, postulating an etiological association with this subtype of ESCC [40].

A 2014 meta-analysis of 132 studies evaluating HPV infection in the context of esophageal SCC showed an increased risk associated, especially with HPV-16 infection in Asian countries [41].

19.2.3 Diagnosis

Most patients in India present at advanced stages of disease [42, 43]. The available investigations for diagnosis and staging of esophageal cancer in India include upper gastrointestinal endoscopy and biopsy, contrast-enhanced computed tomography (CECT) scan of the thorax and upper abdomen, fused positron emission tomography—CT (PET-CT) scan, endoscopic ultrasonography (EUS), and fiberoptic bronchoscopy. The usual workup followed in India in the diagnostic and staging process of a patient suspected to have esophageal cancer includes endoscopic mapping of the disease, histopathological confirmation, and staging using contrast-enhanced computed tomography (CECT) of the thorax and abdomen. Additional diagnostic methods such as endoscopic ultrasound and positron emission tomography with or without computed tomography (PET/PET-CT) are used in select institutions where the infrastructure and expertise are available. Fiberoptic bronchoscopy is used to rule out involvement of the trachea-bronchial tree in patients with upper and middle third tumors planned for curative treatment.

19.2.3.1 Endoscopy

Flexible upper gastrointestinal endoscopy visualizing the esophagus from the cricopharynx to the gastroesophageal junction, the stomach, and the duodenum is essential to map the extent of the disease, aids in planning the treatment (surgery/intraluminal brachytherapy), and is helpful in obtaining a tissue diagnosis by biopsy of the abnormal areas and tumor. In the authors' institute and in several other centers, this is also used to simultaneously introduce a nasogastric tube for enteral feeding in patients with grade 3 or more dysphagia.

Several studies have been done in India on cytological and histological diagnosis of esophageal cancer on endoscopy. One study evaluated the utility of brush cytology and its correlation with biopsy in 100 patients with upper gastrointestinal symptoms [44]. Cytohistopathological correlation was found in more than 80% of the cases, and the study concluded that brush cytology was an effective method for evaluation and screening of upper gastrointestinal lesions and could be utilized for rapid diagnosis with minimal discomfort to the patient [44]. Two other studies compared the sensitivity and specificity of cytology and biopsy in establishing the diagnosis of esophageal cancer [45, 46]. Both studies concluded that cytology increases the diagnostic efficacy but also emphasized that cytology alone cannot be used instead of histology due to a high false positive rate [45, 46]. A small study evaluated 48 patients with esophageal cancer to assess the optimal number of biopsy specimens required to obtain the highest yield [47]. Eight specimens were obtained from each patient; the first two specimens provided a positive diagnosis in 95.8% of cases, and the fifth and sixth specimens increased the positive yield to 100% [47].

19.2.3.2 Endoscopic Ultrasonography

Accurate staging of esophageal cancer is essential to plan treatment. EUS helps to delineate the different layers of the esophageal wall, and it is a useful staging modality in combination with CT and or PET. EUS-guided FNA is useful to get a tissue diagnosis from suspicious lymph nodes, such as the celiac. Complete EUS, however, may not be possible in patients with obstructive growths. Endoscopic mucosal resection can be performed for superficial esophageal cancers restricted to the mucosa without involvement of the lamina propria. Loco-regional staging of the tumor invasion and lymph node involvement done by EUS has been shown to be superior to that by CT. The utility of EUS is not well established in evaluation of the residual esophageal disease after neoadjuvant chemotherapy or chemoradiation, as it cannot reliably differentiate between fibrosis due to inflammation or residual/recurrent disease. However, the use of routine EUS in all patients diagnosed with esophageal cancer is debatable, as the ability to influence treatment decisions in all cases is unproven.

19.2.3.3 Contrast Enhanced Computed Tomography (CECT) Scan of the Thorax and Upper Abdomen

A CECT scan of the thorax and upper abdomen is widely accepted to be the minimum staging investigation for esophageal cancer. CECT scanning in the pretreatment assessment of esophageal cancer in the Indian setting was found to be highly accurate in determination of the tumor "T" stage, invasion of surrounding structures and distant metastases, but not effective in determination of the nodal involvement [48]. The diagnosis of invasion of the tracheobronchial tree was 96% accurate, whereas the invasion of the aorta and pericardium could be predicted in more than 85% of the cases. Previous studies also indicated the utility of computed tomography in patients undergoing surgery for esophageal cancer [49, 50].

19.2.3.4 Positron Emission Tomography (PET/PET-CT)

The addition of CT to PET has resulted in better specificity and sensitivity than either of the modalities alone, as the combined approach gives functional and morphological details in a single investigation. The treatment algorithm for locally advanced esophageal cancer includes neoadjuvant therapy, either chemotherapy alone or in combination with radiotherapy, followed by surgery. Accurate staging is important to avoid unnecessary morbidity due to treatment and futile thoracotomies in metastatic disease. A small study evaluated 28 patients with esophageal carcinoma with contrast-enhanced computed tomography followed by PET/CT after 2 weeks [51]. Nine patients were upstaged by PET/CT compared to CECT, out of which 7 (25%) were correctly upstaged, and 2 (7.14%) were falsely upstaged. They concluded that PET/CT improved their ability to detect distant metastases in 25% of patients that were missed by CECT [51]. Unusual sites of metastases, such as muscular metastases, have been detected without any morphological evidence of disease [52]. In a study of 156 patients conducted at the authors' institution, 16% of patients with esophageal cancer were found to have distant metastases on evaluation with FDG PET/CT. The sensitivity, specificity, positive predictive value, negative predictive value, and accuracy for detecting distant metastases were 83.3%, 98.4%, 92.5%, 96.1%, and 95.3%, respectively [53]. This study established the incorporation of PET/CT in the staging workup of all patients of esophageal carcinoma fit for curative intent therapy in the authors' institution.

The clinical utility and accuracy of various imaging modalities in the diagnosis of esophageal cancer are summarized in Table 19.1.

19.2.4 Staging

TNM staging is one of the most important and reliable prognostic variables. Standardized and accurate staging of cancer is important for uniform reporting and comparison of results from various centers. It also determines whether the intent of treatment is curative or palliative. It is based on clinical examination and

Table 19.1 Clinical usefulness and accuracy of modalities used in staging of esophageal cancer

Modality	Clinical utility	Overall accuracy (%)
Computed tomography (chest, abdomen)	Invasion of local structures (airways, aorta)	≥90%
	Metastatic disease	≥90%
Endoscopy	Local tumor (T) staging (operator dependent)	80%–90%
Ultrasonography (with or without fine-needle aspiration of lymph nodes)	Local nodal (N) staging (operator dependent)	70%–90%
Positron emission tomography	Metastatic disease Assessing response to neoadjuvant therapy	≥90%

information obtained by imaging: CT scan/PET-CT and/or endoscopic ultrasonography (EUS).

The 9th edition of the UICC TNM classification is expected to come into effect from January 2026 [54].

19.2.5 The Tata Memorial Centre Experience

The authors' institution, the Tata Memorial Centre, is the largest tertiary-level cancer hospital in the country and is a high-volume center for treatment of esophageal cancer. Between 1200 and 1300 new patients with esophageal cancer are seen every year, most of them presenting in advanced stage of disease, or in an emaciated condition, precluding potentially curative treatment. Squamous esophageal cancers predominate in a ratio of 80:20, and the commonest location of tumors is in the lower third of the esophagus. The typical diagnostic workup of patients with a good performance status includes a detailed flexible fiberoptic upper gastrointestinal endoscopy with mapping of the disease and biopsy, PET-CT scan with contrast, pulmonary function tests with diffusion coefficient of carbon monoxide (DLCO), and cardiac evaluation. Flexible fiberoptic bronchoscopy is performed in patients with upper and middle third lesions and those with an obvious change of voice; endoscopic ultrasonography is done selectively for patients with low volume disease on CECT scan (to confirm early disease amenable to upfront surgery) or in borderline resectable disease after neoadjuvant therapy. This diagnostic workup is curtailed in patients who are emaciated and not fit for radical therapy and in patients with obviously metastatic disease. Patients who are high risk for surgery due to coexisting comorbidities undergo a thorough cardiopulmonary evaluation and are discussed in a special "high-risk multidisciplinary team" meeting by surgeons, intensivists and critical care specialists, anesthesiologists, and pulmonary physicians to optimize them prior to surgery. The preferred therapeutic approach is discussed in a subsequent section of the chapter.

19.3 Treatment of Squamous Esophageal Cancer in India

19.3.1 Treatment

India is a vast and populous country with significant resource constraints. The wide variation in availability of facilities and technical expertise across different regions has made standardization of treatment a difficult process. While the establishment of 27 Regional Cancer Centres across the country has partially addressed the issue, the urban-rural divide and between-center variability of care are still considerable. Efforts by the authors' institute and the National Cancer Grid (NCG) have culminated in the establishment of uniform esophageal cancer treatment guidelines tailored to the country's varied levels of expertise and availability of infrastructure [55]. One of the core recommendations of the guidelines is establishment of multidisciplinary teams (MDTs) for management of esophageal cancer. While some major cancer centers in India have a multidisciplinary team including a surgical, medical, and radiation oncologist in place, several others do not, and one of the biggest challenges has been to ensure the same standards of care and decision-making regardless of whether the patient initially presents to a surgeon, gastroenterologist, medical, or radiation oncologist. The National Cancer Grid Virtual Tumour Boards propagate the concept of MDT decision making while also serving as a resource for case-based learning [56].

19.3.1.1 Patient Evaluation

The initial evaluation of the patient includes assessment of physical (ECOG performance) status, oral hygiene, nutrition, and cardiopulmonary status. This is particularly important in the Indian scenario, where patients generally present in an advanced stage and in poor general health. Generally, only patients who are ECOG performance score (PS) of 0 or 1 are selected for radical treatment. Assessment of oral hygiene is necessary because of the high prevalence of tobacco chewing in India [27, 30], and the possibility of co-existing oropharyngeal malignancy. Since most patients present with significant dysphagia and some degree of nutritional impairment, assessment of nutritional status and early institution of rehabilitation are key. Malnutrition is found to be an independent risk factor for severe morbidity after esophageal surgery (HR 3.07) [57]. The enteral route is the preferred route of nutritional rehabilitation due to its inherent advantages of keeping the gut in use, as well as the ease of administration and relatively low complication rate compared to parenteral nutrition [58]. All patients considered for radical treatment undergo extensive evaluation of cardiopulmonary status including pulmonary function tests (PFT), 2D Echocardiography, and in select cases, stress cardiac testing. Pulmonary rehabilitation is started at the outset for all patients planned for radical treatment with the active involvement of the chest physician and physiotherapists. A Japanese study showed that institution of chest physiotherapy at least 7 days prior to surgery decreased the rate of post-esophagectomy pulmonary complications from 24.3% to 6.4% [59]. Early institution of chest physiotherapy, tobacco and alcohol cessation are routinely advocated as soon as a diagnosis of esophageal cancer is made.

19.3.1.2 Principles of Management

Broadly, decisions regarding treatment are based on the anatomical location and stage of disease and the performance status of the patient. The authors' repeated emphasis on the performance status of the patient is primarily because poor general health precludes potentially curative treatment in considerable proportion of patients in India. Concurrent radical chemoradiation is the preferred therapeutic strategy for lesions in the upper third of the esophagus, i.e., within 5 cm of the cricopharynx, while surgery is the preferred treatment for lesions in the middle and lower third of the esophagus. Early-stage lesions (T1/T2, N0) are usually treated by surgery alone for middle and lower third lesions. Endoscopic mucosal resection (EMR) and Endoscopic Submucosal Dissection (ESD), though less morbid procedures, are not widely practiced in India primarily since very few patients present at a stage amenable to the procedure and the limited availability of expertise across the country. Patients with locally advanced disease (T3/T4, N+) undergo multimodality treatment, generally with neoadjuvant chemotherapy [60, 61] or neoadjuvant chemoradiotherapy followed by surgery. Patients with metastatic disease are usually treated with palliative radiotherapy, palliative chemotherapy, esophageal stenting, or a combination.

19.3.2 Surgery

Surgery is the preferred modality of treatment for middle and lower third esophageal cancer [62–65]. Most patients in India with early-stage disease (T1/T2, N0) are considered for upfront surgery, while patients with locally advanced disease undergo surgery after neoadjuvant therapy. Rarely, patients with residual disease after radical chemoradiotherapy are taken up for esophagectomy, albeit at the cost of significantly higher postoperative morbidity. In spite of the established role of surgery in the radical treatment of esophageal cancer, there is very little consensus on what constitutes a standard esophagectomy in terms of approach, extent, and template for lymph node dissection. This may, in part, be because esophageal resections in India are performed by surgeons from varied surgical specialties including general surgery, gastrointestinal surgery, thoracic surgery, and surgical oncology.

19.3.2.1 Approach

Transthoracic esophagectomy predominantly by a modified McKeown three-stage procedure is the standard approach by most thoracic surgeons and surgical oncologists, while most general and gastrointestinal surgeons prefer a transhiatal approach, particularly for lower third tumors [62–65]. In a single-institutional series of 367 transhiatal esophagectomies performed over a period of 18 years, the five-year overall survival was 38% with a postoperative mortality rate of 12% [62]. Both approaches are widely practiced in India, though there is an increasing trend toward the transthoracic approach in high-volume oncology centres [64, 66]. In these centers, transhiatal resection is performed in limited numbers as a compromise surgery in patients with poor pulmonary function or extensive pulmonary fibrosis precluding transthoracic resection.

19.3.2.2 Lymphadenectomy

Lymphadenectomy for esophageal cancer is a controversial topic in India, as in many other parts of the world [67]. Surgical oncologists who predominantly perform transthoracic esophagectomies place more emphasis on extensive lymph nodal clearance. Infracarinal nodal dissection or a standard two-field dissection is the standard template for dissection by most surgeons performing a transthoracic esophagectomy. In India, very few centers with high volumes of esophageal surgery practice elective three-field lymphadenectomy routinely. The increase in lymph node yield with more radical lymphadenectomy needs to be balanced against an increased postoperative morbidity, primarily with recurrent laryngeal paresis and pulmonary complications [66]. In contrast, the lymph node yield achieved by a transhiatal resection is low and is usually limited to the periesophageal lymph nodes. However, as mentioned in the previous section, transhiatal resections are usually performed only as a compromise surgery in high-volume centers.

19.3.2.3 Minimally Invasive Surgery

Surgeons in India were early to adopt minimally invasive esophagectomy. A few high-volume centers have published data showing better results with a minimally invasive approach with respect to pulmonary morbidity and operative blood loss [64, 68–70]. A prospective study comparing minimally invasive esophagectomy with open esophagectomy [70] demonstrated comparable results in terms of lymph node yield (9.5 vs 7.3), duration of surgery (312 min vs 262 min), average blood loss (276 mL vs 313 mL), and morbidity (26.5% vs 28.6%). A larger series [68] of 463 thoracoscopic esophagectomies demonstrated a lower morbidity rate (16%) and postoperative mortality rate (0.9%). The results of the TIME trial and the more recent MIRO trial have reiterated the benefit of minimally invasive esophageal surgery on short-term postoperative outcomes [71, 72]. The 3-year follow-up of the TIME trial showed a trend toward improved overall and disease-free survival with the minimally invasive approach [71]. With this evidence, the superiority of minimally invasive esophagectomy with respect to short-term outcomes and equivalence if not superiority, in long-term oncological outcomes have been established. This has reflected in the evolving trend of esophageal surgery in India, with most centers offering the minimally invasive approach. The safety of thoraco-laparoscopic esophagectomy has also been established in the older patient population in India [73].

Different surgical groups in India use different patient positions for thoracoscopic esophagectomy with lateral, prone, and more recently, semi-prone positions based on surgeon preference. The prone or semi-prone position offers the advantage of not requiring lung isolation for thoracoscopy, whereas the lateral position offers better exposure to the superior mediastinum for radical lymph node dissection. The authors' preference is to perform MIS esophagectomy through the lateral approach.

Robotic surgery for esophageal cancer has been increasingly performed in India over the past decade [74–76]. A series of 83 robotic esophageal resections showed comparable postoperative outcomes to thoracoscopic esophagectomy with no conversion. The docking and operating time decreased significantly as experience increased [74]. Retrospective studies comparing robot-assisted to open esophagectomy showed improved perioperative outcomes with the robotic procedure [75]. Propensity score matched comparisons between thoracolaparoscopic and robotic approaches showed comparable results with increased cost for the robotic procedure [76] Equivalent long-term oncological outcomes with robotic resections as compared to open surgery have been shown in recent reports [77]. However, no distinct advantage over thoracoscopic esophagectomy has been demonstrated. Especially in the Indian scenario, where the cost of robotic instruments and other consumables may exceed that of any benefit in terms of hospital stay, the advantages of robotic esophagectomy over thoraco-laparoscopy need careful consideration.

19.3.2.4 Reconstruction

The stomach is the preferred conduit for reconstruction, and in cases where the stomach is not available, the colon is the next preferred alternative. The posterior mediastinum is the most commonly used route of reconstruction; the retrosternal route being used only when the patient is being considered for postoperative radiotherapy to the mediastinum or when the surgeon adopts an abdomen-first approach to a transthoracic esophagectomy. A small, randomized study of 49 patients comparing posterior mediastinal versus retrosternal conduit placement [78] found both routes to have comparable outcomes. The anastomosis is usually performed in the neck either by a stapled or handsewn technique [79]. Both techniques are widely practiced in India, depending upon surgeon preference and cost constraints. Our own preference is to perform a triangulated stapled anastomosis. Some clinical trials on anastomotic technique are described in a subsequent section of the chapter.

19.3.3 Multimodality Management

India has promoted multimodality management in esophageal cancer in the last two decades. In view of the strength of evidence supporting neoadjuvant therapy currently, patients with locally advanced potentially operable esophageal cancer are treated with either neoadjuvant chemotherapy [60, 61] or neoadjuvant chemoradiotherapy. The common chemotherapy regimens include doublets consisting of cisplatin with 5-fluorouracil or cisplatin with paclitaxel, while a few centers use triplets of cisplatin, 5-fluorouracil, and either paclitaxel or docetaxel, which have superior response rates at the cost of higher morbidity. The commonly followed schedule is to administer three cycles at three weekly intervals, followed by reassessment with CT scan imaging and surgery between 4 and 6 weeks after the last cycle of chemotherapy. The CROSS and the NEOCRTEC trials have established the role of neoadjuvant chemoradiation in esophageal SCC. Both trials have shown advantage with this approach in terms of survival, pathological complete response, and R0 resection rates [80, 81]. Considering this evidence, the use of neoadjuvant chemoradiotherapy has increased substantially in India. The most commonly used protocol is the CROSS protocol, i.e., radiation 41.4 Gy in 23 fractions of 1.8 Gy over 5 weeks with concurrent weekly chemotherapy, paclitaxel 50 mg/m^2, and carboplatin at AUC 2. However, despite improved cancer-specific outcomes, this approach has shown an increase in severity of postoperative complications and one-year mortality as seen in the NeoRes trial, which needs to be considered while adopting this approach [82].

Postoperative radiotherapy or chemoradiotherapy is not practiced as a routine after esophagectomy. The use of adjuvant radiotherapy is restricted to patients with positive resection margins and occasionally, patients with significant residual metastatic lymphadenopathy after neoadjuvant chemotherapy. In spite of evidence supporting the use of adjuvant immunotherapy in patients with residual disease after neoadjuvant chemoradiation [83], very few patients in India receive Nivolumab due to the prohibitive cost of therapy.

19.3.4 Chemoradiotherapy

Chemoradiotherapy is the primary modality of treatment for upper third esophageal cancers and locally advanced middle and lower third cancers that are unresectable. It is also the treatment of choice in patients who are medically inoperable or unwilling to undergo surgery. The most widely practiced and well-tolerated regimen includes radiotherapy to 66 Gy in 33# in 6.5 weeks with concurrent weekly cisplatin 35 mg/m^2, 5–6 cycles [84]. In institutes with facilities for intraluminal brachytherapy, the radiation regimen may be changed to teletherapy 50 Gy in 25# in 5 weeks, followed by 2# of high-dose-rate intraluminal brachytherapy of 12 Gy after 2 weeks, the chemotherapy regimen remaining the same. Several concurrent chemotherapy regimens are practiced including 3 weekly cisplatin and 5-fluorouracil, and three weekly paclitaxel and cisplatin, along with standard doses of radiation. Pretherapy fiberoptic bronchoscopy in cancers of the upper and middle third is done to rule out airway involvement.

19.3.5 Palliative Therapy

The emphasis of management in patients presenting with metastatic esophageal cancer is on early palliation of dysphagia. Patients with metastatic disease but grade 3 or less dysphagia are treated with palliative radiotherapy, chemotherapy with or without stenting [85]. Patients with absolute dysphagia who need immediate palliation are treated with esophageal stents, most commonly self-expanding metal stents [86]. A few centers offer intraluminal radiotherapy for metastatic and locally advanced esophageal cancer and have been found to offer faster and sustained palliation of dysphagia [87]. Rarely, patients with bulky disease obstructing the tracheobronchial tree as well as the esophagus are treated with double stents, i.e., tracheal and esophageal stents.

19.3.6 The Tata Memorial Centre Experience

At the authors' institute, patients with early (T1 or T2 with N0) disease are treated with primary surgery, while those with more advanced (T3 or T4a or N+) disease are treated with neoadjuvant chemotherapy (NACT) or chemoradiotherapy (NACTRT) followed by surgical resection. Over 3500 surgeries have been performed for esophageal cancer over the last 20 years. The preferred choice of surgery is a transthoracic three-stage esophagectomy, while transhiatal esophagectomy is occasionally performed as a compromise procedure in patients with borderline fitness or extensive pulmonary fibrosis. Elective three-field lymphadenectomy is done in all patients with supracarinal disease and those with radiologically or metabolically metastatic supracarinal lymphadenopathy. Patients without these features were considered for randomization to a trial comparing standard two-field with elective radical three-field lymphadenectomy. Minimally invasive esophagectomy (thoracoscopy and/or laparoscopy) is performed in approximately half the patients undergoing transthoracic esophagectomy. The preferred conduit is the stomach and the posterior mediastinum, the most common route of reconstruction. Esophagogastric anastomosis is performed in the neck by a triangulated stapled anastomosis. A nasojejunal tube is placed intraoperatively for postoperative enteral feeding.

Preoperative evaluation includes a detailed history and examination, assessment of functional capacity by stair climbing or a six-minute walk test, and blood investigations including a complete blood count, coagulation profile, and renal and liver function tests. All patients undergo pulmonary function testing in the form of spirometry and diffusion capacity for carbon monoxide, and cardiac evaluation with an electrocardiogram and resting echocardiography. Patients with cardio-pulmonary risk factors (ischemic heart disease, limited functional capacity, or poor performance on spirometry) may be considered for either stress echocardiography or a formal cardio-pulmonary exercise test to determine peak oxygen consumption and anaerobic threshold. Patients considered high risk for postoperative complications are discussed in a multidisciplinary clinic consisting of anesthesiologists, surgeons, and pulmonary physicians, for optimization prior to surgery.

Preoperative preparation includes chest physiotherapy, incentive spirometry, and nutritional rehabilitation along with smoking cessation. Anti deep vein thrombosis (DVT) prophylaxis is started 12 hours prior to surgery and continued postoperatively. Prophylactic antibiotics are given preoperatively and repeated once after 3 h intraoperatively and are not continued routinely in the postoperative period.

Anesthesia management: All patients undergoing open surgery receive thoracic epidural analgesia (unless contraindicated), while we avoid it for MIS esophagectomy (unless specifically indicated in patients who cannot receive other multimodal analgesia). For thoracoscopic and robotic surgery, we use either double-lumen tubes or bronchial blockers for lung isolation. In addition to standard monitors, we use invasive arterial pressure monitoring for all cases. Fluid therapy is optimized and is guided by hemodynamic parameters, urine output, and serial arterial lactate measurements. We have increasingly started intraoperative nerve monitoring, especially while performing three-field lymphadenectomy [88, 89], necessitating the use of monitoring tubes and avoidance of muscle relaxants. We also use Indo Cyanine Green (ICG) in MIS esophagectomy to facilitate identification of the thoracic duct (including variant anatomy) and gastric conduit vascularity.

Most patients are extubated immediately postoperatively on table and shifted to a recovery ward rather than the intensive care unit. Physiotherapy and active mobilization are started soon after shifting to the recovery ward. Postoperative analgesia is multimodal and combines epidural (for open surgery), local anesthetics with systemic paracetamol, and nonsteroidal anti-inflammatory agents. Enteral (nasojejunal) feeding is started the morning after surgery and stepped up gradually to full enteral feeds by the evening of the second postoperative day. The nasogastric tube is clamped on the second postoperative day and removed by the same evening if the chest radiograph shows no gastric tube dilatation. Routine laryngoscopy examination is done to check the vocal cord status on the 4th postoperative day, and oral liquids are started on the 5th postoperative day. Contrast swallows are not done prior to starting orals, and patients are on full solid feeds by the 8th postoperative day. Uncomplicated patients are discharged by the 9th or 10th postoperative day.

The postoperative major morbidity and mortality are 22.1% and 4.7%, respectively. Common postoperative complications include pulmonary complications (26.6%), anastomotic leaks (12%), vocal cord paresis (25.1%), and thoracic duct injuries (3.3%, of which 1.1% required surgical re-exploration). Patients who have postoperative vocal cord palsy are evaluated by Fibreoptic Endoscopic Evaluation of Swallowing (FEES) to guide speech and swallowing therapy, and graded introduction of feeds. Our management of anastomotic leaks depends on the magnitude of the leak and the hemodynamic stability of the patient. Minor leaks are usually managed conservatively, with surgical intervention reserved for major leaks with hemodynamic compromise, or gastric tube ischemia/necrosis. We have increasingly used endoscopic vacuum therapy to shorten the duration for healing of leaks [90].

19.4 Research in Esophageal Cancer in India

Research on esophageal cancer in India has a long history. The main areas of focus in esophageal cancer research have been the possible etiological factors and associations with squamous esophageal cancer, the choice of primary treatment for the disease, modifications in surgical technique, the role of neoadjuvant and adjuvant treatment, and palliative treatment options.

19.4.1 Epidemiology Research

Epidemiological research from the Kashmir valley, which is a high-incidence area for squamous esophageal cancer, established that low socio-economic status was an independent risk factor [15]. A large case-control study, matched for age, sex, and geographic area, showed a strong inverse association between higher education and wealth status and ESCC risk. The same study also established the probable etiological role of "hookah" smoking and "nass chewing" on esophageal squamous cell cancer with odds ratios of 1.85 and 2.88, respectively [17]. In a small study evaluating the prevalence of human papillomavirus (HPV) strains in ESCC, researchers found that a high proportion (87%) of patients with ESCC harbored high-risk HPV strains [39]. While association between HPV strains and ESCC is already established, and the study supported the hypothesis of persistent oncogenic viruses in cancer development, a larger study would be required to firmly establish causation. In a study of epigenetic, genetic, and environmental interactions in ESCC, significantly higher methylation frequencies were noted in tobacco chewers compared to nontobacco users for all the four genes (p16, DAPK, BRCA1, and GSTP1) studied [34]. Betel quid chewing, alcohol consumption, and a null GSTT1 genotype had maximum risk for ESCC without promoter hypermethylation, whereas tobacco chewing, smoking, and null GSTT1 variants were found to be associated with ESCC with promoter hypermethylation on logistic regression analysis [34].

19.4.2 Primary Treatment

One of the two randomized trials [91, 92] comparing surgeries with radical radiotherapy for localized esophageal cancer, was conducted in the authors' institute. Although this trial was primarily designed to evaluate quality of life in patients treated with surgery or radiotherapy, it established that surgery was superior to radiotherapy even for overall survival [91]. The study randomized 99 patients to either surgery alone ($n = 47$) or radiotherapy alone ($n = 52$). Outcomes with respect to disease-specific symptoms, which were the primary outcome, were consistently superior in the surgery arm; specifically, the quality of swallowing, which is an important endpoint of treatment of esophageal cancer, was superior in the surgery arm compared to radiotherapy. The secondary endpoint of survival was vastly superior in the surgery arm compared to the radiotherapy arm ($p = 0.002$) [91].

19.4.3 Neoadjuvant Therapy

A randomized trial conducted in the authors' institution compared two commonly used neoadjuvant chemotherapy regimens—platinum (cisplatin or carboplatin) combined with either 5-fluorouracil or Paclitaxel [93]. The trial showed superior toxicity profile and pathological response rates with the Paclitaxel combination, with equivalent overall survival [93]. A small, randomized trial compared quality of life (QOL) outcomes after transhiatal esophagectomy with or without neoadjuvant chemotherapy [59]. Utilizing the validated EORTC QLQ C-30 and OES-18 questionnaires, the authors showed that quality of life (QOL) improved after surgery in all patients in functional, global health, and symptom scales; in addition, the results showed an improved QOL in patients treated with neoadjuvant chemotherapy and surgery compared to those with surgery alone [61]. In another series reporting on outcomes following neoadjuvant chemoradiation for esophageal cancer, 76.6% patients completed neoadjuvant treatment and proceeded to surgery. Of these, 93.4% underwent R0 resection with a pathological complete response in 37.2%. 1- and 2- year survival was reported to be 76% and 62.8% respectively [94]. In a series from Chennai, 64% patients undergoing neoadjuvant chemoradiation received surgery, of which 38% had a pathological complete response. There were no mortalities in the 90-day period [95]. Similar outcomes were reported from other centres [96, 97]. All these centers used radiation doses between 41.4 and 45 Gy. This data clearly shows a trend toward preference for neoadjuvant chemoradiation in esophageal SCC in India.

19.4.4 Surgical Trials

Several trials have been conducted on surgical techniques and variations therein. These include the use of pedicled omentum to reinforce esophagogastric anastomosis [98], modifications of the anastomotic technique [99], and the route of reconstruction [8]. In addition, observational studies on minimally invasive esophagectomy [64, 68–70, 73] and robotic esophagectomy [74–76] have also been performed.

A small randomized trial [8] was performed on 49 patients to compare outcomes between the anterior mediastinal (retrosternal) ($n = 24$) and the posterior mediastinal ($n = 25$) routes of reconstruction. The duration (235 vs 225 min) and blood loss (531 vs 538 mL) of surgery were similar in the two groups. Similarly, there were no significant differences between the retrosternal and posterior mediastinal routes respectively in immediate postoperative pulmonary (45.8% vs 48%) or cardiac (25% vs 20%) complication rates, anastomotic leaks (16.7% vs 16%), hospital stay (15 vs 17 days), and mortality (12.5% vs 4%) [78]. Long-term outcomes including stricture rate, dysphagia, aspiration, reflux, and weight loss, were also similar in the two groups [78]. In a small study involving patients who underwent esophagectomy with a cervical anastomosis, patients were randomized into either no pyloric drainage or pyloroplasty with gastric emptying as the primary endpoint [100]. The study demonstrated significant delay in gastric emptying in both the groups though it was less pronounced in the pyloroplasty group. The sequelae of delayed gastric emptying were seen in both groups, and the authors concluded that the intrathoracic stomach causes delayed gastric emptying and pyloroplasty failed to prevent its occurrence [100].

19.4.4.1 Anastomotic Technique

A randomized trial [89] was performed to evaluate whether the addition of a pedicled omental wrap on the esophagogastric anastomosis would decrease the incidence of anastomotic leaks. Patients undergoing radical esophagectomy (63% Ivor-Lewis and 37% transhiatal esophagectomy) were randomized to conventional anastomosis (manual end-to-side esophagogastric) with (n = 97) or without an omental wrap (n = 97). The anastomotic leak rate was significantly lower (3.1% vs 14.4%, p = 0.005) in patients who had the omental wrap [98]. This difference was seen in both the Ivor Lewis and the transhiatal esophagectomy groups. Another randomized trial was conducted to evaluate whether a wide cross-sectional area at the anastomotic site would lead to lower rates of anastomotic leaks and strictures [99]. One hundred patients were randomized to the control arm (end-to-side esophagogastric anastomosis on the anterior gastric all without removal of the crescent) or the experimental arm (end-to-side anastomosis after removal of a crescent from the anterior gastric wall). Anastomotic leak rates (4.3% vs 20.8%, p = 0.03) and strictures (8.5% vs 29.2%, p = 0.02) were significantly lower with the modified (wider anastomotic) technique [99]. A randomized trial comparing a side-to-side stapled anastomosis to a handsewn technique had anastomotic leaks and strictures as the primary and secondary endpoints, respectively [79]. Out of 174 patients randomized, anastomotic leak rates were similar in the two groups (14/87 vs 16/87, p = 0.33); however, postoperative strictures were significantly lower (17/82 vs 7/81, p = 0.045) in the stapled anastomosis [79].

19.4.4.2 Perioperative Management

Two relatively large, randomized trials of perioperative management were conducted in the authors' institute. The first, a randomized trial, evaluated whether it was safe to shorten the duration of nasogastric drainage after esophagectomy [101]. One hundred and fifty patients undergoing modified McKeown three-stage or transhiatal esophagectomy with gastric tube reconstruction were randomly allocated to either conventional (6–10 days) or shortened (2 days) nasogastric drainage. The primary composite endpoint was anastomotic leaks and/or pulmonary complications and was found to be similar (18.7% vs 21.3%) in the two groups; patient discomfort scores were significantly lower in the early removal arm [101]. The trial established that it was feasible and safe to remove the nasogastric drainage tube 2 days after esophagectomy and a neck anastomosis without any adverse effects [101]. The authors performed another randomized trial to evaluate the impact of restricted intraoperative and postoperative fluid administration on major postoperative pulmonary complications [102]. The study initially planned to recruit 320 patients, but was prematurely terminated after 183 patients were accrued on the advice of an independent data monitoring committee. Eligible patients were randomized to either conventional (liberal) fluid administration or restricted fluids intra- and post-operatively. At the planned interim analysis after 183 patients were accrued, the major postoperative complication rates were identical, and the DSMC felt that continuing the trial would be futile as the likelihood of demonstrating an important difference between the two groups was very low [102].

A randomized trial evaluating the role of intraoperative Indocyanine green fluorescence angiography (ICG-FA) versus visual assessment (VA) demonstrated that the ICG-FA group had substantially lower anastomotic leaks after McKeown esophagectomy [103]. A small, randomized trial compared feeding jejunostomy (FJ) with nasojejunal (NJ) tube feeding and concluded that the NJ group had better self-reported physical domain QOL score with no difference in the complications or tube efficacy between the two groups [104]. Enhanced Recovery After Surgery protocols have shown improved short-term outcomes after esophagectomy, like in other major gastrointestinal surgery [105]. Guidelines for perioperative management in esophageal surgery have been given by the ERAS society [106].

19.4.5 Palliative Treatment

A randomized trial conducted at the authors' institution compared palliative chemotherapy using weekly Paclitaxel with best supportive care (BSC) with BSC alone in patients with advanced unresectable/metastatic esophageal cancer that were not amenable to curative-intent treatment [107]. The trial demonstrated that palliative chemotherapy improved overall survival with manageable toxicity [107]. Another phase 2/3 randomized trial was stopped after the phase 2 results showed no benefit and a trend toward poorer outcomes with the use of oral metronomic chemotherapy in patients who underwent definitive chemoradiation for unresectable esophageal cancer [108]. A randomized trial evaluated whether the combined treatment of esophageal stenting followed by radiotherapy was superior to stenting alone in advanced inoperable esophageal cancer [85]. The study, which randomized 84 patients, concluded that the combination of self-expandable metal stenting followed by 30 Gray radiation (10 fractions, over 2 weeks) offered longer dysphagia relief (7 vs 3 months, $p = 0.002$), and prolonged survival (median 180 vs 120 days, $p = 0.009$) compared to stenting alone [85].

19.4.6 Ongoing Research

There are several ongoing trials on various aspects of esophageal cancer treatment. A large ($n = 700$) randomized trial has completed recruitment in the authors' institution, evaluating the role of radical lymphadenectomy in operable esophageal cancer [109]. Patients with operable esophageal cancer were randomized intraoperatively (after confirming operability and absence of gross supracarinal lymphadenopathy) to either standard two-field or radical three-field lymphadenectomy; survival results are expected in 2026. Another large ($n = 840$) randomized trial [110, 111] was conducted in multiple centers in India in collaboration with the Medical Research Council, UK, to evaluate the role of adjuvant Aspirin after radical treatment of esophageal cancer—recruitment is complete, and survival results are expected in 2027/28.

19.5 Future Directions

Treatment for esophageal cancer in India has so far been carried out in institutions with a wide range of experience in managing this disease without an organizational framework. Challenges to improve overall patient outcomes in esophageal cancer include the wide disparity in quality of cancer care provision, availability of qualified, trained experts in all parts of the country, and the relative lack of infrastructure. Healthcare provision in India is multitiered, with only basic medical facilities at a primary health center level, while tertiary level treatment centers have state-of-the-art infrastructure and highly qualified medical and paramedical staff, especially in apex government and private institutions. Future efforts will include widespread dissemination of evidence-based treatment guidelines for management of esophageal cancer, training adequate manpower, centralization of treatment, wider adoption of multidisciplinary treatment teams and multimodality treatment protocols, creation of a collaborative network, and standardized data capture.

The lack of a cooperative working group to meet the above challenges was felt to be a lacuna in the system. The creation of the National Cancer Grid in India has filled this gap with several initiatives aimed at reducing disparities in the quality of cancer care in the country. Some of these initiatives include development of resource-stratified evidence-based guidelines, virtual multidisciplinary tumor boards, quality assurance programs for surgical pathology, pooled procurement of cancer medicines, and augmenting human resources and support for cancer research. The authors also agree on the need for collaborative research in squamous esophageal cancers amongst countries like Japan, China, Korea, Iran, and India where they are far more common than adenocarcinomas. Possible questions to answer include the role of neoadjuvant immunotherapy, personalized therapy to guide the choice of neoadjuvant treatment, the ideal surgical approach, the extent of lymphadenectomy, and quality of life issues.

References

1. Siegel R, Naishadham D, Jemal A. Cancer statistics. CA Cancer J Clin. 2012;62:10–29.
2. https://gco.iarc.who.int/media/globocan/factsheets/populations/356-india-fact-sheet.pdf. Accessed 14 Aug 2025.
3. Kamangar F, Dores GM, Anderson WF. Patterns of cancer incidence, mortality and prevalence across five continents: defining priorities to reduce cancer disparities in different geographic regions of the world. J Clin Oncol. 2006;24:2137–50.
4. Vaughan TL, Davis S, Kristal A, Thomas DB. Obesity, alcohol and tobacco as risk factors for cancer of the esophagus and gastric cardia: adenocarcinoma versus squamous cell carcinoma. Cancer Epidemiol Biomarkers Prev. 1995;4:85–92.
5. Devesa SS, Blot WJ, Fraumeni JF Jr. Changing patterns in the incidence of esophageal and gastric carcinoma in the United States. Cancer. 1998;83:2049–53.
6. Vizcaino AP, Moreno V, Lambert R, Parkin DM. Time trends incidence of both major histologic types of esophageal carcinomas in selected countries, 1973–1995. Int J Cancer. 2002;99:860–8.

7. Bhome R, Desai D, Abraham P, Joshi A, Gupta T, Bhaduri A, et al. Esophageal adenocarcinoma versus squamous cell carcinoma: retrospective hospital-based analysis of a 12-year temporal trend. Indian J Gastroenterol. 2012;31:340–2.
8. Tony J, Kumar SK, Thomas V. Time trends and pathological profile of carcinoma lower oesophagus and gastro-oesophageal junction over the last 20 years-an experience from South India. Trop Gastroenterol. 2007;28:113–6.
9. Cherian JV, Sivaraman R, Muthusamy AK, Jayanthi V. Carcinoma of the esophagus in Tamil Nadu (South India): 16-year trends from a tertiary center. J Gastrointestin Liver Dis. 2007;16:245–9.
10. Pandith AA, Siddiqi MA. Burden of cancers in the valley of Kashmir: 5 year epidemiological study reveals a different scenario. Tumour Biol. 2012;33:1629–37.
11. Phukan RK, Chetia CK, Ali MS, Mahanta J. Role of dietary habits in the development of esophageal cancer in Assam, the north-eastern region of India. Nutr Cancer. 2001;39:204–9.
12. Khan NA, Teli MA, Mohib-UlHaq M, Bhat GM, Lone MM, Afroz F. A survey of risk factors in carcinoma esophagus in the valley of Kashmir, Northern India. J Cancer Res Ther. 2011;7:15–8.
13. Mir MM, Dar NA. Esophageal cancer in Kashmir (India): an enigma for researchers. Int J Health Sci (Qassim). 2009;3:71–85.
14. Sehgal S, Kaul S, Gupta BB, Dhar MK. Risk factors and survival analysis of the esophageal cancer in the population of Jammu, India. Indian J Cancer. 2012;49:245–50.
15. Dar NA, Shah IA, Bhat GA, Makhdoomi MA, Iqbal B, Rafiq R, et al. Socioeconomic status and esophageal squamous cell carcinoma risk in Kashmir, India. Cancer Sci. 2013;104:1231–6.
16. Dar NA, Islami F, Bhat GA, Shah IA, Makhdoomi MA, Iqbal B, et al. Poor oral hygiene and risk of esophageal squamous cell carcinoma in Kashmir. Br J Cancer. 2013;109:1367–72.
17. Dar NA, Bhat GA, Shah IA, Iqbal B, Makhdoomi MA, Nisar I, et al. Hookah smoking, nass chewing, and oesophageal squamous cell carcinoma in Kashmir, India. Br J Cancer. 2012;107:1618–23.
18. Nayar D, Kapil U, Joshi YK, Sundaram KR, Srivastava SP, Shukla NK, et al. Nutritional risk factors in esophageal cancer. J Assoc Physicians India. 2000;48:781–7.
19. Nandakumar A, Anantha N, Pattabhiraman V, Prabhakaran PS, Dhar M, Puttaswamy K, et al. Importance of anatomical subsite in correlating risk factors in cancer of the oesophagus—report of a case-control study. Br J Cancer. 1996;73:1306–11.
20. Ganesh B, Talole SD, Dikshit R. Tobacco, alcohol and tea drinking as risk factors for esophageal cancer: a case-control study from Mumbai, India. Cancer Epidemiol. 2009;33:431–4.
21. Chitra S, Ashok L, Anand L, Srinivasan V, Jayanthi V. Risk factors for esophageal cancer in Coimbatore, southern India: a hospital-based case-control study. Indian J Gastroenterol. 2004;23:19–21.
22. Gupta PC, Ray CS. Smokeless tobacco and health in India and South Asia. Respirology. 2003;8:419–31.
23. Znaor A, Brennan P, Gajalakshmi V, Mathew A, Shanta V, Varghese C, et al. Independent and combined effects of tobacco smoking, chewing and alcohol drinking on the risk of oral, pharyngeal and esophageal cancers in Indian men. Int J Cancer. 2003;105:681–6.
24. Sankaranarayanan R, Duffy SW, Padmakumary G, Nair SM, Day NE, Padmanabhan TK. Risk factors for cancer of the oesophagus in Kerala, India. Int J Cancer. 1991;49:485–9.
25. Srivastava M, Kapil U, Joshi YK, Nayar D, Chattopadhyaya TK, Shukla NK, et al. Nutritional risk factors in carcinoma esophagus. Nutr Res. 1995;15:177–85.
26. Joshi SC, Saxena SR, Satyawali VN, Joshi A, Nigam P, Singh VK, et al. Oesophageal carcinoma—a study of risk factors (emphasis on nutrition) in a teaching hospital of Kumaon region of Uttarakhand. J Assoc Physicians India. 2009;57:631–5.
27. Rani M, Bonu S, Jha P, Nguyen SN, Jamjoum L. Tobacco use in India: prevalence and predictors of smoking and chewing in a national cross sectional household survey. Tob Control. 2003;12:e4.
28. Akhtar S. Areca nut chewing and esophageal squamous cell carcinoma risk in Asians: a meta-analysis of case-control studies. Cancer Causes Control. 2013;24:257–65.

29. Bennett LA, Campillo C, Chandrashekar CR, Gureje O. Alcoholic beverage consumption in India, Mexico, and Nigeria: a cross-cultural comparison. Alcohol Health Res World. 1998;22:243–52.
30. Neufeld KJ, Peters DH, Rani M, Bonu S, Brooner RK. Regular use of alcohol and tobacco in India and its association with age, gender and poverty. Drug Alcohol Depend. 2005;77:283–91.
31. Sinha R, Anderson DE, McDonald SS, Greenwald P. Cancer risk and diet in India. J Postgrad Med. 2003;49:222–8.
32. Siddiqui MA, Tricker AR, Kumar R, Fazili Z, Preussmann R. Dietary sources of N nitrosamines in a high-risk area for oesophageal cancer—Kashmir, India. IARC Sci Publ. 1991;105:210–3.
33. Mir MM, Dar NA, Gochhait S, Zargar SA, Ahangar AG, Bamezai RN. p53 mutation profile of squamous cell carcinomas of the esophagus in Kashmir (India): a high-incidence area. Int J Cancer. 2005;116:62–8.
34. Talukdar FR, Ghosh SK, Laskar RS, Mondal R. Epigenetic, genetic and environmental interactions in esophageal squamous cell carcinoma from northeast India. PLoS One. 2013;8:e60996.
35. Gaur D, Arora S, Mathur M, Nath N, Chattopadhaya TK, Ralhan R. High prevalence of p53 gene alterations and protein overexpression in human esophageal cancer: correlation with dietary risk factors in India. Clin Cancer Res. 1997;3:2129–36.
36. Murtaza I, Mushtaq D, Margoob MA, Dutt A, Wani NA, Ahmad I, et al. A study on p53 gene alterations in esophageal squamous cell carcinoma and their correlation to common dietary risk factors among population of the Kashmir valley. World J Gastroenterol. 2006;12:4033–7.
37. Syrjänen K. HPV infections and oesophageal cancer. J Clin Pathol. 2002;55:721–8.
38. Liyanage S, Segelov E, Garland S, Tabrizi S, Seale H, et al. The role of human papillomaviruses in esophageal squamous cell carcinoma. Asia Pac J Clin Oncol. 2013;9:12–28.
39. Vaiphei K, Kochhar R, Bhardawaj S, Dutta U, Singh K. High prevalence of human papillomavirus in esophageal squamous cell carcinoma: a study in paired samples. Dis Esophagus. 2013;26:282–7.
40. Gupta N, Barwad A, Rajwanshi A, Kochhar R. Prevalence of human papilloma virus in esophageal carcinomas: a polymerase chain reaction-based study. Acta Cytol. 2012;56:80–4.
41. Hardefeldt HA, Cox MR, Eslick GD, et al. Association between human papilloma virus (HPV) and oesophageal squamous cell carcinoma: a meta-analysis. Epidemiol Infect. 2014;142:1119–37.
42. Ali I, Wani WA, Saleem K. Cancer scenario in India with future perspectives. Cancer Therapy. 2011;8:56–70.
43. Dinshaw KA, Rao DN. Hospital cancer registry annual report 1996. Division of Epidemiology & Biostatistics. Mumbai: Published by Tata Memorial Hospital; 2000. p. 43.
44. Karmarkar P, Wilkinson A, Manohar T, Joshi A, Mahore S. Diagnostic utility of endoscopic brush cytology in upper gastrointestinal lesions and its correlation with biopsy. IOSR J Dent Med Sci. 2013;5:32–6.
45. Sharma P, Misra V, Singh PA, Misra SP, Gupta SC. A correlative study of histology and imprint cytology in the diagnosis of gastrointestinal tract malignancies. Indian J Pathol Microbiol. 1997;40:139–46.
46. Batra M, Handa U, Mohan H, Sachdev A. Comparison of cytohistologic techniques in diagnosis of gastroesophageal malignancy. Acta Cytol. 2008;52:77–82.
47. Lal N, Bhasin DK, Malik AK, Gupta NM, Singh K, Mehta SK. Optimal number of biopsy specimens in the diagnosis of carcinoma of the oesophagus. Gut. 1992;33:724–6.
48. Sharma OP, Chandermohan, Mashankar AS, Ganguly M, Sarangi L, Patange VB, et al. Role of computed tomography in preoperative evaluation of esophageal carcinoma. Ind J Cancer. 1994;31:12–8.
49. Chowdhury V, Gulati P, Kakkar A, Aranya RC. Computed tomography evaluation of esophageal carcinoma. Indian J Cancer. 1992;29:172–6.
50. Sharma OP, Subnani S. Role of computerized tomography imaging in staging oesophageal carcinoma. Semin Surg Oncol. 1989;5:355–8.

51. Kumar P, Damle NA, Bal C. Role of F18-FDG PET/CT in the staging and restaging of esophageal cancer: a comparison with CECT. Indian J Surg Oncol. 2011;2:343–50.
52. Mallarajapatna GJ, Kallur KG, Ramanna NK, Susheela SP, Ramachandra PG. PET/CT-guided percutaneous biopsy of isolated intramuscular metastases from postcricoid cancer. J Nucl Med Technol. 2009;37:220–2.
53. Purandare NC, Pramesh CS, Karimundackal G, et al. Incremental value of F18-FDG PET/CT in therapeutic decision – making of potentially curable esophageal adenocarcinoma. Nuc Med Comm. 2014;35(8):864–9.
54. https://www.uicc.org/news-and-updates/25-7-announcements/9th-edition-uicc-tnm-classification-malignant-tumours-now-available. Accessed 14 Aug 2025.
55. https://www.ncgindia.org/assets/ncg-guidelines-2019/ncg-guidelines-for-thoracic-cancer-2019.pdf. Accessed 14 Aug 2025.
56. https://www.ncgindia.org/key-initiatives/virtual-tumor-board. Accessed 14 Aug 2025.
57. Yoshida N, Baba Y, Shigaki H, et al. Preoperative nutritional assessment by controlling nutritional status (CONUT) is useful to estimate postoperative morbidity after esophagectomy for esophageal cancer. World J Surg. 2016;40:1910–7.
58. Parshad R, Misra MC, Joshi YK, Kapur BM. Role of enteral hyperalimentation in patients of carcinoma oesophagus. Indian J Med Res. 1993;98:165–9.
59. Inoue J, Ono R, Makiura D, et al. Prevention of postoperative pulmonary complications through intensive preoperative respiratory rehabilitation in patients with esophageal cancer. Dis Esophagus. 2013;26:68–74.
60. Lone GN, Sheikh AA, Sheikh ZA, Baba KM, Qurieshi MA, Mufti GN, et al. Role of preoperative chemotherapy in squamous cell carcinoma of esophagus in Kashmir, a cancer belt – a pilot study. Asian Pac J Cancer Prev. 2011;12:465–70.
61. Kataria K, Verma GR, Malhotra A, Yadav R. Comparison of quality of life in patients undergoing transhiatal esophagectomy with or without chemotherapy. Saudi J Gastroenterol. 2012;18:195–200.
62. Rao YG, Pal S, Pande GK, Sahni P, Chattopadhyay TK. Transhiatal esophagectomy for benign and malignant conditions. Am J Surg. 2002;184:136–42.
63. Gupta NM. Oesophagectomy without thoracotomy: first 250 patients. Eur J Surg. 1996;162:455–61.
64. Subramanyeshwar RT, Raju KVVN, Patnaik SC, Saksena AR, Pratap RR, Rayani BK, et al. Minimally invasive esophagectomy the standard of care: experience from a tertiary care cancer center from India. Indian J Surg Oncol. 2021;12:335–49.
65. Kawoosa NU, Dar AM, Sharma ML, Ahangar AG, Lone GN, Bhat MA, et al. Transthoracic versus transhiatal esophagectomy for esophageal carcinoma: experience from a single tertiary care institution. World J Surg. 2011;35:1296–302.
66. Ranganathan P, Jiwnani S, Ashok A, Purwar P, Karimundackal G, Parab S, et al. Predicting pulmonary complications after esophagectomy: a retrospective cohort study. Ind J Cancer. 2025;62:135–41.
67. Lerut T, Coosemans W, DeLeyn P, Decker G, Deneffe G, Van Raemdonck D. Is there a role for radical esophagectomy? Eur J Cardiothorac Surg. 1999;16 Suppl 1:S44–7.
68. Rajan PS, Vaithiswaran V, Rajapandian S, Senthilnathan P, Praveenraj P, Palanivelu C. Minimally invasive oesophagectomy for carcinoma oesophagus—approaches and options in a high volume tertiary centre. J Indian Med Assoc. 2010;108:642–4.
69. Palanivelu C, Prakash A, Senthilkumar R, Senthilnathan P, Parthasarathi R, Rajan PS, et al. Minimally invasive esophagectomy: thoracoscopic mobilization of the esophagus and mediastinal lymphadenectomy in prone position—experience of 130 patients. J Am Coll Surg. 2006;203:7–16.
70. Kothari KC, Nair CK, George PS, Patel MH, Gatti RC, Gurjar GC. Comparison of esophagectomy with and without thoracotomy in a low-resource tertiary care center in a developing country. Dis Esophagus. 2011;24:583–9.

71. Straatman J, van der Wielen N, Cuesta MA, et al. Minimally invasive versus open esophageal resection: three year follow-up of the recently reported randomized controlled trial, the TIME trial. Ann Surg. 2017;266:232–6.
72. Mariette C, Markar S, Dabakuyo-Yonli B, et al. Hybrid minimally invasive vs. open esophagectomy for patients with esophageal cancer: long-term outcomes of a multicenter, open-label, randomized phase III controlled trial, the MIRO trial. N Eng J Med. 2019;380:152–62.
73. Puntamberkar S, Kenawadekar R, Pandit A, et al. Minimally invasive esophagectomy in the elderly. Indian J Surg Oncol. 2013;4:326–31.
74. Puntambekar SP, Kenawadekar R, Kumar S, et al. Robotic transthoracic esophagectomy. BMC Surg. 2015;15:47.
75. Sayed AI, Goel S, Aggarwal A, Singh S. Robot assisted minimally invasive esophagectomy: safety, perioperative morbidity and short-term oncological outcome-a single institution experience. J Robot Surg. 2022;16:517–25.
76. Balasubramanian S, Chittawadagi B, Misra S, Ramakrishnan P, Chinnusamy P. Propensity matched analysis of short term oncological and perioperative outcomes following robotic and thoracolaparoscopic esophagectomy for carcinoma esophagus-the first Indian experience. J Robot Surg. 2022;16:97–105.
77. Van der Sluis PC, van der Horst S, May Anne M, et al. Robot-assisted minimally invasive thoracolaparoscopic esophagectomy versus open transthoracic esophagectomy for resectable esophageal cancer: a randomized controlled trial. Ann of Surg. 2019;269:621–30.
78. Khiria LS, Pal S, Peush S, Chattopadhyay TK, Deval M. Impact on outcome of the route of conduit transposition after transhiatal oesophagectomy: a randomized controlled trial. Dig Liver Dis. 2009;41:711–6.
79. Saluja SS, Ray S, Pal S, et al. Randomized trial comparing side-to-side stapled and hand-sewn esophagogastric anastomosis in neck. J Gastrointest Surg. 2012;16:1287–95.
80. Shapiro J, van Lanschot JJB, Hulschof MCC, et al. Neoadjuvant chemoradiotherapy plus surgery versus surgery alone for oesophageal or junctional cancer (CROSS): long-term results of a randomised controlled trial. Lancet Oncol. 2015;16:1090–8.
81. Yang H, Liu H, Chen Y, et al. Neoadjuvant chemoradiotherapy followed by surgery versus surgery alone for locally advanced squamous cell carcinoma of the esophagus (NEOCRTEC5010): a phase III multicenter, randomized, open-label clinical trial. J Clin Oncol. 2018;36:2796–803.
82. Klevebro F, von Dobeln GA, Wang N, et al. A randomized clinical trial of neoadjuvant chemotherapy versus neoadjuvant chemoradiotherapy for cancer of the esophagus or gastro-esophageal junction. Ann Oncol. 2016;27:660–7.
83. Kelly RJ, Ajani JA, Kuzdzal J, Zander T, Van Cutsem E, Piessen G, CheckMate 577 Investigators, et al. Adjuvant nivolumab in resected esophageal or gastroesophageal junction cancer. N Engl J Med. 2021;384:1191–203. Erratum in: N Engl J Med. 2023; 388: 672.
84. Kumar S, Dimri K, Khurana R, Rastogi N, Das KJ, Lal P. A randomised trial of radiotherapy compared with cisplatin chemo-radiotherapy in patients with unresectable squamous cell cancer of the esophagus. Radiother Oncol. 2007;83:139–47.
85. Javed A, Pal S, Dash NR, Ahuja V, Mohanti BK, Vishnubhatla S, et al. Palliative stenting with or without radiotherapy for inoperable esophageal carcinoma: a randomized trial. J Gastrointest Cancer. 2012;43:63–9.
86. Madhusudhan C, Saluja SS, Pal S, Ahuja V, Saran P, Dash NR, et al. Palliative stenting for relief of dysphagia in patients with inoperable esophageal cancer: impact on quality of life. Dis Esophagus. 2009;22:331–6.
87. Sharma V, Mahantshetty U, Dinshaw KA, Deshpande R, Sharma S. Palliation of advanced/recurrent esophageal carcinoma with high-dose-rate brachytherapy. Int J Radiat Oncol Biol Phys. 2002;52:310–5.
88. Gopinath SK, Jiwnani S, Valiyuthan P, Parab S, Niyogi D, Tiwari V, et al. Intraoperative nerve monitoring during minimally invasive esophagectomy and 3-field lymphadenectomy: safety, efficacy, and feasibility. J Chest Surg. 2023;56:336–45.

89. Nadkarni S, Jiwnani S, Reddy VS, Niyogi D, Tiwari VK, Karimundackal G, et al. Robotic esophagectomy and 3-field lymphadenectomy with intraoperative nerve monitoring. Multimed Man Cardiothorac Surg. 2022;2022. https://doi.org/10.1510/mmcts-2022-067.
90. Sundaram S, Puri R, Niyogi D, Tiwari V, Mahajan A, Kale A, et al. Modified low-cost EndoVac is safe and efficacious for treatment of postoperative leaks even at low pressures. Surg Endosc. 2025;20:1–6.
91. Fok M, McShane J, Law SYK, Wong J. Prospective randomized study on radiotherapy and surgery in treatment ofoesophageal carcinoma. Asian J Surg. 1994;17:223–9.
92. Badwe RA, Sharma V, Bhansali MS, Dinshaw KA, Patil PK, Dalvi N, et al. The quality of swallowing for patients with operable esophageal carcinoma: a randomized trial comparing surgery with radiotherapy. Cancer. 1999;85:763–8.
93. Noronha V, Patil VM, Menon N, Joshi A, Shah MJ, Singh A, et al. Phase III randomized trial comparing neoadjuvant paclitaxel plus platinum with 5-fluorouracil plus platinum in esophageal or gastroesophageal junction squamous cell carcinoma. J Natl Cancer Inst. 2025;117:58–75.
94. Goel A, Shah SH, Selvakumar VPP, et al. Robot-assisted Mckeown esophagectomy is feasible after neoadjuvant chemoradiation. Our initial experience. Indian J Surg. 2018;80:24–19.
95. Krishnamurthy A, Mohanraj N, Radhakrishnan V, et al. Neoadjuvant chemoradiation for locally advanced resectable carcinoma of the esophagus: a single center experience from India with a brief review of the literature. Indian J Cancer. 2017;54:646–51.
96. Bajwa HK, Singareddy R, Reddy MM, et al. Preoperative chemoradiation in carcinoma esophagus: experience from a tertiary cancer center in India. Ind J Med Ped Oncol. 2018;39:272–5.
97. Nusrath S, Thammineedi SR, Raju KVVN, Patnaik SC, Saksena AR, Karthik J, et al. Factors associated with pathologic complete response following neoadjuvant chemoradiation and esophagectomy for carcinoma of esophagus and gastroesophageal junction. J Surg Oncol. 2023;127:48–55.
98. Bhat MA, Dar MA, Lone GN, Dar AM. Use of pedicled omentum in esophagogastric anastomosis for prevention of anastomotic leak. Ann Thorac Surg. 2006;82:1857–62.
99. Gupta NM, Gupta R, Rao MS, Gupta V. Minimizing cervical esophageal anastomotic complications by a modified technique. Am J Surg. 2001;181:534–9.
100. Chattopadhyay TK, Gupta S, Padhy AK, Kapoor VK. Is pyloroplasty necessary following intrathoracic transposition of stomach? Results of a prospective clinical study. Aust N Z J Surg. 1991;61:366–9.
101. Mistry RC, Vijayabhaskar R, Karimundackal G, Jiwnani S, Pramesh CS. Effect of short-term vs prolonged nasogastric decompression on major postesophagectomy complications: a parallel-group, randomized trial. Arch Surg. 2012;147:747–51.
102. Pramesh CS, Patil V, Karimundackal G, Jiwnani S, Kulkarni AP, Divatia JV et al. Impact of perioperative fluid restriction on postoperative pulmonary complications following esophagectomy for cancer – a parallel-group randomized controlled trial. Presented at the 13th World Congress of the International Society for Diseases of the Esophagus, Venice, 2012.
103. Thammineedi SR, Patnaik SC, Reddy P, Saksena AR, Shukla S, Schissel ME, et al. Indocyanine green fluorescence angiography versus visual assessment for assessing perfusion of gastric conduit and esophageal stump in post esophagectomy patients: a pilot randomized controlled study. J Surg Oncol. 2025;132:45–53.
104. Agarwal L, Dash NR, Pal S, Madhusudhan KS, Mani V. Single-center randomized trial comparing feeding jejunostomy with nasojejunal tube placement in patients undergoing transhiatal esophagectomy post-neoadjuvant therapy for esophageal cancer. J Gastrointest Cancer. 2024;55:1282–90.
105. Ramakrishnan P, Saini S, Arora A, Khurana G. Impact of enhanced recovery protocols on short-term outcomes in esophagectomy: a retrospective cohort study from Cancer Research Institute, Uttarakhand, India. World J Surg. 2023;47:2968–76.
106. Low DE, Allum W, de Manzoni G, et al. Guidelines for perioperative care in esophagectomy: enhanced recovery after surgery (ERAS®) society recommendations. World J Surg. 2019;43:299–330.

107. Noronha V, Patil VM, Menon N, Goud S, Singh A, Shah M, et al. Phase III randomized trial comparing palliative systemic therapy to best supportive care in advanced esophageal/GEJ cancer. Int J Cancer. 2024;155:2232–45.
108. Noronha V, Patil VM, Menon NS, Joshi A, Goud S, More S, Kannan S, Pawar A, Nakti D, Yadav A, Shah S, Mahajan A, Janu A, Kumar R, Tibdewal A, Mummudi N, Agarwal JP, Banavali SD, Prabhash K. Oral metronomic chemotherapy after definitive chemoradiation in esophageal squamous cell carcinoma: a randomized clinical trial. Esophagus. 2022;19:670–82.
109. Pramesh CS, Mistry RC, Karimundackal G, Jiwnani S. Three field radical esophagectomy versus two field esophagectomy – a prospective randomized trial. Registered at Clinicaltrials.gov; Identifier NCT00193817. Last accessed at Clinicaltrials.gov on 14th Aug 2025.
110. Coyle C, Cafferty FH, Rowley S, MacKenzie M, Berkman L, Gupta S, ADD-ASPIRIN Investigators, et al. ADD-ASPIRIN: a phase III, double-blind, placebo controlled, randomised trial assessing the effects of aspirin on disease recurrence and survival after primary therapy in common non-metastatic solid tumours. Contemp Clin Trials. 2016;51:56–64.
111. Joharatnam-Hogan N, Cafferty F, Hubner R, Swinson D, Sothi S, Gupta K, Add-Aspirin Trial Management Group, et al. Aspirin as an adjuvant treatment for cancer: feasibility results from the Add-Aspirin randomised trial. Lancet Gastroenterol Hepatol. 2019;4:854–62.

Korean Experiences

20

Dae Joon Kim, Min Hee Hong, and Da Hyun Chung

20.1 Esophageal Cancer in Korea

According to the Korean Central Cancer Registry, 277,523 new cases of cancer were reported in Korea in 2021. Of these, 2954 cases (1.06%) were esophageal cancer. The crude incidence rate for esophageal cancer was 5.8 per 100,000 population, and the age-standardized incidence rate was 5.5 per 100,000 population [1]. The male-to-female ratio was 7:1, and incidence was highest at age 60–69 years (38.1%), followed by age 70–79 years (27.8%) and 50–59 years (17.1%). Histologically, 90.1% of esophageal cancer cases are squamous cell carcinoma, and 2.2% are adenocarcinoma [2]. The incidence of esophageal cancer in Korea is relatively low in comparison with that in Japan and China, and the age-standardized incidence rate decreased from 8.2 per 100,000 population in 1999 to 5.5 in 2021 [1].

The epidemiology of esophageal cancer in Korea is documented in several reports. For instance, Choi et al. (2017) reported that light drinking of just one alcoholic drink a day is associated with increased risks of esophageal, gastric, and colorectal cancers [3]. They also reported that underweight was a risk factor for esophageal squamous cell carcinoma (ESCC) and that alcohol

D. J. Kim (✉)
Division of General Thoracic Surgery, Department of Thoracic and Cardiovascular Surgery, Yonsei University College of Medicine, Seoul, Republic of Korea
e-mail: kdjcool@yuhs.ac

M. H. Hong
Division of Medical Oncology, Department of Internal Medicine, Yonsei University College of Medicine, Seoul, Republic of Korea
e-mail: minhee-hong@yuhs.ac

D. H. Chung
Division of Gastroenterology, Department of Internal Medicine, Yonsei University College of Medicine, Seoul, Republic of Korea
e-mail: jungdh@yuhs.ac

Y. Kitagawa et al. (eds.), *Esophageal Squamous Cell Carcinoma*,
https://doi.org/10.1007/978-981-92-2611-5_20

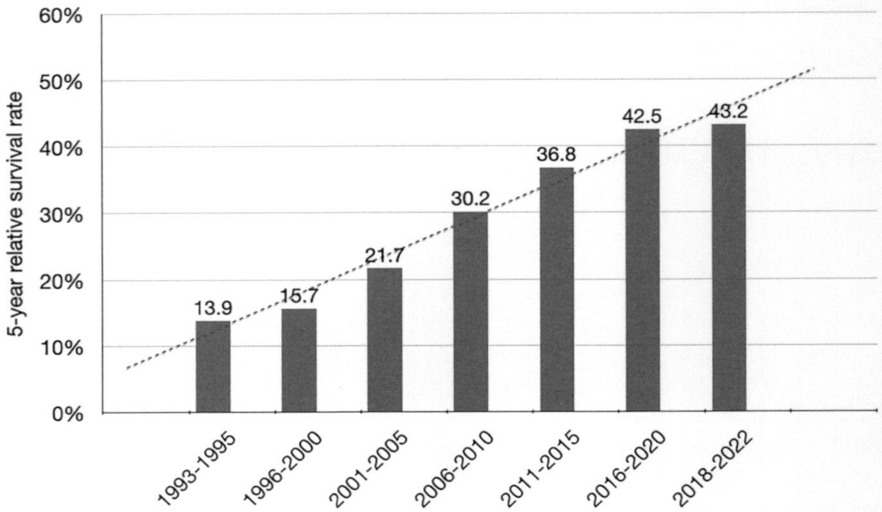

Fig. 20.1 Five-year relative survival rates of patients with esophageal cancer in Korea, 1993–2017

consumption acts synergistically to elevate that risk [4]. After analyzing the Kanghwa cohort, a strong dose-response relationship was reported between volume of alcohol drinking and development of esophageal cancer [5]. Another study reported that alcohol, smoking, and the aspartate aminotransferase to alanine aminotransferase ratio were independently associated with increased risk of esophageal cancer [6].

As Fig. 20.1 shows, the 2018–2022 5-year relative survival rate for esophageal cancer of 43.2% increased over time because of the early detection by the National Cancer Screening Program of Korea [2]. According to the Surveillance, Epidemiology, and End Results summary staging system, the 5-year relative survival rates for localized, regional, and distant diseases were 74.5%, 35.8%, and 7.4%, respectively.

20.2 Diagnosis and Staging

Since the introduction of a nationwide screening program to detect gastric cancer in 1999, esophageal cancer has been diagnosed at earlier stages. In 2021, the proportion of localized, regional, and distant diseases were 36.9%, 37.0%, and 18.0%, respectively (unknown 8.0%) [2]. Diagnosis is mainly by esophagogastroduodenoscopy (EGD) and biopsy, while esophagography is rarely performed. For the staging work-up, EGD, endoscopic ultrasound sonography (EUS), chest and abdominal-pelvic computed tomography (CT), and positron emission tomography (PET)-CT are routinely performed. Bronchoscopic examination is indicated only when airway invasion is suspected.

In recent decades, the growing use of endoscopic treatment for superficial esophageal cancer has underscored the importance of accurate T staging using EUS. Jung et al. (2014) evaluated the diagnostic accuracy of EUS in 126 patients with superficial esophageal cancer [7]. Their findings showed that EUS with a high-frequency catheter probe provided a high accuracy in assessing invasion depth (78.9%), though this accuracy declined for tumors ≥3 cm. For nodal staging and detection of distant metastases, PET-CT scan has been performed routinely in all patients, as it has been covered by the National Health Insurance System in Korea since 2006. Jeong et al. (2018) reported that, in early T-stage esophageal cancers (Tis, T1a, T1b, and T2), the sensitivity, specificity, and accuracy of PET-CT scan in discriminating N0 from node-positive disease were 88.9%, 38.7%, and 73.1%, respectively [8]. In a previous report, a significant proportion of nodal metastases were found to be too small to be detected by PET-CT scan. Among 85 patients who underwent preoperative PET-CT, nodal upstaging was evident postoperatively in 29 (34.1%) patients due to the small size of metastatic foci (mean, 4.47 ± 0.35 mm) in lymph nodes [9]. PET-CT is also used in predicting the response after neoadjuvant concurrent chemoradiation therapy (CCRT), or prognosis after definitive CCRT [10–12]. Currently, PET-CT combined with EUS constitutes the most critical modality for establishing optimal treatment strategy.

The 8th edition of the American Joint Committee on Cancer (AJCC) staging system and corresponding lymph node map are commonly adopted in most institutions [13–15]. However, regarding the lymph node map, some institutions adopted the 12th edition of the Japanese Classification System [16], as it provides a more accurate and detailed description of each lymph node station. Although both staging systems classify supraclavicular lymph node metastasis (LNM) as distant disease, it is often considered potentially curable by most surgeons by administering appropriate multimodality treatment. Cho et al. (2017) reported treatment outcomes in patients with supraclavicular LNM, and they suggested that supraclavicular LNM was not a risk factor for progression-free or overall survival [17]. In our institution, supraclavicular lymph nodes are classified as regional, and the standard treatment approach for patients with supraclavicular LNM includes neoadjuvant CCRT followed by surgical resection.

20.3 Endoscopic Treatment for Superficial Esophageal Cancer

20.3.1 Techniques and Results

In Korea, nationwide cancer screening programs and widespread use of upper gastrointestinal endoscopy for screening have led to an increased rate of superficial ESCC (SESCC) diagnosis [18]. Consequently, the number of endoscopic resections (ER) for SESCC has also been rising [19]. Several international clinical guidelines on ER for superficial esophageal cancer have been established [20, 21]. However, the incidence of early stage esophageal cancer and availability of procedural techniques and medical resources differ significantly across countries and regions. Thus, Korea has published its own guidelines, considering local epidemiologic characteristics, clinical patterns, and healthcare system [22]. According to the Korean guideline, ER is recommended for SESCC without evidence of distant or LNM and without obvious submucosal invasion. It is well established that LNM in esophageal cancer correlates closely with the depth of tumor invasion [23, 24]. Thus, the SESCC depth of invasion must be accurately determined before performing ER for SESCC. Korea guidelines recommend EUS to define SESCC stage and magnifying endoscopy with narrow band imaging for the depth of invasion before endoscopic treatment. However, since preprocedural depth evaluation is not always accurate, and considering the high morbidity and mortality associated with esophagectomy, ER may be considered the initial treatment option in the absence of definitive evidence of submucosal invasion. While ER offers the benefit of esophageal preservation, patients must be carefully selected because there is still a possibility of LNM.

A recent Korean study showed that among patients with SESCC without definite submucosal invasion, no significant difference was found in long-term survival between those who underwent ER and those who received esophagectomy. Moreover, the rate of posttreatment complications was significantly higher in the surgical group [25]. In addition, Korean guidelines recommend endoscopic submucosal dissection (ESD) rather than endoscopic mucosal resection (EMR) for en bloc and curative resection for SESCC confined to the mucosa. Although EMR is relatively easy to perform and is associated with low risk of complications, en bloc resection is difficult by EMR, especially for large lesions; thus, high local recurrence rates after EMR have been reported [26, 27]. Therefore, although ESD is a technically challenging procedure, when considering a high en bloc resection rate and low risks of local recurrence, ESD is an appropriate treatment strategy for SESCC. However, resection technique is generally determined by the size of the lesion, along with additional factors such as the patient's clinical status and endoscopist's experience.

For patients with mucosal defects involving >75% of the esophageal circumference after ESD, Korean guidelines recommend oral steroid therapy or local steroid injection to prevent esophageal stricture. For oral steroid therapy, prednisolone is usually started at 30 mg daily within 1–2 days after the procedure, followed by a tapering over 2–12 weeks [28, 29]. Local steroid injections are also effective treatment options and have a 70% preventive effect against esophageal strictures, which has a rate of 11% in patients administered local steroid injections [30]. Given the potential for esophageal perforation and other adverse events of local steroid injections, their usage should be reserved for patients with mucosal defects involving >75% of the esophageal circumference, who are at high-risk of developing strictures.

20.3.2 Additional Treatment After ESD: Definitive Chemoradiation and Other Treatments

The Korean guidelines stratify additional treatment need according to the depth of tumor invasion and presence or absence of lymphovascular invasion. If the tumor is confined to the lamina propria, completely resected en bloc, and shows no lymphovascular invasion, no additional treatment is required due to the extremely low risk of LNM [31, 32]. When the tumor invades the muscularis mucosa without lymphovascular invasion, the risk of LNM remains low, and close follow-up without additional treatment may be considered. This is because, in mucosa-confined esophageal cancers, tumors invading the muscularis mucosa carry a higher risk of LNM compared to those limited to the lamina propria (8.0%–27.0% vs. 0.0%–8.7%). In cases of piecemeal resection, follow-up strategies should account for the potential inaccuracy of histopathological evaluation. Long-term follow-up studies from Korea demonstrated that ER for SESCC limited to the mucosa resulted in no esophageal cancer-related deaths, supporting its role as a safe and effective treatment option [33, 34]. When the post-ESD pathology reveals submucosal invasion, lymphovascular invasion, or a positive vertical margin—indicating a higher risk of LNM—the resection is classified as non-curative, and additional treatment is recommended. This is because histopathological evaluations of esophagectomy specimens with regional lymph node dissection revealed an association between submucosal invasion in esophageal cancer and LNM, with reported LNM rates of 26.0%–53.8%. Notably, even when invasion is limited to the upper third of the submucosa, LNM has been observed in 8.3%–53.1% of cases [35–42].

It remains unclear whether salvage esophagectomy following non-curative ESD shows better outcomes than those of primary esophagectomy in patients with T1 esophageal cancer. The study conducted in Korea demonstrated short- and long-term clinical outcomes between salvage esophagectomy following noncurative ESD and primary esophagectomy with no difference in LNM, overall survival, disease-specific survival, and recurrence-free survival [43]. Overall, adverse events did not differ significantly between groups, but early complications were more frequent in the primary surgery group (50% vs. 20.6%, $p = 0.021$). Therefore, considering the substantial risks of morbidity and mortality with esophagectomy, initial treatment with ESD for SESCC can be a highly favorable treatment strategy.

Although some studies suggest that undifferentiated tumors may be associated with an increased risk of LNM, others do not support this association [31, 32, 39, 42]. Thus, per the Korean guidelines, undifferentiated histology alone cannot be considered a definitive criterion for non-curative resection; further studies are needed to draw firm conclusions.

In Korea, guidelines, esophagectomy with regional lymph node dissection is the standard approach following non-curative ER. However, given the substantial associated postoperative morbidity (30%–40%) and mortality (1%–2%) [44–46], the patient's overall condition must be carefully evaluated before surgery. Recent studies have shown favorable outcomes with chemoradiation therapy in this setting, suggesting its potential as an alternative treatment strategy for non-curative ER [47–52].

To date, no prospective randomized clinical trials have directly compared esophagectomy and chemoradiation therapy in patients with non-curative ER. However, two phase III multicenter randomized controlled trials are currently underway—one in Korea (ClinicalTrials.gov identifier: NCT03306901, ASSURE trial) and another in China [53]. The outcomes of these studies are expected to help establish the optimal additional treatment strategy for patients with SESCC who undergo non-curative ER.

20.4 Surgery

20.4.1 Analysis of Surgical Treatment Based on the Health Insurance Review and Assessment (HIRA) Data

In Korea, all citizens are covered under the National Health Insurance System, and the HIRA service, a subsidiary organization, is responsible for evaluating the quality and volume of medical services. From 2007 to 2014, HIRA released several nationwide reports assessing the volume-outcome relationship of major surgical procedures, including esophagectomy.

The earliest report, analyzing cases from 2005 to 2006, identified 1272 esophagectomy procedures performed across 76 hospitals. A key finding was that hospitals performing ≥21 cases over 2 years—defined as high-volume centers—had significantly lower operative mortality (2.07%) compared to low-volume centers (6.20%). These institutions also demonstrated shorter hospital stays (26.3 vs. 30.6 days) and lower complication rates. In this period, 13 high-volume hospitals (17.1%) accounted for 68.3% of all esophagectomy procedures.

A follow-up report in 2014 analyzing data from 2012 to 2013 showed an increase to 1751 esophagectomy cases across 82 centers. Again, high-volume centers (now 16 hospitals, 19.5%) performed 73.7% of procedures and continued to show superior outcomes, including operative mortality (3.26% vs. 8.68%); average hospital stay (25.7 vs. 38.0 days); and treatment costs, which were significantly lower in high- than low-volume centers. Notably, most high-volume centers were located in the Seoul metropolitan area, indicating a clear centralization of care.

Despite these findings, no updated data has been published by HIRA since 2014. Moreover, their reports excluded procedures not reimbursed by the national insurance system, such as robotic esophagectomy. Given the increasing adoption of robotic techniques and a shift toward early stage detection, the actual national statistics on esophagectomy may be underrepresented. These limitations underscore the urgent need for a comprehensive, nationwide registry to accurately capture current practices, outcomes, and trends in esophageal cancer surgery in Korea.

20.4.2 Surgical Approaches

Figure 20.2 shows the number of open or video-assisted thoracic surgery (VATS) esophagectomies performed in 2023 by administrative region in Korea, indicating that most procedures were performed in the Seoul metropolitan area. Traditionally, the open Ivor-Lewis esophagectomy was the preferred approach in most institutions, whereas the McKeown esophagectomy was typically reserved for patients with upper thoracic ESCC or for creating a cervical anastomosis in patients

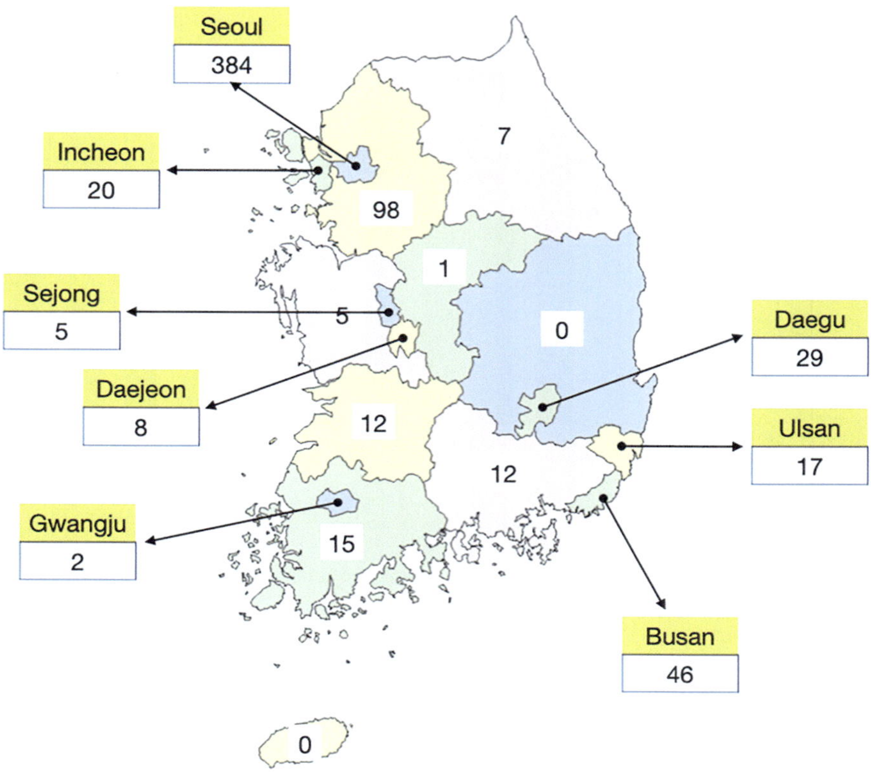

Fig. 20.2 The number of open or video-assisted thoracic surgery (VATS) esophagectomy in 2023 by the administrative region in Korea

undergoing VATS esophagectomy. In a propensity score-matched study comparing Ivor-Lewis esophagectomy with McKeown procedure for middle to lower thoracic ESCC, their mean number of dissected mediastinal lymph nodes was comparable, and no significant differences were observed in overall or disease-free survival [54]. In the last decade, there has been a transition from open esophagectomy (OE) to minimally invasive esophagectomy (MIE), with robot-assisted thoracoscopic esophagectomy (RATE) as the preferred MIE technique in Korea (Fig. 20.3).

20.4.3 Extent of Resection and Lymphadenectomy

Most institutions follow the National Comprehensive Cancer Network guidelines, which recommend dissecting at least 15 lymph nodes to ensure adequate lymphadenectomy. Although the Japanese guidelines have recently gained attention, their concept of D1, D2, or D3 lymphadenectomy has not been widely adopted in the surgical community.

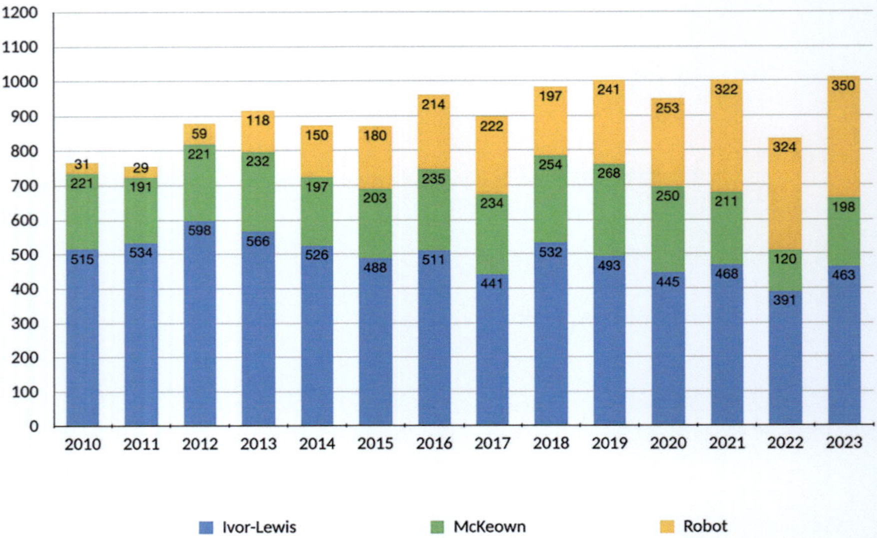

Fig. 20.3 Annual trends in esophageal cancer surgeries by approach in Korea (2010–2023)

Two-Field Lymphadenectomy (2-FL) Versus Three-Field Lymphadenectomy (3-FL)

For Ivor-Lewis esophagectomy, the predominant approach in Korea, the 2-FL is the widely accepted standard procedure. Shim et al. analyzed 91 patients with upper thoracic ESCC and showed significant differences in long-term survival outcomes between those who underwent 2-FL ($n = 34$) and 3-FL ($n = 57$) [55]. For the 2-FL and 3-FL groups, the 5-year overall survival was 52% vs. 44% ($p = 0.65$), while the 5-year disease-free survival was 39% vs. 38%, respectively ($p = 0.97$). The authors concluded that, without preoperative evidence of cervical LNM, cervical lymph node dissection may not provide additional survival benefit. In addition, a retrospective study of 611 patients who underwent 3-FL found that supraclavicular LNM was not an independent prognostic factor for overall survival in multivariate analysis [56]. A recent 2025 report suggests that selective right recurrent laryngeal nerve (RLN) lymph node dissection may be considered for cT1N0 ESCC [57]. Among 658 patients with cT1N0 ESCC, right RLN node dissection was performed in 88 and omitted in 570. According to their 1:2 ratio propensity score-matched analysis, overall survival (77.2% vs. 77.9%, $p = 0.94$) and recurrence-free interval (72.1% vs. 72.8%) did not differ significantly. They suggested that selective right RLN node dissection could be an acceptable approach in early-stage ESCC.

En Bloc Versus Non-en Bloc Resection

Although the concept of en bloc esophagectomy (EBE) was introduced for thoracic esophageal cancer in the early 1980s, it has not been widely adopted due to its increased postoperative morbidity and unclear oncologic benefit. Furthermore, with recent advances in neoadjuvant CCRT, interest in EBE has significantly declined, including in Korea.

20.4.4 Minimally Invasive Esophagectomy

Since we first performed RATE in July 2006, it has served as the distinctive mainstay of MIE in Korea, as Fig. 20.3 illustrates. At our institution, among 112 esophagectomies performed in 2018, 48.1% were by robotic assistance, while 23.5% were via VATS. We reported the oncologic outcomes of RATE in thoracic ESCC by analyzing 115 patients undergoing total mediastinal lymphadenectomy without neoadjuvant therapy in 2017 [58]. The 3-year overall survival and freedom from recurrence rates were 94.4% and 96.2% for stage I; 86.2% and 80.1% for stage II; and 77.8% and 79.5% for stage IIIA disease, respectively. Na et al. (2022) conducted a propensity score–matched study comparing RATE and OE in 272 patients with ESCC and showed fewer major complications with RATE, including shorter hospital stay and higher number of retrieved lymph nodes [59]. While overall recurrence rates were similar, RATE achieved significantly better 5-year overall survival (75.1% vs. 57.9%, $p = 0.002$) and regional nodal control (81.4% vs. 62.7%, $p = 0.003$) compared to OE. Kwon et al. (2025) reported a propensity score-matched analysis comparing RATE ($n = 443$) and OE ($n = 443$) [60]. After matching, 65.5% had pathologic stage I disease, and approximately 29% received neoadjuvant therapy. RATE was associated with a higher 5-year overall survival (70.4% vs. 61.8%, $p < 0.01$) and freedom from recurrence rate (62.8% vs. 55.8%, $p = 0.004$) compared to OE. Recently, Lee et al. (2025) reported the first series of MIE using the da Vinci single-port robotic system (Intuitive Surgical Inc., Sunnyvale, CA, USA) [61]. The single-port system was introduced through the 4 cm working window at the subcostal area, with a 12-mm assistant port placed at the eighth intercostal space. They suggested that single-port esophagectomy is technically feasible, although larger studies are needed to validate its safety and efficacy.

20.4.5 Severance Hospital Experiences

We have been performing McKeown esophagectomy with 3-FL for thoracic ESCC. Regarding the extent of lymphadenectomy, we adopted D3 dissection according to the 11th edition of the Japanese classification of esophageal cancer [62]. This aggressive surgical approach is applied even in cases of superficial ESCC. In our previous study comparing total mediastinal lymphadenectomy with traditional lymph node dissection for pT1 ESCC, the 3-year overall and disease-free survival rates were better in the mediastinal lymphadenectomy group (95.1% vs. 83.3% and 92.3% vs. 73.7%, respectively) [63]. For locally advanced ESCC, we performed EBE including thoracic duct resection. We reported that skeletonizing EBE enabled the identification and removal of lymphatic metastases along the thoracic duct and facilitated sufficient circumferential resection margins,

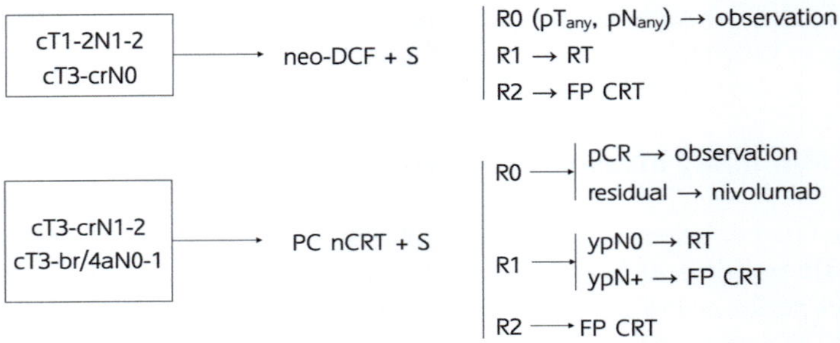

Fig. 20.4 Institutional treatment algorithm for locally advanced ESCC. *cT3-cr* completely resectable cT3, *cT3-br* borderline resectable cT3, *RT* radiation therapy, *CRT* chemoradiation therapy

leading to improved locoregional control and prolonged disease-free survival, particularly in patients with pT2–3 ESCCs [64]. Currently, we employ neoadjuvant chemotherapy using the DCF regimen, based on the JCOG1109 (NeXT) study, for patients with cT1–2N1–2 or completely resectable cT3N0 ESCC. For more advanced cases, we adopt neoadjuvant CCRT using the CROSS regimen, as illustrated in Fig. 20.4.

With the growing adoption of definitive CCRT as part of esophagus-preserving strategies and the emerging role of immunotherapy in advanced esophageal cancer, the use of salvage esophagectomy for residual or recurrent disease is expected to increase.

20.5 Multimodality Treatments

20.5.1 Definitive Chemoradiation and Other Treatment

As described earlier, the Republic of Korea has a unique health care system that covers all citizens universally [65]. It also means that the government is the only health care payer; thus, out-of-pocket costs are minimal. Furthermore, off-label prescriptions are strictly banned by the government, and doctors follow the approved indications and conduct medical practice according to the reimbursement system.

Generally, based on global and various other guidelines, the combination of 5-fluorouracil (5-FU) and cisplatin is most widely used and considered the standard regimen for CCRT. Although studies using S-1 or docetaxel-based regimens have been conducted, these were small-scale phase II trials and did not lead to widespread approval or clinical adoption [66, 67]. In contrast, the capecitabine/cisplatin regimen has gained clinical acceptance owing to its convenient administration and supportive findings from small-scale Korean studies [68, 69] (Table 20.1).

Table 20.1 Results from capecitabine-based clinical trials on definitive chemoradiotherapy for esophageal squamous cell carcinoma in the Republic of Korea

Study	Regimen	*N*	Outcome
Lee et al. Pilot study [68]	Capecitabine: 825 mg/BSA twice daily for 14 days Cisplatin 60 mg/BSA on day 1 Every 3 weeks Radiation: 2.0 Gy fraction/day to 60 Gy	9	ORR: 100% CR: 66.7% PR: 33.3%
Lee et al. [69]	Induction chemotherapy: 2 cycles, every 3 weeks Capecitabine 1000 mg/BSA twice daily for 14 days Cisplatin 60 mg/BSA on day 1 Concurrent chemoradiotherapy Weekly capecitabine 800 mg/BSA twice daily on days 1–5. Weekly Cisplatin 30 mg/BSA on day 1. Radiation: 54 Gy	74	ORR: 54% Median TTP: 7.8 months Median OS: 12.0 months

BSA body surface area, *ORR* objective response, *CR* complete response, *PR* partial response, *TTP* time to progression, *OS* overall survival

20.5.2 Neoadjuvant Therapy

For many years, neoadjuvant CCRT has been the standard approach for locally advanced ESCC. Similar to the definitive treatment, combined 5-fluorouracil (5-FU) and cisplatin was historically the most widely used regimen for neoadjuvant CCRT. However, since the provision of reimbursement for the CROSS regimen (weekly paclitaxel and carboplatin) in 2021, it has become one of the most commonly adopted regimens due to its ease of administration [70]. In addition, alternative regimens such as capecitabine combined with cisplatin are also utilized following several Korean clinical trials (Table 20.2). Furthermore, neoadjuvant chemotherapy without radiation, particularly the DCF regimen (docetaxel, cisplatin, and 5-FU), has been increasingly utilized [71]. It is noteworthy that the choice of neoadjuvant therapy varies across institutions and remains non-standardized. Recently, a phase II single-arm multicenter trial investigated the feasibility of adding perioperative pembrolizumab to the CROSS regimen in patients with clinical stage II or III ESCC [72]. Despite a manageable safety profile and promising biomarker insights, the trial failed to meet its primary endpoint, with a pathologic complete response (pCR) rate of only 23.1% (95% confidence interval [CI]: 10.7%–42.4%) in both primary tumors and lymph nodes. These results suggest that while combining immune checkpoint inhibitors with CCRT is feasible, further studies are required to optimize patient selection and improve clinical outcomes.

Table 20.2 Results from clinical trials on neoadjuvant treatment for esophageal squamous cell carcinoma in Republic of Korea

Study	Regimen	*N*	Outcome
Lee et al. (Phase II) [80]	Two courses of induction: Cisplatin 60 mg/^{2} day 1 and 5-FU 1000 mg/m^2 days 2–6 Radiotherapy: 48 Gy/4 weeks	88	Esophagectomy rate: 79% mOS: 18 months 5-year OS rate: 23%
Lee et al. (Phase III) [81]	Arm A: Surgery alone Arm B: Chemoradiation then surgery Cisplatin 60 mg/m^2 day 1 and 5-FU 1000 mg/m^2 days 2–6 Radiation: 45.6 Gy/1.2 Gy twice a day	101	mOS: 27.3 and 28.2 months ($p = 0.69$) ORR: 86%, CR: 21%, pathologic CR: 43% in CRT group
Chang et al. (Phase II) [82]	S-1: 70 mg/m^2 days 1–4 and days 22–35 Cisplatin: 75 mg/m^2 days 1 and 22 Radiotherapy: 50.4 Gy, 1.8 Gy/fraction	60	Esophagectomy rate: 42% Pathologic CR: 60% (in resected patients) 2-year PFS and OS rate: 48% and 65%
Yoon et al. (Phase II) [83]	Arm A: ICT then CRT, followed by surgery Arm B: CRT alone followed by surgery ICT: Oxaliplatin 130 mg/m^2 day 1 and S-1 40 mg/m^2 twice daily days 1–4, every 3 weeks, total 2 cycles CRT: Oxaliplatin 130 mg/m^2 day 1 and S-1 30 mg/m^2 twice daily 5 days/week, radiotherapy: 46 Gy, 2 Gy/day	97	Esophagectomy rate: 72.1% Pathologic CR: 23.4% and 38% (in intended patients) 2-year PFS rate: 58.4% and 58.6% 2-year OS rate: 60.7% and 63.7%

5-FU 5-fluorouracil, *mOS* median overall survival, *ORR* objective response, *CR* complete response, *CRT* chemoradiotherapy, *PFS* progression-free survival, *ICT* induction chemotherapy

20.5.3 Adjuvant Therapy

In patients who undergo upfront surgery without neoadjuvant therapy, fluoropyrimidine-based adjuvant chemotherapy is commonly administered, particularly with lymph node involvement or other high-risk pathological features. This approach aims to reduce the risk of recurrence and improve long-term outcomes. Shim et al. (2022) conducted a Korean phase III randomized trial and demonstrated that adjuvant chemotherapy with capecitabine and cisplatin, compared to surgery alone, reduced early recurrence, although it did not improve long-term disease-free survival. This supports the use of capecitabine/cisplatin as an alternative to 5-FU/cisplatin in the adjuvant setting [73].

For patients treated with neoadjuvant CCRT followed by surgery, adjuvant nivolumab is recommended for those who do not achieve a pCR (non–ypT0N0). This recommendation is based on the results of the CheckMate 577 trial, which demonstrated a significant improvement in disease-free survival with the use of nivolumab as adjuvant therapy in this setting [74]. Given the high risk of recurrence in these patients, the addition of immune checkpoint inhibitors in the adjuvant setting has become an important component of standard care.

20.5.4 Palliative Chemotherapy

For many years, first-line systemic therapy for advanced or metastatic ESCC consisted of cytotoxic doublet regimens such as 5-FU/cisplatin, capecitabine/cisplatin, and, in some centers, docetaxel/cisplatin. However, these regimens yielded an objective response rate of approximately 30% and a median overall survival of <1 year [75, 76]. With the emergence of immune checkpoint inhibitors, combining programmed death-1 (PD-1) inhibitors (pembrolizumab or nivolumab) with platinum-based chemotherapy has become a standard first-line option for programmed death ligand-1 (PD-L1) positive patients. In phase III trials (KEYNOTE-590 and CheckMate-648), these regimens improved median overall survival from approximately 10 months to 12–13 months in all patients, and further extended survival to 13–15 months in PD-L1–positive subgroups, with an approximately 15–20 percentage points increase in objective response rates [77, 78]. Additionally, a chemotherapy-free regimen combining nivolumab and ipilimumab was approved in the Republic of Korea, offering an alternative option for selected patients based on the CheckMate-648 trial results. In June 2025, tislelizumab was approved for first-line use regardless of PD-L1 expression, offering a new option for broader patient populations [79]. Tislelizumab can be combined with paclitaxel/cisplatin, and due to its convenient administration, its clinical use is expected to increase. However, as of 2025, reimbursement limitations in certain regions restrict the broad use of these regimens in all patients.

For patients who had not received immunotherapy as part of first-line treatment, PD-1 inhibitors are recommended as second-line therapy, regardless of PD-L1 expression. In contrast, for patients previously treated with immune checkpoint inhibitors, cytotoxic monotherapy, such as irinotecan, docetaxel, or paclitaxel, is commonly recommended as second-line treatment.

References

1. Korean Central Cancer Registry. Annual report of cancer statistics on Korea in 2022. 2025 [cited 2025 Jun 2]. Available from: https://cancer.go.kr/lay1/S1T639C641/contents.do.
2. National Cancer Information Center. Information on esophageal cancer. 2024 [cited 2025 Jun 2]. Available from: https://www.cancer.go.kr/lay1/program/S1T211C223/cancer/view.do?cancer_seq=4277&menu_seq=4282.
3. Choi YJ, et al. The relationship between drinking alcohol and esophageal, gastric or colorectal cancer: a nationwide population-based cohort study of South Korea. PLoS One. 2017;12(10):e0185778.
4. Choi YJ, et al. Joint effects of low body mass index and alcohol consumption on developing esophageal squamous cell cancer: a Korean nationwide population-based cohort study. Asian Pac J Cancer Prev. 2017;18(7):1881–7.
5. Jung SH, et al. Population based study of the association between binge drinking and mortality from cancer of oropharynx and esophagus in Korean men: the Kangwha cohort study. Asian Pac J Cancer Prev. 2014;15(8):3675–9.

6. Kimm H, Kim S, Jee SH. The independent effects of cigarette smoking, alcohol consumption, and serum aspartate aminotransferase on the alanine aminotransferase ratio in Korean men for the risk for esophageal cancer. Yonsei Med J. 2010;51(3):310–7.
7. Jung JI, et al. Clinicopathologic factors influencing the accuracy of EUS for superficial esophageal carcinoma. World J Gastroenterol. 2014;20:6322–8.
8. Jeong DY, et al. Surgically resected T1- and T2-stage esophageal squamous cell carcinoma: T and N staging performance of EUS and PET/CT. Cancer Med. 2018;7(8):3561–70.
9. Park SY, et al. Relationship between the size of metastatic lymph nodes and positron emission tomographic/computer tomographic findings in patients with esophageal squamous cell carcinoma. World J Surg. 2015;39(12):2948–54.
10. Han S, et al. Prognostic and predictive values of interim (18)F-FDG PET during neoadjuvant chemoradiotherapy for esophageal cancer: a systematic review and meta-analysis. Ann Nucl Med. 2021;35(4):447–57.
11. Lee S, et al. (18)F-FDG PET/CT parameters for predicting prognosis in esophageal cancer patients treated with concurrent chemoradiotherapy. Technol Cancer Res Treat. 2021;20:15330338211024655.
12. Park JK, Kim JJ, Moon SW. A study about different findings of PET-CT between neoadjuvant and non-neoadjuvant therapy: SUVmax is not a reliable predictor of lymphatic involvement after neoadjuvant therapy for esophageal cancer. J Thorac Dis. 2016;8(5):784–94.
13. Rice TW, et al. Recommendations for clinical staging (cTNM) of cancer of the esophagus and esophagogastric junction for the 8th edition AJCC/UICC staging manuals. Dis Esophagus. 2016;29(8):913–9.
14. Rice TW, et al. Recommendations for pathologic staging (pTNM) of cancer of the esophagus and esophagogastric junction for the 8th edition AJCC/UICC staging manuals. Dis Esophagus. 2016;29(8):897–905.
15. Rice TW, et al. Recommendations for neoadjuvant pathologic staging (ypTNM) of cancer of the esophagus and esophagogastric junction for the 8th edition AJCC/UICC staging manuals. Dis Esophagus. 2016;29(8):906–12.
16. Mine S, et al. Japanese classification of esophageal cancer, 12th edition: part I. Esophagus. 2024;21(3):179–215.
17. Cho WK, et al. Supraclavicular and/or celiac lymph node metastases from thoracic esophageal squamous cell carcinoma did not compromise survival following neoadjuvant chemoradiotherapy and surgery. Oncotarget. 2017;8(2):3542–52.
18. Jung HK, et al. Treatment pattern and overall survival in esophageal cancer during a 13-year period: a nationwide cohort study of 6,354 Korean patients. PLoS One. 2020;15(4):e0231456.
19. Min YW. Endoscopic treatment for esophageal cancer. Korean J Gastroenterol. 2018;71(3):116–23.
20. Kitagawa Y, et al. Esophageal cancer practice guidelines 2022 edited by the Japan esophageal society: part 1. Esophagus. 2023;20(3):343–72.
21. Pimentel-Nunes P, et al. Endoscopic submucosal dissection for superficial gastrointestinal lesions: European Society of Gastrointestinal Endoscopy (ESGE) guideline – update 2022. Endoscopy. 2022;54(6):591–622.
22. Park CH, et al. Clinical practice guideline for endoscopic resection of early gastrointestinal cancer. Clin Endosc. 2020;53(2):142–66.
23. Ancona E, et al. Prediction of lymph node status in superficial esophageal carcinoma. Ann Surg Oncol. 2008;15(11):3278–88.
24. Spataro J, et al. Early esophageal cancer: a gastroenterologist's disease. Dig Dis Sci. 2019;64(11):3048–58.
25. Min YW, et al. Comparison of endoscopic submucosal dissection and surgery for superficial esophageal squamous cell carcinoma: a propensity score-matched analysis. Gastrointest Endosc. 2018;88(4):624–33.
26. Ishihara R, et al. Comparison of EMR and endoscopic submucosal dissection for en bloc resection of early esophageal cancers in Japan. Gastrointest Endosc. 2008;68(6):1066–72.

27. Takahashi H, et al. Endoscopic submucosal dissection is superior to conventional endoscopic resection as a curative treatment for early squamous cell carcinoma of the esophagus (with video). Gastrointest Endosc. 2010;72(2):255–64, 264.e1–2.
28. Kataoka M, et al. Efficacy of short period, low dose oral prednisolone for the prevention of stricture after circumferential endoscopic submucosal dissection (ESD) for esophageal cancer. Endosc Int Open. 2015;3(2):E113–7.
29. Zhou G, et al. Efficacy of prednisone for prevention of esophageal stricture after endoscopic submucosal dissection for superficial esophageal squamous cell carcinoma. Thorac Cancer. 2017;8(5):489–94.
30. Nagami Y, et al. Locoregional steroid injection prevents stricture formation after endoscopic submucosal dissection for esophageal cancer: a propensity score matching analysis. Surg Endosc. 2016;30(4):1441–9.
31. Eguchi T, et al. Histopathological criteria for additional treatment after endoscopic mucosal resection for esophageal cancer: analysis of 464 surgically resected cases. Mod Pathol. 2006;19(3):475–80.
32. Choi JY, et al. Feasibility of endoscopic resection in superficial esophageal squamous carcinoma. Gastrointest Endosc. 2011;73(5):881–9, 889.e1–2.
33. Park HC, et al. Ten-year experience of esophageal endoscopic submucosal dissection of superficial esophageal neoplasms in a single center. Korean J Intern Med. 2016;31(6):1064–72.
34. Song BG, et al. Endoscopic submucosal dissection under general anesthesia for superficial esophageal squamous cell carcinoma is associated with better clinical outcomes. BMC Gastroenterol. 2018;18(1):80.
35. Akutsu Y, et al. The overall prevalence of metastasis in T1 esophageal squamous cell carcinoma: a retrospective analysis of 295 patients. Ann Surg. 2013;257(6):1032–8.
36. Tachibana M, et al. Clinicopathological features of superficial squamous cell carcinoma of the esophagus. Am J Surg. 1997;174(1):49–53.
37. Endo M, et al. Clinicopathologic analysis of lymph node metastasis in surgically resected superficial cancer of the thoracic esophagus. Dis Esophagus. 2000;13(2):125–9.
38. Araki K, et al. Pathologic features of superficial esophageal squamous cell carcinoma with lymph node and distal metastasis. Cancer. 2002;94(2):570–5.
39. Bollschweiler E, et al. High rate of lymph-node metastasis in submucosal esophageal squamous-cell carcinomas and adenocarcinomas. Endoscopy. 2006;38(2):149–56.
40. Kim DU, et al. Risk factors of lymph node metastasis in T1 esophageal squamous cell carcinoma. J Gastroenterol Hepatol. 2008;23(4):619–25.
41. Moriya H, et al. Lymphatic tumor emboli detected by D2–40 immunostaining can more accurately predict lymph-node metastasis. World J Surg. 2011;35(9):2031–7.
42. Yamashina T, et al. Long-term outcome and metastatic risk after endoscopic resection of superficial esophageal squamous cell carcinoma. Am J Gastroenterol. 2013;108(4):544–51.
43. Kim M, et al. Outcomes of primary esophagectomy and esophagectomy after endoscopic submucosal dissection for superficial esophageal squamous cell carcinoma: a propensity-score-matched analysis. Cancers (Basel). 2023;15(23):5542.
44. Ra J, et al. Postoperative mortality after esophagectomy for cancer: development of a preoperative risk prediction model. Ann Surg Oncol. 2008;15(6):1577–84.
45. Chang AC, et al. Outcomes after transhiatal and transthoracic esophagectomy for cancer. Ann Thorac Surg. 2008;85(2):424–9.
46. Connors RC, et al. Comparing outcomes after transthoracic and transhiatal esophagectomy: a 5-year prospective cohort of 17,395 patients. J Am Coll Surg. 2007;205(6):735–40.
47. Motoori M, et al. Comparison between radical esophagectomy and definitive chemoradiotherapy in patients with clinical T1bN0M0 esophageal cancer. Ann Surg Oncol. 2012;19(7):2135–41.
48. Kawaguchi G, et al. The effectiveness of endoscopic submucosal dissection followed by chemoradiotherapy for superficial esophageal cancer. Radiat Oncol. 2015;10:31.
49. Ikeda A, et al. Endoscopic submucosal dissection (ESD) with additional therapy for superficial esophageal cancer with submucosal invasion. Intern Med. 2015;54(22):2803–13.

50. Hamada K, et al. Efficacy and safety of endoscopic resection followed by chemoradiotherapy for superficial esophageal squamous cell carcinoma: a retrospective study. Clin Transl Gastroenterol. 2017;8(8):e110.
51. Kurokawa Y, et al. A phase II trial of combined treatment of endoscopic mucosal resection and chemoradiotherapy for clinical stage I esophageal carcinoma: Japan Clinical Oncology Group Study JCOG0508. Jpn J Clin Oncol. 2009;39(10):686–9.
52. Minashi K, et al. Efficacy of endoscopic resection and selective chemoradiotherapy for stage I esophageal squamous cell carcinoma. Gastroenterology. 2019;157(2):382–390.e3.
53. Yang Y, et al. Esophagectomy versus definitive chemoradiotherapy for patients with clinical stage N0 and pathological stage T1b esophageal squamous cell carcinoma after endoscopic submucosal dissection: study protocol for a multicenter randomized controlled trial (Ad-ESD Trial). Trials. 2020;21(1):603.
54. Park SY, et al. Comparison of the oncologic outcomes for patients with middle to lower esophageal squamous cell carcinoma undergoing surgical treatment using the Ivor-Lewis or McKeown operation. Ann Surg Oncol. 2024;31(12):7750–8.
55. Shim YM, Kim HK, Kim K. Comparison of survival and recurrence pattern between two-field and three-field lymph node dissections for upper thoracic esophageal squamous cell carcinoma. J Thorac Oncol. 2010;5(5):707–12.
56. Park SY, et al. Clinical and pathologic supraclavicular lymph node metastases in esophageal squamous cell carcinoma treated by esophagectomy with three-field lymph node dissection. Ann Surg Oncol. 2024;31(5):3399–408.
57. Kwon Y, et al. Clinical implications of selective right paratracheal lymph node dissection in patients with early-stage esophageal cancer: propensity score-matched analysis. Eur J Surg Oncol. 2025;51(8):110095.
58. Park SY, et al. The oncologic outcome of esophageal squamous cell carcinoma patients after robot-assisted thoracoscopic esophagectomy with total mediastinal lymphadenectomy. Ann Thorac Surg. 2017;103(4):1151–7.
59. Na KJ, et al. Robotic esophagectomy versus open esophagectomy in esophageal squamous cell carcinoma: a propensity-score matched analysis. J Robot Surg. 2022;16(4):841–8.
60. Kwon Y, et al. Long-term oncologic outcomes of robot-assisted versus conventional open esophagectomy for esophageal cancer: propensity-score matched anaylsis. Eur J Surg Oncol. 2025;51(5):109591.
61. Lee JH, et al. Single-port robot-assisted minimally invasive esophagectomy using the single-port robotic system via the subcostal approach: a single-center retrospective study. Cancers (Basel). 2025;17(7):1052.
62. Japan Esophageal Society. Japanese classification of esophageal cancer, 11th edition: part I. Esophagus. 2017;14(1):1–36.
63. Park SY, et al. Extent of mediastinal lymphadenectomy and survival in superficial esophageal squamous cell carcinoma. J Gastrointest Surg. 2017;21(10):1584–90.
64. Kim HE, et al. Skeletonizing en bloc esophagectomy revisited: oncologic outcome in association with the presence of thoracic duct lymph nodes. Ann Surg Oncol. 2022;29(8):4909–17.
65. Kim DS. Introduction: health of the health care system in Korea. Soc Work Public Health. 2010;25(2):127–41.
66. Cho SH, et al. Concurrent chemoradiotherapy with S-1 and cisplatin in advanced esophageal cancer. Dis Esophagus. 2008;21(8):697–703.
67. Shim HJ, et al. A phase II study of concurrent chemoradiotherapy with weekly docetaxel and cisplatin in advanced oesophageal cancer. Cancer Chemother Pharmacol. 2012;70(5):683–90.
68. Lee SJ, et al. Definitive chemoradiotherapy with capecitabine and cisplatin in patients with esophageal cancer: a pilot study. J Korean Med Sci. 2009;24(1):120–5.
69. Lee SS, et al. Capecitabine and cisplatin chemotherapy (XP) alone or sequentially combined chemoradiotherapy containing XP regimen in patients with three different settings of stage IV esophageal cancer. Jpn J Clin Oncol. 2007;37(11):829–35.
70. Shapiro J, et al. Neoadjuvant chemoradiotherapy plus surgery versus surgery alone for oesophageal or junctional cancer (CROSS): long-term results of a randomised controlled trial. Lancet Oncol. 2015;16(9):1090–8.

71. Kato K, et al. Doublet chemotherapy, triplet chemotherapy, or doublet chemotherapy combined with radiotherapy as neoadjuvant treatment for locally advanced oesophageal cancer (JCOG1109 NExT): a randomised, controlled, open-label, phase 3 trial. Lancet. 2024;404(10447):55–66.
72. Hong MH, et al. A phase II trial of preoperative chemoradiotherapy and pembrolizumab for locally advanced esophageal squamous cell carcinoma (ESCC). J Clin Oncol. 2019;37(15_suppl):4027.
73. Shim YM, et al. The efficacy of adjuvant chemotherapy with capecitabine and cisplatin after surgery in locally advanced esophageal squamous cell carcinoma: a multicenter randomized phase III trial. Dis Esophagus. 2022;35(1):doab040.
74. Kelly RJ, et al. Adjuvant Nivolumab in resected esophageal or gastroesophageal junction cancer. N Engl J Med. 2021;384(13):1191–203.
75. Bleiberg H, et al. Randomised phase II study of cisplatin and 5-fluorouracil (5-FU) versus cisplatin alone in advanced squamous cell oesophageal cancer. Eur J Cancer. 1997;33(8):1216–20.
76. Lee J, et al. A phase II study of capecitabine and cisplatin (XP) as first-line chemotherapy in patients with advanced esophageal squamous cell carcinoma. Cancer Chemother Pharmacol. 2008;62(1):77–84.
77. Sun JM, et al. Pembrolizumab plus chemotherapy versus chemotherapy alone for first-line treatment of advanced oesophageal cancer (KEYNOTE-590): a randomised, placebo-controlled, phase 3 study. Lancet. 2021;398(10302):759–71.
78. Doki Y, et al. Nivolumab combination therapy in advanced esophageal squamous-cell carcinoma. N Engl J Med. 2022;386(5):449–62.
79. Xu J, et al. Tislelizumab plus chemotherapy versus placebo plus chemotherapy as first-line treatment for advanced or metastatic oesophageal squamous cell carcinoma (RATIONALE-306): a global, randomised, placebo-controlled, phase 3 study. Lancet Oncol. 2023;24(5):483–95.
80. Lee JL, et al. Efficacy of neoadjuvant chemoradiotherapy in resectable esophageal squamous cell carcinoma--a single institutional study. Acta Oncol. 2003;42(3):207–17.
81. Lee JL, et al. A single institutional phase III trial of preoperative chemotherapy with hyperfractionation radiotherapy plus surgery versus surgery alone for resectable esophageal squamous cell carcinoma. Ann Oncol. 2004;15(6):947–54.
82. Chang H, et al. A prospective phase II trial of S-1 and cisplatin-based chemoradiotherapy for locoregionally advanced esophageal cancer. Cancer Chemother Pharmacol. 2014;73(4):665–71.
83. Yoon DH, et al. Randomized phase 2 trial of S1 and oxaliplatin-based chemoradiotherapy with or without induction chemotherapy for esophageal cancer. Int J Radiat Oncol Biol Phys. 2015;91(3):489–96.

Chinese Experiences 21

Lijie Tan and Han Tang

21.1 Introduction

Esophageal cancer has a poor prognosis, leading to about 187,000 deaths, a little decrease in China annually, and most of them are esophageal squamous cell carcinoma (ESCC) [1]. In 1940, Dr. Wu performed the first esophageal resection, pioneering the surgical treatment for esophageal cancer in China. Since then, Chinese doctors have been investigating and exploring the optimal strategy for treatment of esophageal cancer. Over the past decades, multimodality treatment for esophageal cancer, showing a survival benefit, has become the mainstream in China, and individualized comprehensive therapy is recommended by Clinical Practice Guidelines for the Diagnosis and Treatment of Esophageal Cancer [2]. The diagnostic and therapeutic flow in China is shown in Fig. 21.1. In this chapter, we summarize the experiences and advances in the treatment of ESCC in the era of multimodality management in China. In the first section, we provide an overview of endoscopic treatment of ESCC. In the second section, we address commonly used surgical techniques for ESCC, with a particular focus on surgical approach, especially robot-assisted esophagectomy and inflatable video-assisted mediastinoscopic transhiatal esophagectomy. In the third section, we discuss perioperative therapy for ESCC, including neoadjuvant and adjuvant therapy, as well as systematic therapy for ESCC.

L. Tan (✉) · H. Tang
Department of Thoracic Surgery, Zhongshan Hospital, Fudan University, Shanghai, China
e-mail: tan.lijie@zs-hospital.sh.cn

Y. Kitagawa et al. (eds.), *Esophageal Squamous Cell Carcinoma*,
https://doi.org/10.1007/978-981-92-2611-5_21

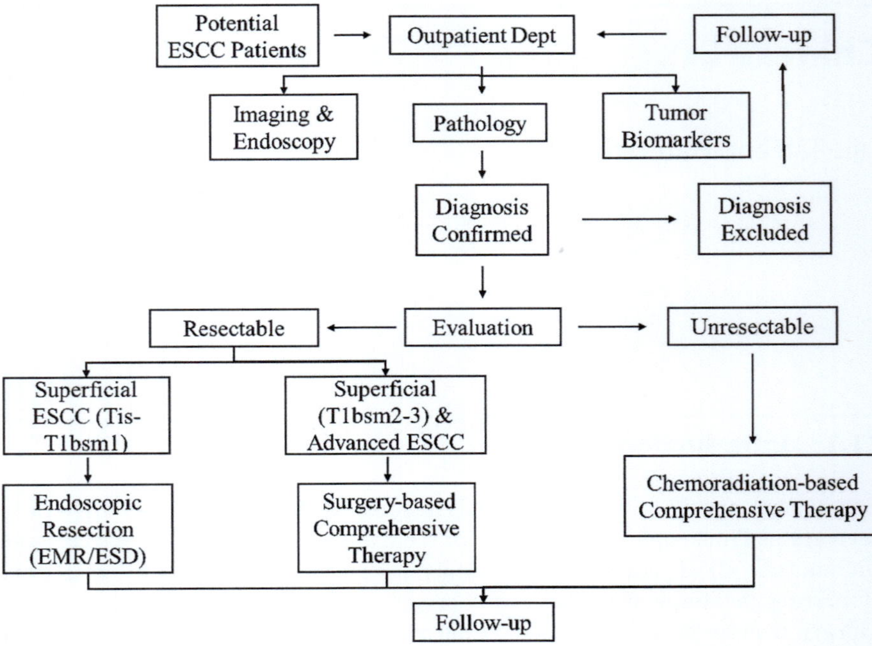

Fig. 21.1 Flow chart of diagnosis and therapy for ESCC. EMR, endoscopic mucosal resection; ESD, endoscopic submucosal dissection; T1bsm1, submucosa invasion less than depth of 200um; T1bsm2-3, submucosa invasion more than depth of 200um. Download from Clinical Practice Guidelines for the Diagnosis and Treatment of Esophageal Cancer in China (2018 Edition) in the official website of National Health Commission of the People's Republic of China

21.2 Epidemiology

Esophageal cancer, with an estimated 511,000 new cases and 445,000 deaths, ranks 11th in the incidence and seventh in mortality of all cancers globally in 2022 [3]. Notably, almost half of the cases occur in China. According to reports from the National Central Cancer Registry of China (NCCRC), this disease ranks as the seventh most frequently diagnosed cancer and the fifth leading cause of cancer death with 224,000 new cases and 187,500 deaths in China in 2022, a small decline in the last 5 years [1]. Notably, 90% of these cases are squamous cell carcinoma, and the high-incidence zone includes Fujian Province, Sichuan Province, Chaozhou-Shantou region, as well as regions along the Taihang mountains, such as Henan Province and Shanxi Province. Approximately 75% of cases occur in men, resulting in 3-fold mortality in men compared to that in women. As for the prognosis, it is reported that the age-standardized 5-year relative survival increased to 30.3% by 9.4% from 2003–05 to 2012–15 for esophageal cancer in China, with multidisciplinary treatment being applied [4]

In the past decade, screening programs for esophageal squamous cell carcinoma has been carried out for the high-risk population living in high-prevalence areas of over 45-year-old with family tumor history, especially esophageal or other digestive tract malignancy or other relevant risk factors, such as smoking, heavy alcohol consumption, a history of squamous cancer of the head and neck, and a preference for very hot or pickled food. For these individuals, endoscopy coupled with biopsy of suspicious regions is the recommended screening approach, which has yielded significant benefits in achieving early detection and treatment of esophageal cancer and improved the survival. Therefore, the blueprint guide of "Healthy China 2030", an official goal was set to reduce premature mortality of major noncommunicable diseases by 30% from 2015 to 2030. Esophageal cancer, as one of noncommunicable diseases, also plays a crucial role in achieving this health life indicator.

21.3 Endoscopic Resection

Endoscopic resection (ER), including endoscopic mucosal resection (EMR) and endoscopic submucosal dissection (ESD), is increasingly propagated and has become an important approach for treatment of superficial esophageal cancer in China. Superficial esophageal cancer is categorized as intraepithelial (high-grade dysplasia, Tis), mucosal (T1a), and submucosal (T1b) cancer. Lesions diagnosed as Tis or T1a ESCC without muscularis mucosae invasion are absolute indications for ER, which are extremely rarely associated with lymph node metastasis, and those as T1a ESCC with muscularis mucosae invasion or T1b ESCC invading less than 200um within submucosa are also preferred to be treated via ER; however, due to an increasing risk of lymph nodes metastasis, these represent relative indications for ER [5]. For a superficial lesion involving ≥ 3/4th of the esophageal circumference, ER should be considered deliberately as such lesion is associated with a high risk of development of stenosis after such resection [6, 7]. Decisions on ER approach are based on preoperative evaluation, including endoscopic examination, computed tomography (CT) of the neck, chest, and abdomen, positron emission tomography–CT (PET-CT) [8, 9]. For superficial lesions, endoscopic ultrasound (EUS) plays a key role in determining whether ER is suitable or not, owing to its relatively high accuracy in detecting depth of invasion as well as positive nodes [10, 11]. In addition to preoperative examinations, endoscopically resected specimen also reveals crucial information, and several histopathological parameters, such as irradicality, the presence of lymphovascular invasion, deeper submucosal tumor invasion, and poor differentiation, determine the necessity of additional treatments, including surgery or chemoradiotherapy [12, 13]. The selection among additional treatments should be made after assessing the patient's surgical tolerability. The detailed procedure of ER is shown in Fig. 21.2. If ER is considered radical for superficial lesions, follow-up is carried out every 3 months in the first year, and one time per year in the following years. In addition to endoscopy, other examinations, including CT of neck, thorax, and abdomen, and tumor biomarkers, should also be routinely performed.

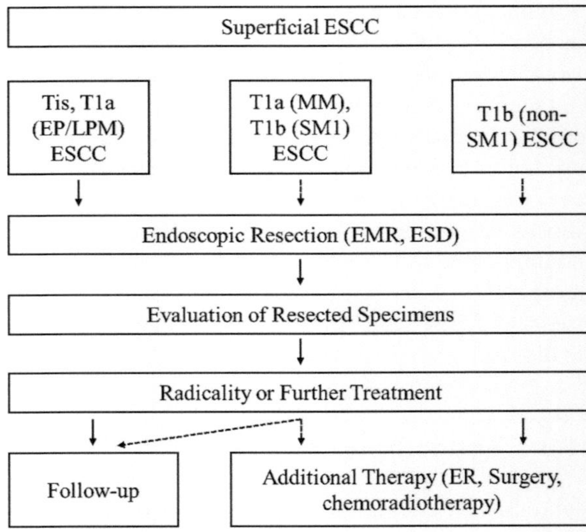

Fig. 21.2 Flow chart of Endoscopic Resection. EP, epithelium; LPM, lamina propria mucosae; MM, muscularis mucosae; SM1, submucosa invasion less than depth of 200 um; EMR, endoscopic mucosal resection; ESD, endoscopic submucosal dissection; ER, endoscopic resection. Download from Clinical Practice Guidelines for the Diagnosis and Treatment of Esophageal Cancer in China (2018 Edition) in the official website of National Health Commission of the People's Republic of China

21.4 Surgery

Esophagectomy remains the most crucial approach for treatment of esophageal cancer in spite of its relatively high perioperative complications. Standard radical surgery typically involves esophagectomy and lymphadenectomy followed by digestive tract reconstruction, commonly using the stomach. The eligibility of a patient for surgical resection strongly depends on the extent of the disease, as long as the general condition of the patient is tolerable of surgery. In China, patients with early stage, not suitable for ER, or locally advanced, non-distant metastatic ESCC (stage $T_{1b\text{-}4a}N_{0\text{–}2}\ M_0$) are considered for surgical resection. Usually, radical resection alone is sufficient for early tumors, and neoadjuvant/adjuvant therapy should be added for locally advanced tumors. The treatment algorithm is shown in Fig. 21.3. Some issues about surgery deserve special attention. This section is divided into 2 parts to clarify the current status and tendency of esophagectomy in China, including surgical approach and lymphadenectomy.

21.4.1 Surgical Approach

Several approaches for the resection of esophageal cancer exist, including sweet procedure (left intrathoracic operation), Ivor-Lewis's procedure (intrathoracic anastomosis), McKeown procedure (cervical anastomosis), and transhiatal approach. In China, before 2000, the Sweet approach was the most popular modality, and the 5-year overall survival (OS) remained 30%–40% [14] because of incapability of lymph nodes dissection of upper mediastinum. Nowadays, with the spread and

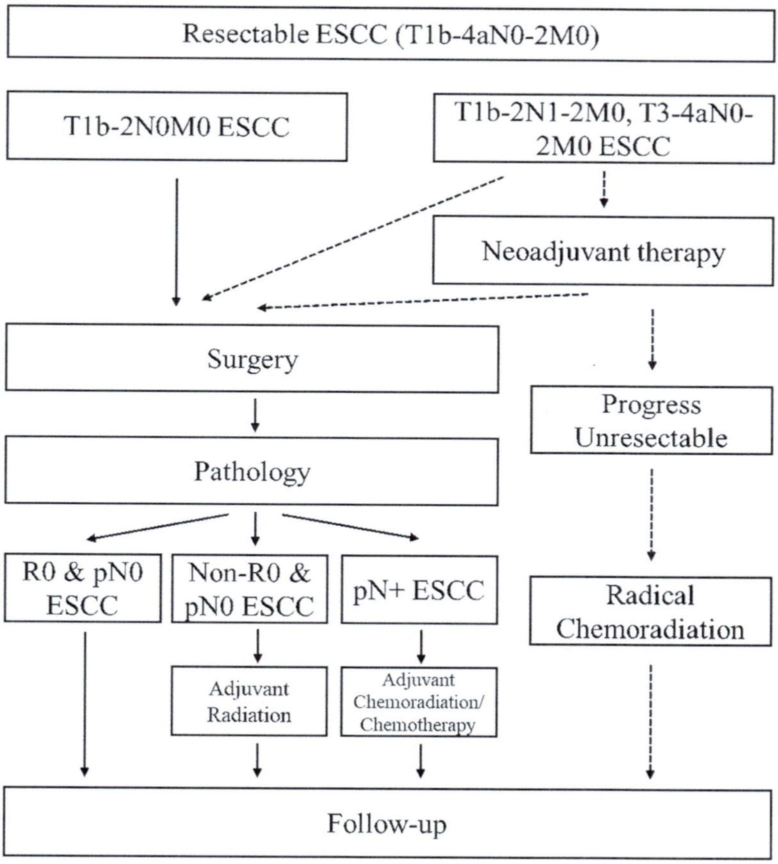

Fig. 21.3 Flow chart of resectable ESCC. Download from Clinical Practice Guidelines for the Diagnosis and Treatment of Esophageal Cancer in China (2018 Edition) in the official website of National Health Commission of the People's Republic of China

popularization of standardized treatment of esophageal cancer, the Ivor-Lewis or McKeown approach through right thoracotomy becomes the mainstream in most medical centers; however, the sweet approach is also performed in some hospitals in the North. In recent years, it has been reported that the 5-year OS raised to 50% [15, 16] after the application of right thoracotomy owing to advantages of dissection of upper mediastinal nodes. Li et al. [17, 18] reported that the right thoracic approach was associated with increased survival in ESCC patients without increasing postoperative complications compared with the left thoracic approach (Sweet procedure) in a single central, prospective, randomized trial. Therefore, it is of great significance to spread and expand the usage of Ivor-Lewis or McKeown approach to take the place of the sweet approach in the whole nation by the Committee. As for the issue of the selection between Ivor-Lewis and McKeown approaches, surgeons make the personalized operative plan and choose the most suitable procedure for individuals according to preoperative evaluation of primary tumor and potential metastatic lymph node locations. Generally, McKeown procedure is used for upper or middle esophageal tumors, Ivor-Lewis procedure for middle or lower tumors in China.

With the rapid advancement of thoracoscopic techniques, there has been a transition from open chest procedures to minimally invasive esophagectomy in China. As is known to all, minimally invasive esophagectomy (MIE) has great advantages in reducing postoperative complications, especially pulmonary complications, without compromised long-term survival [19, 20]; therefore, it is performed in more and more hospitals in China. As the thoracoscopic part is particularly difficult to master, especially when performing an intrathoracic anastomosis, hybrid esophagectomy with laparoscopic gastric mobilization and open right thoracotomy is also performed by surgeons in some low-volume centers, who avoid the challenges in completing their thoracoscopic learning phase owing to insufficient caseload. The MIRO trial demonstrated that the hybrid esophagectomy resulted in a lower incidence of intraoperative and postoperative major complications, specifically pulmonary complications, than OE without compromising survival [21], so hybrid esophagectomy could be an option for surgeons in the low-volume centers.

In the past few years, robot-assisted minimally invasive esophagectomy (RAMIE) has emerged as a novel optional approach for patients, but it is not widely performed and widespread in large medical centers due to its high cost in China. Robotic assistance allows for stable 3-dimensional, magnified view and articulated instruments, enabling precise dissection with 7° of freedom of movement. Since its introduction, RAMIE has been shown to be a safe and oncologically adequate alternative to OE and conventional MIE in a series of retrospective studies [22–24]. Chinese surgeons also revealed that RAMIE was a safe and feasible alternative surgical approach for ESCC and was associated with shorter operative duration and better lymph node dissection in patients who received neoadjuvant therapy compared to MIE [25]. Besides, the plateau of RAMIE was 25 cases of operative duration and 50 cases of lymphadenectomy [26]. As for the long-term survival, results are pending for further follow-up investigations.

Inflatable video-assisted mediastinoscopy transhiatal esophagectomy (IVMTE) was reported by Dr. Fujiwara for the first time in 2014 [27], then, Dr. Cao performed the surgery in China in 2016 [28], and in recent 10 years, it has gained great attention and has experienced rapid development in China due to its advantages in reducing chest wall trauma and improving postoperative recovery. However, the risk of damaging adjacent structures during surgery within the narrow mediastinal space may increase, such as the aorta, trachea, heart, azygos arch, bronchial arteries, and thoracic duct [29, 30]. Additionally, systematic lymph node dissection is crucial in radical esophagectomy for cancer. Concerns have been raised about the dissection of right recurrent laryngeal nerve lymph nodes and subcarinal lymph nodes, as this might compromise the oncological principles of surgery. Consequently, IVMTE has strict indications, being suitable only for T1 or T2 patients without invasive tumors or mediastinal lymph node metastasis. Besides, due to its extrathoracic approach,

IVMTE is also suitable for patients with severe pleural adhesions or poor respiratory function in China. Notably, Dr. Hu reported a new left-primary and right-auxiliary operation mode in mediastinoscopy-assisted radical esophagectomy to expand its usage [31], and Dr. Lin used the sternal lifting to increase operating space and improve the visual field, reducing the difficulty of subcarinal lymph node dissection [32].

21.4.2 Extent of Lymphadenectomy

Lymph node status is an important prognostic factor in esophageal carcinoma, and radical lymphadenectomy may help determine precise postoperative pathological staging, ensure the integrity and radicality of surgery, and, more importantly, improve the survival of patients after surgery. Therefore, lymphadenectomy is an essential part of radical surgery for esophageal cancer. In order to guide the clinical practice in China, a consensus on thoracic lymphadenectomy was reached by the Esophageal Cancer Committee of the Chinese Anti-Cancer Association with a group of experienced experts in 2017 [33]. The Committee made the consensus, taking into consideration of the experts' clinical experiences and existing evidence mostly from Chinese thoracic surgeons. And on the basis of the consistency with the AJCC/UICC and the JES systems, significant modifications have been made, taking clinical practice into account in China. This consensus is easy to use and will facilitate standardization and unification of mediastinal lymph node dissection in China. The Chinese version of the mediastinal lymph node map and its differences with the AJCC/UICC and JES systems are shown in Figs. 21.4 and 21.5, respectively. In the consensus, it emphasized that all 9 stations of mediastinal lymph nodes (C201–C209) should be en bloc dissected during radical surgery, especially the left and right para-recurrent laryngeal nerve nodes and para-esophageal nodes. With regard to cervical and abdominal lymph node dissection for esophageal cancer, the abdominal lymph node dissection comprises of para-cardial lymph nodes, as well as those located along the lesser gastric curvature, the origin of the left gastric artery, the common hepatic artery, the splenic artery, and the celiac trunk; and the cervical lymph node dissection included bilateral cervical para-recurrent laryngeal nerve nodes, bilateral inferior deep cervical nodes and bilateral supraclavicular nodes.

There is fierce debate over the issue of whether cervical lymph node dissection should be routinely performed in all patients with esophageal cancer all over the world, which is also an important topic in China. It is recommended by the Committee that all patients receive at least a 2-field total lymphadenectomy with 15 or more lymph nodes harvested, as in one clinical trial (NCT01047111), patients receiving total mediastinal lymphadenectomy (including bilateral recurrent laryngeal nerve lymph nodes) had better overall survival and disease-free survival than those with standard mediastinal lymphadenectomy [17]. If tumors are located in the upper third of esophagus, 3-field lymphadenectomy, including cervical lymph nodes, must be performed. The 3-field lymphadenectomy is not a routine procedure in China due to the intensive trauma. In

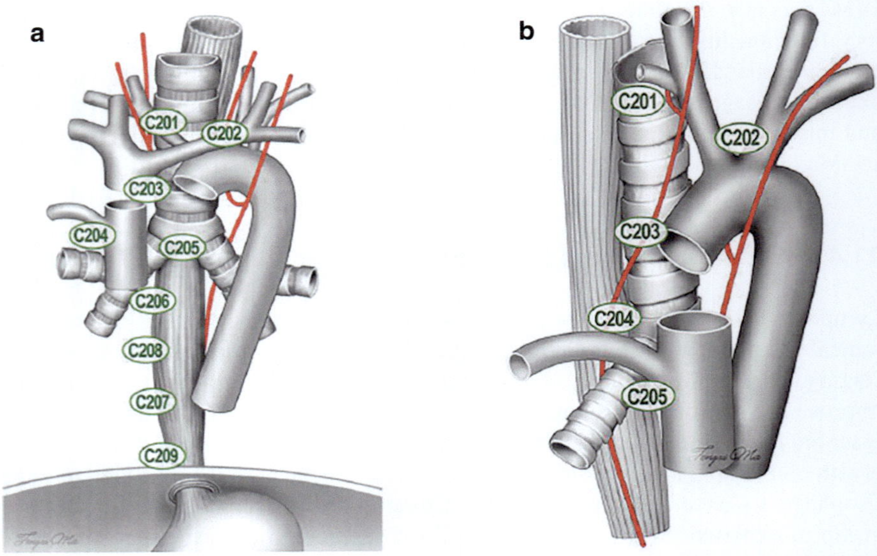

Fig. 21.4 Diagram of the Chinese version of naming and grouping of mediastinal lymph nodes in esophageal cancer: (**a**) anterior view; (**b**) right side view. "C" represents Chinese nomenclature, and "2-" represents thoracic lymph nodes. Station C201, right recurrent laryngeal nerve nodes; Station C202, left recurrent laryngeal nerve nodes; Station C203, upper thoracic paraesophageal lymph nodes; Station C204, right thoracic paratracheal lymph nodes; Station C205, subcarinal lymph nodes; Station C206, middle thoracic paraesophageal lymph nodes; Station C207, lower thoracic paraesophageal lymph nodes; Station C208, inferior pulmonary ligament lymph nodes; Station C209, paradiaphragmatic lymph nodes. Adapted with permission from Dr. Li of REF. [34], AME

order to achieve radical lymph nodes dissection as well as avoid unnecessary dissection, Cancer Hospital, Chinese Academy of Medical Sciences, launched a nationwide trial to find the sentinel lymph node predict the necessity of cervical nodes dissection. The results showed additional cervical lymphadenectomy can be avoided in patients with middle or lower thoracic ESCC and negative right recurrent laryngeal nerve lymph nodes by frozen section treated by upfront surgery [34]. Another trial also revealed 3 field lymphadenectomy (thoracic, abdominal, and neck fields) does not confer a survival advantage over 2 field (thoracic and abdominal fields) lymphadenectomy in patients with tumors located in the middle and distal esophagus [35]. Besides, Dr. Chen proposed 2.5-field lymphadenectomy [36] for all patients with ESCC, the concept of which was to clean up the cervical nodes along the bilateral para-recurrent laryngeal nerve and cervical esophagus through thorax under the thoracoscope, thus avoiding cervical lymphadenectomy. Indeed, it is of great importance that surgeons make the personalized operative plan and modify the extent of lymphadenectomy for individuals according to preoperative evaluation of primary tumor and potential metastatic lymph node location, achieving the utmost benefits for patients.

Region	Chinese system	AJCC/UICC system (18)	JES system (19,20)
Upper mediastinum	Station C201*: Right recurrent laryngeal nerve nodes	Station 2R: Upper right paratracheal lymph nodes	Station 106recR: Right recurrent laryngeal nerve nodes
	Station C202: Left recurrent laryngeal nerve nodes	Station 2L: Upper left paratracheal lymph nodes	Station 106recL: Left recurrent laryngeal nerve nodes
	Station C203: Upper thoracic paraesophageal lymph nodes	Station 8U: Upper thoracic paraesophageal lymph nodes	Station 105: Upper thoracic paraesophageal lymph nodes
	Station C204: Right paratracheal lymph nodes	Station 4R: Right lower paratracheal lymph nodes	Station 106: Thoracic paratracheal lymph nodes ❖ Station 106pre:Pretracheal lymph nodes ❖ Station 106tbR:Right tracheobronchial lymph nodes
	N/A	Station 4L: Left lower paratracheal lymph nodes	Station 106tbL: Left tracheobronchial lymph nodes
		N/A	Station 113: Ligamentum arteriosum lymph nodes
		N/A	Station 114: Anterior mediastinal lymph nodes
	Station C205: Subcarinal lymph nodes	Station 7: Subcarinal lymph nodes	Station 107: Subcarinal lymph nodes
Lower mediastinum	Station C206: Middle thoracic paraesophageal lymph nodes	Station 8M: Middle thoracic paraesophageal lymph nodes	Station 108: Middle thoracic paraesophageal lymph nodes
	Station C207: Lower thoracic paraesophageal lymph nodes	Station 8Lo: Lower thoracic paraesophageal lymph nodes	Station 110: Lower thoracic paraesophageal lymph nodes
	Station C208: Inferior pulmonary ligament lymph nodes	Station 9L: Left lower pulmonary ligament lymph nodes	Station 112L:Posterior mediastinal lymph nodes
		Station 9R: Right inferior pulmonary ligand lymph nodes	Station 112R: Posterior mediastinal lymph nodes
	N/A	N/A	Station 109L:Left main bronchus lymph nodes
			Station 109R:Right main bronchus lymph nodes
	Station C209: Paradiaphragmatic lymph nodes	Station 15:Paradiaphragmatic lymph nodes	Station 111:Supradiaphragmatic lymph nodes

Fig. 21.5 Comparison of the Chinese version of naming and grouping mediastinal lymph nodes with the AJCC/UICC and the JES systems for esophageal cancer. *, "C" represents Chinese standards, and "2-" represents thoracic lymph nodes. AJCC, American Joint Committee of Cancer; UICC, Union for International Cancer Control; JES, Japan Esophageal Society. Adapted with permission from Dr. Li of REF. [34], AME

21.5 Perioperative Therapy

21.5.1 Neoadjuvant Therapy

Neoadjuvant therapy is introduced and recommended for patients with locally advanced resectable ESCC (cT_{1b-2} N_{1-2} or c$T_{3-4a}N_{0-2}$) in China with the publication of CROSS trial [37] and JCOG9907 trial [38]. The direct comparison between the neoadjuvant chemoradiotherapy and chemotherapy is reported in the CMISG1701 trial, and there is no significant difference in long-term survival although a 9% increase in 3-year overall survival rate with the addition of radiotherapy with neoadjuvant chemotherapy (cisplatin and paclitaxel) in c$T_{3-4a}N_{0-1}$ M_0 esophageal squamous cell cancer [39]; therefore, the strategy of neoadjuvant therapy has not been unified among medical centers. Some medical centers adopt neoadjuvant chemoradiotherapy (nCRT), while others prefer neoadjuvant chemotherapy (nCT). Neoadjuvant chemoradiotherapy and chemotherapy are both acceptable according to the conditions of the individual. The three-arm JCOG1109 trial found that triplet therapy (docetaxel plus cisplatin plus fluorouracil) significantly improved median overall survival compared with the cisplatin plus fluorouracil regimen, with higher rates of grade 3 or 4 haematological adverse events [40]. Considering the potential severe adverse events, neoadjuvant platinum triplet therapy is not routinely adopted in China. The platinum-based combination chemotherapy is the standard regimen of nCT, and other agents such as paclitaxel or 5-FU could be added to the regimen according to the clinician's experience in China. Usually, the nCRT regimen is composed of the drugs of nCT with reduced dosages and radiation varying from 40 to 50Gy. Notably, nCRT therapy is mostly applied in large-volume medical centers, and many other hospitals mainly perform nCT in China.

In recent years, the advent of immune checkpoint inhibitors has marked a new frontier in cancer therapy. Preliminary results from phase 1/2 trials have shown promising pathological complete response rates in esophageal squamous cell carcinoma when immune checkpoint inhibitors are combined with neoadjuvant therapies. Notably, the ESCORT-NEO/NCCES01 study, a phase 3, open-label, randomized trial, enrolling 391 patients in China, demonstrated the superior pCR rates in neoadjuvant immunochemotherapy compared to chemotherapy alone for locally advanced ESCC, with a tolerable safety profile [41]. Based on this conclusion, neoadjuvant immunochemotherapy strategy is being adopted more and more in low-volume hospitals in China. Several randomized phase 3 studies are currently underway to distinguish the better strategy among neoadjuvant chemoradioimmunotherapy, immunochemotherapy, and chemoradiotherapy, including NEOCRTEC2101 (NCT05357846), iCROSS (NCT04973306), and KEYSTONE-002 (NCT04807673). As for the locally advanced non-resectable ($T_{4b}N_xM_0$) tumors, induction chemoradiotherapy with reduced doses (40 to 50Gy) is given first, after finishing, take resection if operable, or else, continue chemoradiotherapy.

21.5.2 Adjuvant Therapy

Adjuvant therapy may play an important role in improving prognosis although a network meta-analysis showed no survival benefits [42]. In China, non-R0 resection is the indication of postoperative radiation, and pN+ is the indication of postoperative chemotherapy. In addition, patients with multi-station lymph nodes metastases are recommended to take adjuvant chemoradiotherapy [43, 44]. Single-agent immune checkpoint inhibitors are appealing options in the adjuvant setting due to their reduced toxicity compared with cytotoxic chemotherapy. The CheckMate-577 trial showed efficacy of a 12-month nivolumab course in patients with residual disease after neoadjuvant chemoradiotherapy and esophagectomy. Compared with placebo, adjuvant nivolumab significantly improved diseasefree survival with manageable toxicity and low impact on health-related quality of life, and is now recommended in this setting [45].

21.6 Systemic Therapy

For patients with esophageal cancer ineligible for surgical resection, the standard treatment is definitive chemoradiotherapy, which consists of external beam radiotherapy (50.0–60.0 Gy in 1.8–2 Gy fractions over 5–6 weeks) and concurrent chemotherapy (carboplatin and paclitaxel weekly). Recently, chemoradioimmunotherapy has become a new standard first-line treatment for inoperable or metastatic esophageal cancer, and the selection of chemotherapy drugs and immune checkpoint inhibitors varies across different regions and patient conditions. In China, the combination of paclitaxel and cisplatin is favored, as evidenced by several first-line studies focused on esophageal squamous cell carcinoma. However, the diversity in the choice of PD-1 inhibitors presents a challenge, as there are no head-to-head clinical trials directly comparing the specific efficacies of various PD-1 inhibitors. Thus, treatment decisions for chemotherapy regimens and PD-1 inhibitors in patients with advanced esophageal squamous cell carcinoma should be considered on a patient-specific basis. Owing to the development of immune checkpoint inhibitors in the last decade, therapeutic options have diversified and largely depend on patients' previous treatment history of immunotherapy in first-line therapy. For patients with esophageal squamous cell carcinoma without previous immunotherapy, PD-1 inhibitors, such as pembrolizumab, nivolumab, and tislelizumab, have shown superior efficacy to standard chemotherapy in second-line treatment, according to the KEYNOTE-181, ATTRACTION-3, and RATIONALE-302 trials [46–48].

In China, the treatment compliance of patients is far from satisfactory, especially in patients with neoadjuvant therapy [49]. Some patients refuse to undergo surgery and are likely to take chemoradiotherapy as long as feeling eating well. There were no conclusions about the issue of whether good-response (clinical complete response, cCR) cases should undergo operation or not. The SANO trial, assessing whether active surveillance leads to non-inferior overall survival compared to planned surgery, revealed comparable oncological outcomes, with improved quality of life in the surveillance group [50]. Given the high pathological complete response rates with neoadjuvant chemoradiotherapy in esophageal squamous cell carcinoma populations, investigators have explored the potential of a so-called watch-and-wait approach for patients who respond to treatment in China [51].

In China, comprehensive traditional surgical therapy for esophageal cancer is widely adopted; in the meantime, newly emerging therapies, such as immunotherapy, are also increasingly applied. The diagnosis and therapy of ESCC will be more standardized and individualized, under the guidance of Clinical Practice Guidelines for the Diagnosis and Treatment of Esophageal Cancer.

References

1. Han B, et al. Cancer incidence and mortality in China, 2022. J Natl Cancer Cent. 2024;4(1):47–53.
2. National Health Commission of the People's Republic of China. Clinical practice guidelines for the diagnosis and treatment of esophageal cancer (2018 Edition). Chin J Cancer Res. 2018;31(2):223–58.
3. Bray F, et al. Global cancer statistics 2022: GLOBOCAN estimates of incidence and mortality worldwide for 36 cancers in 185 countries. CA Cancer J Clin. 2024;74(3):229–63.
4. Zeng H, et al. Changing cancer survival in China during 2003–15: a pooled analysis of 17 population-based cancer registries. Lancet Glob Health. 2018;6(5):e555–67.
5. Katada C, et al. Clinical outcome after endoscopic mucosal resection for esophageal squamous cell carcinoma invading the muscularis mucosae–a multicenter retrospective cohort study. Endoscopy. 2007;39(9):779–83.
6. Ono S, et al. Predictors of postoperative stricture after esophageal endoscopic submucosal dissection for superficial squamous cell neoplasms. Endoscopy. 2009;41(8):661–5.
7. Shi Q, et al. Risk factors for postoperative stricture after endoscopic submucosal dissection for superficial esophageal carcinoma. Endoscopy. 2014;46(8):640–4.
8. Lagergren J, et al. Oesophageal cancer. Lancet. 2017;390(10110):2383–96.
9. Lordick F, et al. Oesophageal cancer: ESMO clinical practice guidelines for diagnosis, treatment and follow-up. Ann Oncol. 2016;27(suppl 5):v50–7.
10. Ajani JA, et al. Esophageal and esophagogastric junction cancers, version 1.2015. J Natl Compr Cancer Netw. 2015;13(2):194–227.
11. O'Farrell NJ, et al. Appraisal of staging endoscopic ultrasonography in a modern high-volume esophageal program. World J Surg. 2013;37(7):1666–72.
12. Kim DU, et al. Risk factors of lymph node metastasis in T1 esophageal squamous cell carcinoma. J Gastroenterol Hepatol. 2008;23(4):619–25.
13. Eguchi T, et al. Histopathological criteria for additional treatment after endoscopic mucosal resection for esophageal cancer: analysis of 464 surgically resected cases. Mod Pathol. 2006;19(3):475–80.
14. Zhang R. Current status and progression of surgery in treating esophageal cancer. Chin Cancer. 1999;8:28–9.
15. Peng L, Chen L, Li Q. Ivor Lewis subtotal esophagectomy with two-field lymphadenectomy and prognosis. Chin Oncol. 2003;13:574–6.
16. Wu C, Xue H, Zhu Z. Analysis of the therapeutic effect of esophagectomy with extended 2-field lymph node dissection for esophageal carcinoma. Chin J Oncol. 2009;31:630–3.
17. Li B, et al. Extended right thoracic approach compared with limited left thoracic approach for patients with middle and lower esophageal squamous cell carcinoma: three-year survival of a prospective, randomized, Open-label trial. Ann Surg. 2018;267(5):826–32.
18. Li B, et al. Comparison of Ivor-Lewis vs Sweet esophagectomy for esophageal squamous cell carcinoma: a randomized clinical trial. JAMA Surg. 2015;150(4):292–8.
19. Biere SS, et al. Minimally invasive versus open oesophagectomy for patients with oesophageal cancer: a multicentre, open-label, randomised controlled trial. Lancet. 2012;379(9829):1887–92.
20. Straatman J, et al. Minimally invasive versus open esophageal resection: three-year follow-up of the previously reported randomized controlled trial: the TIME trial. Ann Surg. 2017;266(2):232–6.
21. Mariette C, et al. Hybrid minimally invasive esophagectomy for esophageal cancer. N Engl J Med. 2019;380(2):152–62.
22. Ruurda JP, et al. Robot-assisted minimally invasive esophagectomy for esophageal cancer: a systematic review. J Surg Oncol. 2015;112(3):257–65.

23. van der Sluis PC, et al. Oncologic long-term results of robot-assisted minimally invasive thoraco-laparoscopic esophagectomy with two-field lymphadenectomy for esophageal cancer. Ann Surg Oncol. 2015;22(Suppl 3):S1350–6.
24. van Hillegersberg R, et al. First experience with robot-assisted thoracoscopic esophagolymphadenectomy for esophageal cancer. Surg Endosc. 2006;20(9):1435–9.
25. Yang Y, et al. Robot-assisted versus conventional minimally invasive esophagectomy for resectable esophageal squamous cell carcinoma: early results of a multicenter randomized controlled trial: the RAMIE trial. Ann Surg. 2022;275(4):646–53.
26. Zhang X, et al. Robot assisted esophagectomy for esophageal squamous cell carcinoma. J Thorac Dis. 2018;10(6):3767–75.
27. Fujiwara H, et al. Perioperative outcomes of single-port mediastinoscope-assisted transhiatal esophagectomy for thoracic esophageal cancer. Dis Esophagus. 2017;30(10):1–8.
28. Li GS. Prof. Qingdong Cao: single-port inflatable mediastinoscopy combined with laparoscopy for the radical treatment of esophageal cancer. J Thorac Dis. 2016;8(9):E1108–e1109.
29. Okumura H, et al. Clinical significance of mediastinoscope-assisted transhiatal esophagectomy in patients with esophageal cancer. Langenbeck's Arch Surg. 2015;400(6):699–706.
30. Jin Y, et al. Retrospective comparison of two minimally invasive Esophagectomy in the treatment of esophageal cancer: pneumatic Mediastinoscopy versus Thoracoscopy. J Laparoendosc Adv Surg Tech A. 2019;29(5):638–42.
31. Yuan P, et al. Left-primary & right-auxiliary operation mode in mediastinoscope-assisted radical esophagectomy. Surg Endosc. 2023;37(10):7884–92.
32. Huang JS, et al. Single-port inflatable mediastinoscopy combined with laparoscopic esophagectomy via right cervical auxiliary operating port and sternal lifting: a safe and reliable surgical method. J Thorac Dis. 2025;17(3):1481–90.
33. Li H, et al. Chinese expert consensus on mediastinal lymph node dissection in esophagectomy for esophageal cancer (2017 edition). J Thorac Dis. 2018;10(4):2481–9.
34. Mao Y, et al. Three-field vs two-field lymphadenectomy in thoracic ESCC patients: a multicenter randomized study (NST 1503). J Natl Cancer Cent. 2025;5(2):203–11.
35. Li B, et al. Esophagectomy with three-field versus two-field lymphadenectomy for middle and lower thoracic esophageal cancer: long-term outcomes of a randomized clinical trial. J Thorac Oncol. 2021;16(2):310–7.
36. Chen C. Minimally invasive esophagectomoy–experience from Fujian Medical University. J Clin Surg. 2016;24(7):560–1.
37. van Hagen P, et al. Preoperative chemoradiotherapy for esophageal or junctional cancer. N Engl J Med. 2012;366(22):2074–84.
38. Ando N, et al. A randomized trial comparing postoperative adjuvant chemotherapy with cisplatin and 5-fluorouracil versus preoperative chemotherapy for localized advanced squamous cell carcinoma of the thoracic esophagus (JCOG9907). Ann Surg Oncol. 2012;19(1):68–74.
39. Tang H, et al. Neoadjuvant chemoradiotherapy versus neoadjuvant chemotherapy followed by minimally invasive esophagectomy for locally advanced esophageal squamous cell carcinoma: a prospective multicenter randomized clinical trial. Ann Oncol. 2023;34(2):163–72.
40. Kato K, et al. Doublet chemotherapy, triplet chemotherapy, or doublet chemotherapy combined with radiotherapy as neoadjuvant treatment for locally advanced oesophageal cancer (JCOG1109 NExT): a randomised, controlled, open-label, phase 3 trial. Lancet. 2024;404(10447):55–66.
41. Qin J, et al. Neoadjuvant chemotherapy with or without camrelizumab in resectable esophageal squamous cell carcinoma: the randomized phase 3 ESCORT-NEO/NCCES01 trial. Nat Med. 2024;30(9):2549–57.
42. Pasquali S, et al. Survival after neoadjuvant and adjuvant treatments compared to surgery alone for resectable esophageal carcinoma: a network meta-analysis. Ann Surg. 2017;265(3):481–91.
43. Kang J, H. Z. Current status of research on concurrent chemoradiotherapy after surgery for esophageal cancer. Chin J Radiat Oncol. 2016;25(5):534–8.

44. Jiang Y, Zhao C, Li S. Current status and progress of perioperative treatment of esophageal cancer. Chin Clin Oncol. 2015;20(2):185–9.
45. Kelly RJ, et al. Adjuvant nivolumab in resected esophageal or gastroesophageal junction cancer. N Engl J Med. 2021;384(13):1191–203.
46. Kojima T, et al. Randomized phase III KEYNOTE-181 study of Pembrolizumab versus chemotherapy in advanced esophageal cancer. J Clin Oncol. 2020;38(35):4138–48.
47. Kato K, et al. Nivolumab versus chemotherapy in patients with advanced oesophageal squamous cell carcinoma refractory or intolerant to previous chemotherapy (ATTRACTION-3): a multicentre, randomised, open-label, phase 3 trial. Lancet Oncol. 2019;20(11):1506–17.
48. Shen L, et al. Tislelizumab versus chemotherapy as second-line treatment for advanced or metastatic esophageal squamous cell carcinoma (RATIONALE-302): a randomized phase III study. J Clin Oncol. 2022;40(26):3065–76.
49. Yang H, et al. Neoadjuvant chemoradiotherapy followed by surgery versus surgery alone for locally advanced squamous cell carcinoma of the esophagus (NEOCRTEC5010): a phase III multicenter, randomized, open-label clinical trial. J Clin Oncol. 2018;36(27):2796–803.
50. van der Wilk BJ, et al. Neoadjuvant chemoradiotherapy followed by active surveillance versus standard surgery for oesophageal cancer (SANO trial): a multicentre, stepped-wedge, cluster-randomised, non-inferiority, phase 3 trial. Lancet Oncol. 2025;26(4):425–36.
51. Yang Y, et al. Detecting residual disease after neoadjuvant chemoradiotherapy for oesophageal squamous cell carcinoma: the prospective multicentre preSINO trial. Br J Surg. 2025;112(2):znae342.

Taiwan Experiences

22

Osbert Qi-Yao Leow, Tzu-Yi Yang, and Yin-Kai Chao

22.1 Esophageal Cancer in Taiwan

In recent years, the diagnosis and treatment of esophageal cancer have made significant progress, driven by international and domestic clinical research. However, the challenges posed by esophageal cancer in Taiwan have distinct characteristics and an urgent nature. According to data from the National Cancer Registry, the age-standardized incidence rate of esophageal cancer in Taiwan increased from 3.28 per 100,000 population in 1995 (695 newly diagnosed cases) to 6.51 per 100,000 population in 2022 (2831 newly diagnosed cases), representing more than a fourfold increase over just a few decades. Among these cases, more than 90% are squamous cell carcinoma, with major risk factors including smoking and alcohol consumption. This contrasts markedly with Western countries, where adenocarcinoma predominates and is more closely associated with obesity and gastroesophageal reflux disease, reflecting substantial epidemiological differences.

The distinctive features of esophageal cancer in Taiwan include a marked male predominance (male-to-female ratio exceeding 10:1) and a relatively younger age at onset (with the mean age of male patients approximately 50–60 years). As shown in Fig. 22.1, the incidence rate among men increased steadily over time and remained substantially higher than that among women, who consistently exhibited low and relatively stable incidence rates throughout the study period.

Owing to the lack of obvious symptoms in early-stage esophageal cancer and the absence of effective screening tools, this "occult" nature of the disease results in nearly 70% of patients being diagnosed at advanced stages. As shown in Fig. 22.2, despite a gradual increase in early-stage disease detection, advanced-stage disease (stage III–IV) continues to account for a substantial proportion of newly diagnosed

O. Q.-Y. Leow · T.-Y. Yang · Y.-K. Chao (✉)
Department of Thoracic Surgery, Chang Gung Memorial Hospital-Linkou, Chang Gung University, Taoyuan, Taiwan
e-mail: chaoyk@cgmh.org.tw

Y. Kitagawa et al. (eds.), *Esophageal Squamous Cell Carcinoma*,
https://doi.org/10.1007/978-981-92-2611-5_22

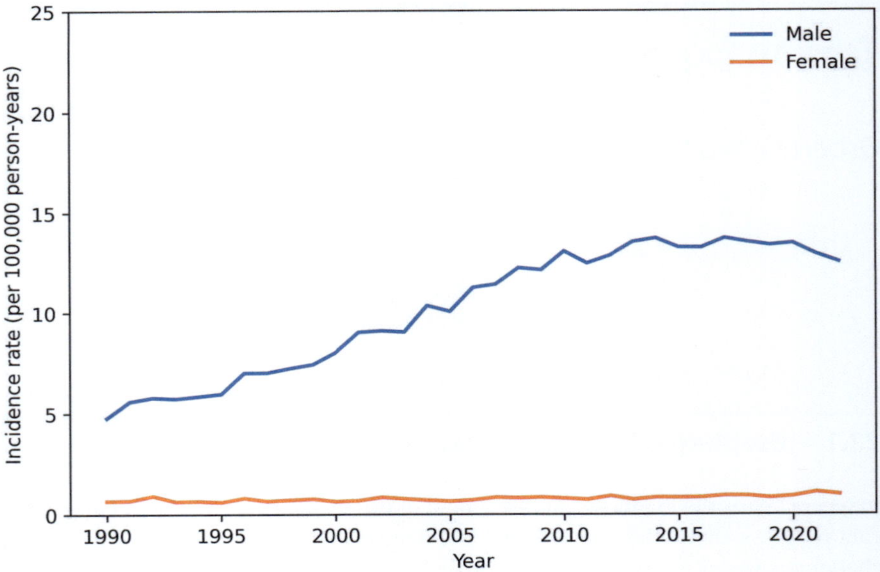

Fig. 22.1 Age-standardized incidence rates of esophageal cancer in Taiwan by sex from 1990 to 2021. The incidence rate among men increased steadily over time and remained markedly higher than that among women, whose incidence rates were consistently low and relatively stable throughout the study period. (Data were obtained from the Taiwan Cancer Registry (TCR))

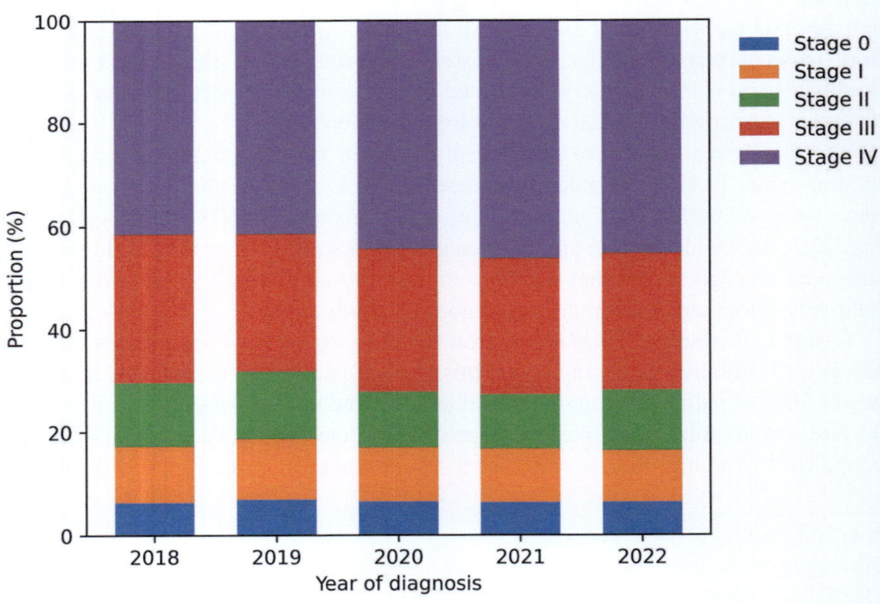

Fig. 22.2 Trends in stage distribution of esophageal cancer at diagnosis in Taiwan from 2018 to 2022, classified according to the American Joint Committee on Cancer (AJCC) 8th edition staging system. Despite a gradual increase in early-stage disease detection, advanced-stage disease (stage III–IV) continues to account for a substantial proportion of newly diagnosed cases. (Data were obtained from the Taiwan Cancer Registry (TCR))

cases. Such stage distribution has a profound impact on patient prognosis. According to data from the Taiwan Cancer Registry, among patients newly diagnosed with esophageal squamous cell carcinoma (ESCC) between 2008 and 2014, the 5-year overall survival rate was only 17%.

22.2 Staging and Preoperative Workup

Figure 22.3 illustrates the staging and treatment algorithm commonly applied in Taiwan. Standard staging workup includes esophagogastroduodenoscopy (EGD), chest and abdominal computed tomography (CT), endoscopic ultrasound (EUS), and positron emission tomography (PET), all of which are reimbursed by Taiwan's National Health Insurance (NHI). EUS is especially valuable for evaluating suspected submucosal lesions, with a reported accuracy of 89% for T-staging [1]. PET has become a standard modality for detecting both locoregional and distant metastases since 2008 [2]. The American Joint Committee on Cancer (AJCC) staging system is universally adopted for both clinical and pathological staging in Taiwan, despite the availability of alternative staging systems developed in Japan and China [3–5].

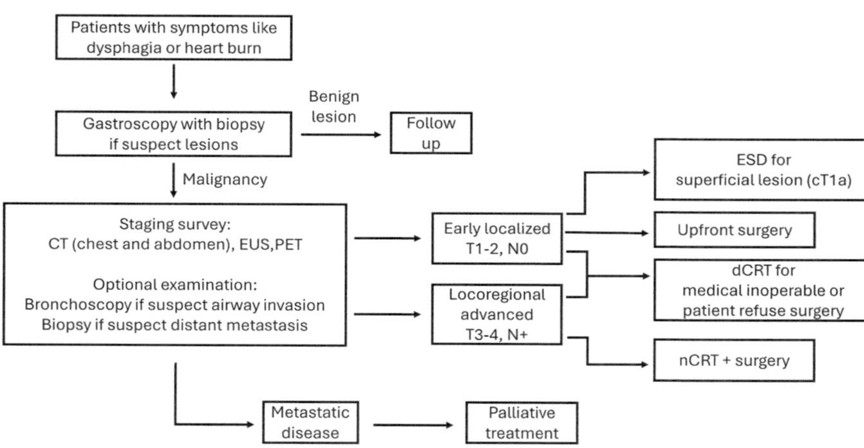

Fig. 22.3 Overview of the staging-based treatment algorithm for esophageal cancer in Taiwan. Clinical staging is performed using EGD, CT, EUS, and PET, with classification according to the AJCC 8th edition staging system. Early-stage disease is managed with endoscopic therapy or surgery, whereas locally advanced resectable disease is treated with neoadjuvant therapy followed by esophagectomy. Definitive chemoradiotherapy or systemic therapy is reserved for unresectable or metastatic disease. (All diagnostic procedures are reimbursed by Taiwan's National Health Insurance (NHI))

22.3 Endoscopic Treatment for Superficial Esophageal Cancer

In line with the NCCN guidelines, endoscopic submucosal dissection (ESD) is recommended for mucosal lesions. Hsu et al. found an over 90% 10-year disease-specific survival rate in patients with superficial ESCC treated with ESD, although the risk of metachronous recurrence warrants surveillance [6]. Yeh et al. conducted a systematic review and meta-analysis, finding no significant difference in overall, disease-specific, or recurrence-free survival between ESD and esophagectomy [7].

Special considerations are needed for patients with comorbidities. For example, anatomical changes from prior head and neck cancer treatment can complicate ESD. However, Ke et al. demonstrated that ESD remains a feasible and effective option in such cases [8]. Similarly, for patients with liver cirrhosis, Tsou et al. found ESD can be performed safely, even in those without severe liver dysfunction [9].

22.4 Principle of Systemic Therapy and Esophagectomy for Resectable ESCC

Since the publication of the CROSS study [10], neoadjuvant therapy followed by surgery has become the standard treatment for patients with locally advanced ESCC in Taiwan. On the other hand, upfront surgery is only reserved for patients who have cT1b-2N0M0 disease. Regarding the type of neoadjuvant therapy, while Japan and Korea prefer chemotherapy alone [11, 12], Taiwan primarily uses chemoradiotherapy (CRT), with radiation dose given at 45–50.4 Gy. As for chemotherapy, commonly used regimens include the CROSS (carboplatin plus paclitaxel) and the PF (cisplatin plus 5-fluorouracil), with regimen selection based on clinical indications and financial considerations. Gao et al. reported that the CROSS regimen was associated with superior survival outcomes and greater cost-effectiveness when compared with PF [13, 14]. The staging-based treatment algorithm for esophageal cancer is shown in Fig. 22.3.

22.5 Special Consideration in Patients with Liver Cirrhosis Who Need Esophagectomy

Because increased alcohol consumption is a shared risk factor for esophageal carcinoma and liver cirrhosis (LC), patients diagnosed with both conditions are not uncommon. The coexistence of these two serious disorders poses significant therapeutic challenges, especially when surgical removal of the esophageal malignancy is considered. The morbidity and mortality rates of patients with LC after esophagectomy may be as high as 87% and 26%, respectively [15]. Preoperative risk assessment in patients with LC undergoing esophagectomy has traditionally relied on the Child–Pugh score. Previous studies have demonstrated that advanced LC (Child–Pugh classes B and C) constitutes a contraindication to esophagectomy.

Accordingly, esophagectomy in patients with LC should be considered only in those with Child–Pugh class A disease. Nevertheless, Child–Pugh class A cirrhosis is a heterogeneous condition, characterized by (i) varying degrees of thrombocytopenia and (ii) the potential presence of asymptomatic esophageal and/or gastric varices.

In this context, frail patients with esophageal cancer and Child–Pugh class A liver cirrhosis (LC) should undergo a comprehensive risk assessment before proceeding with esophagectomy. Data from a tertiary medical center in Taiwan demonstrated that in-hospital mortality was acceptable among patients with Child–Pugh class A LC. However, the burden of postoperative morbidity was significantly higher in patients with LC than in those without LC [16]. Yang et al. further demonstrated that preoperative transient elastography helps predict postoperative pleural effusions in patients with LC [17].

22.6 Extent of Surgical Resection and Lymphadenectomy

Although McKeown esophagectomy remains the most commonly adopted approach across centers in Taiwan, the optimal extent of surgical resection continues to be debated, particularly in patients who have received preoperative therapy. The widespread adoption of neoadjuvant treatment for esophageal cancer has prompted a reevaluation of the longstanding paradigm that improved locoregional control necessarily requires more radical surgery. This question is especially pertinent in patients treated with nCRT.

Findings from several medical centers in Taiwan support the continued relevance of radical surgical approaches even after nCRT [18, 19]. The observed improvement in patient outcomes was primarily attributable to two key factors: an increased rate of negative circumferential resection margins (CRM) and a higher lymph node yield. These advantages are closely associated with the adoption of total meso-esophagectomy (TME), which represents a more aggressive surgical strategy for esophageal cancer.

During TME, surgical dissection is performed in accordance with the anatomical concept of the mesoesophagus—a bilaminar fascial structure located between the anterior surface of the descending aorta and the esophagus. This bi-fascial compartment contains the vascular and lymphatic networks supplying the esophagus. Notably, the TME technique facilitates not only improved CRM clearance but also more extensive lymph node dissection, particularly within the upper mediastinum.

22.7 Reconstruction

Gastric conduit reconstruction is the standard approach, used in 95% of patients at our center. Although it remains debatable whether extracorporeal gastric stapling reduces the rates of conduit necrosis and anastomotic leak [20, 21], in most institutes in Taiwan, mini-laparotomy for gastric tubulization after laparoscopic gastric mobilization is applied, followed by ICG angiography used to confirm perfusion.

Three reconstruction routes are available during McKeown esophagectomy: posterior mediastinal, retrosternal, and subcutaneous. The subcutaneous route is rarely used due to higher risks of anastomotic leakage and cutaneous fistulas. Both of the other two reconstruction routes have their own advantages and potential risks, so individualized strategy for reconstruction is considered [22]. Retrosternal reconstruction, which is created by laparoscopy routinely, is preferred in patients with high recurrence risk or those undergoing palliative surgery [23, 24].

22.8 Minimally Invasive Surgery (Including Thoracoscopic and Robotic Approach)

Recently, invasive esophagectomy (MIE) has gained widespread adoption since the 1990s and has been shown to reduce pulmonary complications [25]. In Taiwan, the utilization of MIE increased from approximately 50% in 2011 to over 80% by 2016 [26]. Current MIE approaches include hybrid and total minimally invasive techniques. Lee et al. reported that single-incision MIE achieved perioperative outcomes comparable to those of conventional approaches while significantly reducing postoperative pain [27]. In addition, MIE is more cost-effective, largely due to shorter intensive care unit stays [28].

Robotic-assisted minimally invasive esophagectomy (RAMIE), first introduced by Kernstine et al. [29], is now performed in several high-volume centers in Taiwan. Several studies have compared RAMIE with thoracoscopic MIE, highlighting their respective perioperative and oncologic outcomes [30–32] (Table 22.1). Notably, the REVATE trial (NCT03713749)—a prospective, multicenter randomized controlled study conducted in high-volume centers across Taiwan and China—demonstrated that RAMIE resulted in significantly higher lymph node yield along the left recurrent laryngeal nerve (RLN) and a lower incidence of RLN palsy compared with thoracoscopic MIE [32].

Table 22.1 Taiwan-based studies comparing RAMIE and MIE

Authors	Study design	Study periods	Study cohorts	Primary findings
Tagkalos et al.	Multicenter, retrospective	2008–2022	RAMIE vs MIE (440:505)	Patients who received RAMIE were more likely to achieve textbook outcome
Chao et al.	Multicenter, retrospective	2015–2022	RAMIE vs MIE (206:371)	RAMIE had lower post-operative pneumonia and recurrent laryngeal nerve palsy rate
Chao et al.	Randomized, multicenter, prospective	2018–2022	RAMIE vs MIE (103:100)	RAMIE leaded to more successful left recurrent laryngeal nerve lymph node dissection than MIE

Abbreviations: *CCI* Charlson comorbidity index, *RAMIE* robot-assisted minimally invasive esophagectomy, *MIE* minimally invasive esophagectomy

Table 22.2 Studies on immunotherapy for ESCC in Taiwan

Authors	Study periods	Study population	Study cohorts	Primary findings
Liu et al	2017–2024	Patients underwent nCRT followed by surgery	Adjuvant IO vs adjuvant CT vs no adjuvant therapy (23:36:68)	Adjuvant IO did not demonstrate a significant survival advantage compared to adjuvant CT
Kao et al	2017–2021	Patients with metastatic unresectable ESCC	Nivo+ CT vs Nivo+ Ipilimumab vs CT (25:7:27)	Nivo+ CT had better OS and PFS than dual IO or standard CT
Guo et al	2018–2022	Patients underwent nCRT followed by surgery	Adjuvant CT+ IO	Adjuvant CT+ IO might be associated with improved 1-year RFS

Abbreviations: *nCRT* neoadjuvant chemoradiotherapy, *IO* immunotherapy, *CT* chemotherapy, *ESCC* esophageal squamous cell carcinoma, *OS* overall survival, *PFS* progression free survival, *RFS* relapse free survival

22.9 Postoperative Adjuvant Therapy After Neoadjuvant Therapy

Despite clinical trials supporting the use of immunotherapy for adjuvant settings [33–35], the routine use of adjuvant immunotherapy remains uncommon. It was not only due to financial constraints but also the inconsistent real-world evidence. Liu et al. reported suboptimal real-world outcomes for adjuvant nivolumab compared to CheckMate 577 [36]. As an alternative, adjuvant chemoradiotherapy was employed, consisting of 20–30 Gy of radiation and chemotherapy regimens similar to those used in nCRT. Recently, Guo et al. reported the phase II trial (NCT03322267) evaluating adjuvant chemoradiotherapy combined with pembrolizumab in patients with locally advanced ESCC who underwent trimodality therapy but had high-risk features for recurrence. The 1-year relapse-free survival (RFS) rate was 60.0%. Median RFS and overall survival (OS) were 14.3 months (95% CI: 9.0–19.5) and 21.6 months (95% CI: 0.0–45.5), respectively [37]. Long-term survival outcome is still awaited (Table 22.2) [36–38].

22.10 Summary

ESCC represents a major health challenge in Taiwan. Over the past two decades, multidisciplinary treatment strategies have led to substantial improvements in survival outcomes. Although protocols vary among institutions, nationwide data collection efforts and prospective studies are currently underway to further optimize patient outcomes.

References

1. Rösch T. Endosonographic staging of esophageal cancer: a review of literature results. Gastrointest Endosc Clin N Am. 1995;5(3):537–47.
2. Chang KY, et al. Modern staging and utility of PET imaging in esophageal cancer management. J Natl Compr Cancer Netw. 2008;6(9):862–9.
3. Amin MB, et al. The Eighth Edition AJCC Cancer Staging Manual: continuing to build a bridge from a population-based to a more "personalized" approach to cancer staging. CA Cancer J Clin. 2017;67(2):93–9.
4. Mine S, et al. Japanese classification of esophageal cancer, 12th edition: part I. Esophagus. 2024;21(3):179–215.
5. Inaba K, et al. Overlap method: novel intracorporeal esophagojejunostomy after laparoscopic total gastrectomy. J Am Coll Surg. 2010;211(6):e25–9.
6. Hsu MH, et al. Long-term outcomes of endoscopic submucosal dissection for superficial esophageal squamous cell carcinoma in Taiwan. BMC Gastroenterol. 2021;21(1):308.
7. Yeh JH, et al. Long-term outcomes of endoscopic submucosal dissection and comparison to surgery for superficial esophageal squamous cancer: a systematic review and meta-analysis. Ther Adv Gastroenterol. 2020;13:1756284820964316.
8. Ke RT, et al. Similar survival after endoscopic submucosal dissection and esophagectomy in early esophageal cancer and synchronous or metachronous head and neck cancer. J Cardiothorac Surg. 2024;19(1):52.
9. Tsou YK, et al. Endoscopic submucosal dissection of superficial esophageal neoplasms is feasible and not riskier for patients with liver cirrhosis. Dig Dis Sci. 2016;61(12):3565–71.
10. van Hagen P, et al. Preoperative chemoradiotherapy for esophageal or junctional cancer. N Engl J Med. 2012;366(22):2074–84.
11. Watanabe M, et al. Outcomes of preoperative chemotherapy with docetaxel, cisplatin, and 5-fluorouracil followed by esophagectomy in patients with resectable node-positive esophageal cancer. Ann Surg Oncol. 2014;21(9):2838–44.
12. Makino T, et al. Utility of initial induction chemotherapy with 5-fluorouracil, cisplatin, and docetaxel (DCF) for T4 esophageal cancer: a propensity score-matched analysis. Dis Esophagus. 2018;31(4). https://doi.org/10.1093/dote/dox130.
13. Gao X, et al. Neoadjuvant carboplatin/paclitaxel versus 5-fluorouracil/cisplatin in combination with radiotherapy for locally advanced esophageal squamous cell carcinoma: a multicenter comparative study. Cancers (Basel). 2022;14(11):2610.
14. Gao X, et al. Treatment burden and cost-effectiveness analysis of the neoadjuvant CROSS regimen in esophageal squamous cell carcinoma: a multicenter retrospective study. Dis Esophagus. 2023;36(11):doad031.
15. Chen YH, et al. Effect of esophageal cancer screening on mortality among patients with oral cancer and second primary esophageal cancer in Taiwan. Am J Otolaryngol. 2023;44(4):103856.
16. Cheng C, et al. Impact of child-pugh class a liver cirrhosis on perioperative outcomes of patients with oesophageal cancer: a propensity score-matched analysis. Eur J Cardiothorac Surg. 2021;59(2):395–402.
17. Yang TY, et al. Preoperative transient elastography in patients with esophageal cancer. Diagnostics (Basel). 2022;12(12):3194.
18. Ng CB, et al. Temporal trends in survival outcomes for patients with esophageal cancer following neoadjuvant chemoradiotherapy: a 14-year analysis. Ann Surg Oncol. 2024;31(10):6652–61.
19. Hsu P-K, et al. Modified en bloc esophagectomy for squamous cell carcinoma after neoadjuvant chemoradiotherapy. Ann Thorac Surg. 2023;115(4):862–9.
20. Crenshaw GD, et al. Extracorporeal gastric stapling reduces the incidence of gastric conduit failure after minimally invasive esophagectomy. Am Surg. 2010;76(8):823–8.

21. McGuire AL, Gilbert S. Transthoracic extracorporeal gastric conduit preparation for minimally invasive Ivor-Lewis esophagectomy. Innovations (Phila). 2015;10(4):236–40; discussion 240.
22. Booka E, et al. What is the best reconstruction procedure after esophagectomy? A meta-analysis comparing posterior mediastinal and retrosternal approaches. Ann Gastroenterol Surg. 2023;7(4):553–64.
23. Yang TY, et al. Survival outcomes of patients with esophageal cancer and post-chemoradiotherapy surgical T4b disease: is palliative resection justified? Ann Surg Oncol. 2024;31(10):6628–34.
24. Horikawa M, et al. Laparoscopic creation of a retrosternal route for gastric conduit reconstruction. Surg Endosc. 2022;36(4):2680–7.
25. Seesing MFJ, et al. Minimally invasive esophagectomy: a propensity score-matched analysis of semiprone versus prone position. Surg Endosc. 2018;32(6):2758–65.
26. Lee YK, et al. Selection of minimally invasive surgical approaches for treating esophageal cancer. Thorac Cancer. 2022;13(15):2100–5.
27. Lee JM, et al. Comparison of single- and multi-incision minimally invasive esophagectomy (MIE) for treating esophageal cancer: a propensity-matched study. Surg Endosc. 2017;31(7):2925–31.
28. Liu CY, et al. Cost-effectiveness of minimally invasive esophagectomy for esophageal squamous cell carcinoma. World J Surg. 2018;42(8):2522–9.
29. Kernstine KH, et al. The robotic, 2-stage, 3-field esophagolymphadenectomy. J Thorac Cardiovasc Surg. 2004;127(6):1847–9.
30. Tagkalos E, et al. Incidence and predictors of textbook outcome after minimally invasive esophagectomy for cancer: a two-center study. Cancers (Basel). 2024;16(6):1109.
31. Chao YK, et al. Robot-assisted minimally invasive oesophagectomy versus thoracoscopic approach: multi-institutional study on short-term outcomes. BJS Open. 2024;8(4):zrae063.
32. Chao YK, et al. Multicentre randomized clinical trial on robot-assisted versus video-assisted thoracoscopic oesophagectomy (REVATE trial). Br J Surg. 2024;111(7):znae143.
33. Kelly RJ, et al. Adjuvant nivolumab in resected esophageal or gastroesophageal junction cancer. N Engl J Med. 2021;384(13):1191–203.
34. Cao Y, et al. Pembrolizumab versus chemotherapy for patients with esophageal squamous cell carcinoma enrolled in the randomized KEYNOTE-181 trial in Asia. ESMO Open. 2022;7(1):100341.
35. Kato K, et al. Nivolumab versus chemotherapy in patients with advanced oesophageal squamous cell carcinoma refractory or intolerant to previous chemotherapy (ATTRACTION-3): a multicentre, randomised, open-label, phase 3 trial. Lancet Oncol. 2019;20(11):1506–17.
36. Liu C, et al. Preliminary real-world outcomes of adjuvant immunotherapy in resected esophageal cancer: a retrospective study from Taiwan. J Chest Surg. 2025;58(4):134–45.
37. Guo JC, et al. Adjuvant chemoradiotherapy plus pembrolizumab for locally advanced esophageal squamous cell carcinoma with high risk of recurrence following neoadjuvant chemoradiotherapy: a single-arm phase II study. Cancer Immunol Immunother. 2024;73(11):230.
38. Ming-Wei, Kao Yao-Hung, Kuo Kun-Chou, Hsieh Ching-Tai, Lee Shih-Chi, Wu Wen-Chi, Yang. Immune checkpoint inhibitor nivolumab combined with chemotherapy improved the survival of unresectable advanced and metastatic esophageal squamous cell carcinoma: A Real-World Experience International Journal of Molecular Sciences. 2023;24(8):7312. https://doi.org/10.3390/ijms24087312.

European Experiences

23

H. C. G. Overtoom and S. S. Gisbertz

23.1 Introduction

Esophageal cancer (EC) is a major global health burden, ranked as the 11th most prevalent cancer type and seventh leading cause of cancer-related mortality [1]. In 2022, more than 500.000 new cases were diagnosed worldwide, with approximately 6% of new diagnoses originating from Europe [1]. The incidence of the two major EC histopathological subtypes varies geographically and is driven by distinct etiological factors [1, 2]. Esophageal squamous cell carcinoma (ESCC) remains the worldwide predominant subtype, accounting for over 90% of cases, meanwhile esophageal adenocarcinoma (EAC) represents the dominant subtype in Western populations [3, 4]. Beyond their histopathological and epidemiological differences, ESCC and EAC are characterized by distinct molecular features, which contribute to differences in prognosis and treatment outcomes [2, 5]. These differences necessitate careful consideration when selecting and tailoring staging and therapeutic strategies. Although overall survival remains poor, the 5-year survival rate of esophageal cancer has improved considerably over the past two decades, largely due to the advances in multimodal treatment strategies, refinements in minimally invasive surgical techniques, and the introduction of new drugs such as immune checkpoint inhibitors [6]. This review provides an overview of current evidence on the epidemiology, staging, and treatment of ESCC in Europe.

H. C. G. Overtoom (✉) · S. S. Gisbertz
Department of Surgery, Amsterdam UMC, Location University of Amsterdam, Amsterdam, The Netherlands

Cancer Center Amsterdam, Cancer Treatment and Quality of Life, Amsterdam, The Netherlands

Amsterdam Gastroenterology Endocrinology Metabolism, Amsterdam UMC, Location University of Amsterdam, Amsterdam, The Netherlands
e-mail: h.c.g.overtoom@amsterdamumc.nl; s.s.gisbertz@amsterdamumc.nl

Y. Kitagawa et al. (eds.), *Esophageal Squamous Cell Carcinoma*,
https://doi.org/10.1007/978-981-92-2611-5_23

23.2 Epidemiology

The European EC patient population generally consists of men over 65 years of age, with EAC histological subtype in approximately 70% of cases [1]. Epidemiological studies confirm the annual EAC incidence increase over recent years, averaging 2.1% in Europe [3, 4]. This rise is expected to persist, although no (inter)national population-wide screening programs for EC have been implemented in Europe due to its relatively limited incidence [3, 4]. The increase in early onset EC (diagnosed before 50 years of age) is particular warranted because of the associated advanced stages at diagnosis and worse survival outcomes [7]. Rates of ESCC have remained stable or declined slightly, particularly in Northern and Western European countries [4].

The incidence of EAC in Europe has largely been attributed to the rising levels of excess body weight, higher numbers of Barrett's esophagus (BE), and increased gastro-esophageal reflux disease (GERD) [8]. Smoking, heavy alcohol consumption, and their synergistic effects are the known major risk factors for ESCC in Western populations, similar to Asian populations [8, 9]. The decline in ESCC incidence, particularly in Western European countries, has been associated with decreasing prevalence of tobacco smoking and alcohol consumption and is expected to continue [3]. Although socioeconomic status (SES) is not correlated with the incidence of esophageal cancer in Europe, it does influence treatment selection and clinical outcome, with higher SES being associated with more favorable outcomes and vice versa [10].

23.3 Prognosis

The average 5-year survival rate across all EC disease stages at diagnosis is approximately 22% [11]. The 5-year survival per histological subtype is estimated at 36% for nonmetastatic EAC, and 27% for nonmetastatic ESCC in Western populations [11, 12]. Overall survival of EC has improved 14% over the last decade, largely attributable to the introduction of targeted immunotherapies, centralization of care, and advances in multimodal treatments, like chemotherapy, radiotherapy, and surgery [3, 11].

23.4 Screening, Centralization, and Cancer Registries

Esophageal cancer is considered a complex disease, with a generally poor prognosis, necessitating management by a specialized multidisciplinary team [13]. The poor prognosis of EC is largely attributed to the high proportion of advanced-stage diagnoses and the high rate of disease dissemination over time, despite curative-intent treatment. This underscores the importance of screening and surveillance modalities in high-risk patients. However, in Europe, screening is recommended only for a subset of patients with Barrett's Esophagus (BE) patients, since nationwide screening programs are less feasible compared to other global regions due to the relatively lower incidence, especially of ESCC [14, 15]. Centralization of care and volume requirements have been introduced to improve outcomes, which have significantly prolonged survival in EC patients [13]. Effective January 1, 2026, the Netherlands has implemented an increased annual treatment threshold of 75 combined esophageal and gastric cancer surgeries in order to further improve patient outcomes. Nevertheless, requirements vary widely across Europe, with 25% of countries lacking any formal criteria, highlighting the need for improvement [16]. European countries with centralized healthcare demonstrate better outcomes due to the standardization of care, increased adherence to guideline-based treatment, and national cancer registries [16, 17].

23.5 Diagnosis and Staging

The primary diagnostic modality for EC is endoscopy with biopsies. According to European guidelines, a minimum of six to eight representative biopsies should be obtained from all suspicious lesions for histopathological assessment [15]. After confirmation of EC, staging is performed by FDG-PET-CT to assess the primary tumor (T), lymph nodes (N), and presence of metastatic disease (M) [18]. Endoscopic or endobronchial ultrasonography is performed on indication to evaluate invasion toward the adjacent structures, or to perform fine needle aspiration of suspected lymph node metastases outside the standard resection or radiotherapy field [19]. Magnetic resonance imaging is generally not indicated for the primary staging of esophageal cancer due to poor image quality resulting from cardiac and respiratory motion; however, ongoing studies aim to address this limitation [20]. Clinical staging with FDG-PET-CT is repeated after neoadjuvant therapy to exclude disease progression (M1) before continuation of curative-intent treatment, and in pathological assessment.

Staging is generally performed according to the eighth edition of the American Joint Committee on Cancer (AJCC) and International Union for Cancer Control (UICC) staging manual [21]. The location of ESCC is categorized as cervical, upper thoracic, middle thoracic, or lower thoracic, defined by the respective anatomical landmarks: the sternal notch, azygos vein, inferior pulmonary vein, and the esophagogastric junction (EGJ) [22]. In adenocarcinoma, the differentiation between esophageal and EGJ-originating cancers is of predominant value, and is determined by location of the lesion's epicenter [22]. Adenocarcinoma epicenters ≤ 2 cm into the gastric cardia are staged as esophageal cancer, whereas more distal epicenters are staged as gastric cancer, according to the eighth AJCC/UICC staging manual [22]. The genetic signature of EGJ-localized carcinomas may provide a more accurate assessment of tumor origin and is expected to be incorporated into the ninth AJCC/UICC staging manual [2, 22].

Several nodal classification systems are used worldwide. In European practice, periesophageal lymph nodes—extending from the cervical to the celiac region—are generally regarded as regional nodes. In the eighth edition of the AJCC/UICC staging system, the distinction between regional and extra-regional lymph nodes is independent of the location of the primary tumor, in contrast to the 12th edition of the Japanese Classification of Esophageal Cancer (JES) [22, 23]. However, nodal staging is comparable, since the 12th edition of the JES, and is now exclusively based on the number of suspected lymph nodes and ranges from N0 to N3. In Europe, extra-regional lymph nodes are classified as metastatic disease (M1) and are therefore not eligible for curative-intent treatment. By contrast, in the JES classification, extra-regional lymph nodes are subdivided into M1a and M1b, depending on the potential therapeutic benefit if resected [22, 23]. The ongoing international TIGER study, investigating the distribution of lymph node metastases, combines the most applied nodal classification systems and aims to globally standardize the staging and surgical management of lymph node metastases in EC [24].

23.6 Pathological and Molecular Typing

Histopathological confirmation of the suspected lesion(s) is required for diagnosing EC, and is performed according to the World Health Organization (WHO) criteria [15, 25]. The ESCC and EAC histological subtypes are distinct in their molecular characteristics, and can be seen as separate disease entities [2, 6]. Notably, differences in ESCC incidence between Western and Asian patients, as well as variations in treatment outcomes such as pathological complete response rates, suggest divergent etiologies and/or genomic alterations [2, 5, 26, 27]. Conflicting data on the genomic alterations in Western versus Asian ESCC patients has prevented consensus on this phenomenon, thus remains an interesting topic of research [2, 26, 27].

Molecular biomarker classifications have increased significantly over the last decade, resulting in more robust prognostic models and individualized targeted treatment options [8, 28]. Programmed cell death-ligand 1 (PD-L1) remains the primary clinically accepted biomarker with therapeutic treatment consequences for ESCC in Europe [19]. Immunohistochemistry (IHC) assessment is recommended in potential candidates for first- or second-line treatment with immune checkpoint inhibitors (ICIs) [15]. PD-L1 expression may be evaluated using three scoring systems: the tumor proportion score (TPS), evaluating the percentage of viable tumor cells showing partial or complete membrane staining; tumor area positivity (TAP) as percentage of area covered by tumor cells with positive staining; or the combined positivity score (CPS), calculated by the number of vital tumor cells with PD-L1 positive plasma membrane staining (including lymphocytes and macrophages). The generally accepted thresholds for PD-L1 positivity are TPS $\geq 1\%$, TAP $\geq 5\%$, or CPS ≥ 10, although cutoff values vary across clinical trials [19].

23.7 Perioperative Management

Diagnosis, staging, and histopathological assessment are complemented by comprehensive medical evaluation for adequate choice of treatment and, if necessary, clinical optimization to enhance perioperative outcomes [29]. This evaluation includes assessing patient operability using the WHO performance status, as well as evaluating pulmonary and cardiac function [19, 30]. Nutritional assessment is performed according to the European Society of Clinical Nutrition and Metabolism (ESPEN), and patients are referred to a dietitian if required [15, 31]. In addition, exercise-based prehabilitation is advised when oxygen uptake is <11 mL/kg/min at the ventilatory anaerobic threshold, and/or <18 mL/kg/min at peak exercise, to reduce postoperative complications and potentially improve oncological outcomes [32].

23.8 Endoscopic Treatment

Endoscopic treatment is a curative treatment option in early EC, although early onset EC is infrequently diagnosed. Endoscopic submucosal dissection (ESD) or endoscopic mucosal resection (EMR) is indicated for superficial (cT1aN0M0), well- or moderately differentiated (G1–G2) ESCC, with diameter ≤20 mm, and without ulceration or suspected lymph node metastases on EUS/PET-CT [8, 33]. Endoscopic treatment for cT1b tumors has been proven feasible but is yet investigated in European ESCC populations [34, 35]. The preferred treatment modality according to the European Society of Gastrointestinal Endoscopy (ESGE) is an en-bloc ESD because of the superior efficacy, higher complete resection rate and lower risk of local recurrences [36]. Esophagectomy with lymphadenectomy is recommended if the deep resection margin after endoscopic treatment is tumor-positive, or in the presence of lymphovascular invasion, although organ-sparing chemoradiotherapy (CRT) may be considered in ESCC [15]. Endoscopic surveillance after endoscopic resection may be optional in high-risk cT1N0 patients, although still under investigation in the PREFER study [35, 37].

Moreover, endoscopic treatment plays a significant role in the management of complications [38]. Endoscopic vacuum therapy has been shown to substantially reduce the need for re-operations in patients with anastomotic leakage [39]. Long-term complications like strictures are also treated endoscopically [38].

23.9 Perioperative Therapy

Neoadjuvant chemoradiotherapy is considered the standard preoperative care in operable patients with resectable, locally advanced ESCC (cT2–4 N0–3 M0) in Europe [19]. The CROSS trial, a landmark study in EC, demonstrated significant long-term survival benefit after neoadjuvant chemoradiotherapy (weekly carboplatin-paclitaxel with 41.4 Gy radiation) followed by surgery compared to surgery alone, with 10-year survival rates of 46% versus 23% ($p = 0.007$), respectively, in the ESCC subgroup [40]. The NeoRes trial, investigating neoadjuvant chemotherapy (nCT) versus neoadjuvant chemoradiotherapy (nCRT), although underpowered for adequate subgroup analysis, suggested improved survival outcomes of ESCC subgroup after nCRT [41]. Consequently, nCRT is the preferred treatment for resectable, locally advanced ESCC in Europe, in contrast to Asian countries, where doublet or triplet chemotherapy is predominantly used preoperatively for operable, resectable ESCC [19, 42].

Definitive chemoradiotherapy (dCRT) is the treatment of choice in cervical locally advanced (T3–T4) ESCC [19]. Patients with non-resectable (non-cervical) ESCC (cT4b or anticipated R1), inoperable conditions, or cervical lymph node metastases are also treated with dCRT, consistent with clinical practice in Asian countries [19, 42]. The standard dCRT radiotherapy (RT) dose is generally 50.4 Gy, combined with either platin/taxane- or platin/fluoropyrimidine-based chemotherapy [19, 43]. In Europe, higher RT doses are not considered to be more effective, and may significantly compromise outcomes of potential salvage surgery [43, 44].

The recently published Dutch SANO trial evaluated the role of active surveillance (AS) in patients with clinically complete response after nCRT, to reduce the rate of futile surgery in patients with a pathological complete response [45]. However, implementation of AS strategies is hindered by several factors: only 9% of patients (69 out of 776) remained eligible for the AS strategy during the study, analyses were based on limited follow-up data of 2 years, and the study lacked statistical power as the non-inferiority margin was based on 5-year survival data [46]. The ongoing NEEDS trial, investigating nCRT followed by surgery versus dCRT with salvage surgery on indication in ESCC patients, is expected to support clinical decision-making regarding the role of AS in the management of ESCC [47].

Immunotherapy is an increasing subject of interest; however, generally not administered in the neoadjuvant curative setting in Europe.

23.10 Surgical Treatment

In Europe, surgical resection with lymphadenectomy is considered the cornerstone of curative-intent treatment in resectable and operable EC patients [15]. Surgery is generally scheduled six to 10 weeks after completion of neoadjuvant therapy in patients without metastases on restaging FDG-PET-CT. Transthoracic approach is generally preferred because of the superior surgical overview, increased R0 rates, higher lymph node yield, and prolonged survival compared to the transhiatal approach [48, 49]. Transcervical approaches without transthoracic access have been introduced in European centers, such as in the MICE study, with the aim of reducing postoperative pulmonary complications [50]. However, their widespread implementation remains limited due to the incidence of recurrent laryngeal nerve palsy and the considerable training demands. The choice of surgical technique is primarily determined by tumor location, favoring either esophagectomy with gastric conduit reconstruction through the Ivor-Lewis procedure with transthoracic anastomosis or the McKeown procedure with cervical anastomosis, independent of histopathological subtype [15]. The Ivor-Lewis procedure is performed for tumors located distal to the tracheal carina, whereas the McKeown procedure is preferred in proximal tumors [15]. Nevertheless, an intrathoracic anastomosis is favored, as cervical anastomoses are associated with a higher risk of anastomotic leakage and laryngeal nerve damage, according to the ICAN trial [51]. The McKeown procedure is considered in case of extended proximal radiotherapy fields or suspected proximal lymph node metastases.

Lymph node metastases are amongst the most important prognostic factors, emphasizing the importance of adequate lymphadenectomy for accurate staging and improved survival [52, 53]. However, significant variation exists in European clinical practice regarding the optimal lymph node dissection, ranging from extended paratracheal dissection in high-volume centers to selective node picking of suspected lymph node metastases [54]. Moreover, extended lymphadenectomy can be complex and is also associated with increased morbidity [55]. According to European guidelines, a two-field lymphadenectomy is advised; however, no recommendation is made regarding the optimal extent of dissection due to the lack of consensus. The ongoing international TIGER study, investigating the distribution patterns of lymph node metastases in over 5000 patients, aims to support the standardization of lymphadenectomy and achieve international consensus on its optimal extent [24]. Cervical lymph node dissection, as part of the three-field lymphadenectomy, is generally not performed in European countries, in contrast to Asian countries [24, 55]. Generally, if a patient has cervical metastases, these (and the primary tumor and other suspected lymph nodes) are treated with definitive chemoradiotherapy [15]. Moreover, no international consensus has been reached on the resection versus preservation of the thoracic duct (TD) during esophagectomy. Although survival outcomes are conflicting, TD resection has been associated with increased LN yield, but further investigation is warrented [56].

Minimally invasive techniques, including robotic-assisted approaches, are considered superior to open surgery, as demonstrated by multiple trials—including TIME, MIRO, and ROBOT—which reported reduced complications, increased lymph node yield, and improved long-term overall survival [57–59].

Intraoperative visual enhancement techniques have been increasingly investigated and applied over the past decade. These techniques allow individualized assessment of factors influencing surgical outcomes including tissue perfusion, anastomotic tension, and fluorescence-guided surgery. Indocyanine green (ICG) fluorescence is a safe, multipurpose tracer that has very promising applications in EC surgery. ICG fluorescence quantification is feasible for the intraoperative perfusion assessment of the anastomosis and gastric conduit, which, although still in development, could help prevent anastomotic leakage [60, 61]. Furthermore, ICG has demonstrated feasibility for sentinel node-navigated surgery and ICG-guided lymphadenectomy after endoscopic submucosal injections [37, 62]. This technology, although histopathological correlation is still unknown, could lead to patient-tailored lymphadenectomy based on ICG fluorescence of tumor-draining lymph nodes.

Patients with incomplete response to dCRT or local relapse during surveillance are eligible for salvage surgery [19, 44]. However, salvage procedures are associated with significant morbidity, including anastomotic leakage in 25% of cases, four times higher chance of developing conduit necrosis, and more than three times higher 30-day/in-hospital mortality, based on a European cohort study with mixed histological subtypes [44, 63]. This complex procedure is therefore deemed to be performed by specialized EC centers to minimize adverse outcomes.

23.11 Postoperative Management

The postoperative outcomes are optimized through the implementation of the Enhanced Recovery After Surgery (ERAS) protocol [64]. The ERAS principles—preoperative counselling, optimized analgesia, early mobilization, and nutritional support—have been associated with reductions in length of stay, reduced complications, improved functional recovery, and higher patient-reported quality of life in high-volume European centers [64–66]. The ERAS protocols allow for center-specific conceptualization of the ERAS principles, which can be adapted to institutional logistics and clinical context. The Amsterdam UMC, for instance, incorporated a specific early mobilization target of 100 m on postoperative day one to guide postoperative recovery [67].

23.12 Follow-Up

The majority of esophageal cancer recurrences occur within the first 2 years following multimodal curative-intent treatment [68]. There is no conclusive evidence that regular follow-up after initial therapy improves survival, except in patients eligible for local treatment of loco-regional recurrence, like salvage surgery following dCRT [15, 68]. Consequently, follow-up visits should focus on symptom assessment, nutrition status, and psychosocial support [15].

23.13 Adjuvant Therapy

In contrast to clinical practice in Asian countries, adjuvant chemotherapy is generally not administered after nCRT + surgery with curative intent in Europe for ESCC [19, 42].

Immunotherapy is currently under evaluation in the adjuvant setting. The Checkmate577 trial showed the significant benefit of adjuvant nivolumab in ESCC patients with residual disease after nCRT in their interim analysis, and subsequently was implemented in most of the European countries [69]. However, recently published long-term survival data showed no overall statistical difference, and general outcomes of the control group were worse compared to populations with similar characteristics [69, 70]. This led to the withdrawal of the indication for adjuvant nivolumab in ESCC patients with residual disease after nCRT in some of the European countries, like the Netherlands, although final conclusions based on the recently published data are under evaluation.

23.14 Palliative Treatment

Immune checkpoint inhibitors have a central role in the treatment of advanced and metastatic ESCC in Europe, depending on PD-L1 assessment. Negative or unknown PD-L1 tumors opt for platinum-fluoropyrimidine chemotherapy (ChT) with either tislelizumab or nivolumab [15]. Tumors with PD-L1 TAP score ≥5% opt for combination of tislelizumab and platinum doublet chemotherapy based on the RATIONALE-306 study [19, 71]. Patients with PD-L1 TPS ≥1% are eligible for either nivolumab-ChT or nivolumab-ipilimumab therapy, while patients with PD-L1 CPS ≥10 may opt for pembrolizumab-ChT (platinum or fluoropyrimidine) [15, 72]. Taxane or irinotecan ChT is considered as second-line or subsequent-line systemic treatment [73]. Regimes including toripalimab, are generally not used in European clinical practice since applicability in European population is still under evaluation [19].

23.15 Future Implications

Future patient-tailored staging and treatment strategies are expected to significantly improve outcomes in esophageal cancer. Advances in imaging modalities—such as ultrasmall superparamagnetic iron oxides as MRI contrast agents combined with motion-compensated MRI sequences—may enhance both prognostic assessment and staging accuracy on an individual patient basis. Genomic and preclinical models, including esophagus-on-a-chip systems, enable evaluation of treatment susceptibility profiles, thereby significantly increasing treatment efficacy in individual patients [74]. Moreover, noninvasive methods for response assessment or follow-up, such as circulating tumor DNA, though still under investigation, have the potential to reduce disease burden and facilitate timely diagnosis and intervention [75]. In addition, image-guided radiotherapy or surgery, standardized lymphadenectomy, and enhanced visualization techniques, including fluorescence-guided surgery, could further improve treatment-related outcomes.

23.16 Summary

Esophageal squamous cell carcinoma is a malignant disease with dismal prognosis. Management requires specialized multidisciplinary teams to ensure accurate staging, optimal treatment selection, and comprehensive patient care. Staging and treatment selection are increasingly supported by individualized histopathological assessment, including biomarker analysis, to guide targeted therapeutic strategies. Over recent decades, outcomes in ESCC have improved significantly due to advances in targeted and multimodal therapies, refined surgical techniques, perioperative optimization, and centralization with volume-based care requirements. Future improvements are expected through the improvement of staging modalities, patient-tailored management based on preclinical susceptibility profiles, additional targeted therapies, enhanced intraoperative visualization techniques, and personalized surgical lymphadenectomy.

References

1. Bray F, Laversanne M, Sung H, Ferlay J, Siegel RL, Soerjomataram I, et al. Global cancer statistics 2022: GLOBOCAN estimates of incidence and mortality worldwide for 36 cancers in 185 countries. CA Cancer J Clin. 2024;74(3):229–63.
2. Cancer Genome Atlas Research Network, et al. Integrated genomic characterization of oesophageal carcinoma. Nature. 2017;541(7636):169–75.
3. Arnold M, Laversanne M, Brown LM, Devesa SS, Bray F. Predicting the future burden of esophageal cancer by histological subtype: international trends in incidence up to 2030. Am J Gastroenterol. 2017;112(8):1247–55.
4. Rumgay H, Arnold M, Laversanne M, Whiteman DC, Thrift AP, Wei W, et al. International trends in esophageal squamous cell carcinoma and adenocarcinoma incidence. Am J Gastroenterol. 2021;116(5):1072–6.
5. Gao X, Overtoom HCG, Eyck BM, Huang SH, Nieboer D, van der Sluis PC, et al. Pathological response to neoadjuvant chemoradiotherapy for oesophageal squamous cell carcinoma in Eastern versus Western countries: meta-analysis. Br J Surg. 2024;111(5):znae083.
6. Yang H, Wang F, Hallemeier CL, Lerut T, Fu J. Oesophageal cancer. Lancet. 2024;404(10466):1991–2005.
7. Codipilly DC, Sawas T, Dhaliwal L, Johnson ML, Lansing R, Wang KK, et al. Epidemiology and outcomes of young-onset esophageal adenocarcinoma: an analysis from a population-based database. Cancer Epidemiol Biomarkers Prev. 2021;30(1):142–9.
8. Rustgi AK, El-Serag HB. Esophageal carcinoma. N Engl J Med. 2014;371(26):2499–509.
9. Abnet CC, Arnold M, Wei WQ. Epidemiology of esophageal squamous cell carcinoma. Gastroenterology. 2018;154(2):360–73.
10. Bus P, Aarts MJ, Lemmens VE, van Oijen MG, Creemers GJ, Nieuwenhuijzen GA, et al. The effect of socioeconomic status on staging and treatment decisions in esophageal cancer. J Clin Gastroenterol. 2012;46(10):833–9.
11. van Putten M, de Vos-Geelen J, Nieuwenhuijzen GAP, Siersema PD, Lemmens V, Rosman C, et al. Long-term survival improvement in oesophageal cancer in the Netherlands. Eur J Cancer. 2018;94:138–47.
12. van Laarhoven H, Verhoeven R, van Berge Henegouwen M, Mohammad NH, van Hillegersberg R, Slingerland M, et al. Real-world outcomes of the CROSS regimen in patients with resectable esophageal or gastro-esophageal junction adenocarcinoma: a nationwide cohort study in the Netherlands. EClinicalMedicine. 2025;80:103067.
13. Visser MR, van Berge Henegouwen MI, van Hillegersberg R. Centralization and quality control in esophageal cancer surgery: a way forward in Europe. Dis Esophagus. 2024;37(9):doae035.
14. Shaheen NJ, Falk GW, Iyer PG, Gerson LB. ACG clinical guideline: diagnosis and management of Barrett's esophagus. Am J Gastroenterol. 2016;111(1):30–50; quiz 1.
15. Obermannová R, Alsina M, Cervantes A, Leong T, Lordick F, Nilsson M, et al. Oesophageal cancer: ESMO clinical practice guideline for diagnosis, treatment and follow-up. Ann Oncol. 2022;33(10):992–1004.
16. Visser MR, Voeten DM, Gisbertz SS, Ruurda JP, Achiam MP, Nilsson M, et al. Western European variation in the organization of esophageal cancer surgical care. Dis Esophagus. 2024;37(9). https://doi.org/10.1093/dote/doae033.
17. Grilli R, Violi F, Bassi MC, Marino M. The effects of centralizing cancer surgery on post-operative mortality: a systematic review and meta-analysis. J Health Serv Res Policy. 2021;26(4):289–301.
18. van Vliet EP, Heijenbrok-Kal MH, Hunink MG, Kuipers EJ, Siersema PD. Staging investigations for oesophageal cancer: a meta-analysis. Br J Cancer. 2008;98(3):547–57.
19. Puhr HC, Prager GW, Ilhan-Mutlu A. How we treat esophageal squamous cell carcinoma. ESMO Open. 2023;8(1):100789.
20. Lee SL, Yadav P, Starekova J, Christensen L, Chandereng T, Chappell R, et al. Diagnostic performance of MRI for esophageal carcinoma: a systematic review and meta-analysis. Radiology. 2021;299(3):583–94.

21. Rice TW, Gress DM, Patil DT, Hofstetter WL, Kelsen DP, Blackstone EH. Cancer of the esophagus and esophagogastric junction-major changes in the American Joint Committee on Cancer eighth edition cancer staging manual. CA Cancer J Clin. 2017;67(4):305–17.
22. Rice TW. Esophagus and esophagogastric junction. Springer; 2017.
23. Mine S, Tanaka K, Kawachi H, Shirakawa Y, Kitagawa Y, Toh Y, et al. Japanese classification of esophageal cancer, 12th edition: part I. Esophagus. 2024;21(3):179–215.
24. Hagens ERC, van Berge Henegouwen MI, van Sandick JW, Cuesta MA, van der Peet DL, Heisterkamp J, et al. Distribution of lymph node metastases in esophageal carcinoma [TIGER study]: study protocol of a multinational observational study. BMC Cancer. 2019;19(1):662.
25. Nagtegaal ID, Odze RD, Klimstra D, Paradis V, Rugge M, Schirmacher P, et al. The 2019 WHO classification of tumours of the digestive system. Histopathology. 2020;76(2):182–8.
26. Zhang R, Li C, Wan Z, Qin J, Li Y, Wang Z, et al. Comparative genomic analysis of esophageal squamous cell carcinoma among different geographic regions. Front Oncol. 2022;12:999424.
27. Deng J, Chen H, Zhou D, Zhang J, Chen Y, Liu Q, et al. Comparative genomic analysis of esophageal squamous cell carcinoma between Asian and Caucasian patient populations. Nat Commun. 2017;8(1):1533.
28. Liu Z, Zhao Y, Kong P, Liu Y, Huang J, Xu E, et al. Integrated multi-omics profiling yields a clinically relevant molecular classification for esophageal squamous cell carcinoma. Cancer Cell. 2023;41(1):181–95.e9.
29. Moran J, Guinan E, McCormick P, Larkin J, Mockler D, Hussey J, et al. The ability of prehabilitation to influence postoperative outcome after intra-abdominal operation: a systematic review and meta-analysis. Surgery. 2016;160(5):1189–201.
30. Yates JW, Chalmer B, McKegney FP. Evaluation of patients with advanced cancer using the Karnofsky performance status. Cancer. 1980;45(8):2220–4.
31. Cederholm T, Barazzoni R, Austin P, Ballmer P, Biolo G, Bischoff SC, et al. ESPEN guidelines on definitions and terminology of clinical nutrition. Clin Nutr. 2017;36(1):49–64.
32. Rayner CJ, Bartlett DB, Allen SK, Wooldridge T, Seymour T, Sunshine S, et al. Prehabilitation during neoadjuvant chemotherapy results in an enhanced immune response in esophageal adenocarcinoma tumors: a randomized controlled trial. J Sport Health Sci. 2025;14:101063.
33. Shaheen NJ, Sharma P, Overholt BF, Wolfsen HC, Sampliner RE, Wang KK, et al. Radiofrequency ablation in Barrett's esophagus with dysplasia. N Engl J Med. 2009;360(22):2277–88.
34. Merkow RP, Bilimoria KY, Keswani RN, Chung J, Sherman KL, Knab LM, et al. Treatment trends, risk of lymph node metastasis, and outcomes for localized esophageal cancer. J Natl Cancer Inst. 2014;106(7):dju133.
35. Chan MW, Nieuwenhuis E, Jansen M, Belghazi K, Nagengast WB, Westerhof J, et al. Endoscopic follow-up of radically resected submucosal adenocarcinoma in Barrett's esophagus: early results of an ongoing prospective, international, multicenter cohort registry (prefer trial). Gastrointest Endosc. 2022;95(6):AB415–AB6.
36. Pimentel-Nunes P, Libânio D, Bastiaansen BAJ, Bhandari P, Bisschops R, Bourke MJ, et al. Endoscopic submucosal dissection for superficial gastrointestinal lesions: European Society of Gastrointestinal Endoscopy (ESGE) guideline – update 2022. Endoscopy. 2022;54(6):591–622.
37. Frederiks CN, Overwater A, Bergman J, Pouw RE, de Keizer B, Bennink RJ, et al. Feasibility and safety of tailored lymphadenectomy using sentinel node-navigated surgery in patients with high-risk T1 esophageal adenocarcinoma. Ann Surg Oncol. 2023;30(7):4002–11.
38. Wichmann D, Fusco S, Werner CR, Voesch S, Duckworth-Mothes B, Schweizer U, et al. Endoscopic management for post-surgical complications after resection of esophageal cancer. Cancers (Basel). 2022;14(4):980.
39. Ubels S, Verstegen MHP, Klarenbeek BR, Bouwense S, van Berge Henegouwen MI, Daams F, et al. Treatment of anastomotic leak after oesophagectomy for oesophageal cancer: large, collaborative, observational TENTACLE cohort study. Br J Surg. 2023;110(7):852–63.
40. Eyck BM, van Lanschot JJB, Hulshof M, van der Wilk BJ, Shapiro J, van Hagen P, et al. Ten-year outcome of neoadjuvant chemoradiotherapy plus surgery for esophageal cancer: the randomized controlled CROSS trial. J Clin Oncol. 2021;39(18):1995–2004.

41. Klevebro F, von Döbeln GA, Wang N, Johnsen G, Jacobsen AB, Friesland S, et al. A randomized clinical trial of neoadjuvant chemotherapy versus neoadjuvant chemoradiotherapy for cancer of the oesophagus or gastro-oesophageal junction. Ann Oncol. 2016;27(4):660–7.
42. Kitagawa Y, Ishihara R, Ishikawa H, Ito Y, Oyama T, Oyama T, et al. Esophageal cancer practice guidelines 2022 edited by the Japan esophageal society: part 1. Esophagus. 2023;20(3):343–72.
43. Hulshof M, Geijsen ED, Rozema T, Oppedijk V, Buijsen J, Neelis KJ, et al. Randomized study on dose escalation in definitive chemoradiation for patients with locally advanced esophageal cancer (ARTDECO study). J Clin Oncol. 2021;39(25):2816–24.
44. Markar S, Gronnier C, Duhamel A, Pasquer A, Théreaux J, Du Rieu MC, et al. Salvage surgery after chemoradiotherapy in the management of esophageal cancer: is it a viable therapeutic option? J Clin Oncol. 2015;33(33):3866–73.
45. van der Wilk BJ, Eyck BM, Wijnhoven BPL, Lagarde SM, Rosman C, Noordman BJ, et al. Neoadjuvant chemoradiotherapy followed by active surveillance versus standard surgery for oesophageal cancer (SANO trial): a multicentre, stepped-wedge, cluster-randomised, non-inferiority, phase 3 trial. Lancet Oncol. 2025;26(4):425–36.
46. Markar SR, Van Berge Henegouwen M, Bruns C, Ferri L, van Hillegersberg R, Hofstetter W, et al. SANO trial: innovations, risks, and unanswered questions. Lancet Oncol. 2025;26(7):e338.
47. Nilsson M, Olafsdottir H, Alexandersson von Döbeln G, Villegas F, Gagliardi G, Hellström M, et al. Neoadjuvant chemoradiotherapy and surgery for esophageal squamous cell carcinoma versus definitive chemoradiotherapy with salvage surgery as needed: the study protocol for the randomized controlled NEEDS trial. Front Oncol. 2022;12:917961.
48. Kutup A, Nentwich MF, Bollschweiler E, Bogoevski D, Izbicki JR, Holscher AH. What should be the gold standard for the surgical component in the treatment of locally advanced esophageal cancer transthoracic versus transhiatal esophagectomy. Ann Surg. 2014;260(6):1016–22.
49. Mertens AC, Kalff MC, Eshuis WJ, Van Gulik TM, Van Berge Henegouwen MI, Gisbertz SS. Transthoracic versus transhiatal esophagectomy for esophageal cancer: a nationwide propensity score-matched cohort analysis. Ann Surg Oncol. 2021;28(1):175–83.
50. Vercoulen R, van Veenendaal L, Kramer IF, Hutteman M, Shiozaki A, Fujiwara H, et al. Minimally Invasive transCervical oEsophagectomy (MICE) for oesophageal cancer: prospective cohort study (IDEAL stage 2A). Br J Surg. 2024;111(7):znae160.
51. van Workum F, Verstegen MHP, Klarenbeek BR, Bouwense SAW, van Berge Henegouwen MI, Daams F, et al. Intrathoracic vs cervical anastomosis after totally or hybrid minimally invasive esophagectomy for esophageal cancer: a randomized clinical trial. JAMA Surg. 2021;156(7):601–10.
52. Visser E, Markar SR, Ruurda JP, Hanna GB, van Hillegersberg R. Prognostic value of lymph node yield on overall survival in esophageal cancer patients: a systematic review and meta-analysis. Ann Surg. 2019;269(2):261–8.
53. Henckens SPG, Hagens ERC, van Berge Henegouwen MI, Meijer SL, Eshuis WJ, Gisbertz SS. Impact of increasing lymph node yield on staging, morbidity and survival after esophagectomy for esophageal adenocarcinoma. Eur J Surg Oncol. 2023;49(1):89–96.
54. van Rijswijk AS, Hagens ERC, van der Peet DL, Henegouwen MIV, Gisbertz SS. Differences in esophageal cancer surgery in terms of surgical approach and extent of lymphadenectomy: findings of an international survey. Ann Surg Oncol. 2019;26(7):2063–72.
55. Schuring N, van Berge Henegouwen MI, Gisbertz SS. History and evidence for state of the art of lymphadenectomy in esophageal cancer surgery. Dis Esophagus. 2024;37(4):doad065.
56. Nijssen DJ, van der Aa DC, Ali M, Kazemier G, Jamaludin FS, Eshuis WJ, et al. Resection vs. ligation vs. preservation of the thoracic duct during esophagectomy for cancer: a systematic review and meta-analysis. Cancers (Basel). 2025;17(6):967.
57. Straatman J, van der Wielen N, Cuesta MA, Daams F, Roig Garcia J, Bonavina L, et al. Minimally invasive versus open esophageal resection: three-year follow-up of the previously reported randomized controlled trial: the TIME trial. Ann Surg. 2017;266(2):232–6.
58. Tagkalos E, van der Sluis PC, Berlth F, Poplawski A, Hadzijusufovic E, Lang H, et al. Robot-assisted minimally invasive thoraco-laparoscopic esophagectomy versus minimally invasive esophagectomy for resectable esophageal adenocarcinoma, a randomized controlled trial (ROBOT-2 trial). BMC Cancer. 2021;21(1):1060.

59. Nuytens F, Dabakuyo-Yonli TS, Meunier B, Gagnière J, Collet D, D'Journo XB, et al. Five-year survival outcomes of hybrid minimally invasive esophagectomy in esophageal cancer: results of the MIRO randomized clinical trial. JAMA Surg. 2021;156(4):323–32.
60. Nijssen DJ, Joosten JJ, Osterkamp J, van den Elzen RM, de Bruin DM, Svendsen MBS, et al. Quantification of fluorescence angiography for visceral perfusion assessment: measuring agreement between two software algorithms. Surg Endosc. 2024;38(5):2805–16.
61. Joosten JJ, Slooter MD, van den Elzen RM, Bloemen PR, Gisbertz SS, Eshuis WJ, et al. Perfusion assessment by fluorescence time curves in esophagectomy with gastric conduit reconstruction: a prospective clinical study. Surg Endosc. 2023;37(8):6343–52.
62. Müller DT, Schiffmann LM, Reisewitz A, Chon SH, Eckhoff JA, Babic B, et al. Mapping the lymphatic drainage pattern of esophageal cancer with near-infrared fluorescent imaging during robotic assisted minimally invasive Ivor Lewis esophagectomy (RAMIE)-first results of the prospective ESOMAP feasibility trial. Cancers (Basel). 2023;15(8):2247.
63. Visser MR, Voeten DM, Gisbertz SS, Ruurda JP, van Hillegersberg R, van Berge Henegouwen MI. Outcomes of salvage surgery for esophageal carcinoma: a nationwide cohort study from the Dutch upper GI cancer audit. Ann Surg Oncol. 2025;32(4):2687–97.
64. Low DE, Allum W, De Manzoni G, Ferri L, Immanuel A, Kuppusamy M, et al. Guidelines for perioperative care in esophagectomy: enhanced recovery after surgery (ERAS(®)) society recommendations. World J Surg. 2019;43(2):299–330.
65. Kennelly P, Davey MG, Griniouk D, Calpin G, Donlon NE. Evaluating the impact of enhanced recovery after surgery protocols following oesophagectomy: a systematic review and meta-analysis of randomised clinical trials. Dis Esophagus. 2025;38(1):doae118.
66. van Vulpen JK, Hiensch AE, van Hillegersberg R, Ruurda JP, Backx FJG, Nieuwenhuijzen GAP, et al. Supervised exercise after oesophageal cancer surgery: the PERFECT multicentre randomized clinical trial. Br J Surg. 2021;108(7):786–96.
67. Schuring N, Geelen SJG, van Berge Henegouwen MI, Steenhuizen SCM, van der Schaaf M, van der Leeden M, et al. Early mobilization after esophageal cancer surgery: a retrospective cohort study. Dis Esophagus. 2023;36(6):doac085.
68. Schuring N, Stam WT, Plat VD, Kalff MC, Hulshof M, van Laarhoven HWM, et al. Patterns of recurrent disease after neoadjuvant chemoradiotherapy and esophageal cancer surgery with curative intent in a tertiary referral center. Eur J Surg Oncol. 2023;49(10):106947.
69. Kelly RJ, Ajani JA, Kuzdzal J, Zander T, Cutsem EV, Piessen G, et al. Adjuvant nivolumab in resected esophageal or gastroesophageal junction cancer (EC/GEJC) following neoadjuvant chemoradiotherapy (CRT): first results of overall survival (OS) from CheckMate 577. J Clin Oncol. 2025;43(16_suppl):4000.
70. Lin Y, Liang HW, Liu Y, Pan XB. Nivolumab adjuvant therapy for esophageal cancer: a review based on subgroup analysis of CheckMate 577 trial. Front Immunol. 2023;14:1264912.
71. Xu J, Kato K, Raymond E, Hubner RA, Shu Y, Pan Y, et al. Tislelizumab plus chemotherapy versus placebo plus chemotherapy as first-line treatment for advanced or metastatic oesophageal squamous cell carcinoma (RATIONALE-306): a global, randomised, placebo-controlled, phase 3 study. Lancet Oncol. 2023;24(5):483–95.
72. Sun JM, Shen L, Shah MA, Enzinger P, Adenis A, Doi T, et al. Pembrolizumab plus chemotherapy versus chemotherapy alone for first-line treatment of advanced oesophageal cancer (KEYNOTE-590): a randomised, placebo-controlled, phase 3 study. Lancet. 2021;398(10302):759–71.
73. Chen YX, Wang ZX, Jin Y, Zhao Q, Liu ZX, Zuo ZX, et al. An immunogenic and oncogenic feature-based classification for chemotherapy plus PD-1 blockade in advanced esophageal squamous cell carcinoma. Cancer Cell. 2023;41(5):919–32.e5.
74. Pal S, Shimshoni E, Torres SF, Kong M, Tai K, Sangwan V, et al. Patient-derived esophageal adenocarcinoma organ chip: a physiologically relevant platform for functional precision oncology. J Transl Med. 2025;23(1):577.
75. Liu Z, Yang Y, Liu J, Zhang H, Yu H, Han Y, et al. Personalized circulating tumor DNA (ctDNA) analysis in predicting residual disease after neoadjuvant chemoradiotherapy (nCRT) for esophageal squamous cell carcinoma (ESCC). J Clin Oncol. 2023;41(16_suppl):e16062–e.

The North American Experiences

24

Nicolas Zhou, Kyle G. Mitchell, and Wayne L. Hofstetter

Abbreviation

CPS	Combined positive score
CT	Computed tomography
ctDNA	Circulating tumor DNA
DFS	Disease-free survival
EAC	Esophageal adenocarcinoma
EGD	Esophagogastroduodenoscopy
EMR	Endoscopic mucosal resection
ESCC	Esophageal squamous cell carcinoma
ESD	Endoscopic submucosal dissection
EUS	Endoscopic ultrasound
LVI	Lymphovascular invasion
MIE	Minimally invasive esophagectomy
MSI	Microsatellite instability
NBI	Narrow band imaging
OS	Overall survival
pCR	Pathologic complete response
PET	Positron emission tomography
PFS	Progression free survival
QoL	Quality of life
TPS	Tumor proportion score

N. Zhou · K. G. Mitchell · W. L. Hofstetter (✉)
Department of Thoracic and Cardiovascular Surgery, University of Texas MD Anderson Cancer Center, Houston, TX, USA
e-mail: nzhou@mdanderson.org; KGMitchell@mdanderson.org; WHofstetter@mdanderson.org

Y. Kitagawa et al. (eds.), *Esophageal Squamous Cell Carcinoma*,
https://doi.org/10.1007/978-981-92-2611-5_24

24.1 Introduction

Esophageal squamous cell carcinoma (ESCC) remains a significant global health concern, accounting for the majority of esophageal cancer cases worldwide, though its epidemiologic profile in North America is distinct and evolving. Over the recent decades, the incidence of ESCC has steadily declined, a trend largely attributed to decreasing rates of tobacco and alcohol use, which are its primary etiologic factors. Population-based analyses reveal that the age-adjusted incidence rate of ESCC in the United States dropped from 3.06 per 100,000 in 1975 to 1.15 per 100,000 in 2018, in stark contrast to the rising incidence of esophageal adenocarcinoma, which now predominates in the region [1]. At MD Anderson Cancer Center, we typically perform about 80 resections per year, with 15% being ESCC, with no change in that trend over a 20-year period. Nevertheless, ESCC remains clinically important due to its aggressive biology, frequent late-stage presentation, and worldwide incidence [1–3].

The North American approach to ESCC is characterized by a specialized, multidisciplinary model of care that incorporates advanced staging and patient-centered shared decision-making. Tumor profiling is used to gauge the potential effect of immunotherapy [4–7]. Centralization of surgical care to high-volume centers is encouraged, allowing patients to take advantage of multidisciplinary teams that are dedicated to esophageal cancer and can optimize treatment outcomes.

Treatment of ESCC is stage-specific and multimodal, with distinct strategies for early stage, locoregionally advanced, and metastatic disease. Endoscopic therapy has become the standard of care in early intramucosal disease, while neoadjuvant chemoradiation followed by surgery is the most common Western therapy for locoregionally advanced disease. In the metastatic setting, recent advances in immunotherapy have broadened therapeutic options and improved survival outcomes, particularly in tumors with high PD-L1 expression but also for all patients with ESCC. Across all stages, the North American paradigm emphasizes a collaborative treatment strategy that engages the patient in shared decision-making, ensuring individualized care plans that reflect both evidence-based guidelines and patient preferences.

24.2 Diagnostic Approaches

The diagnostic evaluation of ESCC is a comprehensive process that begins with a thorough history and physical examination. Early stage disease is often asymptomatic, while more advanced disease typically presents with progressive dysphagia, unintentional weight loss, and occasionally odynophagia. For mid-esophageal tumors, potential airway involvement should be carefully assessed, as it may manifest as cough, hemoptysis, increased sputum production, recurrent pneumonias, voice changes, or be clinically silent. Additionally, ulcerated tumors may cause gastrointestinal bleeding, presenting with anemia-related symptoms such as fatigue and/or pallor [8].

Initial laboratory testing typically includes a complete blood count, comprehensive metabolic panel, and nutritional markers. These are routinely obtained to evaluate for anemia, nutritional status, and organ function. These parameters not only provide a baseline for monitoring but may also help predict perioperative risk and treatment tolerance.

Endoscopic evaluation plays a central role in both diagnosis and staging. Upper endoscopy allows for direct visualization and biopsy of the lesion [8–11]. During endoscopy, it is essential to document the proximal and distal extent of the tumor from the incisors, its relationship to the gastroesophageal junction, and its length and circumferential extent. Endoscopic ultrasound (EUS) provides high-resolution imaging of the esophageal wall layers and adjacent lymph nodes, enabling more precise T and N staging. EUS-guided fine-needle aspiration of suspicious lymph nodes enables cytologic confirmation, correlates with PET-CT findings, and improves overall staging accuracy.

The detection of early or flat mucosal lesions may be missed using standard white-light imaging. Thus, advanced endoscopic techniques are routinely used. These include chromoendoscopy using Lugol's iodine or acetic acid, filtered light to enhance visualization of mucosal and vascular patterns, or confocal laser endomicroscopy for real-time in vivo histologic assessment. Among these, filtered light has shown value in identifying high-grade dysplasia and superficial tumors, making it especially useful in early stage disease surveillance and diagnosis [8, 12–15].

Cross-sectional imaging of the chest, abdomen, and pelvis with high-resolution, contrast-enhanced computed tomography (CT) is routinely performed to evaluate for locoregional extension and distant spread [8]. PET-CT is recommended for staging intermediate or higher stage tumors, as it is more sensitive than CT alone for detecting distant metastases, and areas of FDG-avid regional disease can be targeted for radiation therapy. Magnetic resonance imaging may provide additional information in select cases—particularly for suspected metastases to the liver, brain, adrenal glands, or bone.

For tumors located in the upper or mid-esophagus, fiberoptic bronchoscopy should be performed to assess for tracheal or bronchial invasion [15], which may render a tumor unresectable and therefore significantly impact treatment strategy. Airway involvement correlates with increased morbidity and decreased survival and may be the decisive factor in determining operability in a subset of patients [8, 16].

The diagnostic workup for ESCC requires a comprehensive, multidisciplinary approach, integrating clinical assessment, advanced imaging (CT, PET-CT), and endoscopic staging (including EUS and, when indicated, bronchoscopy). This integrated strategy ensures accurate staging and enables tailored, evidence-based management for patients with ESCC.

$$TPS = \frac{Number\ of\ PD-L1-staining\ tumor\ cells}{Total\ number\ of\ viable\ tumor\ cells} \text{x}100$$

$$CPS = \frac{Number\ of\ PD-L1-staining\ tumor\ cells, lymphocytes, and\ macrophages}{Total\ number\ of\ viable\ tumor\ cells} \text{x}100$$

Fig. 24.1 TPS and CPS formula. TPS: Tumor proportion score; CPS: Combined positive score

24.3 Molecular Evaluation

In the diagnosis and management of ESCC, the most clinically relevant molecular markers with therapeutic and prognostic implications are PD-L1 expression and microsatellite instability (MSI). These biomarkers predict the effectiveness of immunotherapy and provide overall prognosis [17–19]. Approximately 54% of ESCC patients exhibit positive PD-L1 expression, 57% demonstrate high tumor mutational burden, and 1% show microsatellite instability [17]. High PD-L1 expression is associated with improved prognosis and higher potential benefit from immune checkpoint inhibitors [20], while MSI-high status, though rare in ESCC, predicts favorable response to combined immunotherapy and potentially poor response to CXRT [17, 21, 22].

PD-L1 expression is quantified using two scoring systems: the Tumor Proportion Score (TPS) and the Combined Positive Score (CPS), which incorporate tumor and immune cell staining (Fig. 24.1). A CPS ≥10 or TPS ≥1% has been utilized as the threshold for selecting patients who would derive the greatest benefit from immunotherapy in combination with chemotherapy, in accordance with American Society of Clinical Oncology guidelines [18].

HER2 gene amplification is found to be present in 10% by immunohistochemistry and 8.6% positive in follow up in-situ hybridization techniques [23]. However, unlike in adenocarcinoma, the clinical significance of HER2 expression in ESCC remains unclear due to a lack of robust, high-quality evidence.

In summary, CPS is a validated, clinically actionable biomarker for guiding immunotherapy in ESCC. As our understanding of tumor biology evolves, molecular profiling is increasingly becoming a routine component of personalized ESCC care.

24.4 Early Disease Management

Early stage ESCC, including Tis to T1b lesions, may be amenable to endoscopic therapy, which can serve both diagnostic staging and curative potential. T1a tumors, confined to the mucosa, are subclassified into m1 (epithelium), m2 (lamina propria), and m3 (muscularis mucosae). T1b tumors, which invade the submucosa, are further stratified based on depth: sm1 (<500 μm), sm2 (500–1000 μm), and sm3 (>1000 μm).

Endoscopic ultrasound (EUS), typically performed alongside esophagogastroduodenoscopy (EGD), is employed to assess depth of invasion and lymph node involvement. EUS is the most sensitive modality for locoregional staging of early ESCC, with pooled sensitivity and specificity of 84% and 91%, respectively, for T1a disease, and 83% and 89%, respectively, for T1b disease. Overall T-staging accuracy of 79% [11]. However, EUS has limitations in distinguishing early stage lesions, particularly T1a from T1b. Studies indicate that 38% of clinical T1b and 76% of clinical T2 tumors may be over-staged, potentially leading to overtreatment [24, 25]. Importantly, attempting endoscopic resection first does not preclude more aggressive therapy. Patients with unfavorable final pathology (e.g., deeper invasion or lymphovascular invasion (LVI)) can still proceed to multimodality treatment including esophagectomy, chemoradiation, or both, preserving the principle of oncologic safety while minimizing overtreatment.

For EUS mucosal and superficial submucosal tumors, diagnostic endoscopic resection is the preferred initial strategy. Endoscopic mucosal resection (EMR) is generally suitable for lesions <15 mm that are well-demarcated and non-ulcerated [26, 27]. On the other hand, EMR for larger lesions often results in piecemeal resection, limiting the ability to assess deep (vertical) and lateral margins. Endoscopic submucosal dissection (ESD) enables en bloc resection regardless of lesion size, offering superior histologic assessment of depth, margins, and LVI—but requires longer procedural time and steeper learning curve [26, 27].

Post-resection histopathologic features including depth of invasion, LVI, tumor grade, and lesion length, guide subsequent management [28]. This is particularly relevant in ESCC T1b tumors, where the risk of nodal metastasis is significantly higher than in similar depth tumors with adenocarcinoma histology. For T1a lesions, the risk of lymph node metastasis is <1% for m1–m2 disease, but increases to approximately 8% for m3, likely due to a higher incidence of LVI [29]. One study reported a 5-year metastasis rate of 46.7% in mucosal ESCC with LVI, compared to just 0.7% in those without [29].

Endoscopic treatment is now recognized as the cornerstone of therapy for appropriately selected early stage ESCC, particularly for lesions limited to m1 and m2 layers. Selected m3 tumors may also be managed endoscopically in highly selected patients, with close multidisciplinary evaluation (Fig. 24.2). Both EMR and ESD play integral roles, and their selection should be guided by lesion characteristics, technical expertise, and institutional resources.

Data from high-volume centers, particularly in Japan, demonstrate excellent results with ESD, including en bloc resection rates >95% [30, 31], curative resection rates of 100% [29], and 5-year disease-specific survival exceeding 90% for superficial ESCC [29, 31, 32]. EMR, while more limited, also provides favorable outcomes with low complication rates in small, noninvasive lesions. Increasingly, Western studies have mirrored these findings [28, 33], affirming the safety and efficacy of endoscopic therapy in well-resourced healthcare systems.

In the North American experience, endoscopic resection offers a minimally invasive, organ-preserving alternative to esophagectomy for early ESCC. With proper patient selection, it achieves diagnostic accuracy, curative intent, and excellent long-term outcomes, making it a central component of contemporary ESCC treatment algorithms.

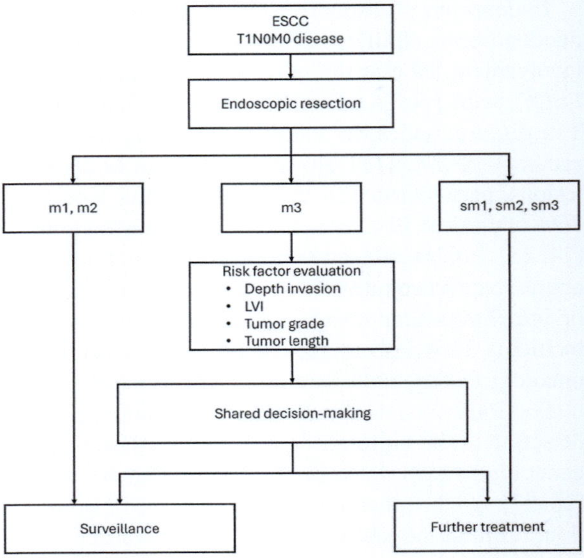

Fig. 24.2 Treatment algorithm for ESCC early stage T1N0M0 disease. ESCC: Esophageal squamous cell carcinoma; T1a tumors are further classified into m1 (epithelium), m2 (lamina propria), and m3 (muscularis mucosae). T1b tumors are further classified into sm1 (<500 μm), sm2 (500–1000 μm), and sm3 (>1000 μm)

24.5 Locoregionally Advanced Disease

Patients with locoregionally advanced ESCC are routinely discussed in a multidisciplinary tumor board setting, where treatment strategies are tailored based on tumor characteristics, patient comorbidities, surgical candidacy, and patient preferences. The CROSS trial [34, 35] remains the cornerstone of current treatment algorithms, demonstrating a 49% pathologic complete response (pCR) rate for ESCC using concurrent chemoradiation with 41.4 Gy and carboplatin/paclitaxel, establishing trimodality therapy as the standard of care. This result also supports the use of bimodality therapy (chemoradiation alone) in patients who are elderly or medically frail, offering a potentially curative, organ-sparing alternative to trimodality therapy.

Two randomized controlled trials have directly compared bimodality and trimodality therapy in ESCC. The Stahl trial [36] randomized patients to chemoradiation followed by surgery versus definitive chemoradiation. Two-year survival rates were 39.9% (95% CI: 29.4–50.4%) in the surgical group versus 35.4% (95% CI: 25.2–45.6%) for the definitive chemoradiation group. Although the authors concluded equivalence, interpretation is limited by several trial design limitations, including a high cross-over rate, a perioperative mortality rate of 11%, and statistical irregularities [37, 38].

In modern North American practice, the standard approach typically begins with neoadjuvant chemoradiation to 50.4 Gy, based on the INT-0123 trial, which showed no survival benefit or local control from dose escalation beyond this threshold [39]. For patients with residual disease following chemoradiation, esophagectomy is strongly recommended if they remain a surgical candidate. However, management of patients who achieve clinical complete response remains controversial. The FFCD 9102 trial [40] attempted to address this question. Patients who achieved cCR after chemoradiation (46 Gy or split-course 15 + 22 Gy) were randomized to undergo either surgery or continued chemoradiation. Two-year survival was 34% in the surgery arm and 40% in the chemoradiation arm (HR 0.90, $P = 0.44$). However, several shortcomings limit the trial's generalizability: the perioperative mortality rate was 9%, compared to 2% in CROSS [35] and just 0.5% in the NEOCRTEC5010 trial [41]. Additionally, the R0 resection rate in FFCD was only 75%, far below the 92% in CROSS and 98% in NEOCRTEC, likely contributing to a 33.6% locoregional recurrence rate in the surgical arm and increased mortality.

Our institutional experience [42] aligns more closely with CROSS and NEOCRTEC (Fig. 24.3) supporting the principle that, in surgically fit patients, trimodality therapy offers the best chance for locoregional disease control and long-term survival.

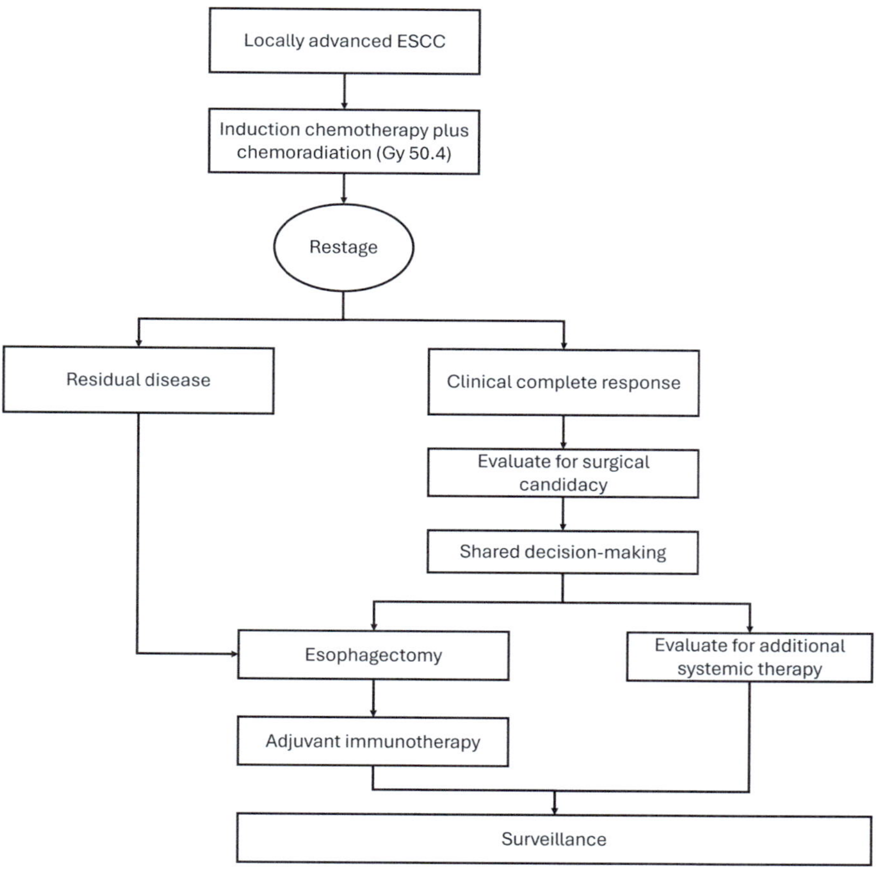

Fig. 24.3 Treatment algorithm for locoregionally advanced ESCC. ESCC: Esophageal squamous cell carcinoma

24.6 Salvage Esophagectomy

In the Western experience with esophageal adenocarcinoma (EAC), selective salvage esophagectomy following failure of definitive chemoradiation has demonstrated acceptable survival and complication rates [43, 44]. However, this strategy does not directly translate to ESCC. Our institutional data show that patients with ESCC undergoing salvage esophagectomy face significantly higher morbidity and worse overall survival (OS) [45].

In our experience, 71.4% of salvage patients experience major morbidity, including major pulmonary complications reported in 40% of cases, major cardiovascular events in 48.6%, anastomotic leak rates between 11% and 25%, and 30-day mortality rate of 8.6% [45]. These data support a highly selective approach to salvage esophagectomy in ESCC patients who have failed chemoradiation, limited to patients with excellent performance status and a clear benefit-risk profile.

Moreover, tumor characteristics strongly influence outcomes in ESCC, specifically tumor location and tumor biology. In our analysis, tumors located in the upper or mid-esophagus (HR: 2.04, $P = 0.024$) and longer tumor length (HR: 1.18, $P = 0.046$) were associated with worse survival [42], Local recurrences in these regions after definitive chemoradiation pose substantial technical challenges and are associated with increased postoperative morbidity and mortality. While neoadjuvant chemoradiation can elicit excellent tumor responses and offers a reasonable chance of achieving a pathologic complete response, for surgically fit patients with disease in close proximity to or abutting the airway, we tend to favor induction chemotherapy with docetaxel, cisplatin, and 5-fluorouracil (DCF) followed by surgery, as outlined in the JCOG1109 protocol [46]. This approach provides the potential for more definitive local control once they undergo surgical resection without the risk associated with radiation. In appropriately selected individuals, it should be pursued within a shared decision-making framework that considers oncologic benefit, technical feasibility, and patient preference.

24.7 Surgical Principles

The primary objective of surgical resection in ESCC is to achieve an R0 resection and perform an adequate lymphadenectomy, ensuring both locoregional disease control and accurate pathological staging. Oncologic resection requires sufficient proximal and distal margins, along with comprehensive removal of regional lymphatic tissue. While patterns of lymph node metastasis are influenced by factors such as tumor location, depth of invasion, histologic grade, and tumor biology, the precise distribution of lymphatic spread in ESCC remains an ongoing area of study. The TIGER study [NCT03222895] [47] is currently investigating these patterns to provide evidence-based recommendations on the optimal extent of lymphadenectomy.

Historically, three-field lymphadenectomy has been associated with improved locoregional control but carries a higher risk of recurrent laryngeal nerve injury [48, 49]. However, randomized trials have not shown a clear survival advantage with routine three-field dissection [50], leading to variation in clinical practice. In our practice, where most ESCC patients undergo neoadjuvant chemoradiation, we routinely perform a two-field lymphadenectomy. Selective dissection of high paratracheal and cervical nodes is added when there is clinical evidence of nodal involvement, such as FDG-avid nodes on PET/CT or suspicious findings on EUS. This approach balances the goal of achieving complete oncologic resection with minimizing the risk of recurrent laryngeal nerve injury—an especially important consideration in the higher-BMI patient population commonly seen in North America.

In the abdominal field, a D2 lymphadenectomy is routinely performed, involving en bloc removal of lymph nodes along the lesser curvature, paracardial region, celiac axis, splenic artery, left gastric artery, and common hepatic artery. Additionally, all peri-esophageal lymphatic tissue from the hiatus to the proximal extent of the esophageal dissection is resected en bloc to optimize both locoregional clearance and staging accuracy.

24.8 Minimally Invasive Approach

The advent of minimally invasive esophagectomy (MIE) has introduced a technically advanced approach that allows adherence to the same oncologic principles while reducing perioperative morbidity. MIE—whether performed as totally laparoscopic/thoracoscopic, robot-assisted, or hybrid techniques—is safe and feasible in appropriately selected patients [51–53]. In a randomized controlled trial, hybrid MIE was associated with significantly lower postoperative complication rates, particularly Clavien-Dindo grade $\geq$ II events and pulmonary complications, compared to open transthoracic esophagectomy, with no compromise in long-term outcomes such as OS or DFS (disease-free survival) [52].

A critical consideration in the adoption of MIE is the learning curve associated with achieving technical proficiency and consistent outcomes. Studies suggest that 30 to 100 cases may be needed to reach optimal performance, depending on the surgeon's experience and the institutional case volume [54–56]. Notably, more efficient learning and improved outcomes have been documented in high-volume centers (>50 esophagectomies/year). These findings support the ongoing centralization of esophageal surgery in North America, where specialized, high-volume institutions provide access to multidisciplinary expertise, advanced perioperative care, and surgical proficiency—resulting in improved clinical outcomes for patients undergoing esophagectomy.

24.9 Adjuvant Therapy

Historically, adjuvant systemic therapy is a consideration only for patients with residual disease. Adjuvant chemoradiation was reserved for those with R1 or R2 resection who did not receive chemoradiation preoperatively, or for those patients who were presumed to have early disease but were found to have significant regional disease burden on surgical pathology. Recently, the results of the CheckMate-577 demonstrated survival benefit in EGJ cancer treated with neoadjuvant chemoradiotherapy followed by surgical resection, with median DFS of 22.4 months (95% CI: 16.6–34.0) compared to 11.0 months in placebo group [57]. Subgroup analysis suggested greater benefit in patients with CPS >5, and while both histologic subtypes benefited, ESCC appeared to derive greater advantage (29.7 vs. 11 months, HR: 0.61; 95% CI: 0.42–0.88). Thus, adjuvant nivolumab is now the preferred treatment for ESCC patients who have received preoperative chemoradiation followed by surgery with R0 resection who had residual disease at time of surgery [58].

24.10 Surveillance Strategy

Surveillance strategies for ESCC are guided by the NCCN Clinical Practice Guidelines [58] and are tailored based on disease stage, treatment modality, and tumor biology. For patients with early stage disease (TisN0, T1aN0) who have undergone endoscopic resection (EMR or ESD), the recommended surveillance protocol includes endoscopy every 3 months during the first year, every 6 months during the second year, and then annually thereafter indefinitely. For patients who have undergone esophagectomy for early stage disease, routine endoscopic surveillance is not recommended unless the patient develops symptoms; imaging is also not routinely performed in asymptomatic individuals.

For patients with T1bN0 disease, the surveillance protocol involves endoscopy every 3 months in the first year, every 4–6 months in the second year, and then annually thereafter. In cases where recurrent or residual disease is suspected, EUS may be performed concurrently to evaluate depth of involvement and regional nodal disease. In addition, CT scans of the chest, abdomen, and pelvis with intravenous contrast are typically performed every 6 months for the first 2 years, and then continued up to 5 years, provided there are no contraindications.

In patients with locoregionally advanced disease treated with definitive chemoradiotherapy, surveillance involves clinical evaluation—including history, physical examination, and imaging with CT (neck, chest, abdomen ± pelvis) or PET/CT—every 3–6 months for the first 2 years, then every 6–12 months for up to 5 years, and annually thereafter. For those treated with neoadjuvant chemoradiation followed by esophagectomy, a similar surveillance schedule is followed, although it is often tailored based on pathological response, symptom burden, and risk of recurrence. Routine use of endoscopy is not universally recommended for asymptomatic patients after surgery unless clinically indicated.

Emerging data support the potential role of circulating tumor DNA (ctDNA) as a noninvasive biomarker in surveillance. The detection of mutations and altered DNA shed by carcinoma into the circulatory system could be detected in the form of a "liquid biopsy". The presence of ctDNA in patients with ESCC has been associated with worse OS and PFS [59] and its detection may be particularly useful in cases of equivocal imaging findings or uncertain residual disease, as well as for patients who are unable to undergo traditional methods of evaluation and biopsy. Multiple studies have shown ctDNA to be predictive of response to therapy [60, 61] as well as recurrence [60, 62]. Making it a promising tool for future surveillance strategies. The ongoing NEOCRTEC2401 (NCT06561178) trial is currently evaluating the correlation between ctDNA and disease recurrence in ESCC patients who underwent neoadjuvant chemoradiation followed by surgery without achieving a pathologic complete response.

Beyond oncologic monitoring, surveillance should also address survivorship care, including evaluation of nutritional status, promotion of smoking and alcohol cessation, and management of treatment-related complications such as anastomotic strictures, reflux, or delayed gastric emptying. Ultimately, surveillance should be individualized, based on tumor characteristics, treatment course, patient comorbidities, and input from a multidisciplinary care team.

24.11 Metastatic Disease

In metastatic ESCC, PD-L1 testing and MSI status should be established, and molecular profiling should be considered to guide systemic therapy [58].

The current standard management of metastatic ESCC is first-line systemic therapy with a platinum/fluoropyrimidine doublet (e.g., cisplatin or oxaliplatin plus 5-fluorouracil or capecitabine) in combination with a PD-1 immune checkpoint inhibitor. Historically, chemotherapy alone provided limited benefit, with median OS of less than 1 year. The addition of immunotherapy has significantly improved outcomes. The pivotal CheckMate 648 trial demonstrated that nivolumab plus chemotherapy (13.2 vs. 10.7 months, $P = 0.002$), or nivolumab plus ipilimumab (12.7 vs. 10.7 months, $P = 0.01$), improved OS compared to chemotherapy alone in previously untreated metastatic ESCC [63]. Treatment benefit from nivolumab plus chemotherapy or nivolumab plus ipilimumab was significantly higher in those with TPS > 1%.

Similarly, the KEYNOTE-590 [64] and ESCORT-1st [65] trials established the benefit of pembrolizumab or camrelizumab, respectively, in combination with chemotherapy as first-line therapy, though camrelizumab has not yet received FDA (Food and Drug Administration) approval. Dual checkpoint inhibition (nivolumab plus ipilimumab) is an alternative first-line option for patients who are not candidates for chemotherapy or prefer a chemotherapy-free regimen, as supported by CheckMate 648. The choice between immunochemotherapy and dual immunotherapy is influenced by patient comorbidities, preferences, and regulatory approvals [63].

PD-L1 expression, measured by TPS or combined positive score CPS, influences treatment selection and regulatory approval. In the United States, immunotherapy is approved for all-comers regardless of PD-L1 status, but the magnitude of benefit is greater in patients with higher PD-L1 expression (TPS ≥1% or CPS ≥10). In Europe and Asia, approvals are more restrictive, often requiring PD-L1 positivity. Currently, there are many ongoing trials in Asia evaluating the use of neoadjuvant immunotherapy as part of the treatment algorithm in resectable locoregionally advanced ESCC and in the metastatic setting (Table 24.1). The results of these trials will be informative for the role of immunotherapy in the treatment of ESCC.

After progression on first-line immunochemotherapy, second-line options include single-agent immunotherapy (nivolumab or pembrolizumab, depending on prior exposure and PD-L1 status) or standard chemotherapy with taxanes or irinotecan [66]. The benefit of immunotherapy rechallenge after progression on first-line immunochemotherapy is unclear, and standard chemotherapy remains the preferred option in this setting [67].

Targeted therapies have not demonstrated clinical benefit in ESCC and are not standard of care. Phase 3 trials of anti-*EGFR* agents gefitinib [68] and panitumumab [69] have been negative. To date, no known trials of Anti-*HER2* agents against ESCC have been completed and published to our knowledge. For *NTRK* fusion-positive tumors, entrectinib, larotrectinib, or repotrectinib may be useful in certain settings [57].

Table 24.1 Select active phase III ESCC trials

Trial name (NCT #)	Population	Comparison arms	Primary outcome	Locations
JCOG1904 (ARMADILLO) (jRCTs031200067)	T1bN0Mo ESCC with residual disease after chemoradiation and will undergo salvage endoscopic resection	Experimental: Chemoradiation without additional prophylactic irradiation Comparator: Chemoradiation without additional prophylactic irradiation	Progression-free survival	Japan
JCOG2013 (MODERN 3) (jRCT1030220248)	Non-T4 upper and mid-thoracic esophageal cancer underwent esophagectomy	Experimental: Esophagectomy with prophylactic supraclavicular node dissection Comparator: Esophagectomy without prophylactic supraclavicular node dissection	Overall survival	Japan
DISCOVER study (jRCT1071240001)	Esophageal cancer after esophagectomy	Observational	Predicted recurrence-free positive diagnostic rate in postoperative 28-day ctDNA-negative cases	Japan
ESO-Shanghai 26 (NCT06676449)	Locoregionally advanced ESCC	Experimental: PD-1 inhibitor + chemotherapy + TDLN-sparing radiotherapy and chemotherapy Comparator: Chemotherapy + TDLN-sparing radiotherapy	1. Progression-free survival for patients with TDLN V15 $\leq 50\%$ 2. Progression-free survival for all patients	China

(continued)

Table 24.1 (continued)

Trial name (NCT #)	Population	Comparison arms	Primary outcome	Locations
ESO-Shanghai 27 (NCT06964568)	Locoregionally advanced ESCC	Experimental 1: TDLN-sparing radiotherapy + PD-1 inhibitor maintenance therapy Experimental 2: TDLN-sparing radiotherapy and surveillance Experimental 3: Unlimited radiotherapy and PD-1 inhibitor maintenance Comparator: Unlimited radiotherapy and surveillance	1. Progression-free survival for TDLN-sparing radiotherapy followed by PD-1 inhibitor maintenance therapy vs TDLN-sparing radiotherapy followed by surveillance 2. Progression-free survival for PD-1 inhibitor maintenance therapy vs. All patients with surveillance	China
NEOCRTEC2101 (NCT05357846)	Resectable locoregionally advanced ESCC	Experimental: Neoadjuvant chemoradiotherapy + sintilimab Comparator: Neoadjuvant chemoradiotherapy	Overall survival	China
A Study of Neoadjuvant Therapy for the Treatment of Patients With Locoregionally Advanced Esophageal Squamous Cell Carcinoma (NCT06354530)	Resectable locoregionally advanced ESCC	Experimental 1: Neoadjuvant camrelizumab + chemotherapy + anlotinib Experimental 2: Neoadjuvant camrelizumab + concurrent chemoradiotherapy	1. Pathologic complete response 2. Major pathological response	China
iCROSS (NCT04973306)	Resectable locoregionally advanced ESCC	Experimental: Neoadjuvant chemoradiotherapy + tislelizumab followed by esophagectomy Comparator: Neoadjuvant chemoradiotherapy followed by esophagectomy	1. Pathologic complete response 2. Overall survival	China

NICE 2 (NCT05043688)	Resectable locoregionally advanced ESCC	Experimental: 1. Neoadjuvant camrelizumab + chemotherapy 2. Camrelizumab + chemoradiotherapy Comparator: Neoadjuvant chemoradiotherapy	1. Event-free survival (tumor progression/recurrence/death)	China
Local Therapy for Oligometastatic ESCC Patients Treated with PD-1 Inhibitor (NCT06190782)	Oligometastatic ESCC	Experimental: PD-1 inhibitor +/− chemotherapy combined with local therapy Comparator: PD-1 inhibitor +/− chemotherapy alone	Progression-free survival	China
IDeate-Esophageal01 (NCT06644781)	Unresectable or Metastatic ESCC who progressed following treatment	Experimental: Ifinatamab + deroxtecan Comparator: Chemotherapy	Overall survival	USA, Japan, South Korea, Taiwan
Study of Larotinib in unresectable advanced or recurrent esophageal cancer (NCT04415853)	Unresectable locoregionally advanced or metastatic ESCC with EGFR overexpression	Experimental: larotinib Comparator: Irinotecan/ Tegafur	Overall survival	China

ESCC esophageal squamous cell carcinoma, *TDLN* tumor draining lymph nodes-sparing

24.12 Quality of Life and Survivorship

The treatment of ESCC, whether via surgery or chemoradiation, carries significant implications for patients' long-term quality of life (QoL). Historically, the high morbidity and mortality associated with esophagectomy precluded meaningful analysis of postoperative quality of life, but with advances in surgical techniques, perioperative care, and the adoption of multimodal therapy, patient-reported outcomes have become increasingly central to treatment evaluation [70]. Esophagectomy, especially when performed with curative intent, remains a physically and psychologically demanding procedure with well-documented short- and long-term QoL consequences.

Immediately following esophagectomy, patients commonly experience sharp declines in physical, role, and social functioning. Symptoms such as fatigue, pain, dyspnea, reflux, diarrhea, and dysphagia often peak within the first 6 weeks to 3 months postoperatively. Although some degree of recovery in function occurs by 6–12 months, most patients do not return to their baseline QoL levels, and a proportion continue to experience persistent issues even 5–10 years after surgery [70, 71]. Long-term survivors may continue to face challenges such as altered eating patterns, weight loss, dumping syndrome, and psychological stress including anxiety, depression, and fear of recurrence. Notably, the development of lasting symptoms after esophagectomy (LASER symptoms) [72] such as pain in chest scars, low mood and reduced energy, additional heartburn, diarrhea unrelated to eating, and bloating/cramps after eating is now a validated model to assess for significant QoL impairments in post-esophagectomy patients [73].

MIE including robot-assisted have shown some QoL benefits over open procedures, particularly in reducing early postoperative pain and accelerating return to physical activity and social function at an earlier period of 4–6 weeks after surgery [74]. However, even with these approaches, symptoms like reflux and dysphagia may persist, and some studies suggest that differences in global QoL between MIE and open esophagectomy may diminish after the first year [75, 76].

In comparison, chemoradiation therapy, which may be used definitively or as part of a neoadjuvant regimen, also affects QoL, albeit in different domains. Patients undergoing CRT often report temporary declines in global health, fatigue, eating difficulties, and emotional well-being during treatment. However, evidence from the CROSS trial [34, 35] and subsequent studies suggests that these impairments often resolve posttreatment, and CRT does not appear to have lasting adverse effects on QoL when compared to surgery alone. Moreover, while CRT avoids the anatomical disruption of surgery, it may still lead to long-term swallowing difficulties and radiation-induced fibrosis in some cases.

Importantly, QoL is not only a reflection of physical symptoms but also serves as a predictor of survival [70, 71]. Poor preoperative or early postoperative QoL, particularly in domains such as fatigue, appetite loss, and physical functioning, has been associated with decreased long-term survival in multiple studies. This underscores the need for routine, validated QoL assessments—using tools like the EORTC QLQ-C30 and OES18—in both clinical trials and practice to identify patients at risk and to inform shared decision-making.

Overall, both esophagectomy and chemoradiation can offer curative treatment for ESCC, but at the cost of considerable and lasting impact on patients' quality of life. As survival continues to improve, the importance of addressing survivorship issues—nutritional support, physical rehabilitation, and psychosocial care—must become an integral part of the care continuum for ESCC patients.

24.13 Conclusion

ESCC remains a formidable malignancy with a complex clinical course requiring nuanced, multidisciplinary management. In North America, treatment has evolved to incorporate a highly individualized and stage-specific approach, emphasizing shared decision-making, tumor biology, and clinical context.

For early stage ESCC, endoscopic resection offers a curative, organ-preserving alternative in well-selected patients, while locoregionally advanced disease is best managed with trimodality therapy in appropriate surgically fit patients, as supported by landmark trials like CROSS. Salvage esophagectomy remains a high-risk but occasionally appropriate option for highly selected patients with residual or recurrent disease following definitive chemoradiation.

Surgical resection, particularly with minimally invasive techniques, must adhere to rigorous oncologic principles, including R0 resection and systematic lymphadenectomy. Advances in perioperative care, patient selection, and centralization of surgery have improved outcomes. In addition, adjuvant immunotherapy now offers additional survival benefit in patients with residual disease postsurgery.

For metastatic disease, the integration of PD-1 checkpoint inhibitors into front-line regimens has revolutionized treatment. Immunotherapy, either alone or in combination with chemotherapy, has become the new standard, though long-term disease control remains a clinical challenge.

Surveillance protocols, including emerging tools like ctDNA, aim to detect recurrence early while addressing broader survivorship needs such as nutrition, function, and psychological well-being. Given the lasting impact of ESCC treatment on quality of life, patient-reported outcomes should be central to therapeutic decisions, not ancillary.

Looking forward, the future of ESCC care lies not only in extending survival, but in improving the quality of that survival—through precision therapies, early detection, holistic survivorship care, and patient shared decision-making embedded within a robust multidisciplinary framework.

References

1. Rodriguez GM, DePuy D, Aljehani M, et al. Trends in epidemiology of esophageal cancer in the US, 1975-2018. JAMA Netw Open. 2023;6(8):e2329497.
2. Rustgi AK, El-Serag HB. Esophageal carcinoma. N Engl J Med. 2014;371(26):2499–509.
3. Sheikh M, Roshandel G, McCormack V, et al. Current status and future prospects for esophageal cancer. Cancers (Basel). 2023;15(3):765.

4. Shah MA, Kennedy EB, Catenacci DV, et al. Treatment of locally advanced esophageal carcinoma: ASCO guideline. J Clin Oncol. 2020;38(23):2677–94.
5. Waters JK, Reznik SI. Update on management of squamous cell esophageal cancer. Curr Oncol Rep. 2022;24(3):375–85.
6. Lordick F, Mariette C, Haustermans K, et al. Oesophageal cancer: ESMO Clinical Practice Guidelines for diagnosis, treatment and follow-up. Ann Oncol. 2016;27(suppl 5):v50–7.
7. Codipilly DC, Wang KK. Squamous cell carcinoma of the esophagus. Gastroenterol Clin N Am. 2022;51(3):457–84.
8. Varghese TK Jr, Hofstetter WL, Rizk NP, et al. The Society of Thoracic Surgeons guidelines on the diagnosis and staging of patients with esophageal cancer. Ann Thorac Surg. 2013;96(1):346–56.
9. DaVee T, Ajani JA, Lee JH. Is endoscopic ultrasound examination necessary in the management of esophageal cancer? World J Gastroenterol. 2017;23(5):751–62.
10. Wang KK, Wongkeesong M, Buttar NS, et al. American Gastroenterological Association medical position statement: role of the gastroenterologist in the management of esophageal carcinoma. Gastroenterology. 2005;128(5):1468–70.
11. Luo LN, He LJ, Gao XY, et al. Endoscopic ultrasound for preoperative esophageal squamous cell carcinoma: a meta-analysis. PLoS One. 2016;11(7):e0158373.
12. Muto M, Minashi K, Yano T, et al. Early detection of superficial squamous cell carcinoma in the head and neck region and esophagus by narrow band imaging: a multicenter randomized controlled trial. J Clin Oncol. 2010;28(9):1566–72.
13. Uedo N, Fujishiro M, Goda K, et al. Role of narrow band imaging for diagnosis of early-stage esophagogastric cancer: current consensus of experienced endoscopists in Asia-Pacific region. Dig Endosc. 2011;23(Suppl 1):58–71.
14. Kumagai Y, Inoue H, Nagai K, et al. Magnifying endoscopy, stereoscopic microscopy, and the microvascular architecture of superficial esophageal carcinoma. Endoscopy. 2002;34:369–75.
15. Riedel M, Hauck RW, Stein HJ, Mounyam L, Schulz C, Schömig A, Siewert JR. Preoperative bronchoscopic assessment of airway invasion by esophageal cancer: a prospective study. Chest. 1998;113(3):687–95. https://doi.org/10.1378/chest.113.3.687. PMID: 9515844.
16. Old OJ, Isabelle M, Barr H. Staging early esophageal cancer. Adv Exp Med Biol. 2016;908:161–81.
17. Li S, Yu Y, Xu Y, Zhou Y, Huang J, Jia J. Clinicopathological characteristics and the relationship of PD-L1 status, tumor mutation burden, and microsatellite instability in patients with esophageal carcinoma. BMC Cancer. 2025;25(1):576.
18. Shah MA, Kennedy EB, Alarcon-Rozas AE, et al. Immunotherapy and targeted therapy for advanced gastroesophageal cancer: ASCO guideline. J Clin Oncol. 2023;41(7):1470–91.
19. Zhou N, Hofstetter WL. Prognostic and therapeutic molecular markers in the clinical management of esophageal cancer. Expert Rev Mol Diagn. 2020;20(4):401–11.
20. Yoon HH, Jin Z, Kour O, et al. Association of PD-L1 expression and other variables with benefit from immune checkpoint inhibition in advanced gastroesophageal cancer: systematic review and meta-analysis of 17 phase 3 randomized clinical trials. JAMA Oncol. 2022;8(10):1456–65.
21. Petrelli F, Ghidini M, Ghidini A, Tomasello G. Outcomes following immune checkpoint inhibitor treatment of patients with microsatellite instability-high cancers: a systematic review and meta-analysis. JAMA Oncol. 2020;6(7):1068–71.
22. Marabelle A, Le DT, Ascierto PA, et al. Efficacy of pembrolizumab in patients with non-colorectal high microsatellite instability/mismatch repair-deficient cancer: results from the phase II KEYNOTE-158 study. J Clin Oncol. 2020;38(1):1–10.
23. Egebjerg K, Garbyal RS, Hasselby JP, et al. Prevalence of HER2 overexpression and amplification in squamous cell carcinoma of the esophagus: a systematic review and meta-analysis. Crit Rev Oncol Hematol. 2021;161:103339.
24. Dhupar R, Rice RD, Correa AM, et al. Endoscopic ultrasound estimates for tumor depth at the gastroesophageal junction are inaccurate: implications for the liberal use of endoscopic resection. Ann Thorac Surg. 2015;100(5):1812–6.

25. Akutsu Y, Kato K, Igaki H, et al. The prevalence of overall and initial lymph node metastases in clinical T1N0 thoracic esophageal cancer: from the results of JCOG0502, a prospective multicenter study. Ann Surg. 2016;264(6):1009–15.
26. ASGE Standards of Practice Committee, Al-Haddad MA, Elhanafi SE, Forbes N, et al. American Society for Gastrointestinal Endoscopy guideline on endoscopic submucosal dissection for the management of early esophageal and gastric cancers: methodology and review of evidence. Gastrointest Endosc. 2023;98(3):285–305.e38.
27. ASGE Standards of Practice Committee, Forbes N, Elhanafi SE, Al-Haddad MA, et al. American Society for Gastrointestinal Endoscopy guideline on endoscopic submucosal dissection for the management of early esophageal and gastric cancers: summary and recommendations. Gastrointest Endosc. 2023;98(3):271–84.
28. Nelson DB, Dhupar R, Katkhuda R, et al. Outcomes after endoscopic mucosal resection or esophagectomy for submucosal esophageal adenocarcinoma. J Thorac Cardiovasc Surg. 2018;156(1):406–13.
29. Yamashina T, Ishihara R, Nagai K, et al. Long-term outcome and metastatic risk after endoscopic resection of superficial esophageal squamous cell carcinoma. Am J Gastroenterol. 2013;108(4):544–51.
30. Ishihara R, Iishi H, Uedo N, et al. Comparison of EMR and endoscopic submucosal dissection for en bloc resection of early esophageal cancers in Japan. Gastrointest Endosc. 2008;68(6):1066–72.
31. Konishi H, Urabe Y, Nakamura T, et al. Long-term prognosis after endoscopic submucosal dissection for esophageal cancer in older adult patients. BMC Gastroenterol. 2024;24:164.
32. Nagami Y, Ominami M, Shiba M, et al. The five-year survival rate after endoscopic submucosal dissection for superficial esophageal squamous cell neoplasia. Dig Liver Dis. 2017;49(4):427–33.
33. McCarty JC, Parker RK, Vidri RJ, et al. A retrospective cohort study of endoscopic therapy and esophagectomy for stage 1 esophageal cancer: less is more. Gastrointest Endosc. 2020;92(1):23–30.
34. Van Hagen P, Hulshof MC, CROSS study group. Preoperative chemoradiotherapy for esophageal or junctional cancer. N Engl J Med. 2012;366(22):2074–84.
35. Shapiro J, van Lanschot JJB, CROSS Study Group. Neoadjuvant chemoradiotherapy plus surgery versus surgery alone for oesophageal or junctional cancer (CROSS): long-term results of a randomised controlled trial. Lancet Oncol. 2015 Sep;16(9):1090–8.
36. Stahl M, Stuschke M, Lehmann N, et al. Chemoradiation with and without surgery in patients with locally advanced squamous cell carcinoma of the esophagus. J Clin Oncol. 2005;23(10):2310–7. Erratum in: J Clin Oncol. 2006;24(3):531.
37. Zhou N, Lee KH, Pedroza C, et al. Bayesian post-hoc analysis of chemoradiation with and without surgery in patients with locally advanced squamous cell carcinoma of the esophagus. J Thorac Cardiovasc Surg. 2022;164(3):688–693.e1.
38. Ruhstaller T, Mueller A, Koeberle D, et al. Is there really enough evidence to abandon surgery after radiation chemotherapy in esophageal cancer? J Clin Oncol. 2005;23:8547–8.
39. Minsky BD, Pajak TF. INT 0123 (Radiation Therapy Oncology Group 94-05) phase III trial of combined-modality therapy for esophageal cancer: high-dose versus standard-dose radiation therapy. J Clin Oncol. 2002;20(5):1167–74.
40. Bedenne L, Michel P, Bouché O. Chemoradiation followed by surgery compared with chemoradiation alone in squamous cancer of the esophagus: FFCD 9102. J Clin Oncol. 2007;25(10):1160–8.
41. Yang H, Liu H, Chen Y, et al. (NEOCRTEC5010): a phase III multicenter, randomized, open-label clinical trial. J Clin Oncol. 2018;36(27):2796–803.
42. Zhou N, Mitchell KG, Corsini EM, et al. Analysis of trimodal and bimodal therapy in a selective-surgery paradigm for locally advanced oesophageal squamous cell carcinoma. Br J Surg. 2021;108(10):1207–15.

43. Swisher SG, Moughan J, Komaki RU, et al. Final results of NRG oncology RTOG 0246: an organ-preserving selective resection strategy in esophageal cancer patients treated with definitive chemoradiation. J Thorac Oncol. 2017;12(2):368–74.
44. Marks JL, Hofstetter W, Correa AM, et al. Salvage esophagectomy after failed definitive chemoradiation for esophageal adenocarcinoma. Ann Thorac Surg. 2012;94(4):1126–32.
45. Mitchell KG, Nelson DB, Corsini EM, et al. Morbidity following salvage esophagectomy for squamous cell carcinoma: the MD Anderson experience. Dis Esophagus. 2020;33(3):doz067.
46. Kato K, Machida R, Ito Y, et al. Doublet chemotherapy, triplet chemotherapy, or doublet chemotherapy combined with radiotherapy as neoadjuvant treatment for locally advanced oesophageal cancer (JCOG1109 NExT): a randomised, controlled, open-label, phase 3 trial. Lancet. 2024;404(10447):55–66.
47. Hagens ERC, van Berge Henegouwen MI, van Sandick JW, et al. Distribution of lymph node metastases in esophageal carcinoma [TIGER study]: study protocol of a multinational observational study. BMC Cancer. 2019;19(1):662.
48. Orringer MB, Marshall B, Iannettoni MD. Transhiatal esophagectomy: clinical experience and refinements. Ann Surg. 1999;230(3):392.
49. Altorki N, Kent M, Ferrara C, et al. Three-field lymph node dissection for squamous cell and adenocarcinoma of the esophagus. Ann Surg. 2002;236(2):177–83.
50. Nishihira T, Hirayama K, Mori S. A prospective randomized trial of extended cervical and superior mediastinal lymphadenectomy for carcinoma of the thoracic esophagus. Am J Surg. 1998;175(1):47–51.
51. Luketich JD, Pennathur A, Franchetti Y, et al. Minimally invasive esophagectomy: results of a prospective phase II multicenter trial-the eastern cooperative oncology group (E2202) study. Ann Surg. 2015;261(4):702–7.
52. Mariette C, Markar SR, Fédération de Recherche en Chirurgie (FRENCH) and French Eso-Gastric Tumors (FREGAT) Working Group. Hybrid minimally invasive esophagectomy for esophageal cancer. N Engl J Med. 2019;380(2):152–62.
53. Müller-Stich BP, Probst P, Nienhüser H, et al. Meta-analysis of randomized controlled trials and individual patient data comparing minimally invasive with open oesophagectomy for cancer. Br J Surg. 2021;108(9):1026–33.
54. Prasad P, Wallace L, Navidi M, et al. Learning curves in minimally invasive esophagectomy: a systematic review and evaluation of benchmarking parameters. Surgery. 2022;171(5):1247–56.
55. Claassen L, Hannink G, Esophagectomy Learning Curve Collaborative Group. Learning curves of Ivor Lewis totally minimally invasive esophagectomy by hospital and surgeon characteristics: a retrospective multinational cohort study. Ann Surg. 2022;275(5):911–8.
56. Helminen O, Kauppila JH, Saviaro H, et al. Minimally invasive esophagectomy learning curves with different types of background experience. J Thorac Dis. 2021;13(11):6261–71.
57. Kelly RJ, Ajani JA, CheckMate 577 Investigators. Adjuvant nivolumab in resected esophageal or gastroesophageal junction cancer. N Engl J Med. 2021;384(13):1191–203. Erratum in: N Engl J Med. 2023;388(7):672.
58. Ajani JA, D'Amico TA, Bentrem DJ, et al. Esophageal and esophagogastric junction cancers, version 3.2025, NCCN clinical practice guidelines in oncology. JNCCN; 2025.
59. Ng HY, Ko JMY, Lam KO, et al. Circulating tumor DNA dynamics as prognostic markers in locally advanced and metastatic esophageal squamous cell carcinoma. JAMA Surg. 2023;158(11):1141–50.
60. Morimoto Y, Matsuda S, Kawakubo H, et al. Tumor burden monitoring with circulating tumor DNA during treatment in patients with esophageal squamous cell carcinoma. Ann Surg Oncol. 2023;30(6):3747–56.
61. Jia R, Zhao CH, Li PS, et al. Post-radiation circulating tumor DNA as a prognostic factor in locally advanced esophageal squamous cell carcinoma. Oncol Lett. 2021;21(1):68.
62. Wang X, Yu N, Cheng G, et al. Prognostic value of circulating tumour DNA during post-radiotherapy surveillance in locally advanced esophageal squamous cell carcinoma. Clin Trans Med. 2022;12(11):e1116.

63. Doki Y, Ajani JA, Kato K, et al. Nivolumab combination therapy in advanced esophageal squamous-cell carcinoma. N Engl J Med. 2022;386(5):449–62.
64. Sun JM, Shen L, Shah MA, et al. KEYNOTE-590 Investigators. Pembrolizumab plus chemotherapy versus chemotherapy alone for first-line treatment of advanced oesophageal cancer (KEYNOTE-590): a randomised, placebo-controlled, phase 3 study. Lancet. 2021;398(10302):759–71.
65. Luo H, Lu J, Bai Y, et al. ESCORT-1st Investigators. Effect of camrelizumab vs placebo added to chemotherapy on survival and progression-free survival in patients with advanced or metastatic esophageal squamous cell carcinoma: the ESCORT-1st randomized clinical trial. JAMA. 2021;326(10):916–25.
66. Hirano H, Kato K. Systemic treatment of advanced esophageal squamous cell carcinoma: chemotherapy, molecular-targeting therapy and immunotherapy. Jpn J Clin Oncol. 2019;49(5):412–20.
67. Puhr HC, Prager GW, Ilhan-Mutlu A. How we treat esophageal squamous cell carcinoma. ESMO Open. 2023;8(1):100789.
68. Dutton SJ, Ferry DR, Blazeby JM, et al. Gefitinib for oesophageal cancer progressing after chemotherapy (COG): a phase 3, multicentre, double-blind, placebo-controlled randomised trial. Lancet Oncol. 2014;15(8):894–904.
69. Moehler M, Maderer A, Thuss-Patience PC, et al. Cisplatin and 5-fluorouracil with or without epidermal growth factor receptor inhibition panitumumab for patients with non-resectable, advanced or metastatic oesophageal squamous cell cancer: a prospective, open-label, randomised phase III AIO/EORTC trial (POWER). Ann Oncol. 2020;31(2):228–35.
70. DeSouza M, Donohoe CL, Dolan JP. Quality of life after esophagectomy. In: Esophageal cancer: diagnosis and treatment. Springer; 2018. p. 169–80.
71. Toh Y, Morita M, Yamamoto M, et al. Health-related quality of life after esophagectomy in patients with esophageal cancer. Esophagus. 2022;19:1–10.
72. Markar SR, Zaninotto G, Castoro C, et al. Lasting symptoms after esophageal resection (LASER): European multicenter cross-sectional study. Ann Surg. 2022;275(2):e392–400.
73. Paine H, Chidambaram S, Johar A, et al. LAsting Symptoms after Oesophageal Resectional Surgery (LASORS): multicentre validation cohort study. Br J Surg. 2025;112(2):znae319.
74. Kauppila JH, Xie S, Johar A, et al. Meta-analysis of health-related quality of life after minimally invasive versus open oesophagectomy for oesophageal cancer. Br J Surg. 2017;104(9):1131.
75. Maas KW, Cuesta MA, van Berge Henegouwen MI, et al. Quality of life and late complications after minimally invasive compared to open esophagectomy: results of a randomized trial. World J Surg. 2015;39(8):1986–93.
76. Parameswaran R, Blazeby JM, Hughes R, et al. Health-related quality of life after minimally invasive oesophagectomy. Br J Surg. 2010;97(4):525–31.

South America Experiences

25

Flavio Roberto Takeda

25.1 Introduction

Esophageal cancer remains one of the most aggressive and lethal malignancies worldwide, with an estimated 604,100 new cases and 544,100 deaths annually in 2020. It ranks as the sixth leading cause of cancer-related mortality, with most cases being squamous cell carcinoma (85%) [1]. In Brazil, esophageal cancer is the sixth most common cause of cancer-related death in both sexes, excluding nonmelanoma skin cancer [2].

Between 1996 and 2016, data from DATASUS (Brazilian national registry system) recorded 122,763 deaths attributable to esophageal cancer (ICD-10 code C15) in Brazil. Of these, 29,542 occurred in the state of São Paulo, representing nearly one-quarter of the national total. A significant proportion of these cases can be associated with referral to tertiary and quaternary healthcare centers specialized in the management of such tumors [2]. Over the last 13 years, the incidence of esophageal cancer in the Hospital das Clínicas of the University of São Paulo has risen markedly, from 15% to 32.5% [3]. Furthermore, in 2016, the National Cancer Institute (INCA) projected 7950 new cases in men and 2860 in women, corresponding to estimated risks of 8.04 per 100,000 men and 2.76 per 100,000 women [2].

In Brazil, squamous cell carcinoma (SCC) constitutes the predominant histological subtype, accounting for approximately 76% of cases, followed by adenocarcinoma. A study conducted at the São Paulo State Cancer Institute (ICESP) reported that, between 2009 and 2011, among 565 patients diagnosed with esophageal cancer, nearly 80% had SCC, and approximately 63% presented with unresectable disease at diagnosis [3].

F. R. Takeda (✉)
University of Sao Paulo School of Medicine, Sao Paulo, Brazil

Esophageal Complex Diseases Division of Rede D'Or, Rio de Janeiro, Brazil

Y. Kitagawa et al. (eds.), *Esophageal Squamous Cell Carcinoma*,
https://doi.org/10.1007/978-981-92-2611-5_25

25.2 Surgical Approach

Patients are placed under general anesthesia with epidural analgesia, orotracheal intubation using a selective tube to permit exclusion of ventilation to the right hemithorax, central venous catheterization, and invasive arterial blood pressure monitoring. The prone position is adopted with appropriate stabilization on the operating table (Fig. 25.1).

Thoracoscopy is performed in the right hemithorax with the placement of five trocars (Fig. 25.2). Following discontinuation of ventilation to this side, the first 12-mm auxiliary trocar in the posterior axillary line was inserted. Subsequent trocars were positioned under direct vision after the establishment of an intrathoracic CO_2 pressure of 8 mmHg. Four 8 mm trocars were arranged along a semicircular line extending from the medial border of the scapula to the posterior right costal margin, and the fifth was inserted near the spine at the midpoint of this line.

Dissection is performed from the lower to the upper mediastinum, allowing en bloc resection of the esophagus and lower periesophageal lymph nodes, including periaortic and supradiaphragmatic pericardial chains (Fig. 25.3). Right and left infracarinal lymphadenectomy was then completed, with exposure of the main bronchi at the carina (Fig. 25.4).

The azygos vein arch was isolated and divided using a 60-mm endoscopic stapler with a vascular cartridge, followed by dissection of the upper third of the thoracic esophagus.

Particular attention was given to clipping the thoracic duct at its origin near the right diaphragmatic crus and the intercostal vessels (Fig. 25.5). A Penrose drain was applied to facilitate mobilization and retraction of the esophagus, enhancing

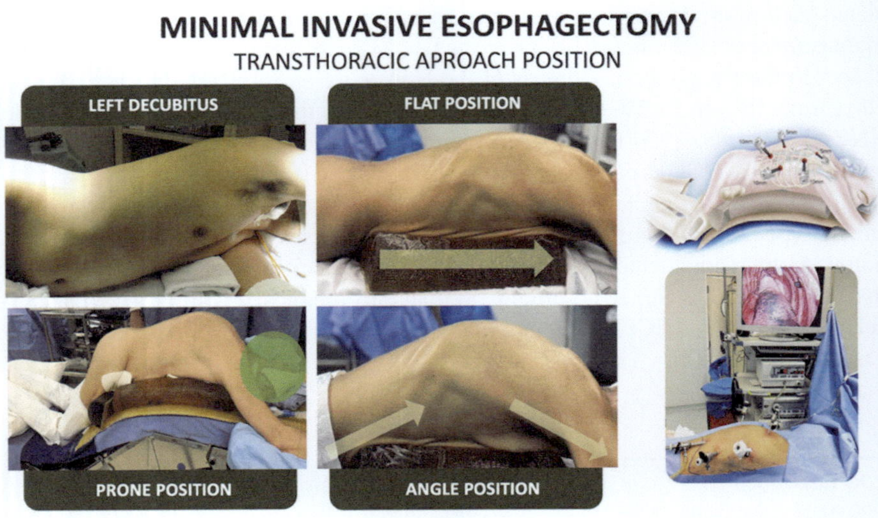

Fig. 25.1 Prone positioning by transthoracic esophagectomy technique for patients with middle and distal squamous cell carcinoma of the esophagus

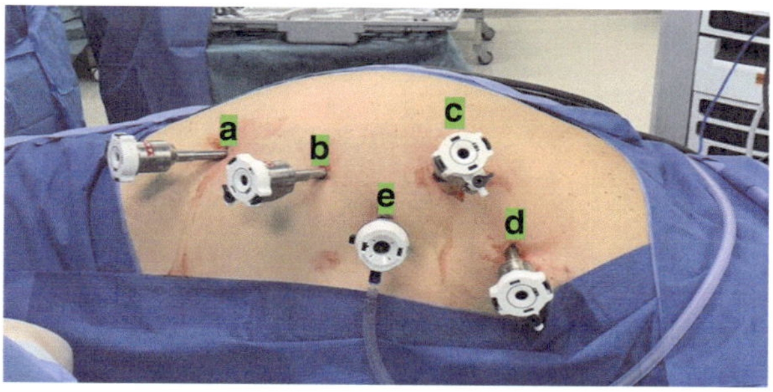

Fig. 25.2 Trocar positioning by transthoracic esophagectomy technique for patients with middle and distal squamous cell carcinoma of the esophagus. (A) 8 mm trocar in the posterior midscapular line in the penultimate intercostal space; (B) 8 mm trocar in the posterior axillary line 10 cm below the scapula; (C) 8 mm trocar near the inferior border of the scapula; (D) 8 mm trocar in the posterior axillary line and inferior border of the scapula; (E) 12 mm auxiliary trocar in the posterior axillary line

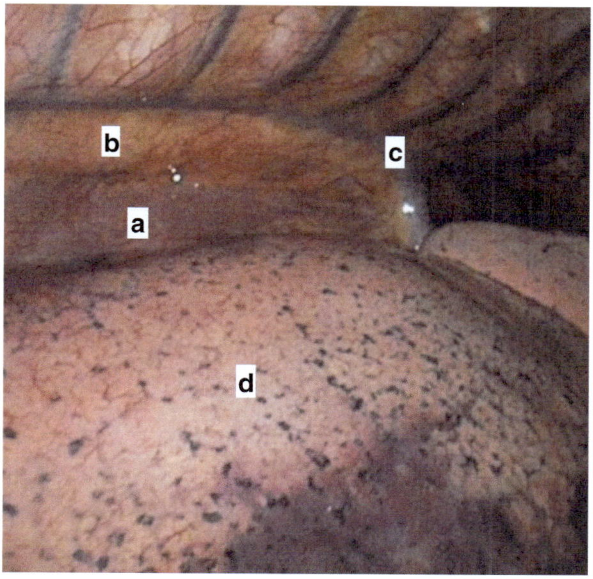

Fig. 25.3 Initial visualization of the surgical field by transthoracic esophagectomy technique by thoracoscopy for patients with adenocarcinoma of the esophagogastric junction. (A) Esophagus, (B) descending aorta, (C) azygos vein, and (D) lower lobe of the right lung [4]

exposure of mediastinal structures. This drain was subsequently exteriorized at the cervical field to aid retrieval. A tubular chest tube with a water seal was placed through the distal trocar site. All ports were closed with musculoaponeurotic and skin sutures, and dressings were applied. Patients were then repositioned supine for the cervical phase, with repositioning of the orotracheal tube if required. If pleural opening was suspected, or in distal tumors requiring intentional pleural entry, a chest drain (pigtail or tubular with water seal) was inserted in the left hemithorax.

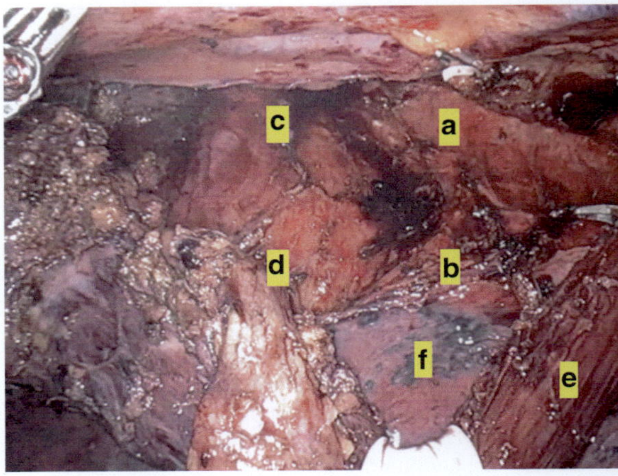

Fig. 25.4 Appearance after infracarinal lymphadenectomy by transthoracic esophagectomy technique by thoracoscopy for patients with esophagogastric junction adenocarcinoma. (A) Left main bronchus, (B) right main bronchus, (C) left pulmonary vein, (D) right pulmonary vein, (E) esophagus, and (F) right lung

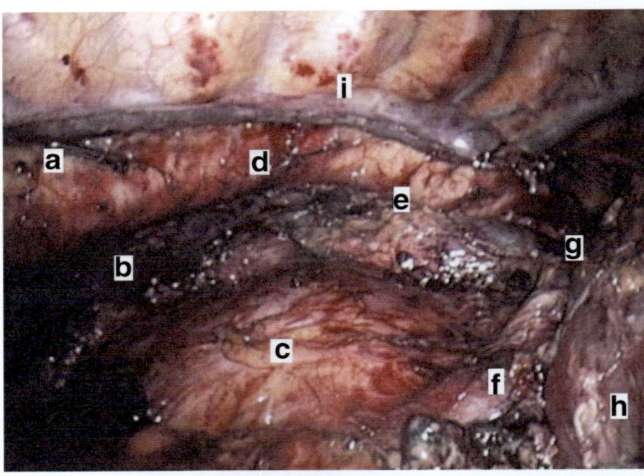

Fig. 25.5 Final mediastinal appearance after esophagectomy with lymphadenectomy using the transthoracic esophagectomy technique by thoracoscopy for patients with esophagogastric junction adenocarcinoma. (A) Clipped thoracic duct, (B) left parietal pleura, (C) left atrium, (D) descending aorta, (E) left main bronchus, (F) right main bronchus, (G) carina, (H) esophagus, (I) azygos vein [4]

The abdominal phase was performed either laparoscopically or with a hand-assisted technique. The stomach was mobilized along the greater curvature while preserving the arcade from the right gastroepiploic vessels. Division of the lesser curvature was achieved through ligation of the left gastric vessels. Lymphadenectomy of the celiac trunk was systematically performed in cases of adenocarcinoma at the esophagogastric junction. A small right subcostal incision, extending one of the trocar sites, was used for specimen extraction with polar gastrectomy. The esophagus was divided at the cervical level, and the specimen was retrieved by traction of a nasogastric tube attached to the esophageal stump, serving as a guide for gastric conduit transposition. The isoperistaltic gastric tube was constructed extracorporeally using mechanical staplers, with reinforcement of staple lines by oversuturing. This technique was selected to optimize conduit caliber, as narrower conduits have been associated with higher rates of postoperative dysphagia. Once pneumoperitoneum was reestablished, cervical traction of the conduit was performed under laparoscopic vision to prevent axial twisting [4].

For the cervical phase, a left transverse cervicotomy was performed 2 cm above the clavicle, extending from the sternal notch to the medial border of the sternocleidomastoid muscle. The skin, subcutaneous tissue, platysma, prethyroid, and omohyoid muscles were sequentially divided. Through the medial border of the sternocleidomastoid, the cervical esophagus was identified and isolated with meticulous preservation of the recurrent laryngeal nerve. Dissection proceeded distally to connect with the previously mobilized thoracic esophagus (via the Penrose drain). Following division of the esophagus, the gastric conduit was transposed, and esophagogastric anastomosis was performed. The current technique consists of a side-to-side stapled anastomosis, followed by transverse stapling and reinforcement of staple lines. A novel protocol under investigation involves microsurgical arterial and venous anastomosis between the gastric conduit and cervical vessels to enhance conduit perfusion and reduce the risk of anastomotic fistula. Cervical drainage was routinely employed, most frequently with a Penrose drain [4].

Reconstruction following esophagectomy is typically achieved through esophagogastroplasty, which involves mobilization of the stomach, or part of it, through the mediastinum for anastomosis with the cervical esophagus. Mobilization requires ligation of the left gastric artery, the left gastroepiploic artery, and the short gastric vessels, with perfusion of the gastric conduit subsequently maintained predominantly by the right gastroepiploic arcade and, in some cases, by the right gastric artery when its preservation does not compromise conduit mobility [5]. From a reconstructive standpoint, the gastric conduit can be conceptualized as a pedicled flap with four potential vascular pedicles: the right and left gastroepiploic arteries and the right and left gastric arteries. Construction of the gastric tube necessitates ligation of three of these pedicles (the left gastric, the left gastroepiploic, and frequently the right gastric arteries). Consequently, the fundic segment used for anastomosis may be relatively hypoperfused, increasing the risk of ischemia in an area distant from the right gastroepiploic pedicle [6, 7].

The most relevant complications of esophagectomy are anastomotic strictures and fistulas. Operative mortality rates vary between 4.2% and 19.3%, with postoperative morbidity reported in 46%–52% of cases. The principal causes of mortality include pulmonary complications, disease progression, and anastomotic leakage [8, 9]. Esophagogastric anastomotic fistulas occur in 3.5%–21.5% of procedures and account for 9%–50% of surgery-related deaths [10, 11]. Although rare, gastroaortic and tracheo-esophageal fistulas have been described, representing severe and therapeutically challenging complications [12, 13].

In Brazilian series, the incidence of cervical esophagogastric anastomotic fistulas has ranged from 9.2% in benign conditions to 24% in esophageal or cardia carcinoma [14]. These fistulas constitute critical prognostic determinants in the postoperative course of esophagectomized patients. Multiple studies have investigated their pathogenesis, and evidence suggests that fistula development is not primarily related to the surgical technique, type of suture, or material employed. Instead, ischemia of the gastric conduit, induced by mobilization and tubularization, as well as mechanical tension at the anastomotic site, appears to be the major contributing factors [9–12]. Ischemia results in tissue hypoxia, which compromises healing and predisposes to leakage [15]. Tension is associated with the extent of esophageal resection and the length obtained during gastric conduit construction. The technique described by Akiyama et al. [16], which includes mobilization of the entire greater curvature from the fundus to the prepyloric region while preserving the entry of the Latarget nerve along the lesser curvature, generally provides sufficient length for cervical anastomosis, even in tall patients [15].

25.2.1 Transhiatal Esophagectomy

Transhiatal esophagectomy can be performed using a minimally invasive approach, combining laparoscopic abdominal access with cervicotomy, gastric conduit reconstruction, and cervical anastomosis. In adenocarcinoma of the esophagogastric junction tumors, comparative analyses between open transhiatal resection and thoracoscopic approaches have demonstrated a higher number of lymph nodes retrieved with thoracoscopy (31.8 vs. 20.7; $p < 0.001$) and improved survival in early stage disease (up to stage IIB). Overall survival and disease-free survival, however, did not differ significantly between the two techniques. Both approaches are associated with low mortality and morbidity rates consistent with the complexity of the procedure. Advances in laparoscopic transhiatal techniques may be particularly advantageous for patients with esophagogastric junction tumors who present elevated surgical risk [17, 18].

25.2.2 Results

Between 2009 and 2019, a total of 345 esophagectomies with cervical anastomosis were performed. Anastomotic leakage was identified in 46 patients (13.3%). The predominant sites of spontaneous fluid drainage were the cervical region (38/46, 82.6%), the upper mediastinum (4/46, 8.7%), and the entire mediastinum associated with mediastinitis (4/46, 8.7%). The median interval to clinical presentation was 5.6 days (range, 2–8). Importantly, two patients developed clinically evident fistula despite negative findings on contrast swallow radiography. Upper endoscopy was not systematically employed for the assessment of anastomotic defects; its use was restricted to therapeutic dilation in cases with refractory healing beyond 14 days. Partial necrosis of the proximal gastric conduit and anastomosis was estimated in four cases (8.7%), whereas complete necrosis of the gastric tube occurred in one patient (2.1%) with a history of liver transplantation [4].

At our institution, cervical anastomosis is performed systematically. In Brazil, approximately 77% of esophageal carcinoma cases are squamous cell type, and the choice of esophagogastric anastomotic site is influenced by the extent of oncological margins. Achieving an adequate proximal margin frequently necessitates a cervical anastomosis following esophagectomy. Huang et al. demonstrated that, in patients with middle thoracic esophageal cancer, radical esophagectomy with cervical anastomosis was associated with more extensive lymphadenectomy compared with intrathoracic anastomosis [19]. Notably, cervical anastomosis did not increase postoperative mortality and was associated with improved 5-year survival rates [4]. Furthermore, long-term quality of life is not adversely affected by cervical anastomosis. Wormald et al. reported no significant differences between cervical and intrathoracic anastomosis regarding functional or symptom scores, including overall health status, dysphagia, odynophagia, and swallowing dysfunction [20].

25.3 Discussion and Perspectives

The tradition of Brazilian surgery in the management of esophageal diseases can be traced back to 1977, with the seminal publications of Professor Henrique Walter Pinotti at the Hospital das Clínicas, Faculty of Medicine, University of São Paulo (USP) [21]. At that time, transhiatal esophagectomy was the most frequently performed procedure, although it carried a surgical morbidity rate of approximately 40%. Subsequent international collaborations, particularly with Japanese institutions, introduced the three-field esophagectomy described by Akiyama in 1981 [22], marking a shift toward conventional transthoracic approaches in Brazil. In the early 2000s, under the leadership of Professors Ivan Cecconello and Rubens Sallum, the advent of minimally invasive techniques allowed esophagectomy to be performed with outcomes comparable to those achieved with open surgery.

In Brazil, esophageal squamous cell carcinoma (ESCC) remains the predominant histological subtype, contrasting with the increasing prevalence of adenocarcinoma in North America and parts of Europe. The incidence of ESCC is heterogeneously distributed, with higher rates historically observed in the South and parts of the Southeast, reflecting region-specific exposures and socioeconomic determinants. Classical risk factors—tobacco and alcohol—intersect with cultural practices such as the chronic ingestion of very hot beverages (chimarrão/maté), nutritional deficiencies, poor oral health, and delayed diagnosis. In addition, legacy conditions such as Chagas-related megaesophagus and caustic strictures have shaped the patient profile in Brazilian tertiary centers. This epidemiological context has historically influenced national expertise, particularly favoring the use of cervical anastomoses, as in the McKeown technique. Over the past two decades, advances in minimally invasive and robotic surgery have further refined esophageal dissection, contributing to significant improvements in morbidity and mortality.

For resectable, locally advanced ESCC (cT2–T4a, any N), the current standard of care is neoadjuvant chemoradiotherapy (CRT) followed by surgical resection. The CROSS regimen (weekly carboplatin/paclitaxel with 41.4 Gy) demonstrated improved R0 resection rates, overall survival, and remarkably high pathologic complete response (pCR) rates in ESCC. For cervical esophageal tumors, or in patients unfit for surgery, definitive CRT remains a guideline-concordant organ-preserving strategy, with salvage esophagectomy reserved for persistent or recurrent localized disease in highly specialized centers. The USP experience has underscored the importance of careful patient selection and meticulous postoperative management to mitigate the heightened morbidity associated with salvage procedures in previously irradiated fields [23].

For patients with metastatic or unresectable disease, first-line systemic therapy now integrates PD-1 inhibitors with platinum/fluoropyrimidine chemotherapy in eligible populations, reflecting results from pivotal phase III trials. In Brazil, pragmatic adaptations to this regimen must consider disparities in access across public and private healthcare systems [24].

Among surgical complications, anastomotic fistula remains the most severe and feared event after esophagectomy with gastric conduit reconstruction, leading to increased morbidity, mortality, and prolonged hospitalization. Despite technological advances, the vascular perfusion of the proximal gastric conduit continues to represent the fundamental limitation of esophagogastric anastomosis. In this setting, recent work by Takeda and collaborators has introduced the innovative application of supercharged microanastomosis—a technique adapted from reconstructive plastic surgery. By establishing microvascular arterial and venous anastomoses between the gastric conduit and cervical vessels, this approach significantly enhances perfusion and drainage at the anastomotic site [25].

The rationale is evident: ischemia constitutes the primary determinant of anastomotic leakage. By improving arterial inflow and mitigating venous congestion, supercharged microanastomosis directly addresses the pathophysiological basis of fistula formation. Early clinical experience from USP demonstrates that this adjunct not only reduces fistula incidence but also promotes faster healing, decreases the need for reoperations, and reduces nutritional and economic burdens.

Beyond its immediate surgical benefits, this technique has broader implications for the global management of esophageal cancer. In Brazil, where squamous cell carcinoma predominates and cervical anastomoses are frequently employed, the risk of leakage is particularly relevant. By successfully incorporating microsurgical principles into complex oncologic resections, this line of research establishes a paradigm shift at the intersection of gastrointestinal and reconstructive surgery. In sum, the studies on supercharged microanastomosis represent an important advance in reducing the burden of anastomotic fistulas and highlight how interdisciplinary innovation can redefine surgical standards, improving both patient outcomes and quality of life.

References

1. Morgan E, Soerjomataram I, Rumgay H, Coleman HG, Thrift AP, Vignat J, Laversanne M, Ferlay J, Arnold M. The global landscape of esophageal squamous cell carcinoma and esophageal adenocarcinoma incidence and mortality in 2020 and projections to 2040: new estimates from GLOBOCAN 2020. Gastroenterology. 2022;163(3):649–658.e2. https://doi.org/10.1053/j.gastro.2022.05.054. Epub 2022 Jun 4. PMID: 35671803.
2. Ministério da Saúde. Estimativa 2016: incidência de câncer no Brasil/Instituto Nacional de Câncer José Alencar Gomes da Silva. Rio de Janeiro: INCA; 2015. p. 42–3.
3. Tustumi F, Takeda FR, Kimura CM, Sallum RA, Ribeiro U Jr, Cecconello I. Esophageal carcinoma: is squamous cell carcinoma different disease compared to adenocarcinoma? A transversal study in a quaternary high volume hospital in Brazil. Arq Gastroenterol. 2016;53(1):44–8.
4. Takeda FR, Sallum RAA, Fernandes FA, Cecconello I. McKeown—cervical anastomosis in minimally invasive esophagectomy. Ann Esophagus. 2021;4:19. https://doi.org/10.21037/aoe-20-103.
5. Thomas P, Giudicelli R, Gossot D, Cattan P, Bricot R. Gastric pull-up: isoperistaltic gastric tube for esophageal replacement. Ann Thorac Surg. 1979;28(2):112–7.
6. Schilling MK, Redaelli C, Friess H, Büchler MW. Anastomotic leakage after esophageal resection: current aspects of pathophysiology, diagnosis and therapy. Chirurg. 1997;68(6):521–30.
7. Urschel JD, Blewett CJ, Young JE, Miller JD, Bennett WF. Ischemic complications after esophagectomy: incidence and risk factors. Ann Thorac Surg. 1997;64(3):702–6.
8. van Lanschot JJ, Hulscher JB, de Boer AG, et al. Randomized comparison of transhiatal and transthoracic esophagectomy with extended en bloc lymphadenectomy for adenocarcinoma of the esophagus. J Thorac Cardiovasc Surg. 2001;121(6):1089–94.
9. Whooley BP, Law S, Murthy SC, Alexandrou A, Wong J. Analysis of reduced hospital stay after esophagectomy: identification of modifiable factors. Arch Surg. 2001;136(2):174–8.
10. Alvarez JA, Baldonedo RF, Bear IG, Solís JA, Fresno MF, Jorge JI. Anastomotic leak after esophageal resection: incidence, management, and impact on outcome. Ann Thorac Surg. 2001;72(2):524–30.
11. Griffin SM, Shaw IH, Dresner SM. Early complications after Ivor Lewis subtotal esophagectomy with two-field lymphadenectomy: risk factors and management. J Am Coll Surg. 2001;193(2):186–93.
12. Buskens CJ, Hulscher JB, Fockens P, Obertop H, van Lanschot JJ. Benign tracheo-neo-esophageal fistulas after subtotal esophagectomy. Ann Thorac Surg. 2001;72(1):221–4.
13. Navarro RA, Bueno J, Ramos R, Villanueva AG, Menéndez R, Cordero PJ, et al. Gastroaortic fistula after esophagectomy: an unusual and devastating complication. Ann Thorac Surg. 2001;71(3):1014–6.
14. Zilberstein B, Cecconello I, Alves L, Pinotti HW. Esophagogastric anastomotic fistula: incidence, diagnosis, treatment and prognosis. Rev Hosp Clin Fac Med Univ São Paulo. 1994;49(1):9–12.
15. Low DE, Kuppusamy MK, Alderson D, et al. Benchmarking complications associated with esophagectomy. Ann Surg. 2019;269(2):291–8.
16. Akiyama H, Tsurumaru M, Udagawa H, Kajiyama Y. Radical lymph node dissection for cancer of the thoracic esophagus. Ann Surg. 1978;188(3):309–16.
17. Takeda FR, Obregon CA, Navarro YP, Moura DTH, Ribeiro U Jr, Aissar Sallum RA, Cecconello I. Thoracoscopic esophagectomy is related to better outcomes in early adenocarcinoma of esophagogastric junction tumors. World J Gastrointest Endosc. 2021;13(8):319–28. https://doi.org/10.4253/wjge.v13.i8.319. PMID: 34512879; PMCID: PMC8394183.
18. Takeda FR, Ramos MFKP, Pereira MA, Sallum RAA, Ribeiro U Jr, Nahas SC, Cecconello I. Tumor size predicts worse prognosis in esophagogastric junction adenocarcinoma. Updates Surg. 2022;74(6):1871–9. https://doi.org/10.1007/s13304-022-01313-6. Epub 2022 Jul 1. PMID: 35776245.

19. Huang PM, Yang SM, Ko WJ, Chen JS, Lee YC. Cervical esophagogastrostomy after radical esophagectomy for middle-third esophageal carcinoma: comparison with intrathoracic anastomosis. J Thorac Cardiovasc Surg. 2001;142(6):1332–7. https://doi.org/10.1067/mtc.2001.118824.
20. Wormald JC, Bennett J, Pepper C, McCulloch P, Parsons SL, Catton JA. Quality of life after minimally invasive and open esophagectomy: results from a multicenter randomized controlled trial. Ann Surg Oncol. 2014;21(9):3061–8. https://doi.org/10.1245/s10434-014-3723-4.
21. Pinotti HW, Pollara WM, Raia AA. Transhiatal esophagectomy without thoracotomy. Surgery. 1977;82(4):576–83.
22. Akiyama H, Tsurumaru M, Kawamura T, Ono Y. Principles of surgical treatment for carcinoma of the esophagus: analysis of lymph node involvement. Ann Surg. 1981;194(4):438–46. https://doi.org/10.1097/00000658-198110000-00009.
23. Takeda FR, Tustumi F, de Almeida Obregon C, Yogolare GG, Navarro YP, Segatelli V, Sallum RAA, Ribeiro U Jr, Cecconello I. Prognostic value of tumor regression grade based on Ryan score in squamous cell carcinoma and adenocarcinoma of esophagus. Ann Surg Oncol. 2020;27(4):1241–7. https://doi.org/10.1245/s10434-019-07967-8. Epub 2019 Oct 29. PMID: 31664618.
24. Victor CR, Fujiki FK, Takeda FR, Hoff PMG, de Castria TB. Safety and effectiveness of chemotherapy for metastatic esophageal cancer in a Community Hospital in Brazil. J Glob Oncol. 2019;5:1–10. https://doi.org/10.1200/JGO.19.00103. PMID: 31365299; PMCID: PMC6775989.
25. Takeda FR, Tutihashi R, Tustumi F, Sallum RAA, de Freitas Busnardo F, Ribeiro U Jr, Cecconello I. Supercharged cervical anastomosis for esophagectomy and gastric pull-up. J Thorac Cardiovasc Surg. 2021;162(3):688–697.e3. https://doi.org/10.1016/j.jtcvs.2020.06.021. Epub 2020 Jun 26. PMID: 32739161.

Index

Y. Kitagawa et al. (eds.), *Esophageal Squamous Cell Carcinoma*,
https://doi.org/10.1007/978-981-92-2611-5

MIX
Papier aus verantwortungsvollen Quellen
Paper from responsible sources
FSC® C105338

If you have any concerns about our products,
you can contact us on
ProductSafety@springernature.com

In case Publisher is established outside the EU,
the EU authorized representative is:
Springer Nature Customer Service Center GmbH
Europaplatz 3, 69115 Heidelberg, Germany

Printed by Libri Plureos GmbH
in Hamburg, Germany